Anonymus

The Chemist & Druggist

Anonymus

The Chemist & Druggist

ISBN/EAN: 9783741172403

Manufactured in Europe, USA, Canada, Australia, Japa

Cover: Foto ©Lupo / pixelio.de

Manufactured and distributed by brebook publishing software
(www.brebook.com)

Anonymus

The Chemist & Druggist

[SUPPLEMENT ONLY.]

Chem. & Drugg. Aust. Suppl.
Vol. 2, no. 23: 83-90, (March, 1880)

THE
Chemist & Druggist.

WITH AUSTRALASIAN SUPPLEMENT.

(Published under direction of the Pharmaceutical Society of Victoria.)

No. 23. { PUBLISHED ON THE 15TH OF EVERY MONTH. }
Registered for Transmission as a Newspaper. **MARCH, 1880.** { SUBSCRIPTION, 15s. PER ANNUM, INCLUDING DIARY, POST FREE.

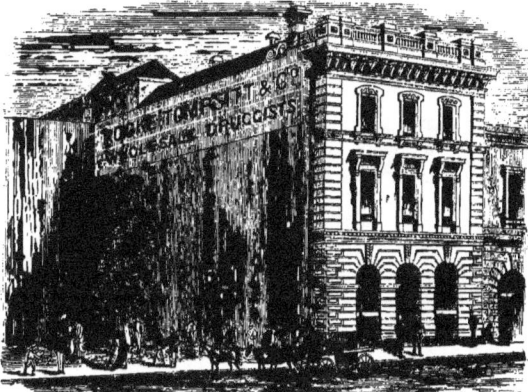

The Chemist and Druggist.

WITH AUSTRALASIAN SUPPLEMENT.

OFFICE: MUTUAL PROVIDENT BUILDINGS, COLLINS STREET WEST.
Published on the 15th of each Month.

THIS Journal is issued gratis to all paid-up Members of the PHARMA-CEUTICAL SOCIETY OF VICTORIA, and to non-members at Fifteen Shillings per annum, payable in advance. A copy of *The Chemists and Druggists' Diary*, published annually, is forwarded post free to every subscriber.

Advertisements, remittances, and all business communications to be addressed to THE HONORARY SECRETARY OF THE PHARMACEUTICAL SOCIETY, MELBOURNE.

SCALE OF CHARGES FOR ADVERTISEMENTS:

	Per annum.		Per annum.
One Page	.. £8 0 0	Quarter Page	.. £3 0 0
Half do.	.. 5 0 0	Business Cards	.. 2 0 0

Special rates for wrapper and pages preceding and following literary matter. Advertisements of Assistants Wanting Situations, 2s. 6d. each.

Advertisements for insertion in the current month should be sent to the office before the 10th.

COMMUNICATIONS for the EDITORIAL department of this journal should be addressed to THE EDITOR, MUTUAL PROVIDENT BUILDINGS, COLLINS STREET WEST, MELBOURNE.

No notice can be taken of anonymous communications. Whatever is intended for insertion must be authenticated by the name and address of the writer—not necessarily for publication, but as a guarantee of good faith.

NOTICE.

IN accordance with the resolution passed at the Annual Meeting, a Special Meeting of the Members of the Pharmaceutical Society will be held at the Mutual Provident Buildings, Collins-street, on Friday, the 7th May, at eight o'clock p.m., to receive the Report of the Council in reference to the proposed Alteration in the Constitution and Laws of the Society.

HARRY SHILLINGLAW,
Hon. Sec.
14th April, 1880.

BIRTH.
BLACKETT.—On the 25th March, at 126 Gertrude-street, Fitzroy, the wife of C. R. Blackett of a son.

DEATH.
PERKINS.—On the 16th March, at his residence, Piper-street, Kyneton, Ebenezer Perkins, aged forty-nine years.

PHARMACY IN NEW ZEALAND.

A MOVEMENT to form a Pharmaceutical Society of New Zealand, inaugurated at the commencement of last year, has, we are glad to learn, progressed very favourably, so that by the end of October the number of members who had joined, exclusive of associates and apprentices, was upwards of one hundred. The head-quarters of the new society have been fixed at Wellington, with local committees in Auckland, Christchurch, and Dunedin, and its first president is Mr. Charles D. Barraud.

Notwithstanding the success that has been attained, a large number of chemists and druggists in business, amounting to one-third, have not yet joined the society, and in the prospect of an attempt being made to obtain a Pharmacy Act for the colony a vigorous effort is being made to induce these to join the common cause.

In anticipation of the meeting of the colonial Parliament a bill has been drafted, based on the Victoria Pharmacy Act, which is said to work well, and which in its turn was founded on the Pharmacy Acts of Great Britain. The main provisions would render examinations compulsory in New Zealand and "introduce means for systematic technical education." There are strong hopes of passing this bill, since the Wellington committee has been assured that it will command the cordial support of the Legislature as a measure calculated to afford important protection to the community and as being in accord with the views of a commission at present sitting on high-class education.—*Pharmaceutical Journal.*

The Month.

THE Registrar-General has recently registered a number of trade marks as follows :—A representation of a crucible, with the word "Salamander" on it, on behalf of the Patent Plumbago Crucible Company, of Battersea, in England. The Holman Liver Pad Company, of New York, are registered as the proprietors of two marks in respect of surgical pads—viz., the word "Holman," and the representation of the bust of a man wearing a pad upon the stomach, as shown in the large hills posted about the city ; and the representation of a man seated in a chair with his feet in a bath, in respect of preparations to be put in baths for curative or medicinal purposes.

The tenders of Messrs. Rocke, Tompsitt and Co., for the supply of medicines, instruments, &c., and photo-lithographic chemicals, to the Government of Victoria for the year 1880-81, has been accepted by the Tender Board.

At a recent meeting of the committee of the Melbourne Hospital the chairman stated that the resolution recently passed by the committee prohibiting the patients using ale and porter bottles for carrying their medicine had caused a very serious inconvenience to some of the patients, who had been compelled to leave the institution without their medicine in consequence of not having proper bottles. He considered that the previous resolution should be rescinded. Mr. Garton also was of the opinion that the patients should not be put to such inconvenience, as many of them could not obtain proper bottles, and gave notice that he would move at the next meeting of the committee that the previous resolution be rescinded.

The following name has been added to the list of legally qualified medical practitioners, registered under the provisions of the Medical Practitioners Statute, 1865 :—Henry Pelham Gordon, Penshurst, M.R.C.S. Eng., 1866. Additional qualification registered—J. G. Beaney, M.D. Univ. Melb., 1879., a.e.g.

The produce of the Murray fisheries has greatly fallen off, owing to the lowness of the rivers. Now most of the fish is caught in the Moira Lakes. Leeches are caught in abundance in the lakes, and a local tradesman has taken a contract to supply Messrs. Felton, Grimwade and Co. with 250,000 leeches; 50 lbs. weight have already been sent down.

A meeting of the creditors of Messrs. W. H. Ford and Co., of Swanston-street, Melbourne, was held at the office of Mr. J. Bickerton, Queen-street, on the 5th April; Mr. Couche in the chair. Mr. Ford submitted a statement of his assets and liabilities, which showed a deficiency of over £3000. Mr. Grimwade proposed that Messrs. Couche and J. Hemmons be appointed to investigate the estate, and to report at a future meeting to be called. The proposal was carried unanimously.

There have been several business changes lately to note. Mr. John Ross is now carrying on, at No. 63 Collins-street, the business formerly conducted by Mr. Gibson; Mr. J. F. F. Grace has purchased the business of Mr. H. Bewley, at St. Arnaud; Mr. R. B. Bridge, of Bright, has left that place for Euroa.

Mr. C. R. Blackett (president of the Pharmaceutical Society) has been appointed a Royal Commissioner for the Melbourne International Exhibition.

SYDNEY EXHIBITION AWARDS.—The following supplementary report has been published :—"Chemicals.—Victoria—Jos. Bosisto, Richmond, essential oil, first; Cuming, Smith and Co., Melbourne, chemicals and mineral acids, first; Felton, Grimwade and Co., Melbourne, chemicals and mineral acids, first; Apollo Stearine Candle Company, Melbourne, candles, &c., first; A. Borthwick, Melbourne, varnishes and paints, second.

Meetings.

THE PHARMACY BOARD OF VICTORIA.

THE monthly meeting of the board was held at the Royal Society's Hall on the 10th March, 1880 ; present—Messrs. Bosisto, Brind, Bowen, Holdsworth, Kennedy, Kruse, and Lewis.

The registrar produced the return made to him by the returning officer of the members elected on the 5th February, 1880, in accordance with the seventh section of the regulations.

On the motion of Mr. Lewis, Mr. H. Brind took the chair.

Appointment of President.—The chairman proposed Mr. Joseph Bosisto, M.L.A., as president ; seconded by Mr. Bowen, and carried unanimously.

The President then took the chair.

Appointment of Treasurer.—Mr. Brind proposed that Mr. George Lewis be appointed treasurer, and referred in complimentary terms to the manner in which Mr. Lewis had performed the duty during the last three years. The motion was seconded by Mr. Kennedy, and carried unanimously.

The minutes of the previous meeting were then read and confirmed.

Applications for Registration.—The following were approved :—Alfred Richmond, Richmond ; Albert Charles Dunn, Nagambie (provisional certificate) ; Henry Simonds, Richmond (certificate from Pharmaceutical Society, Great Britain).

Renewals of Certificates under the Sale and Use of Poisons Act.—Tong On, Harrietville ; Hoy Ling, Vaughan ; Sun Lee On, Omeo ; Ho Lim Sin, Swift's Creek ; Sun Hi On, Buckland ; Morgan W. Edwards, Lubeck (new certificate).

Apprentices' Indentures Registered.—John Shrigley, Clunes ; Frank H. Cole, Fitzroy ; Edward H. Morrison, Sandhurst ; Duncan Shaw, Collingwood.

Appointment of Examiners.—The following were appointed examiners for the modified examination for the year 1880 :— Mr. Joseph Bosisto, honorary examiner *Materia Medica;* Mr. C. R. Blackett, Pharmacy and Latin ; Mr. Wm. Johnson, Chemistry.

Names Erased from the Register.—John Summers, Nagambie ; George Page, Violet Town ; certificates of their deaths having been received from the deputy-registrar of births and deaths.

Correspondence.—A letter was received from W. P. Green, of Geelong, stating that he had returned to the colony, and requesting that his name might be restored to the register. A similar communication was also received from R. D. Murray, Ararat. In these cases the applicants had left the colony; and, in accordance with the provisions of the 13th section of the Act, letters had been written to them to their last known address, and no answer having been received, their names had been erased from the register. The board decided that they must comply with the provisions of the 13th section of the Act before their names could be restored to the register. The following communications were dealt with :—From the hon. secretary Medical Society of Victoria ; the police, Omeo and Harrietville ; Sun Lu On, Jane Summers, Mrs. Coates ; registrars School of Mines, Ballarat and Sandhurst ; from the police, Ballarat, Eganstown, Omeo, Warrnambool, and Smythesdale ; A. J. Owen, manager National Bank ; deputyregistrars Violet Town and Nagambie ; R. B. Bridge, Arthur Power, M. Shanasy, Clemes and Bartleman ; police, Benalla and Fitzroy ; secretary Medical Board.

The Eighth Preliminary Examination.—The examiners forwarded their report of the candidates passed.

Financial and routine business brought the meeting to a close.

THE PHARMACEUTICAL SOCIETY OF VICTORIA.

THE monthly meeting of the society was held at the Mutual Provident Building, Collins-street, on Friday, the 2nd April ; present—Messrs. Blackett, Lewis, Hooper, Bowen, Thomas, Huntsman, Macgowan, Baker, and Jones.

Mr. G. Lewis moved that Mr. Thomas Huntsman take the chair.

Appointment of Office-bearers.—Mr. Lewis said he felt great pleasure; in proposing that the retiring officers be re-elected. The year would be a most eventful one, as the Exhibition would no doubt attract many visitors to the colony. The following were unanimously elected :—Messrs. C. R. Blackett, president ; William Bowen, vice-president ; Messrs. Henry Gamble, treasurer ; Harry Shillinglaw, honorary secretary.

The president then took the chair, and briefly expressed his thanks for the honour conferred upon him.

The vice-president also said he felt gratified at the honour done him by re-electing him vice-president.

The minutes of the previous meeting were then read and confirmed.

An apology was received from Mr. Gamble, who was unable to be present.

Election of New Members.—The following new members, proposed at the last meeting, were duly elected :—Messrs. F. E. Sloper, Sydney ; P. J. Walsh, Hillston, N.S.W ; R. J. Poulton, Fitzroy ; James Pendlebury, Emerald Hill ; and David Clark, Warwick, Queensland. Mr. H. G. M'Burney, of Benalla, was also nominated as a member.

Removal of Offices.—Mr. J. C. Jones said he desired to know why and by whose authority the offices of the society had been removed from the Royal Society's Hall.

The president explained that the society were sub-tenants

and that in consequence of the removal of the offices of the Pharmacy Board the society had also to remove.

Mr. Jones complained that the Pharmacy Board had exercised an undue influence over the affairs of the society, and he moved that a committee be appointed to secure suitable premises. He thought the society was not in a position to spend money in paying high rent for accommodation they did not want. The motion was not seconded.

Mr. Bowen said that no proposition had yet been made to the society from the Pharmacy Board, who had taken the rooms, and if the society did not want the accommodation offered after the next meeting of the Pharmacy Board some definite proposition would be made, when it would be time enough to then consider the matter.

Proposed Amendment of the Constitution and Laws.— A committee of the whole council considered the proposed alterations submitted by Mr. Brownscombe, and agreed upon certain amendments to be submitted to a general meeting of the society on the 7th May next.

Alteration of Time of Meeting.—Mr. Macgowan gave notice that he would at the next meeting move that the meeting of the council be held at three o'clock p.m. in lieu of eight o'clock p.m.

Finance.—In the absence of the hon. treasurer, the hon. secretary submitted a statement of the position of the society for the current year. The statement showed the financial position of the society to be in a very satisfactory condition.

Correspondence.—Communications were received from the following:—The Secretary Pharmaceutical Society, Great Britain, forwarding the calendar for 1880; A. Power, A. R. Dix, David Clark, Professor Maish, E. P. Jones, J. Henzenroeder, Max Brown, R. G. Evans, George Wilson (Deniliquin), Charles V. Florence, E. L. Marks, R. Hughes, S. H. Henshall, E. Beythein, A. B. Jefferson, J. De Castro, T. Phillips, E. H. Jackson, D. Lerew, C. A. Rundle, Warner and Scott, J. Whittle, P. J. Walsh, G. Wilson (Portland), Max Pincus, E. Fyvie, W. H. Eager, F. Wheeler, J. Brownscombe, J. Holdsworth, G. F. Chamberlin, R. Cowl.

Scientific Summary.

FROM the *Pharmaceutical* and other journals this month we have very few matters of interest or novelty to report.

To a limited number of persons, sneezing appears to be a pleasant operation, but those who find it excessively disagreeable will be glad to learn of a simple and cheap remedy, made known in the *British Medical Journal* by Mr. S. M. Bradley, surgeon to the Royal Infirmary at Manchester. It consists in placing a loose plug of cotton wool in the nostrils. In hay fever, in a dusty atmosphere, or in those stages of catarrh in which a cold atmosphere is irritating to the mucous membrane of the nose, this simple application is said to give immediate relief.

An Italian correspondent of the *Lancet* calls attention to an insidious and frightfully fatal disease called "pellaga," of which no less than 97,000 Italians are said to be dying at the present time, the number of victims representing 3·62 per 1000 of the whole population, and in the infected departments, especially in Lombardy and Venice, a higher proportion than ever occurred during the worst cholera epidemic in France. The disease usually runs a slow course, like consumption. Its cause is believed to be the exclusive consumption as food of maize in a deteriorated condition, and the unhealthy state of the hovels in which the rustics live.

Under proper treatment it would seem that aconite is by no means one of the most fatal poisons. In the *British Medical Journal* for 27th December an account is given of recovery after taking a teaspoonful of linimentum aconiti, a quantity nearly equal in strength to an ounce of the B.P. tincture. It cannot be too widely known that after an emetic has been given, or the stomach-pump used, the antidotes to

aconite poisoning which have been found most effectual are strong stimulants, such as ether, brandy, ammonia, &c.

In *New Remedies* for this month a new suppository mould is described and figured, which has the advantage of compressing the suppositories while the mould is opened, and thus preventing their breakage when made of cacao butter or other material of a friable character.

In a note upon vanillin, in the *Chemiker-Zeitung* (18th and 25th December), by Messrs. Haarmann and Reimer, regret is expressed that consumers of vanilla have been so slow in adopting the use of the vanillin prepared artificially by the oxidation of coniferin. On more than one occasion, however, statements have been quoted in this journal which, if correct, would fully explain this, to the effect that the artificial vanillin does not truly represent all the aromatic principle of vanilla. Nevertheless, in the present article the authors maintain that the artificial vanillin is not to be distinguished from the natural principle for which vanilla is valued, it being identical in melting point, crystalline form, smell, taste, and chemical reactions, whilst it can be produced much more cheaply. The amount of vanillin in vanilla varies from ½ to 2 per cent., and it is estimated that the annual consumption of vanilla amounts to at least 50,000 kilograms yearly, at a cost of £150,000. This the authors claim would be fully represented by 1000 kilograms of vanillin, costing £70,000.

At a recent meeting of the Chemical Society Dr. Pavy brought forward a modification in connection with the test for sugar by the reduction of cupric oxide, which promises to be of service where the test is only occasionally used. In order to obviate the inconveniences accompanying the keeping of the usual test solution for any considerable time, he has sought for a method of bringing a mixture of the dry ingredients into a coherent mass, so that they might be kept in solid form. This has now been effected under his directions by means of pressure, and the product is a sort of pellet, which, when placed in about 3 c.c. of water, and heat applied, yields the clear deep blue liquid constituting the ordinary cupric test solution.

The death is announced of Dr. William Budd, formerly of Bristol, whose name will long be honourably remembered in association with the investigation of the nature of typhoid fever.

SANDHURST.

SCHOOL OF MINES AND INDUSTRIES, BENDIGO.

AT the late meetings of administrative council the reports from the various instructors were highly satisfactory, and showed that a steady progress was continued to be made. The new chemistry lecture class shows a roll of 27, and the other classes are equally promising.

Tenders were opened for a partition in mathematical and mining class-room, and for fencing off the school's ground. The lowest tender—that of J. Waugh—was accepted. The architect was further instructed to advertise for tenders for additional fencing, and for outhouses, together with library, shelving, and presses.

The council resolved to prepare an exhibit for the International Melbourne Exhibition of cakes of gold, representing one year's yield of the Bendigo mines. The proper representation of the lines of reef was discussed, and various suggestions made. The method to be adopted was left for further consideration after inquiries were made respecting the practicability of each proposal.

The purchase of Exhibition cases, of a student's microscope, and other minor requirements were authorised. The microscope will be of special importance for the *materia medica* students.

Amongst the donations acknowledged with thanks were the *Science Directories*, from the Science and Art Department, South Kensington; the *Chemistry of Agriculture*, from R. W. E. M'Ivor, Esq., the author; the *Quarterly Journal of the Microscopical Society of Victoria*; and *The Chemist and Druggist, with Australasian Supplement*.

Mr. Vaplan's motion with regard to the salary question having been brought forward, a sub-committee, consisting of Messrs. Mendell, Hosking, Vahland, Ross, and the president, were appointed to bring up a report at the next meeting.

Accounts having been passed for payment to the amount of £116 10s. 2d., the meeting closed.

BALLARAT.

BALLARAT DISTRICT CHEMISTS' ASSOCIATION.

THE monthly general meeting of the association was held at Lester's Hotel, Sturt-street, on Wednesday night, 17th March. There was a fair attendance of members ; Mr. J. T. Thomas, of Melbourne, a member of the Pharmaceutical Council, was present as a visitor. The President (Mr. T. P. Palmer) occupied the chair, and called upon the hon. sec. to read the minutes of the previous meeting, which were confirmed.

Mr. Macgowan, hon. sec., then gave a *résumé* of the business transacted at the annual meeting of the Pharmaceutical Society, held in Melbourne on 12th March ; and stated as it had happened there were for members of the Pharmaceutical Council six vacancies and six nominations, he had been elected a member without a contest.

Mr. Towl introduced the subject of dispensing for Friendly Societies, and remarked upon the low prices at which chemists sometimes tendered for dispensing ; and gave notice of his intention to bring forward a motion at the next meeting for fixing a minimum price for all future tenders.

Mr. Macgowan stated that in an interview which he had had with Mr. Shillinglaw, hon. sec. of the Pharmaceutical Society, that gentleman had very kindly offered to lend the association some of the leading English, American, and foreign periodicals and journals for perusal, the same to be returned in a month or six weeks.

There being no further matters of business to bring forward, the meeting closed with the usual vote of thanks to the chair.

The next meeting of the association will be held on Wednesday, 21st April, at nine p.m.

For the period of the year from 1st April to 31st October the chemists of Ballarat will close their establishments at nine p.m.

Notes and Abstracts.

ANILINE RED IN WINE.—Brunner has given a new test for the presence of aniline red in wine. Digest the wine with a piece of stearin. After cooling, the latter will be found to be coloured violet.

PROTECTION OF IRON CASTINGS.—Rub 1 part of graphite to a powder, add 4 parts of sulphate of lead, 1 part of sulphate of zinc, and 16 parts of linseed oil varnish ; mix well and boil. This forms a varnish which no weather will wash off.

BALSAM OF PERU IN PRURITUS.—Dr. Auerbach, of Berlin, has for some time past treated pruritus by balsam of Peru with the greatest success. After the first rubbing into the part affected, great relief is obtained, and in a few days a cure results.

GROWTH OF VINES FROM SEED.—Dr. A. Blankenhorn maintains that the constitution of European vines is exhausted, owing to their continued propagation by layers and cuttings. He recommends propagation by seed as a defence against the *phylloxera*.

BLACK POLISH ON IRON.—For those who wish to obtain that beautiful deep black polish on iron or steel which is so much sought after, all that is required is to boil 1 part of sulphur in 10 parts of oil of turpentine, the product of which is a brown sulphuric oil of disagreeable smell. This should be put on the outside as lightly as possible, and heated till the required black polish is obtained.

DISGUISING THE ODOUR OF IODOFORM (see also *Am. Jour. Pharm.*, 1879, p. 190).—The addition of oil of peppermint was successfully resorted to by Vulpius. Dr. Lindemann prefers oil of cloves and balsam of Peru, and prescribes two parts of the balsam to one pint of iodoform. Iodoform ointment is prepared either with lard, glycerin, ointment, or soft paraffine ; and a liquid preparation is made with glycerine, alcohol, or collodion, as follows :—

R Iodoform ... ... 1·0
Balsam of Peru ... ... 2·0
Lard (or glycerine ointment or soft paraffine 8·0
Or, R Iodoform ... ... 1·0
Balsam of Peru ... ... 3·0
Alcohol (or glycerine or collodion) ... ... 12·0

Mix, in both cases, the iodoform first with the balsam and then add the vehicle.—*Pharm. Ztg.*, 25th Oct., 1879, p. 663 ; *Allg. Med. Central Ztg.*

NEW METHOD OF CAPSULING BOTTLES.—The London *Chemist and Druggist* says :—A new system of capsuling bottles has come into fashion from France. It is much more rapid than the method of affixing lead capsules, and some may think that it gives more elegant effects. The medium for forming the capsulage is a viscous volatile liquid, into which the top of the bottle is dipped, and immediately withdrawn with a slight rotatory motion. It leaves a transparent capsule, and the effect is better if a label bearing a monogram or trademark had been previously attached to the top of the bottle. We find the following formula for the liquid, given by M. Soulan, of St. Emilion :—

	Parts.
Yellow resin	20
Ether	40
Collodion	60
Fuchsine or other tint, q. s.	

FUCUS VESICULOSUS (ANTI-FAT).—Now that this remedy is so universally used for the reduction of obesity, it may interest the profession to recall to mind another use found for it in 1826. Lacnnec having observed that on the coast of Brittany, where the air is more humid, but at the same time milder and more equable than in the interior of France, the number of phthisical patients was comparatively small ; and having also seen that young men from Brittany became consumptive during their sojourn in large cities, and recovered on returning to their native province, came to the conclusion that the peculiar atmosphere of the sea coast had something to do in these results. He, therefore, tried to imitate it, in some measure, by placing near the beds of the patients certain fresh marine plants. He brought together, into two small wards, a number of phthisical patients, and surrounded their beds with the *fucus vesiculosus*, causing them to drink also an infusion of the same plant. None appeared to suffer from this mode of treatment, as long as the fresh *fucus* could be procured. The cough became less frequent, the breathing less confined, the expectoration less in quantity. In the greater number the hectic fever ceased, and *the progress of emaciation was arrested*. In 1826 the *fucus* caused fattening and arrest of emaciation ; now it produces emaciation, or rather it reduces bulk, according to testimony of many writers, who, perhaps, do not take into account the diet they adopt, or the hygiene they follow, as being a more important factor in the matter. We do not hear now of *fucus* in consumption. In fifty-three years' time shall we hear of anti-fata.—*Med. Press and Circ., Dublin.*

REMARKABLE EXPLOSIONS.—Attention was recently directed in the French Academy to a case of explosion of carbonic acid which occurred in July last in one of the coal pits of Rochebelle (Gard). The coal strata there are much dislocated, and the carbonic acid generated plentifully in the neighbourhood, and finding its way through natural passages, seems to have accumulated in certain parts with sufficient tension to explode with two loud detonations, driving a large quantity of fine coal into the galleries. Three men were asphyxiated, and two others were only able to throw themselves in a swooning state into the cage and be hauled up. That no flame was present (as in explosions of fire damp) is proved by the absence of burns on the bodies of the victims, the fact that blasting cartridges did not go off, &c. The gas is thought to have arisen from sulphuric acid (produced through oxidation of a stratified mass of pyrites) dissolving in subterranean waters, and finding its way down to triassic limestone. In the works of M. Kuhlmann lately an alembic of platina, about 90 centimètres diameter, used for producing daily some 6000 to 7000 kilogrammes of concentrated sulphuric acid, was exploded, the component pieces being shattered and thrown out, with bricks of the fireplace, 20 to 30 mètres in different directions. Fortunately a slight hissing was observed a few seconds previously, so that the workmen had time to escape a terrible fate. The nature of the explosion M. Kuhlmann supposes to be as follows :—This platinum apparatus was being cleaned ; some 30 to 40 kilogrammes of concentrated sulphuric acid had been left in it ; on this some water had been admitted through the siphon, and the whole had been gently heated three or four hours. It is known that mixing sulphuric acid with water produces a good deal of heat ; in the present instance combination is thought to have taken place instantaneously at a pretty high temperature, generating a large amount of vapour. From *data* furnished by Fabre and Silberman, it appears that 40 kilogrammes of acid at 18 deg., with water, is capable of producing instantaneously 18 to 20 cubic mètres of vapour, and this is sufficient to explode a platinum vessel of about 300 litres capacity, and only 2 to 3 mm. thickness. As the combination occurred at about 100 deg., the force would be greater. M. Kuhlmann has repeated the explosion several times in laboratory experiments, and he finds that it always occurs with great violence where the quantity of water is at least ten equivalents for one of acid. In presence of the difficulty of mixing these two substances, which have a very great affinity, but the density of which is so different that they may remain several hours one on the other without mixture and consequent combination, the need of cautious management is obvious.

Correspondence.

TO CORRESPONDENTS.

WE have received a letter from Mr. W. J. Brownscombe; but as at the last meeting of the council the proposed amended rules were discussed, and a decision arrived at, which will be reported to the special meeting summoned for 7th May, there is no necessity for its publication.—ED.

To the Editor of The Australasian Supplement to the Chemist and Druggist.

SIR—I will deem it a great favour if any of your correspondents can inform me of the best compound for coating pills. I have one of Cartner's patent pill-coaters, but fail to turn out pills coated to my satisfaction. I have tried French chalk and liquid gum, sugar and ditto, a mixture of French chalk and sugar and ditto, also albumen and chalk and sugar, but cannot succeed.—Yours, &c. AMBITION.

To the Editor of The Australasian Supplement to the Chemist and Druggist.

SIR—My attention has just been called to a notice of the recent milk adulteration case in your issue of February. I am made to state that colonial milk "was inferior in quality to that produced in England." This I am sure I did not say; and that I had "found that the percentage of water was from 94 to 95." What I desired to convey to the court was that, in my opinion, Wanklyn's milk standard is too high; judged by it several samples of genuine milk analysed in the museum laboratory showed only from 94 to 95 per cent. of pure *milk*—not water.

Will you kindly correct the report in your next issue? and oblige, yours very truly, J. COSMO NEWBERY.
Melbourne, 22nd March, 1880.

MEDICAMENTA ARCANA.

To the Editor of The Australasian Supplement to the Chemist and Druggist.

SIR—With your permission I wish to have a little talk with my fellow-pharmacists, trusting it will be for our mutual benefit; and the subject of our conversation shall be the "Proprietary Medicine Trade."

For years I have watched with regret the importation of this description of medicine from England, France, America, and elsewhere, not only as a loss of revenue to the druggist, but a tacit depreciation of his abilities.

Many of us were in the business prior to our arrival here, and can look back with pleasure at the paucity of patent medicines sold in our time; in fact, can remember that we had our own preparations, and always recommended them in place of "patents." Why? Because on our own articles we could depend, and also that we made a better profit on their sale. But here I find pharmacists (?) lower themselves to tout the preparations of others instead of placing before their patients a remedy produced by their own knowledge of their profession, and, in most instances, better qualified to suit their case than the imported nostrums that inundate our colony. Are they so deficient in the knowledge of the drugs they dispense that they consider it safer and better to recommend So-and-so's essence, or What-d'ye-call-em's syrup, &c.? Why should we have chlorodyne, pectorals, pills, salts, &c., forced on us for sale? Surely the pharmacists of the present day are capable of producing articles as good and in many cases better than this imported legion of medicaments. Let us, I ask, bestir ourselves. Have we not amongst us men

of genius enough to teach something to our brother chemists over the sea, and raise the status of pharmacy by supplying those wants from among ourselves, and thereby relieve us from paying duties and percentages, profits here and there, on this flood of foreign productions? Let our wholesale houses help us, and make the necessary bottles, &c., for putting up our own proprietary articles, and let us be a more independent colony in this matter.

I would suggest, Mr. Editor, that the Pharmaceutical Society should allow samples of colonial preparations to be forwarded for their inspection, and that they publish their opinion on them, and endeavour to eradicate from our prescriptions—"Chlorodyne" (Collis Brown's), "Nepenthe" (Squire's), "Pill, Antib." (Cockle's); "Try one bottle Eno's Fruit Salt"; "Get a box of Kram's Pills;" "Liq. Bismuthi" (Sch's.); and others too numerous to mention in this catalogue.

Having so far ventilated the subject, I trust someone else may be found ready to assist and relieve us from encumbering our shelves with expensive articles that ought to be the legitimate production of the pharmacist himself, and prevent the importation of the trash forced upon us through the advertising medium.—Yours truly, EMANCIPATOR.

THE "DRUGGING OF ANIMALS ACT."

AT the annual meeting of the Pharmaceutical Society, Mr. Graham Mitchell, F.R.C.V.S., a member of the society, brought under notice the desirability of having some measure similar to "Drugging of Animals Act," now in force in England, pass during the next Parliament. For the information of our readers we publish the Act at present in operation in England, and shall be glad of any suggestions, as no doubt this Act might be considerably improved on. The absence of qualified veterinary surgeons in many country districts makes it desirable to provide that medicines should be supplied by only qualified pharmacists.

AN ACT TO PREVENT THE ADMINISTRATION OF POISONOUS DRUGS TO HORSES AND OTHER ANIMALS. 1ST JUNE, 1876. (39 VICT., CAP. 13.)

Whereas it is expedient to make provision against the practice of administering poisonous drugs to horses and other animals by disqualified persons, and without the knowledge and consent of the owners of such horses and animals:

Be it enacted by the Queen's most Excellent Majesty, by and with the advice and consent of the Lords Spiritual and Temporal, and Commons, in this present Parliament assembled, and by the authority of the same, as follows:

1. If any person wilfully and unlawfully administers to or causes to be administered to or taken by any horse, cattle, or domestic animal any poisonous or injurious drug or substance, he shall (unless some reasonable cause or excuse is shown on his behalf) be liable, on summary conviction, to a penalty not exceeding five pounds, or, at the discretion of the court, to imprisonment, with or without hard labour, for any term not exceeding one month in the case of a first offence, or three months in the case of a second or any subsequent offence.

2. Nothing in this Act shall extend to any person being owner or acting by authority of the owner of the horse, cattle, or other animal to which any drug or substance is administered.

3. Nothing in this Act shall exempt a person from liability to any greater or other punishment under any other Act or law, so that he be not more than once punished for the same offence.

4. Any offence against this Act may be prosecuted in the manner provided by the Summary Jurisdiction Acts before two justices of the peace.

5. This Act shall not extend to Scotland or to Ireland.

6. This Act may be cited as the "Drugging of Animals Act, 1876."

A PAYING HOSPITAL.

WE some time ago drew attention to this subject in the columns of this journal. In America we find "invalid hospitals" in healthy localities increasing away from the centres of population, which have proved a great success, and are gradually increasing. This want has been long felt in Australia, where there is great difficulty for strangers and bachelors obtaining good nursing, without which doctoring is of very little use. Many cases have come under our observation lately where slight illnesses have culminated into serious and even fatal results, in consequence of patients not knowing where to find the comforts necessary for their recovery. We are aware that suitable premises have been offered in one suburb (St. Kilda) on favourable terms ; and we would suggest that a public meeting should be called with the view of forming a limited company. We trust that no attempt to increase the Melbourne Hospital nuisance will meet with support. It has been hinted that a wing added to the hospital would be sufficient. To this we are utterly opposed. Without fresh air, thorough drainage, and strict sanitary conditions, we may " throw physic to the dogs." We are glad to find the subject has been taken up with interest by several of our leading medical men. At a recent meeting of the Melbourne Hospital Dr. Gillbee moved the following resolution :—" That in the opinion of this committee a self-supporting hospital would be the means of meeting a serious want ; that it would be of great service in preventing much of the hospital abuse which at present exists ; that it would meet the case of many classes of people who at present when attacked by illness experience great difficulty in obtaining relief, and who will be able by the help of a paying hospital to procure for a payment within their means the medical attendance, skilled nursing, and home comforts which they may need ; and that this committee solicit for this scheme the support of the public and the medical profession."

RUST IN WHEAT.

THE *Rochester Express* of 26th March writes :—" Our attention was called yesterday to a branch of native industry in the establishment of Mr. G. F. Chamberlin, our local chemist. It appears that for some time past Mr. Chamberlin has turned his attention to the discovery of a preventive for rust in wheat, and last year he succeeded in producing what he estimated would be successful. It was tested, and a crop sown with wheat dressed with Mr. Chamberlin's carbolic preparation proved to be entirely free from that pest, whereas, outside the prepared lot, even in the same paddock, undressed grain was found to be full of it. The carbolic preventive, he assures us, has been calculated with great care, the proportion being reduced to the capacity of one grain of wheat before he finally determined on the strength of the compound. The great difficulty Mr. Chamberlin had to contend with seems to have been the impregnation of the plant by the dressing of the grain, but in this he has succeeded beyond expectation, for the effects may be recognised in the parent germ even after the plant has been produced. Mr. Chamberlin has forwarded his carbolic preventive to Queensland as a trial for the £1000 bonus to be given by the Government for a cheap remedy. He has also sent the result of last year's experiments to Adelaide, at the request of that Government."

SIMPLE METHOD OF PREPARING A SOLUTION OF THE DOUBLE IODIDE OF BISMUTH AND POTASSIUM FOR USE AS AN ALKALOIDAL REAGENT.

(BY J. C. THRESH.)

ALTHOUGH it has been long known that a solution of the iodide of bismuth and potassium forms an exceedingly delicate reagent for detection of alkaloids, yet, on account of the trouble involved in making such a solution, it is not frequently employed ; moreover, in the majority of text-books it is not even mentioned.

Such a solution may almost instantly be prepared as follows :—

Take of—

Liq. bismuthi, B.P.	℈j.
Pot. iodid.	℥iss.
Acid. hydrochlor.	℥iss.

Mix.

The resulting fluid is of a rich orange colour, and when added to cold solutions containing an alkaloid, produces immediately an orange red precipitate, which appears to be almost totally insoluble in cold water, though somewhat readily soluble therein when hot. In point of delicacy, it is at least equal to the solution of phosphomolybdic acid, which is both troublesome and difficult to properly prepare. One part of strychnia may be detected in 500,000 of water, and one of morphia in 20,000. All the other alkaloids examined fall between these extremes.

In presence of other organic matter I am inclined to think this reagent is more reliable as an indicator of the presence of an alkaloid than any of the solutions used for that purpose. It appears also to be applicable for volumetrically estimating the strengths of alkaloidal solutions, and the author is at present engaged in devising such a process.

SANITAS, A LATE ANTISEPTIC.

THIS is a London product. The composition and method of preparing it have been described in the London *Chemist and Druggist* as follows :—

" A number of medical and scientific gentlemen and others assembled at the works of the Sanitas Company (Limited) to see the process of manufacture of this interesting product and the perfected methods which have now been arrived at. Mr. C. T. Kingzett, F.C.S., explained the process of manufacture and the principles on which this is founded with all clearness. A continuous blast of hot air is forced through pipes carried through the building, and provided with sub-pipes conducting into 20 or 30 large earthenware carboys, each capable of holding about 100 gallons. These carboys each contain about 80 gallons of water, and 15 gallons of turpentine floating on its surface. The hot air is brought into the liquid at about the point where the water and the turpentine are in contact. The carboys stand in vats of hot water, which keep their contents warm, and the air, as it is discharged, passes upwards through the turpentine, gradually oxidizing it, and throwing down into the water certain soluble products of the decomposition. There is an aperture at the top of the vessel for the escape of the air. After continued action of this kind for about 300 hours, the water is fully charged, and becomes, after filtration, the liquid called by the inventor ' Sanitas.' According to the experiments which Mr. Kingzett carried out for some years on the oxidation of turpentine and essential oils, sanitas would be mainly a solution of peroxide of hydrogen and camphoric acid. To these he considers it owes its antiseptic and disinfectant properties.

" Mr. Kingzett showed some striking experiments to prove the presence of peroxide of hydrogen in sanitas, and afterwards handed round specimens of fish, meat, and other articles of food, some of which had been preserved for months by sanitas ; and he also took a piece of putrid meat, and, immersing it in sanitas, passed it round to the company, who satisfied themselves that all disagreeable odour had been removed. Mr. Haviland, medical officer of health for Northamptonshire, and other gentlemen present, spoke highly of the advantages of sanitas; and a letter was also read from the Duke of Manchester, who had promised to preside on the occasion, but was prevented by neuralgia, saying that he only accepted the position after he had satisfied himself by experiment of the value of the product."

MISCELLANEOUS FORMULÆ.

GLYCERINE CREAM.

Ceresin ...	...	...	...	...	20 parts
Oil sweet almonds	...	...	...	50 „

Melt ; add

Powdered soap	...	...	...	...	10 „
Rose water	...	...	...	...	20 „
Glycerine	...	...	...	...	20 „
Oil of roses, sufficient.					

LACQUER FOR SURGICAL STEEL INSTRUMENTS.

Paraffine	...	...	...	10 parts
Venice turpentine	...	...	...	1 part
Coal tar benzine	...	...	...	50 parts

TRANSPARENT POMATUM.

Paraffine (or ceresin)	...	...	...	15 parts
Castor oil	...	...	...	85 „
Perfume	...	...	...	q. s.

WATERPROOFING OF LEATHER, ETC.

1. | | | | | |
|---|---|---|---|---|
| Lubricating (paraffine) oil... | ... | ... | 2000 parts |
| Raw rapeseed oil | ... | ... | ... | 2000 „ |
| Sperm oil | ... | ... | ... | 500 „ |
| White turpentine | ... | ... | ... | 250 „ |
| Nitrobenzol, sufficient to perfume. | | | | |

2. | | | | | |
|---|---|---|---|---|
| Paraffine oil ... | ... | ... | ... | 1000 parts |
| Rapeseed oil ... | ... | ... | ... | 1000 „ |
| Paraffine | ... | ... | ... | 500 „ |
| Suet ... | ... | ... | ... | 500 „ |
| Resin ... | ... | ... | ... | 500 „ |

IMITATION WHITE WINE VINEGAR.—Filter ordinary vinegar through animal charcoal and paper.

TO RECLAIM SPOILED DISTILLED WATERS.—Add one grain each of alum and borax to every pint.

MAKING FERN PICTURES.

THERE are two ways—the mechanical and the photographical. For the first, take a sheet of strong white paper, and with an atomizer pass over it a spray of very diluted mucilage, so as to obtain a very thin and slightly sticking film, which will make the picture. The ferns and leaves must have been first pressed in a book, and, after arranging them to suit your taste, cause them to lie as closely to the paper as possible ; fill an atomizer with very diluted India ink, and blow a spray over the ferns, more or less in proportion as you want a darker or lighter shade. It is well to do this with intermissions, letting it dry a little, so as to avoid excess of moisture and possibility of running the liquid into drops. When nearly dry, but still a little moist, remove the ferns, which may be used over again several times. For the photographic method, cover a sheet of paper with a weak solution of salt in water and some white of an egg, well beaten; after it is dry, take it into a dark room, and with a tuft of cotton pass over it a solution of nitrate of silver (50 grains to an ounce of water) ; dry it in the dark, and the coat of chloride of silver formed on its surface will receive the impression. Then arrange your ferns between two plates of glass, and cut the paper to the same size as the glass plates ; place it under them and expose to the sun, in the same way as a photographer prints a portrait. Watch it until dark enough, and before removing the paper from the glass take it into a dark room. Here place the picture in a solution of hyposulphite of soda, which will dissolve the chloride of silver, but leave the decomposed material (finely divided black silver) which forms the black back-ground, while the shadow of the leaves will be white.

REMEDIES FOR CHILBLAINS.

THE following applications will he found quite useful to cure chilblains, or at least to greatly relieve the pain and itching. The first ones are for the unbroken, and the last for broken chilblains.

The first is a *liniment*, made as follows :—

Sulphuric acid	...	...	...	1 drachm.
Spirit of turpentine	...	...	1	,,
Olive oil	...	...	...	3 drachms.

Mix the oil and turpentine first, then gradually add the acid. To he rubbed in two or three times a day.

The two others are *ointments* :—

(1)
Lard	...	...	...	...	4 ounces.
Turpentine	...	...	...	...	1 ounce.
Camphor	...	...	...	...	2 drachms.
Oil of rosemary	...	...	...	15 minims.

This ointment to he rubbed in with continued friction.

(2)
Yellow wax	...	...	...	3 ounces.
Olive oil...	...	...	...	3 ,,
Camphorated oil	...	...	...	3 ,,
Goulard extract...	...	...	...	1½ ,,

Melt the wax with the olive oil, then add the camphor oil and Goulard extract.

WATER AND FIRE PROOF PAPER.

A WATER and fire proof paper, lately patented, is made by putting a mixture of ordinary pulp and asbestos reduced to pulp, in the proportion of about two-thirds of the former to one-third of the latter, into a strong solution of common salt and alum. This mixture is put through the engine and then run off through a Fourdrinier. The paper thus made is run through a bath of gum shellac, dissolved in alcohol or other suitable volatile solvent of that gum, and subsequently through ordinary calendar rolls, after which the paper is ready to he cut into such sized sheets as may he required for use. The effect of the strong solution of salt and alum upon the paper is to greatly strengthen it, and to increase its fire-resisting qualities. The shellac bath to which it is treated is said to cause the paper to become thoroughly permeated with the gum, so the paper becomes waterproof to such an extent that long boiling in water does not disintegrate it, and the presence of the gum in and upon the surface of the paper seems to present no obstacle to the proper and usual absorption of ink, either printing or writing. Thus, hy the combination of the asbestos, salt, and alum in the paper, it is rendered so far fire-proof that a direct exposure to an intense fire does not burn up the substance of the paper to an extent that interferes with safely handling it; and when exposed to great heat in books, or between metallic plates, a number of sheets together, it is much less injured hy the fire.

The addition of the gum shellac to the paper makes it, for all practical purposes, water-proof, so that if account books, valuable documents, bank bills, and other monetary papers for which this paper is used be subjected to the action of fire and water, either one or both, in a burning building, they will not be injured to such an extent as to destroy their value.—*Scientific American.*

CORK, CORKS, AND CORKSCREWS.

(BY H. G. GLASSPOOLE.)

(Concluded.)

THE British import duty on unmanufactured cork was abolished in the year 1845, and in 1860 the duties on cork ready made and cork squared for rounding, which had been fixed in 1853 at 6d. per lb. and 8s. per cwt. respectively, were repealed.

The imports of cork into the United Kingdom in 1876 were :—

Cork unmanufactured.		Tons.	Value.
From Portugal	...	6267	£172,666
From Spain	...	395	11,413
From Algeria	...	351	7,045
Other countries	...	195	6,391
Total	... ...	7208	£197,515

Cork manufactured.		Lbs.	Value.
From France	...	3,174,431	£267,624
From Portugal	...	2,537,175	147,975
From Spain	...	927,793	72,354
Other countries	...	21,804	1,586
Total	...	6,661,203	£489,539

Ancient Use of Corks, &c.—The cork tree, and the application of its bark to useful purposes, was well known to the Egyptians, Greeks, and Romans. The former used to construct their coffins of this material. Theophrastus, the Greek philosopher, who wrote on botany, &c., four centuries B.C., mentions this tree amongst the oaks, under the name of *phellus*, and says that it has a thick fleshy bark, which must be stripped off every three years to prevent it from perishing. He adds that it was so light as never to sink in water, and on that account might be used for many purposes. Pliny describes the tree under the name of *suber*, and relates everything said by Theophrastus of *phellus*. From his account we learn that the Roman fishermen used it as floats to their nets and fishing tackle, and as buoys to their anchors. The use of these buoys in saving life appears to have been well known to the ancients, for Lucian (*Epist.* 1, 17) mentions that when two men, one of whom had fallen into the sea, and another who jumped after to afford him assistance, both were saved by means of an anchor buoy. The use of this substance in assisting swimmers was not unknown to the Romans. By Plutarchus, in *Vita Camilli*, we are told that when the imperial city was besieged by the Gauls, Camillus sent a Roman to the Capitol, who to avoid the enemy swam the Tiber with corks under him, his clothes being bound upon his head, and was fortunate enough to succeed in the attempt. The use of cork for stoppers was not entirely unknown to the Romans, and instances of its being thus employed may be seen in Cato's *De Re Rustica*, cap. 120 ; but its application to this purpose seems not to have been very common, or cork stoppers would have been oftener mentioned hy authors who have written on agriculture and cookery, and also in the works of ancient poets. The convivial customs of those days had no connection with the bottle, glass bottles being of a much later invention. Instead of having dozens of sparkling champagne or hock, to be liberated from the bottle by the corkscrew, at their feasts, the guests filled their drinking cups of gold, silver, crystal, or beechwood from a two-handled amphora, a kind of earthenware pitcher in which their choice wines used to be kept. The mouths of these vessels were stopped with wood, and covered with a mastic, composed of pitch, chalk, and oil, to prevent air spoiling the wine or evaporation taking place. Columella, who wrote one of the earliest works on agriculture, gives directions for preparing this cement. Pliny, in describing the cork tree, says it is smaller than the oak, and its acorns are of the very worst quality. He tells us the cork tree did not grow throughout Italy, and in no part whatever of Gaul. At the present day it is abundant in France, and Fee states that the acorns of *Q. suber* are of an agreeable flavour, and the hams of Bayonne are said to owe their high reputation from the pigs having fed on the acorns of the cork tree. Some ancient authors speak of the cork tree as the female of the holm oak (*Q. ilex*), and in countries where the holm does not grow they used to substitute the wood of the cork tree, more particularly in cartwrights' work in the neighbourhood of Lacedæmon, &c.

The employment of corks for stoppers of bottles appears to have come into use about the seventeenth century, when glass bottles, of which no mention is made before the fifteenth century, began to be generally introduced. Before that period apothecaries used stoppers of wax, which were not only much more expensive, but far more troublesome.

In 1553, when C. Stephanus wrote his *Prædium Rusticum*, cork stoppers appear to have been very little known in France, for he states that this material was used principally for soles in that country. Another author, writing about the same time, tells us that thin glass flasks, covered with rushes and straw and with tin mouths, which could be stopped sufficiently close without a cork, were used by the higher classes of that period.

We do not know when cork and corks began to be generally used in this country, but I find in that very amusing and instructive diary of Mr. Samuel Pepys the following entry :— 14th July, 1666, he states, after having written to the Duke of York for money for the fleet, he went down Thames-street, and there agreed for four or five tons of cork to be sent to the fleet, being a new device to make barricados with instead of junts (old cable) ; but he does not inform us how the device answered. In Evelyn's time (1664) cork was much used by old persons for linings to the soles of their shoes, whence the German name for it, "pantoffelholtz," or slipper wood. The Venetian dames, Evelyn says, used it for their choppings, or high-heeled shoes, to make them appear taller than nature intended they should be. The poor in Spain lay planks of cork by their bedside, to tread on instead of carpets. Sometimes they line the inside of their houses, both with stone, with this bark, which renders them very warm, and corrects the moisture of the air. Loudon relates that in the celebrated convent at Cintra (Portugal) several articles of furniture are made of this tree, which strangers who visit the convent are requested to lift in order that surprise may be excited at their extraordinary lightness. The various uses for the common purposes of every-day life to which this substance is applied are well known. Burnt cork supplies our artists and colour-men with Spanish black. It is largely used for lifeboats, for stuffing life belts, mattresses, &c., to be used at sea in the preservation of life.

Virgin cork, or the outer bark of this tree, is now very much used for window flower-boxes, grottoes, &c. Very thin sections of cork are employed in the manufactory of hats ; these sections are cut by steam machinery 50 to 120 plates to the inch. The shreds and parings of this substance are not wasted, but, being ground into powder and mixed with melted India-rubber, form the basis of many floor coverings, such as kamptulicon—the soft, unresounding material which covers the floor of the reading-room of the British Museum, the floors of the Houses of Parliament, and various other public and private institutions, to prevent the noise occasioned by foot-steps, &c.

Cork was formerly employed in medicine even as far back as the time of Pliny, as he tells us that the bark of the cork tree, pulverised and taken in warm water, arrests hæmorrhage at the mouth and nostrils, and the ashes of it taken in warm wine are highly extolled as a cure for spitting blood. (See Pliny's *Nat. Hist.*, b. 24.) In more modern time powdered cork has been applied as a styptic, and hung about the necks of nurses ; it was thought to possess the power of stopping the secretion of milk. Burnt cork mixed with sugar of lead and lard has been used as an application to piles. (See Pareira's *Materia Medica.*)

When rasped or powdered cork is subjected to chemical solvents, such as alcohol, &c., it leaves 70 per cent of an insoluble substance, called suberine. This, treated with nitric acid, yields the following products :—White fibrous matter, 0·18 ; resin, 14·72 ; oxalic acid, 16·00 ; suberic acid (peculiar acid of cork), 14·2, in 100 parts.

Cork contains tannic acid, which makes it an improper substance for closing vessels containing chalybeate liquids, as the iron is in part absorbed by the cork and blackens it by forming in its substance tannate of iron. The whole of the water may thus become discoloured.

Cork is a nitrogenous substance which, next to cellulose, is the most important constituent of the cell wall. Cellulose, corky substance and fatty matters seem to be found in the same cell, and when the cellulose has been absorbed, the corky substance alone remains. It forms the outermost part of the cell wall, and unites the cells together. (See Balfour's *Class-book of Botany.*)

The bark of many trees resembles cork. There is a variety of *Ulmus campestris suberosa*, the cork-bark elm, which grows in our hedgerows, whose bark assumes something of the external appearance of cork in its softness and elasticity, as well as in its chemical properties ; but as it does not grow to any great thickness, it is not of any value for economic purposes.

The cork tree, *Q. suber*, and its varieties, are to be found growing in many of the botanical, horticultural, and private gardens of England. It was introduced in or before 1699 by the Duchess of Beaufort, and is readily propagated by acorns.

In *Notes and Queries*, series 4, Vol. 5, it is stated that in some parts of Lincolnshire it is believed that cork has the power of keeping off cramp. It is placed between the bed and mattress, or even between the sheets. Cork garters are made by sewing together a series of thin disks of this material between two silk ribbons and worn for the same purpose.

Where the bark of *Quercus suber* cannot be obtained, many substitutes have been found to supply its place among the spongy bark or wood substances of other trees. The wood of *Anona Balustris*, growing in the West Indies, called the alligator's apple, is of such a soft nature that it is frequently used by the negroes, instead of corks, to stop their jugs and calabashes.

The word cork is said to be derived from the Spanish *corcho,* from the Latin *cortex.*

THE CORKSCREW.

That useful instrument, the corkscrew, was unknown to our forefathers two hundred years ago, and was not in common use even at a later date. The mode of extracting a cork in those days was by winding a cloth or handkerchief tightly round it and with a peculiar jerk pulling the stopper out of the bottle. Other ways, no doubt, were also adopted—the teeth, for instance. There is no record that I can find as to who first invented this instrument. It came into use about the beginning of the last century, and was for many years called a "bottlescrew." The earliest mention of the corkscrew is in an amusing poem, entitled "The tale of the Bottlescrue," in a collection of poems by Nicholas Amhurst, published in 1723 (*vide Notes and Queries*, 1856, p. 466), in which the poet gives the legendary origin of the invention. Bacchus is described in the poem, and among other things it is said of him—

> This hand a corkscrew did contain,
> And that a bottle of champagne.

Yet the bottlescrew at that time appears to have been the common name of this useful article, for the poet concludes his tale with the following lines :—

> By me shall Birmingham become
> In future days more famed than Rome ;
> Shall owe to me her reputation
> And serve with bottlescrews the nation.

Corkscrews, like corks, are to be found, in some shape or other, in all parts of the civilised world.

AUTUMN LEAVES.—Prof. Church has discovered the curious fact that autumn leaves—brown, red, &c.—may be restored to their original green tint by heating in water with zinc powder. —*Arch. d. Ph.*

REMOVAL OF SILVER-NITRATE STAINS.—Instead of potassium cyanide, Dr. H. Kaetzer uses a solution of 10 grams ammonium chloride and 10 grams corrosive sublimate in 100 grams distilled water, which must be kept in glass-stoppered bottles. It will readily remove the stains from the skin, linen, wool, and cotton, without injuring the fabric.—*Pharm. Ztg.,* 10th Dec., 1879, p. 767, *fr., Neueste Erf. u. Erfahr.*

FROSTED TIN.—By dipping *tinned* iron, previously heated till the tin begins to melt, into a mixture of 16 parts by weight of muriatic acid, 8 of nitric acid, 24 of water, and 1 or 2 of bicarbonate of potassa, rinsing and treating with a solution of hyposulphite of soda, very beautiful chrystalline designs will be formed.

FELTON, GRIMWADE & CO.,

WHOLESALE DRUGGISTS AND MANUFACTURING CHEMISTS,

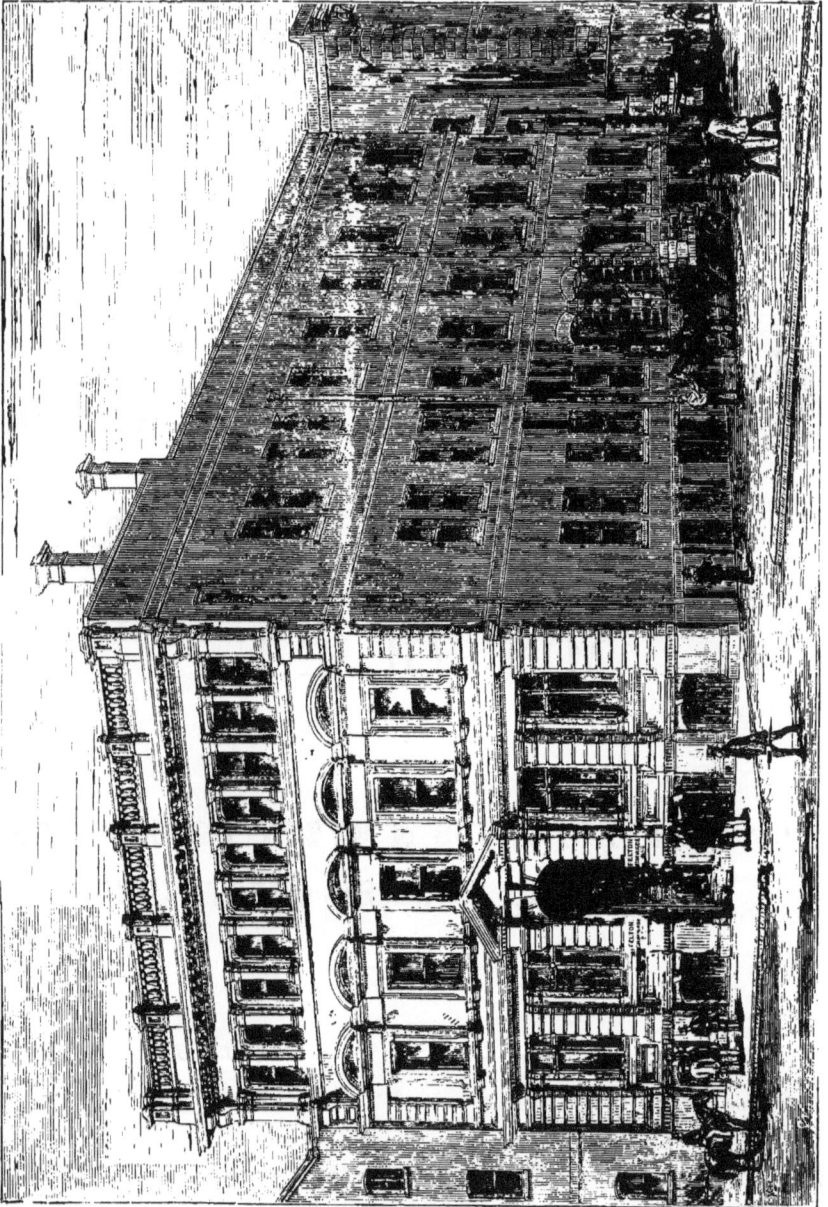

31 & 33 FLINDERS LANE WEST,
MELBOURNE.

N. 2, no. 24: 1-96.
(Apr., 1880).

[SUPPLEMENT ONLY.]

THE
Chemist & Druggist.

WITH AUSTRALASIAN SUPPLEMENT.

(Published under direction of the Pharmaceutical Society of Victoria.)

No. 24. { PUBLISHED ON THE 15TH OF EVERY MONTH. }
Registered for Transmission as a Newspaper.

APRIL, 1880.

{ SUBSCRIPTION, 15s. PER ANNUM, INCLUDING DIARY, POST FREE.

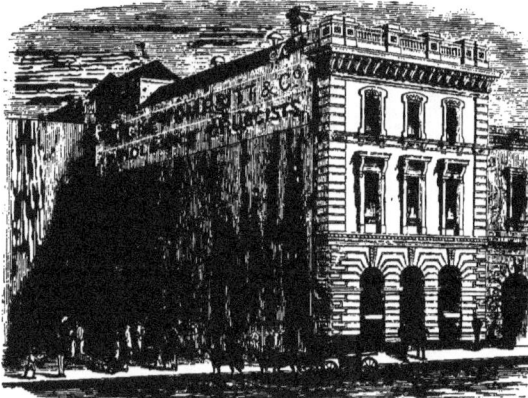

HEMMONS, LAWS & CO.

WHOLESALE DRUGGISTS,

55 & 57

RUSSELL STREET,

MELBOURNE.

INDEX TO LITERARY CONTENTS.

The Chemist and Druggist.

WITH AUSTRALASIAN SUPPLEMENT.

OFFICE: MUTUAL PROVIDENT BUILDINGS, COLLINS STREET WEST.
Published on the 15th of each Month.

THIS Journal is issued gratis to all paid-up Members of the PHARMA-CEUTICAL SOCIETY OF VICTORIA, and to non-members at Fifteen Shillings per annum, payable in advance. A copy of *The Chemists and Druggists' Diary*, published annually, is forwarded post free to every subscriber.

Advertisements, remittances, and all business communications to be addressed to THE HONORARY SECRETARY OF THE PHARMACEUTICAL SOCIETY, MELBOURNE.

SCALE OF CHARGES FOR ADVERTISEMENTS:

	Per annum.		Per annum.
One Page	£8 0 0	Quarter Page	.. £3 0 0
Half do.	5 0 0	Business Cards	.. 2 0 0

Special rates for wrapper and pages preceding and following literary matter. Advertisements of Assistants Wanting Situations, 2s. 6d. each.

Advertisements for insertion in the current month should be sent to the office before the 10th.

COMMUNICATIONS for the EDITORIAL department of this Journal should be addressed to THE EDITOR, MUTUAL PROVIDENT BUILDINGS, COLLINS STREET WEST, MELBOURNE.

No notice can be taken of anonymous communications. Whatever is intended for insertion must be authenticated by the name and address of the writer—not necessarily for publication, but as a guarantee of good faith.

DEATHS.

JESSOP.—On the 15th August, 1877, at his father's residence, 57 Wellington-road, Rhyl, North Wales, Edmond James Jessop (formerly chemist, Prahran), aged twenty-five years, of phthisis.

LONGSTAFF.—On the 4th May, at Victoria-street, Ballarat, Joseph Long-staff, aged forty-five years.

PROCTOR.—On 21st April, at the Ballarat Hospital, John Cameron Proctor, aged fifty-five.

The Month.

THE Governor-in-Council has appointed Mr. Bosisto, M.P., and Mr. C. R. Blackett as members of the commission for promoting technological and industrial education. The Hon. F. S. Dobson, LL.D., M.L.C., and Mr. W. C. Kernot, M.A., of the Melbourne University, have also been appointed.

Mr. Joseph Bosisto, M.L.A., has been appointed a member of the council of the Ballarat School of Mines, *vice* Sir C. Gavan Duffy, resigned.

At the meeting of the Victorian branch of the British Medical Association, held on the 16th April, a lengthy discussion took place with respect to the advisability of establishing paying hospitals in Melbourne. The chairman, Mr. Gillbee, strongly urged the desirability of providing such institutions, and mentioned that a company was in course of formation which will carry out the project. Plans of a large hospital suitable for the purpose were submitted, and after a short discussion the meeting unanimously passed a motion in favour of the project in question, which will probably be brought before the public in a more tangible form shortly.

From the *Argus* of the 15th April we extract the following : —"The announcement in our advertising columns of the death of Edmond James Jessop, formerly chemist, of Prahran, is one to which peculiar interest attaches. Jessop was supposed to have been drowned in the Yarra in 1875. He did not meet with that fate, however, but went clandestinely to the old country, where he died at his father's residence, in North Wales, in 1877. His widow, who resides in Melbourne, did not receive intelligence of the death until the last English mail came in.

The half-yearly meeting of the Australian Health Society was held at the Town Hall on the 21st April, the Mayor of Melbourne being in the chair. Among those present there were seven members of the medical profession. The mayor, in his introductory remarks, referred to the services the society had rendered to the community in the way of spreading a knowledge of the laws of health. There was no report presented, this meeting being only intended to bring the members together, and to draw attention to the society and its operations, and to afford an opportunity for submitting some questions for discussion. A paper was read by Mr. Thomas Brodribb on "Trained Nurses," in which he insisted specially on the need of a better class of nurses, and on the desirability of providing some means for the systematic training of those wishing to follow nursing as a profession. Several of those present, including medical men, spoke of the great want of good nurses in Melbourne. Mrs. J. Webster then read a paper on "The Smoke Nuisance in Melbourne," and insisted on action being taken before the citizens became so much accustomed to the annoyance that they would cease to recognise it, and before vested interests became powerful. Votes of thanks to those who had prepared papers, and to the mayor for taking the chair, closed the proceedings, the chairman expressing the opinion that no society or institution in the city did more genuine work in proportion to its means than the Australian Health Society.

The Microscopical Society of Victoria held its monthly meeting on the 29th April. There was a fair attendance of members, and Mr. E. Bage was proposed as a new member. The president, Mr. T. S. Ralph, read translations of three interesting papers from the transactions of the Belgian Microscopical Society—viz., "On Staining with Picric Acid," "On Preserving Infusoria by Means of Osmic Acid," and "On the Thallus of Diatoms." The latter occasioned considerable discussion, during which several points were raised of interest to microscopists. Mr. J. R. Y. Goldstein described and figured a new genus in the class Polyzoa, and named it Stirpsaria, in the family Bicellariadæ ; also two new species of Serialaria—viz., S. immensa and S. intermedia. A collection of diatomaceous deposits, being a donation from Dr. Hector, of New Zealand, was then distributed amongst the members, and a pleasant *conversazione* terminated the proceedings.

The general public is, perhaps, more interested than it has yet realised in the decision given recently by the Court of Appeal in the action brought by the Pharmaceutical Society of Great Britain against the London and Provincial Supply Association. The suit was instituted in order to try the right of the defendant company to keep a store for the sale of drugs, in spite of its not being registered for that purpose, as required by the statute known as the Pharmacy Act. The court has decided—subject, of course, to an appeal to the House of

Lords—in favour of the right of the association to act as sellers of drugs and poisons, apparently on the one ground that the Pharmacy Act requires all "persons" intending to carry on the business of druggists to be duly registered, and that a company is not a person. It is hardly worth while to inquire into the correctness or incorrectness of the law thus laid down by the three Judges of Appeal, as the case will, in all probability, be taken to a higher tribunal; but, if such is the present state of the law, there can be very little doubt that it calls for immediate alteration. Nothing can be more unfair than that a number of persons should be able to club together for the sale of certain articles of commerce, and, by simply calling themselves an "association," escape the burdens and duties laid on the shoulders of the private trader. The case becomes even stronger when it is remembered that it is not everybody who is qualified to be a dispenser of poisonous drugs. The Pharmacy Act was intended to protect purchasers, and if it is found that, by a mere legal technicality, the public is deprived of the security of having duly qualified dealers in drugs, there is little doubt that the attention of Parliament should be directed to the matter.—*London Daily Telegraph,* 19th March, 1880.

There have been a considerable number of business changes lately. Mr. H. A. Glyde, formerly of Beaufort, has purchased the business of Mr. John Reed, St. Arnaud; Mr. Albert Andrews continuing Mr. Glyde's business on his own account at Beaufort. Mr. J. J. Cunningham, formerly of Wodonga, succeeds Mr. R. B. Bridge, of Bright, in the business lately carried on by him at that place; Mr. Bridge goes to Euroa. Mr. J. M. Paul is acting as manager for the widow of the late Mr. J. Summers, of Nagambie. Mrs. Stillings, the widow of the late Mr. J. Stillings, Taradale, has disposed of the business to Mr. W. W. Caught, by whom it will be continued. Mr. C. R. Soppet notifies that he has taken the business formerly carried on by Mr. W. H. Ford, at Robe-street, St. Kilda. Mr. W. J. Marshall, formerly of Kyneton, has removed to 119 Brunswick-street, Fitzroy, where he is managing for Mrs. A. T. Ewing. Mr. G. C. Powell, at one time dispenser of the Melbourne Benevolent Asylum, succeeds Mr. Jas. F. Donaldson in the business formerly carried on by Mr. Donaldson at Footscray.

Meetings.

THE PHARMACEUTICAL SOCIETY OF VICTORIA.

THE monthly meeting of the Council was held at the rooms, 100 Collins-street, on Friday, 7th May, 1880. Present— Messrs. Blackett, Gamble, Ogg, Huntsman, Jones, Baker, Bowen, Shillinglaw, Macgowan, Hooper, and Norris; the president, Mr. C. R. Blacket, in the chair.

Election of New Members.—Messrs. W. H. Eager, of Rae-street, North Fitzroy, and Henry G. M'Burney, Benalla, were elected members.

Removal of Offices.—The president read a communication he had received from the secretary to the Pharmacy Board, stating that the board were willing to give the society the use of the rooms, and all the advantages heretofore enjoyed by the society, for the sum of £25 per annum and 7s. 6d. per month to the caretaker. The president said he felt sorry at the removal from the Royal Society Hall, and he thought the action had not been so well considered as it might have been. He was not now a member of the Pharmacy Board, and did not know, therefore, what had induced them to take the step they had under the circumstances. However, he saw nothing but to accept the offer.

Mr. J. C. Jones said he considered the amount too much. He thought that the accommodation was not wanted; and he moved that the sum of £20 be offered to the Pharmacy Board.

Mr. Norris seconded the motion, remarking that in his opinion all the room they required might be obtained for £5 a year. He had no doubt that a place to meet in might be obtained at the Clarence or some other hotel.

Mr. Bowen said the remarks of the last speaker were paying a very poor compliment to those gentlemen who had taken an active part in the society, and brought it to its present satisfactory condition. It might appear to Mr. Norris a small matter, but to the president, the treasurer, and himself, who knew what a large amount of work was done every month, the proposition of Mr. Norris was quite out of place.

Mr. Hooper felt that the society was in a position to have the accommodation required. It would be a mistake not to have comfortable rooms. Many visitors would be coming to the colony during the Exhibition, who would no doubt like to avail themselves of the rooms. He therefore moved that the offer made by the Pharmacy Board be accepted. This was seconded by Mr. Ogg, and carried, all but Messrs. Jones and Norris voting for the proposition.

Alteration of Time of Meeting.—Mr. J. T. Macgowan, in accordance with the notice given by him at the last meeting, moved that the meetings of the Council shall for the future be held at 3 p.m., instead of 8 p.m. After considerable discussion on the subject, it was decided for the present to make no alteration.

Donation.—Mr. T. H. Walton, Fitzroy, forwarded a donation:—The *Lancet* for 1879, and Vol. 8 of the *Pharmaceutical Journal,* 1848. A vote of thanks was awarded him.

Deputation to the Minister of Lands.—It was resolved that further action be taken in reference to the piece of land promised to the Society by the late Government, and a deputation consisting of the president, vice-president, treasurer, honorary secretary, Messrs. Bosisto, Ogg, and Bowen; and Messrs. Zox, Harris, and Carter, M.L.A.'s, should have an interview with the Minister.

Exhibits.—Mr. Montague Brown, of Emerald Hill, pharmaceutical chemist, forwarded a sample of medicated orange wine, made entirely from fruit. Upon examination it was found to be a well-made and palatable article.

Mr. Graham Mitchell, F.R.C.V.S., also forwarded two samples of darnel (*Lolium temulentum.*)

Financial and routine business brought the meeting to a close.

At the conclusion of the council meeting an adjourned general meeting of the members was held, to receive the report of a committee appointed at the annual meeting to consider certain proposed alterations in the constitution and laws of the society.

The report of the committee was then read; and it was moved by Mr. Bowen, and seconded by Mr. Baker, and carried, that it be received.

Mr. Norris moved that the consideration of the report be postponed for one month, and that a copy be forwarded to every member of the society by post or otherwise. The motion was seconded by Mr. D. E. Morison. Mr. Norris stated that many members were unaware of the meeting; and he thought, if they had known of it, there would have been a better attendance.

Mr. Gamble said he saw no good in following Mr. Norris's suggestion. The meeting was an adjourned one from the annual meeting, had been well advertised both in *The Chemist and Druggist* and the daily papers, and to comply with Mr. Norris's motion would entail considerable expense and labour.

After some remarks from Messrs. Macgowan, Jones, and Morison, Mr. Wm. Bowen moved that the report of the committee be adopted, which was seconded by Mr. Gamble, and carried unanimously.

A vote of thanks to the chairman, Mr. C. R. Blackett, brought the meeting to a close.

Scientific Summary.

FROM the *Pharmaceutical* and other journals we make the following excerpts:—

The present and final number of *Medicinal Plants* contains figures and descriptions of the following plants :—*Canarium commune, Conium maculatum, Coriandrum sativum, Curcurbita Pepo, Crinum asiaticum, Strychnos Ignatii, Pinus Abies, Avena sativa,* and *Hordeum vulgare.* A correct reprint of *Pinus Picea* is also added, a transposition in the text having occurred in that already published in part 38. A systematic list of the contents of the work, an alphabetical index, a list of errata, and the preface, complete the work. Of the immense amount of labour involved in a work of this kind, only those who have to bring a work up to date can have any idea. The vast amount of foreign literature scattered in various publications that has to be consulted, and the balancing or reconciling of contradictory or conflicting statements, render the production of a work like the present, one of considerable labour. No other publication can be said to give so complete and yet succinct an account of the medicinal plants of Great Britain, India, and the United States, and of their products, as this one. It includes no less than eighty-nine natural orders, two hundred and thirty-three genera, and three hundred and six species, the information concerning which is brought up to the present time. The plan adopted, by means of which the whole can be arranged in consecutive systematic order by simply paying attention to the number attached to each species, is a most excellent one, and now that the work can be bound, it will be found that the four handsome volumes which it is intended to make will have their contents arranged in the most convenient manner possible. No pharmaceutical or medical library will be complete without Bentley and Trimen's *Medicinal Plants.*

A note in the *Chemical News*, by Mr. R. H. Ridout (13th February, p. 73), on the products of the slow oxidation of phosphorus, is not without an application to a common form of specialty terminology that reveals anything but the real nature of the preparation. Four or five years since a country practitioner having in consultation with a London specialist been recommended to use an injection of "ozonised water," unsuccessfully tried in various places to obtain a supply. Mr. Ridout being applied to, although aware of the general impression that ozone is insoluble in water, made an experiment by aspirating a current of air over moist phosphorus. An abundant evolution of an oxidising body was thus produced, which was passed through caustic soda to free it from phosphorous vapour, and then through recently distilled water ; but after this action had been continued for six hours the water was found to contain not a trace of any oxidising agent. After this evidence of the insolubility of ozone in water, an application was made to the specialists for a sample, which proved to be a solution of potassium permanganate.

Dr. Vasowicz, in *La Ruche Pharmaceutique*, has detailed some experiments made with a view to ascertain the correctness of the statements of Dr. Jehn that oil of peppermint is coloured red by hydrate of chloral. He shows that in those cases in which the oil was of ascertained purity no colouration took place ; in those in which it was not possible to ascertain the exact purity a yellow colouration occurred.

Ammoniacal glycyrrhizin appears to be steadily making its way upon the Continent. According to the *Journal de Pharmacie*, the French Minister of War has just ordered its definite introduction into the military hospitals, where a preparation containing four decigrammes of glycyrrhizin in a litre of water is to take the place of the old *tisane de reglisse.*

Baron Müeller and L. Rummel describe, in the *Zeitschrift Oest. Ap. Ver.*, a new glucoside obtained from *Gastrolobium bilobum*, an Australian plant, which possesses poisonous properties. It is called "gastrolobin," and is described as a blackish, brittle hygroscopic substance, with an odour and taste resembling that of sassafras, soluble in hot water and alcohol, and precipitated by a watery solution of acetate of lead. It is easily decomposed by mineral acids and partly by organic acids, and is soluble in ammonia with an intense yellow colour. It is not, however, as yet certain that the glucoside is the principle to which the poisonous properties of the plant are due. A poisonous principle has been found also in other species of this genus, and of the allied genera, *Oxylobium* and *Gompholobium*, and also in *Isotropis striata*, Benth.

Another veteran German pharmacist has passed away, in Dr. Augnst Wiggers, Professor of Pharmacy in the University of Gottingen. The deceased was in his seventy-seventh year, and his jubilee was celebrated about two years since. From France, too, the death is reported of M. Baudrimont, Professor of Chemistry to the Faculty of Sciences, Bordeaux, at the age of seventy-four years.

The revived interest in the subject of the artificial production of the diamond, provoked by Mr. Mactear's experiment, has been intensified by the communication made by Mr. Hannay to the Royal Society, at its last meeting in February. Mr. Hannay, continuing his researches in respect to the solubility of solids in gases, made numerous experiments with different forms of carbon in vapours that he thought most probable to act as solvents, in the hope that from one of them the carbon might be redeposited in a crystalline form. These experiments, Mr. Hannay says, were unsuccessful ; but it was noticed that, when a gas containing carbon and hydrogen was heated under pressure in presence of certain metals, its hydrogen was attracted by the metal and the carbon was set free. Ultimately, the operation was conducted in the presence of a "stable nitrogen compound," and, under these conditions, Mr. Hannay says that, "when the whole is near a red heat, and under very high pressure, the carbon is so acted upon by the nitrogen compound that it is obtained in the clear, transparent form of the diamond." At any rate, there seems to be no doubt that some minute crystalline fragments submitted with the paper as the product of such an operation were really identical with the natural diamond. The stable nitrogen compound used was not specified, but Professor Dewar pointed out the analogy between such a reaction and the production of graphite by heating a cyanide in caustic soda to a low red heat. These statements, so interesting to scientific men, are probably not altogether comfortable to diamond owners, but it will be somewhat reassuring to them to learn that the cost of producing diamonds artificially still far exceeds the market value of the product.

How to effect the dissociation of the "elements"—and especially of the metalloids—is a problem still occupying the attention of scientific men. According to *Nature* (11th March), M. Pictet, who two years since liquefied oxygen, starting with the fact that none of the metalloids, with the exception, perhaps, of oxygen, has yet been detected in the sun, infers that their absence is due to dissociation, and proposes to attempt to reproduce the conditions under which this takes place. This he would do by means of an enormous parabolic mirror, in the focus of which the sun's rays should be concentrated upon the metalloids which it is sought to decompose. Some of the data for working out this problem are known, and, assuming that to dissociate bromine would require "a hundred times as much heat (at the temperature of its dissociation point) as water vapour requires (at its dissociation point) to split it up," M. Pictet calculates that a gram of bromine would need 850 calories to resolve it into its elements, and that to dissociate one gram per minute would require that the solar rays should be concentrated by a mirror of at least thirty-five square metres of surface.

Lectures, &c.

AT a meeting of sections B, C, and D, held at the Royal Society's Hall, on the 3rd May, Mr. Blackett read a short paper on "A method of purifying water for domestic and manufacturing purposes." The method is due to Mr. Birkmyre, of South Yarra, and consists of the use of tersulphate of alumina as a precipitant of all organic and earthy matters. It is readily soluble in water, and of a harmless nature, requiring but a small quantity to purify the water, 1 oz being ample for 400 gals. of water, the precipitate formed completely subsiding in twenty-four hours, leaving the water as colourless as if distilled. The alumina combines with the organic matters, and carries down mechanically all earthy matter that may be in suspension. It appears to entirely remove all traces of albuminoid ammonia, which is such a fertile cause of fevers of the typhoid type, and blood disorders, if it exists in any quantity in the water, and which is a substance very apt to contaminate rain-water if the roofs be not clean or the drainage of the premises imperfect. The paper was illustrated by means of experiments, which demonstrated very conclusively the value of the alumina tersulphate as a purifier, and which, although of considerable commercial value in England, is as yet unknown in colonial commerce.

With the view of increasing the utility of the collections in the Technological Museum the superintendent, Mr. Cosmo Newbery, has, with the sanction of the trustees, arranged that special explanations will be given on each Saturday at eleven o'clock. On Saturday, 17th April, Mr. Newbery commenced his course of explanatory lectures on the collection in the Technological Museum. He devoted his remarks to the collections of cereals, Victorian minerals, and ceramic work, explaining the contents of each case in a lucid and interesting manner. His audience was small, but appreciative. The second lecture was delivered on the 24th April. There was a good attendance of ladies and gentlemen, and considerable interest was manifested by those present. Mr. Newbery described the metallurgical section of the museum, commencing with a description of the varieties of minerals with which the metallurgist meets. He showed the way in which the various metals could be recognised, and their physical properties ascertained. Afterwards an adjournment was made to the Library, where several practical experiments were carried out to illustrate the theories expounded. The lecture was the second of a series, which is to be continued weekly, and it seems that the privilege of attending them is highly appreciated judging from the appearance and character of the audience.

The first of a course of three lectures on agricultural chemistry was commenced on the 21st April by Mr. R. W. Emerson MacIvor, F.C.S., in the Industrial and Technological Museum. There was a good attendance. "The soil" was the subject of the lecture, and after explaining its constituents, Mr. MacIvor pointed out that to procure thorough fertility the soil must contain a portion of the thirteen substances which enter into the composition of a plant, and that if one is missing the plant cannot grow. The soil, also, must not be too retentive or too open. In a moist district the farmer will make more profit out of a comparatively open soil than out of a heavy one; but in a dry country like Victoria a loamy or heavy soil is preferable, as it retains sufficient water to meet the requirements of plants in dry weather. The colour of the soil is also important, a dark one absorbing the sun's rays, and being invariably warmer than a light one, which reflects the rays. The warmth of the soil not only accelerates the growth of the plant, but acts beneficially at the early stage of germination. Referring next to drainage, the lecturer pointed out the importance of farmers in this country draining their land in order to open its pores, and allow of an absorption of any rain which may fall. The evaporating power of the Victorian atmosphere is 42 in. per annum, whereas the average rainfall is only 26 in., so that it was manifestly to the advantage of the farmer to drain his land. After describing the composition of subsoils, Mr. MacIvor concluded by a reference to ploughing, advocating thorough and occasionally deep ploughing. The more strictly chemical portion of the lecture was illustrated by various experiments.

BALLARAT.

THE BALLARAT DISTRICT CHEMISTS' ASSOCIATION. THE monthly meeting of the association was held at Lester's Hotel, on Wednesday, 21st April; there was a good attendance. The president, Mr. T. P. Palmer, took the chair at twenty minutes past nine p.m. The minutes of the previous meeting were read and confirmed.

A letter was read from Mr. Holdsworth, of Sandhurst, suggesting the idea of enlarging the number of members of the Pharmacy Council by the appointment of a member thereat from each of the large towns of the colony, such members to be honorary members; and asking the association to inaugurate the matter. In reply, the hon. secretary was instructed to write to Mr. Holdsworth, and recommend that the chemists of Sandhurst and other large towns should do as Ballarat had done, and form themselves into associations, and seek representation on the council by election instead of hon. membership.

Mr. Towl reported the death in the hospital, after a long illness, of Mr. J. C. Proctor, an old Ballarat chemist, who carried on business for many years in Armstrong-street.

According to notice, Mr. Towl brought forward his motion re dispensing for Friendly Societies. The matter was postponed till next meeting, in order to obtain information relative to the working of the Friendly Societies' dispensaries in Melbourne and suburbs.

The hon. secretary stated that he had attended the meeting of the Council of the Pharmaceutical Society on 2nd April, and when the discussion on the alteration of laws and regulations was proceeding had introduced the request of the association re alteration in the method of voting for members of the council— viz., that it should be conducted by ballot instead of proxy papers; but it was not carried, on account of the expense attending the ballot method. Also, to save time and expense to country members, he had given notice of motion to the effect that the council meetings in future be held at three p.m., in lieu of eight p.m.

The subject of the infringement of the price list by members of the association was brought up, and the president and secretary were deputed to wait upon one of the members respecting it. Considerable discussion then took place about the price of several articles not in the price list. The price of trusses was agreed upon as follows:—Single, 6s.; double, 8s. 6d.; patent single, 8s. 6d.; double, 12s. 6d. Higginson's enemas—common, 6s. 6d.; screw, 7s. 6d.; super., 10s. Guard's hair dye, 4s. Members were requested to note any articles they thought it necessary to add to the list by next meeting; after which fresh lists will be printed.

Mr. Whittle again brought forward the question of altering the method of voting for members of the Council of the Pharmaceutical Society, and urged upon the hon. secretary to introduce the subject again at the general meeting on 7th May.

Mr. Whittle also gave notice of motion to alter some of the rules of the association.

Mr. H. Rocke, of Melbourne, was present for a short time.

The customary vote of thanks to the chair brought the meeting to a close.

We regret to record the death of Mr. Joseph Longstaff, chemist, which took place on the 4th of May, at his residence, Victoria-street. The deceased gentleman arrived in Ballarat in the year 1857, and founded the business in Bridge-street, now being carried on by his cousin, Mr. T. Longstaff; but a few years since he purchased the business of Mr. Keogh, wholesale chemist, in Melbourne. The troublesome legal proceedings which arose out of this transaction, coupled with a serious illness, undermined his previous comparatively strong constitution. He returned to Ballarat about three weeks since with a premonition of his early death, and with a desire to end his days where he had spent such a considerable portion of his life, and where he had earned for himself the respect and esteem of all with whom he had come in contact. Mr. Longstaff leaves a widow and five children, who, we are sure, will receive the condolence and sympathy of a very wide circle of friends.—Ballarat Star.

We regret to record the death of Mr. J. C. Proctor, at the Ballarat Hospital, on the 1st April, where deceased had been for some weeks, under treatment for tumor. Mr. Proctor was fifty-five years of age, and brother-in-law to Dr. Stewart, whose dispensary in Armstrong-street the deceased managed for some time. He was also with Mr. Cowl, of Sturt-street, as an assistant intermittently, for some years. The deceased had resided in Ballarat for twenty-seven years, and bore the reputation of being an excellent chemist.

The unpleasant and offensive odour of iodoform is easily overcome by E. Biermann by the addition of from 5 to 8 drops of volatile oil of fennel to 1 gram of iodoform. Its efficacy is really surprising, and far exceeds that of oil of peppermint (see Amer. Jour. Pharm., April, 1879, p. 190) and of balsam of Peru.—Pharm. Ztg.

MY FIRST AQUARIUM.

THE following interesting letter addressed to the *Australasian* on " My First Aquarium," by Mr. C. A. Atkin, will repay perusal :—

I had hoped, from what I have seen recently in the columns of your contemporaries, that the weakness to which I plead guilty, under the above heading, was about to assume some public and practical form in the land of my adoption. The pre-occupations of business, and the political excitement of the period, as well as the ephemeral attractions of older established sources of amusement, are, doubtless, amongst the causes which have retarded the progress here of an institution of such rapid growth and permanent interest as the "Aquarium" has proved at home. Be that as it may, however, I have found time, during the recent holidays, to indulge to a greater extent than usual in the weakness alluded to, and if I felt that I had been guilty of an extravagance, or that you were likely to incur loss by publishing the fact, I should point to the noble institutions which are being rapidly reared for the same object, under the title of "Aquaria," in every part of the civilised world excepting Australia.

" One of the greatest beauties of the study of Nature is generally considered to reside in the brotherly feeling it establishes between men of all nations, of all ages, of all ranks"— are the words I find recorded in the works of a distinguished naturalist who has just passed away from us (the late Count de Castelnau), and few would gainsay that assertion.

But to proceed with my narrative. Some eighteen years ago, after seven spent in this country, I determined to revisit dear old England, and amonst the many lovely spots which invited my attention, Tiverton, in Devonshire, engrossed a special share. There I made the acquaintance of Mr. D——; and in one of the recesses formed by the bay windows of his drawingroom I saw, for the first time, an aquarium.

It was, of course, a miniature one, and occupied a neatly-designed stand, advantageously placed for the reception of the sun's rays, on which so much of the vitality of its inmates depended. The latter, I found, consisted of gold and silver fish, dace, minnows, &c., which disported themselves amongst numerous aquatic plants evidently thoroughly acclimatised, as some of them were in flower, although my friend assured me the water had not been changed for many months, nor would such a precautionary measure be requisite for some length of time to come, unless an accident occurred.

On the chimneypiece of the room we occupied there were several upright vases, containing distinct varieties of water beetles, and in each vase was a specimen of the *Vallisneria spiralis* growing in full vigour ; so that, taken altogether, the scene, to which I had before been a complete stranger, was replete with objects of beauty and interest, so much so, that I at once determined to become the proprietor of a like attractive collection, to take back with me and show to my friends in Australia.

Innocently enough, therefore, I asked my friend where such a collection could be purchased. "Oh !" said he, " it is homemade ; I and my two boys caught most of the specimens of fish and beetles, and we also gathered the water plants from the brooks running through the fields you see around us !"

From that date my enthusiasm (which some, no doubt, regarded as a mild form of mania) in the matter of the aquarium took its departure. I dreamt and talked about what I had seen at my friend's house, and determined, if possible, to construct and possess a similar collection on my return to Australia.

The following brief *résumé* of my subsequent proceedings will show how far I succeeded ; and I will only add, for the encouragement of others, that it has proved a cheap and never-failing source of instruction and amusement both to myself and friends.

My first ambition was to purchase some goldfish to bring back with me to this country, for the date I speak of was, if I mistake not, antecedent to Mr. Geo. Coppin's notion of acclimatising these golden household pets in Australia ; at any rate, I was not aware of their existence here. On addressing myself, however, to one of the dealers in goldfish in London he so disheartened me as to my chances of being able to land them alive that I abandoned the idea and resolved to trust to the River Yarra and the Melbourne swamp for the stock of my projected aquarium.

My Devonshire friend had impressed upon me the importance of first establishing the growth of plants before putting the fish into the aquarium, and I afterwards discovered the importance of this, both as regards fresh and salt water collections.

Soon after my return to Melbourne I commenced operations by paying a visit to the Royal Park, where, at that time, there existed two or three large water-holes, close to the side of the "camel-house," which was erected on that memorable occasion in the history of Australia when the Burke and Wills exploration expedition left Melbourne, and succeeded in crossing the continent as far as Cooper's Creek.

I found all I wanted for a start in one of these water-holes— aquatic plants, beetles, tadpoles, and water-snails.

First, I brought home the plants, then procured some sand, which I well washed, afterwards cleared all the soil from the roots of the plants, and bedded them firmly into the sand ; then, having filled my tank three parts full with water, I allowed it to remain quiescent for a week or two in order that the plants might become established in their new home.

I next made a small hand-net of muslin and cane, and soon caught sufficient specimens to stock my first aquarium.

The tadpoles proved very interesting objects indeed. They had been in my possession some weeks, when first one and then another of them began to develop into the frog. This wonderful transformation scene may be thus described. First, the two fore feet were visible, then the hind ones, and, last of all, the tail, which, after a time, became absorbed, as it were, into the body, when the transformation was complete. At this stage they should be taken out of the aquarium, or a piece of cork or wood, to serve as a raft, should he put into the tank for them to rest upon, otherwise they will drown.

It was remarkable how few of my friends had ever seen a tadpole before, much less noticed the creature when in this transition state, and their undisguised astonishment quite repaid me for all the trouble I had taken up to this time. It also stimulated my desire to show them something more indicative of the obligation under which my Devonshire friend's kindness had placed me, and encouraged me to prosecute my studies in this direction with fresh vigour and enterprise.

About this time I discovered that a feud existed between the beetles and the tadpoles, to such an extent that I was obliged to separate them, or the voracity of the former creatures would soon have exterminated the tadpoles. My next ambition was directed towards obtaining a supply of fish and a larger aquarium. With the simple appliances of a hand-net and fish kettle, I strolled out towards the Melbourne Swamp, where I was amply rewarded for my trouble by a variety of fish, and an amelioration in the class of plants, larvæ, &c.

(To be continued.)

Legal and Magisterial.

AN attempt to commit suicide by poisoning was made on 16th April by a young girl of Italian parentage, named Clementina Alessio, only seventeen years of age, residing at 42 Queensberry-street, Carlton. It appears that she asked a lad to buy some laudanum, of which she took, it is thought, about an ounce. She was brought to the Melbourne Hospital in an insensible state, and upon the necessary remedies being employed for about an hour by Mr. Newman, resident physician, consciousness returned, and she was progressing favourably. It is supposed that disappointment in a love affair was the cause of the attempt.

What would appear to be an attempt to commit suicide in a determined manner was made on the 16th April by a man named Alfred Sayers, aged forty-five years, a resident of Station-street, Richmond. It appears that he deliberately swallowed nearly an ounce of nitric acid, as he states, by mistake, under the impression that he was taking a cooling drink, but as his friends surmise, with the intention of taking his life. He was promptly removed to the Melbourne Hospital, where he was, although in a very precarious condition, progressing favourably towards recovery.

A most determined attempt to commit suicide was made on the evening of the 14th April by a married woman named Ann Kelly, aged thirty years, a resident of Princes-street, Fitzroy. For some reason which could not be ascertained she swallowed nearly an ounce of laudanum, and was almost *in articulo mortis* when the police, having been summoned, arrived at her house, and hurried her off to the hospital,

Messrs. Woinarski and Newman, the resident surgeons, were promptly in attendance, and at once took steps to counteract the effects of the poison. The stomach pump was called into requisition, and the galvanic battery and the administration of antidotes were persevered with for nearly six hours without any symptoms of the patient's return to consciousness. At length the pupils of the eyes became sensible to light, and there was every prospect of a successful result from the treatment adopted. The woman has not yet sufficiently recovered to give any reason for attempting her own life, but it is believed that domestic infelicity and an over-indulgence in intoxicating liquors are the primary causes.

A young woman twenty-one years of age, named Hattie Burt, attempted to commit suicide on the 26th April, by swallowing a quantity of laudanum. She was, however, fortunately discovered, and being promptly removed to the Melbourne Hospital, the requisite antidotes were applied by Dr. Armstrong, one of the resident surgeons, successfully.

A man named Francis Conway was brought to the Melbourne Hospital, on the 3rd May, suffering from the effects of poisoning by strychnine, which it is believed he took with the intention of committing suicide. Under treatment by Dr. Armstrong, resident surgeon, he slightly improved, and hopes are entertained of his recovery. Conway was at one time in the police force, but he retired about three years ago on a pension. It is believed that drink was the cause of the suicidal act.

"BAUNSCHEIDTISM" AGAIN.—Mr. Samuel Fischer, who professes to cure all complaints by means of what he calls "baunscheidtism," summoned W. Dudgeon at the City Police Court for £1, as work and labour done. Mr. Cohen appeared for the plaintiff, and Mr. Hornbuckle for the defence. The latter raised a preliminary objection that the plaintiff was not a registered medical practitioner, but Mr. Webster, P.M., over-ruled this objection. The plaintiff stated in his evidence that he had agreed to charge 10s. for each application of the instrument to the defendant's child; and, in reply to Mr. Hornbuckle, said "the operation was quite a mechanical one." Mr. Hornbuckle inquired if the plaintiff did not use the instrument to make insertions in the skin, and then rub oil on. Plaintiff—"Yes, that is what I do, so that we shall not be mere slaves to doctors." He proceeded to say that the child was suffering from scrofula, and had been poisoned by vaccination. Mrs. Dudgeon was called, and said Fischer promised to cure the child for £2. After the first application he was paid 10s., and the second time was given an I.O.U. for a like amount, which was afterwards paid. The plaintiff, she said, used the instrument to her child after applying it to a man with yellow jaundice, who had since died. He injected oil into the temples of the child, and also into the glands of the neck. After this the child became nearly blind, and she had to place it under other treatment. Mr. Webster said the case was not borne out by the evidence, and he would dismiss it. He believed that Fischer had a perfect right to sue, and the case was only dismissed on its merits.—*Bendigo Advertiser.*

PROSECUTION OF AN UNREGISTERED CHEMIST.

AT the St. Kilda Police Court, on the 7th May, Robert Soppet, carrying on business in Robe-street, was summoned by the police under the 25th section of the Pharmacy Act. Mr. Soppet produced his certificate of qualification from the Pharmaceutical Society of Great Britain, and pleaded that he was ignorant that he had committed any offence. On his arrival in this colony he forwarded his application for registration to the secretary of the Pharmacy Board, but he had not until the 6th of May finally completed the requisite forms, although he had been in the colony eight months. He asked the bench to deal leniently with him; what he had done was in ignorance, and since the summons had been taken out he had completed his registration. The police, therefore, did not wish to press the charge, and the bench fined the defendant 15s. costs.

Notes and Abstracts.

SALICYLIC ACID TAMPONS.—As employed in the German army, they consist of pieces of soft gauze of about 13 or 16 square centimeters, which are loosely tied around 1 or 2 grams of cotton, so as to be readily formed into any desired shape by pressure. One kilo of these tampons is impregnated with a solution of 110 grams of salicylic acid and 40 grams of castor oil in 3½ or 4 litres of 95 per cent. alcohol. They are afterwards dried in a well-ventilated room, and are intended to be used in applying a temporary bandage until the services of a surgeon may be procured. Bernbeck suggests the use of glycerine in place of the castor oil, considering it far preferable. —*Pharm. Ztg.,* 1879.

EXTEMPORANEOUS PREPARATION OF SYRUP OF LICORICE. —Juehling prepares a syrup, equal in strength to that of the German Pharmacopœia, by mixing:—

Essentia liquiritiæ	...	...	...	10·0
Syrupi simplicis	...	...	...	180·0
Mellis depurati...	...	...	...	120·0 M.

Essentia liquiritiæ is made by extracting twice 1000 grams of licorice root with 3000 grams of water, evaporating the infusion to 500 grams, adding 500 grams of alcohol, filtering and evaporating to 333 grams (consistence of honey).—*Pharm. Ztg.,* 1879.

FERRIC HYDRATES.—The trihydrate, $Fe_2(OH)_6$, has never been prepared thus far, according to Tommasi, who mentions the existence of two isomeric, respectively red and yellow, monohydrates, $Fe_2O_2(OH)_2$, and bihydrates, $Fe_2O(OH)_4$, and publishes the following distinctions:—The red bihydrate remains unaltered up to 50° C. and the yellow to 105° C.; the red monohydrate to 92°, and the yellow to 150° C. The red hydrates, when dehydrated, leave as a residue a brown oxide, having the density 5·1, while the yellow hydrates leave a red or reddish-yellow oxide, having the density 3·95. The red hydrates dissolve even in dilute acids, while the yellow are scarcely soluble in concentrated acids. The red hydrates are readily dissolved by ferric chloride solution, and this solution yields, on the addition of sodium sulphate or sulphuric acid, a precipitate of hydrated oxide; the yellow hydrates are insoluble in ferric chloride. The red hydrates are entirely dehydrated by boiling, while the yellow are only reduced to monohydrates. Tommasi considers the combinations of ferric hydrates with ferric salts mere mechanical mixtures, and not chemical compounds.—*Ber. d. Deutsch. Chem. Ges.,* 1879.

INORGANIC CHEMISTRY.—*The Chemical Cause of the Poisonous Nature of Arsenic.*—The old theory proposed by Liebig that arsenous acid, like corrosive sublimate, formed an insoluble compound with albumen, and hence decomposes the animal tissues, has been given up since it has been found experimentally that these supposed albuminates are not formed by the action of arsenous acid or its salts. Binz and Schulz find that arsenic acid, digested with egg-albumen and fibrin of warm-blooded animals, at the temperature of the body, is reduced. They find that the mucous membrane of the stomach, the liver, and the undecomposed protoplasm of plants *reduce* arsenic acid and also *oxidise* arsenous to arsenic acid. The authors find in this alternate oxidation and reduction, which the two arsenic acids undergo when in contact with the albumen molecules, the reason for the decomposing effect which arsenic in its several forms exerts upon the tissue, or, in other words, for its poisonous character. They draw an analogy with the poisonous effects of nitrogen dioxide, which is also a carrier of oxygen, passing into nitrogen tetroxide, and then, in the presence of water, regenerating nitrogen dioxide. Phosphorus and antimony they consider as showing similar characters.—*Ber. der Chem. Ges.*

BENZOATE OF SODA IN DIPHTHERIA.—Dr. Letzerich has successfully treated, with benzoate of soda, twenty-seven cases of diphtheria which came under his care during an epidemic of the disease in Berlin. Of these cases eight were severe, accompanied by high fever, delirium, retention of the urine and fæces, existing often before the extensive local affection had made its appearance. In the blood there were found numerous bacteria and plasma corpuscles from which, by cultivation in veal broth, very large colonies of micrococci became developed. The dose of sodium benzoate for children and adults is to be regulated by the weight of the body. The formula for infants under one year old is:—

R Sodæ benzoat, pur 5·0	or Sodæ benzoat. pur. ʒj.
Aquæ distillat.	Aquæ distillat.
Aquæ menth. ppt. āā 40·0	Aquæ menth. ppt. āā ʒj.
Syrup cort. aurant. 10	Syrup cort. aurant. ʒij. M.
Half a tablespoonful every hour.	

The dose for children between one and three years of age is given at 7-8 grams (two drachms) dissolved in three and a-half ounces of the vehicle, the whole amount being given in the course of the day, in half to one tablespoonful doses.

For children between three and seven years of age, 8-10 grams (2-2¼ drachms), given in the same way. Those over seven years old take 10-15 grams (2½-4 drachms), and for adults the dose is 15-25 grams (2½-6 drachms) daily in 4½ ounces of the vehicle. An unpleasant after-effect has never been observed even in young infants. The diphtheritic membrane was treated with benzoate of soda in powder, being sprinkled on or applied through a glass tube or quill. There is no slough formed, and thereby the danger is averted of its acting as a firm covering under which an energetic development and growth of the organisms can take place. The insufflation was made every three hours in severe cases, in the middle forms two or three times daily. With older children a simple solution of the salt (ten to two hundred) was used as a gargle. The author also recommends this remedy in gastric or intestinal catarrh, particularly of infants, and states that at times the results are surprising in these latter cases. He recommends it likewise in mycotic catarrh of the bladder, and firmly believes in the statement of Klebs that it is to be recommended in all diseases which originate by infection. —*The Boston Med. and Surg. Journ.*, 17th July, 1879; from *Berlin Klini. Wosch.*, 17th February, 1879.

Correspondence.

COATING PILLS.

To the Editor of The Australasian Supplement to the Chemist and Druggist.

SIR—One of your correspondents, signing himself " Ambition," writes asking for the best method of coating pills. Had he placed his name and address (which I would respectfully say by so doing I do not think there would have been any disgrace when seeking information), I would have communicated with him direct. I may say that I have tried chalk, gum, starch, isinglass, sugar, French chalk, gelatine, mucilage, glue, simple syrup, albumen, and arrowroot. In some instances I have used the above separately, and in others combined them, but obtain the best result as follows:—Dissolve one drachm isinglass in one and a-half ounces simple syrup. Pour a small quantity whilst warm upon some pills that have been made, say, a few weeks, and become hard. After shaking them about for a short time, sprinkle over some French chalk. Place them in a flat-bottom tin, and apply a gentle heat. Keep them continually rotating, adding more chalk, if necessary, until dry. I find that the coating neither cracks, nor does it peel off. I had no guide in my first attempt to sugar-coat pills, and if any correspondent is in possession of a better method, maybe he will kindly enlighten his brethren. By following the foregoing, you can turn out a pill that is smooth and glossy.—I remain, sir, &c.,   CHARLES CROSS.
Gawler, Adelaide, S.A., 7th May, 1880.

To the Editor of The Australasian Supplement to the Chemist and Druggist.

SIR—Your correspondent "Ambition" will find the following process answer very well for coating pills, viz.:—
Make a solution of tolu in ether, nearly saturated (the refuse from making syrup of tolu answers equally well, and is more economical). Put the pills into a jar, and moisten thoroughly with the solution; then throw them into French chalk contained in the pill-coater, and after rotating in the usual manner, expose for a short time to allow the coating to dry; then coat twice in succession as follows:—Mix equal parts of fresh mucilage of acacia and water, add two drops of this to each dozen pills, and throw them into French chalk as before; finally remove all the chalk from the coater, and polish the pills by rotating them for some time in the coater.
The object in first coating with the solution of tolu is to prevent the discolouration of the coating, which invariably follows if this is omitted.
During an experience of thirteen years, I have never found the least objection to the use of tolu.
French chalk, or lycopodium, will be found the best for dusting the pills when rolling, as liquorice, and such-like powders, adhere to the pills, increasing their size, and otherwise interfering with coating them satisfactorily.—Yours, &c.,
                                                        PILULA.

To the Editor of The Australasian Supplement to the Chemist and Druggist.

SIR—We have had our attention called to an insertion of a statement in your paper, or journal, purporting to come from the *Bendigo Independent*, in the which a preparation, of which we are owners—viz., Reuter's Life Syrup—is grossly misrepresented as having poisoned an old man in Sandhurst, when the facts in the case pointed conclusively to his having died from "excessive purging," the result of taking the Syrup for diarrhœa, from which he was suffering, and for which the Syrup was not recommended or calculated.
We call your attention to the retraction contained in same *Bendigo Independent* of Wednesday, 17th December, which speaks for itself, and must now ask that, in justice to us, you give this retraction a place as you did the accusation in your issue for November, 1879.
Our representatives are Messrs. P. Falk and Co., Melbourne. —We remain, very respectfully,   BARCLAY AND CO.
New York, 6th March, 1880.
[We have not seen the retraction referred to, and therefore publish the above letter.—ED. *Aust. Sup. C. & D.*]

LOLIUM TEMULENTUM (DRAKE WEED).

To the Editor of The Australasian Supplement to the Chemist and Druggist.

SIR—As large quantities of drake are now being disposed of, and also found largely mixed with cereals, I think that publicity should be given to the fact that darnel seed is highly injurious and poisonous to stock. It is high time that distillers and others should be prevented purchasing the same by auction and in open market. The following reports will, no doubt, be interesting to your readers, through whom the public might be informed of the danger of using darnel for feeding purposes. The recent mortality amongst fowls and other animals may, to a certain extent, have been caused by the admixture of this poison in their food.—Yours truly,
                              GRAHAM MITCHELL, F.R.C.V.S.

" Melbourne, 4th May, 1875.
" F. B. Clapp, Esq.
" Sir—I herewith enclose report of Baron von Müeller, and progress report of Mr. Cosmo Newbery, on the sample of horse-feed you handed to me.
" I have no doubt that the darnel (*Lolium temulentum*) which it contains was the cause of the death and loss of condition which occurred amongst the 'Bus Company's horses.— I have the honour to be, sir, your obedient servant,
                                         "GRAHAM MITCHELL."

"4th May, 1875.
" Graham Mitchell, Esq.
" Dear Sir—I have been unable to detect any mineral or organic poison in the portion of the horse's stomach or in the fluid received from you. The partly-crushed grain used as horse-feed contains a very large quantity of darnel (*Lolium temulentum*), which is noted by most authors as highly poisonous to horses. I think it would be well to institute some experiments with the food, as the matter is of great importance, darnel being a very common weed here.—Yours truly,
                                            "J. COSMO NEWBERY."

" Melbourne, 3rd May, 1875.
" To Graham Mitchell, Esq., Government Veterinary Surgeon.
" Sir—In reply to your letter of the 26th April, I have the honour to inform you that the sample of horse-feed submitted to my inspection consists mainly of a mixture of partly-crushed wheat, barley, and oats, but contains also a considerable portion of darnel (seed of *Lolium temulentum*), a grain well known to be poisonous as well to man as to pastural animals.—I have the honour to be, sir, your obedient servant, "FERD. VON MUELLER, Government Botanist."

" Darnel (*Lolium temulentum*).—A pernicious, deleterious, annual gramineous weed of the rye-grass genus. It infests the wheat fields of Britain and other countries of Europe. Its seeds are about the same size as those of wheat, and are gathered with them in harvesting, and cannot, without much difficulty, be separated from them in the operation of the farm ; and when they are numerous and find their way with the wheat into bread-flour, they prove highly noxious to man, injuring his health, and sometimes producing delirium, stupefaction, and other symptoms of poisoning. The plant has ceased to be plentiful in all good agricultural districts in Britain, but has almost disappeared in some, but it continues to be dismally prevalent in some parts of the Continent, and fearfully deteriorates many an imported sample of foreign wheat."—*Wilson's Rural Cyclopædia.*

"*Lolium temulentum.*—This grass is found principally in cultivated fields, especially among corn, where it is a noxious weed. The seeds, it is said, when eaten, produce vomiting, purging, violent colic, and death; and Linæus states that the seeds, when mixed with bread, produce but little effect unless when eaten hot, but if malted with barley the ale soon occasions intoxication."—*Parnell.*

"*Lolium temulentum* is remarkable as the only species of the family (of grasses) known to possess poisonous properties. . . . The seeds of this grass are extremely deleterious, acting as a narcotic poison, and if taken in small quantities for a long period together, causing a peculiar disease called dry gangrene, resembling that occasioned by the ergot of rye. Some years ago there was reason to suppose it was used by fraudulent brewers to increase the intoxicating effect of their liquor, but its dangerous properties are now too well known to admit of such application being made with impunity, and mention is made of it here only to call attention to the extreme danger of allowing it to grow among corn. Many accidents have occurred from the use of wheat and other grains mingled with darnel, and especially among the peasantry. Christims relates that the whole of the inmates of the Sheffield Workhouse, about forty years ago, were seized with dangerous illness, attributed to the accidental use of corn mixed with darnel seeds, and more recent instances are not wanting."—*Johnson's Useful Plants of Great Britain.*

MANUFACTURE OF OLIVE OIL IN SOUTHERN FRANCE.

(TRANSLATED FROM "PHAR. HANDELSBL.," 14TH JANUARY, BY LOUIS VON OOTZHAUSEN, PH.G.)

IN the establishment of E. Jourdan de Jauffret et Fils, at Salon in the Provence, the manufacture of olive oil necessarily always begins in the first half of November, because the olives become ripe in this season in the Provence, and, when begun, it must be continued night and day for three or four months, the length of the season, of course, depending on the duration of the harvest.

De Jauffret and Son employ eighteen labourers, who are divided into two divisions, working respectively during the day and during the night, and producing daily 1200 kilogrammes of the best oil from 1000 decalitres of olives. The facilities of the establishment are such that the largest harvests of olives can be handled quickly, so as not to necessitate a prolonged storing of olives, which would cause them to ferment, when they yield an inferior oil.

Nevertheless, there are some manufacturers who believe in this fermentation, claiming that it increases the yield, because it assists the separation of the oil from the cellular tissue of the olives. But experience has shown that this increase in yield can only be obtained at the expense of the quality of the oil, and that the larger yield never makes up for the inferiority of the oil.

In the establishment of Jourdan de Jauffret this is avoided. Nevertheless, their manner of preparing the oil is such that fully as much, if not more, is obtained by them as by those allowing the olives to ferment. Before the olives enter the mills they are carefully spread over the floor of the well-ventilated storeroom, where they are allowed to remain for three days, if the wind is from the south, and four or five days, if from the north. The first stage of the manufacture consists in grinding the olives between revolving granite stones; then the mass, enclosed in baskets, is exposed to a slight pressure in an iron press, and yields the so-called virgin oil (*huile vierge*), which has gained the good reputation for the oil of the Provence. The mass in the baskets is then exposed to a stronger pressure, and yields the well-known good oil usually found in commerce. After this second operation the mass is taken from the basket-work, and is again placed into the mills, where it is thoroughly ground up, when it is again packed into baskets and is exposed to the pressure of hydraulic presses.

During this operation the effect of fermentation is made use of by treating the mass with boiling water, in order to facili-

tate the separation of the oil from the cells, which still retain it. Thus, a larger yield is obtained from the olives without interfering with the quality of the greater portion of the oil, since only the last yield is exposed to heat. This oil is always better than the oil obtained from fermented olives, because frequently a rotten odour is produced by fermentation, which is imparted even to the oil expressed first.

The oil expressed with the aid of hot water is known in commerce as fine table-oil. The greatest precautions must be used in the manufacture. Colnmelle even forbids the kindling of fires in the mills during the manufacture, claiming that the smoke of a single lamp may prove injurious to the quality of the oil. This caution is necessary in the older mills. Even at the present time, most mills are underground, and of such a construction that air and light can scarcely penetrate into them, and that foul odours, &c., can scarcely escape from them; besides, most of the mills are revolved by mules, which adds to their uncleanliness.

The olive oil must be preserved with great care, since Th. de Saussure has shown that the absorption of atmospheric oxygen, which is favoured by heat, has a tendency to turn it rancid. The expressed oil is filtered, and immediately transferred into large cooled stoneware jugs, in which it gets cold very soon, and will keep unaltered for two years.

"Waste-oil" (*huile d'enfer*) is the name given to all oil in the Provence which is collected on the surface of the pits. It is treated with caustic soda and with hot water, in order to remove the fatty acids, and then enters commerce as lubricating machine-oil. It is greatly valued for oiling machinery, and also for wool.

SELLING POISON TO CHILDREN.

A MARRIED woman, named Agnes Fulcknor, thirty-eight years of age, was admitted into the Melbourne Hospital, suffering from poison. It appeared that one of her sons returned to his home, Alfred-street, Emerald Hill, at five o'clock in the evening, and noticed that there was something wrong with his mother. On making inquiries he found that she had sent a little girl, seven years of age, to an adjacent chemist's shop for sixpence worth of laudanum. The poison was supplied, and the woman swallowed it. A policeman was called in, and the woman was taken to the hospital, where she was treated. It is not known what caused Mrs. Fulcknor to take the poison. Her husband states that when he last saw his wife she was in cheerful spirits. This is the second case made public lately in which it has been alleged that chemists have supplied poison to children. The matter is, therefore, one which should be noticed by the authorities.

[As the law stands at present, there is nothing to prevent the sale of poisons included in the second part of schedule 1; but it is very improper for any one to sell poisons to young children.—ED. *Aust. Sup. C. & D.*]

Pharmacy Board of Victoria Notices.

THE NINTH PRELIMINARY EXAMINATION of Apprentices will be held at this office on THURSDAY, the 3rd day of JUNE, 1880, at Eleven a.m. The attention of apprentices is directed to Clause 43 of the Regulations to the Act, which obliges indentures to be registered within twelve months of their being executed.

HARRY SHILLINGLAW, Secretary and Registrar.

Office of the Pharmacy Board, Mutual Provident Buildings, Collins-street West, Melbourne.

THE TWELFTH MODIFIED EXAMINATION of Candidates for Registration under the Pharmacy Act will be held at this office on MONDAY, the 7th JUNE, 1880, at Ten o'clock a.m. Candidates must give to the Secretary notice of their intention to present themselves for examination, together with their indentures of apprenticeship and the fee of three guineas, ten days prior to the day.

HARRY SHILLINGLAW, Secretary and Registrar.

Office of the Pharmacy Board, Mutual Provident Buildings, Collins-street West, Melbourne.

FELTON, GRIMWADE & CO.,

WHOLESALE DRUGGISTS AND MANUFACTURING CHEMISTS,

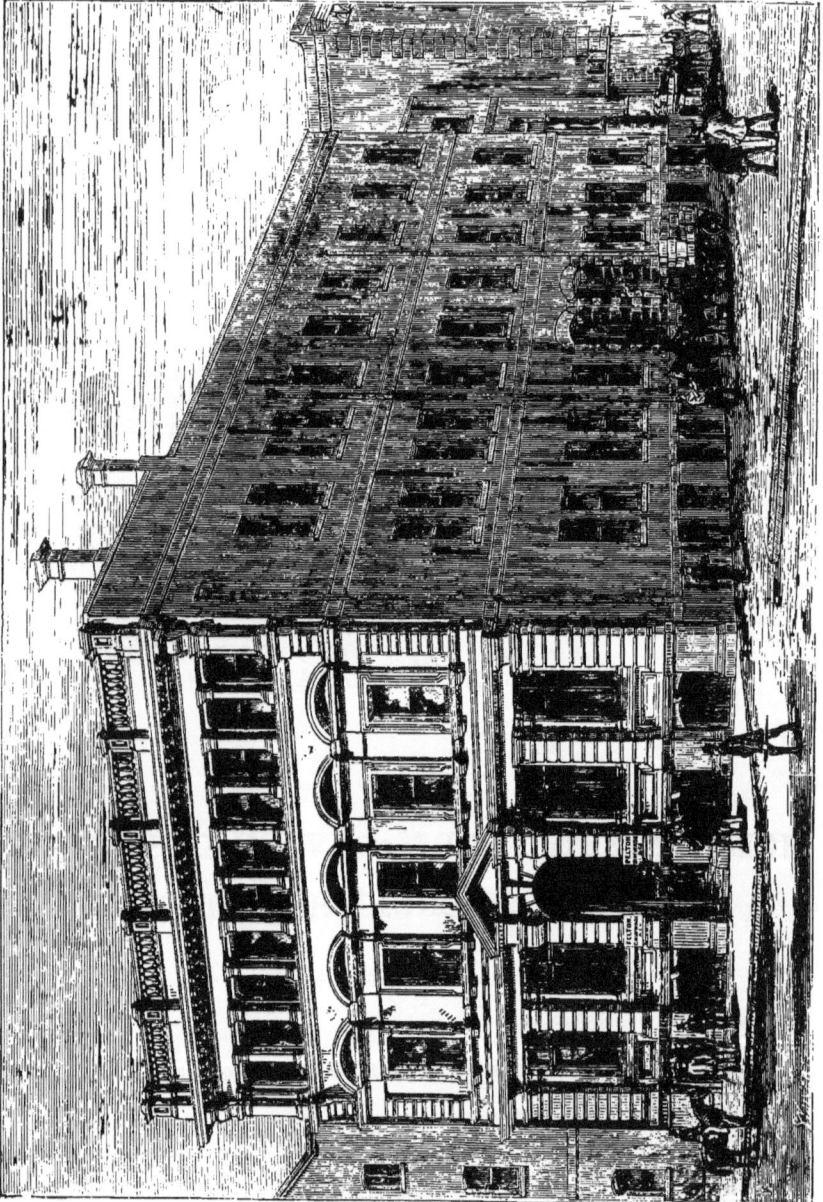

31 & 33 FLINDERS LANE WEST,
MELBOURNE.

[SUPPLEMENT ONLY.]

THE
Chemist & Druggist.

WITH AUSTRALASIAN SUPPLEMENT.

(Published under direction of the Pharmaceutical Society of Victoria.)

No. 25. { PUBLISHED ON THE 15TH OF EVERY MONTH. }
Registered for Transmission as a Newspaper. | MAY, 1880. | { SUBSCRIPTION, 15s. PER ANNUM, INCLUDING DIARY, POST FREE.

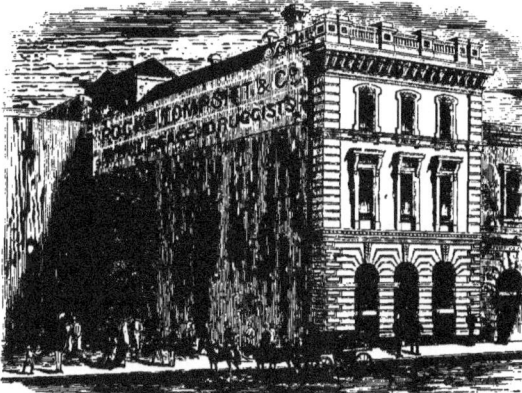
Printed and Published by Mason, Firth & M'Cutcheon, 51 & 53 Flinders Lane West, Melbourne.

The Chemist and Druggist.

WITH AUSTRALASIAN SUPPLEMENT.

OFFICE: MUTUAL PROVIDENT BUILDINGS, COLLINS STREET WEST.

Published on the 15th of each Month.

THIS Journal is issued gratis to all paid-up Members of the PHARMACEUTICAL SOCIETY OF VICTORIA, and to non-members at Fifteen Shillings per annum, payable in advance. A copy of *The Chemists and Druggists' Diary*, published annually, is forwarded post free to every subscriber.

Advertisements, remittances, and all business communications to be addressed to THE HONORARY SECRETARY OF THE PHARMACEUTICAL SOCIETY, MELBOURNE.

SCALE OF CHARGES FOR ADVERTISEMENTS:
	Per annum.		Per annum.
One Page	.. £8 0 0	Quarter Page	.. £3 0 0
Half do.	.. .. 5 0 0	Business Cards	.. 2 0 0

Special rates for wrapper and pages preceding and following literary matter. Advertisements of Assistants Wanting Situations, 2s. 6d. each.

Advertisements for insertion in the current month should be sent to the office before the 10th.

COMMUNICATIONS for the EDITORIAL department of this journal should be addressed to THE EDITOR, MUTUAL PROVIDENT BUILDINGS, COLLINS STREET WEST, MELBOURNE.

No notice can be taken of anonymous communications. Whatever is intended for insertion must be authenticated by the name and address of the writer—not necessarily for publication, but as a guarantee of good faith.

MARRIAGES.
LEWIS—BALDERSON.—On the 5th May, at Trinity Church, Balaclava, by the Rev. Dr. Torrance, Arthur C., second son of Mr. George Lewis, J.P., of Windsor, to Lydia J., third daughter of Mr. R. Balderson, mayor of St. Kilda.

MASON—JACKSON.—On the 16th May, at St. John's Church, by the Rev. J. H. L. Zillmann, George Stephen Mason, of Mason and Son, hatters, Collins-street, to Mary Elizabeth, youngest daughter of Mr. John Jackson, chemist, Jeffcott-street, West Melbourne.

DEATH.
WOOD.—On the 6th inst., at his residence, Cunningham-street, Northcote, Mr. W. B. Wood, aged fifty-two.

LIBRARY.—SPECIAL NOTICE.
The following Periodicals are missing from the Library : — The "Practitioner," January, 1879; "Journal of Science," November and December, 1879, Nos.; "Nature," March and December, 1879, Nos.

Members are invited to examine their Libraries, and if any of the above-mentioned works be found therein, to forward such work or works to the Librarian of the Society.

NOTICE.
Subscriptions for the year 1880 are now due, and members are respectfully requested to remit the same.

THE most important topic of scientific discussion during the past month has been upon the state of the Yan Yean water. For some time the attention of the public has been unpleasantly drawn to this vexed question. The water has been so turbid and disgustingly muddy that a large number, perhaps the greater proportion, of consumers felt reluctant to drink it even after filtration—which, as usually conducted, is of little avail—notwithstanding the assurances we have received from some high scientific authorities that to purify this water is almost wrong, certainly wasteful, as it is argued that the vegetable and suspended organic and mineral matter is very "nourishing." *De gustibus non est disputandum* is an old proverb ; but verily there are some whose sense of taste is so vitiated that they are quite willing to forego the loss of " vegetables," as contained in the Yan Yean pea-soup, preferring clear, bright, "pure" water. " Dirt," Lord Palmerston once said, "is only matter in the wrong place ;" and an increase of six or seven grains of dirt and mud in our potable water would indicate that a great deal of " matter in the wrong place" has got into the reservoir. Whether this result is due to unskilfulness on the part of those who have charge of the works—as Mr. Johnson's letter would seem to show—or not, we think that it is the duty of · the Government to make speedy efforts to effect a complete change in the methods in use, or adopt, as is done in Europe and America, some mode of purification. We know that this is easy enough to talk about, and that the purification by precipitation by alum or lime can be carried out perfectly on a small scale. Even filtration, when conducted properly by means of a "dripstone" or piece of Omaru freestone, as recommended by Mr. Foord, is quite effective. Yet it is said that the economical and engineering difficulties are a serious, if not insuperable, difficulty. But when we know that cities much larger than Melbourne are supplied with water purified by means of lime and filtration, &c., surely the difficulties which have hitherto staggered us might be overcome. As to the objections urged at the Medical Association meeting, we look upon them as,. if not puerile, at least based upon an imperfect conception of the methods proposed to be adopted. We think that our medical friends might assist instead of damping the efforts of water reformers. Drs. Brande and Taylor twenty years ago told us that the Yan Yean water was, in its then state, "unfit for the use of a population." It contained at that time of total solids 11·4 per gallon ; now we find 15·4 grains per gallon as the minimum. Mr. Ellery has, he says, employed lime, in the proportion of 3 grains to a gallon, for many years with perfect success, and with every confidence in its safety ; and how, even if lime is left in solution, anything but benefit could result to the drinker of water thus treated, we, not being believers in the action of infinitesimal doses, treat as a problem beyond our powers. It is, as Mr. Johnson says, to be hoped that as the subject is now being ventilated it will result in good.

The Month.

MR. COSMO NEWBERY delivered another of his interesting lectures on practical chemistry at the Industrial and Technological Museum, on the 22nd May, to a large audience. He dealt briefly with the subject of the methods of extraction of silver by the wet processes, and also continued his descriptions of the collections in the museum. Mr. Rule also continued his description of Tasmanian minerals.

A return moved for by Mr. Bosisto in November last in regard to paying patients in the lunatic asylums of the colony, has been presented to Parliament. It appears that the number of paying patients in all the asylums on the 1st January, 1879, was 207; the number contributing sums equivalent to or in excess of the average weekly cost of maintenance of lunatic patients, 59; and the total amount paid into the Treasury to the master in lunacy for the year 1879, £4594.

The adjourned meeting of those interested in the formation of a Field Naturalists' Club was held on the 17th May, at the Athenæum. Dr. Lucas was voted to the chair. There was a large attendance, and the name decided on was the "Field Naturalists' Club of Victoria." Office-bearers were then elected as follows:—President, Professor M'Coy; vice-presidents, Dr. Lucas and the Rev. J. J. Halley; treasurer, Mr. E. Howitt; secretary, Mr. D. Best; committee, Messrs. F. L. Leith, C. French, J. R. Y. Goldstein, W. J. Kendall, J. Wing, and J. G. Luehmann. The following gentlemen were elected as hon. corresponding members, viz:—The Hon. W. Macleay, of Sydney; Mr. G. Ramsay, director of the Australian Museum, Sydney; Mr. F. G. Waterhouse, director of the Adelaide Museum; the Rev. J. Tenison Woods, Sydney; Mr. A. Howitt, F.G.S., Gippsland. The first field-day was arranged to be held in Studley Park, on Saturday, the 19th June, members to meet at Johnston-street bridge at half-past one p.m.

Mr. Molesworth, at the Assize Court, in the case of Edward Mortensen, tried for manslaughter, suggested that the provisions of the Act for Regulating the Sale of Poisons in Victoria should be so extended as to cause chemists to keep poisonous drugs under lock and key, only dealers in poisons being required to do so at present.

We regret to announce the death of Mr. W. B. Wood, of Bourke-street. The deceased was an old member of the Pharmaceutical Society.

The next quarterly meeting of the members of the society will be held at the rooms on Friday evening, the 2nd July, at half-past eight p.m., at which Mr. J. W. Norris will read a paper on some "Curious Prescriptions."

The *British Medical Journal* is not generally humorous, but this week it has a charming story. In provincial France, it seems, pens and ink are not so common as in Paris, and a doctor of Chalons going to see a country patient could find no materials for his prescription. He wrote, therefore, in charcoal on a barn door. The relations of the sick man being, however, unable to read, far less to transcribe it, were obliged to take the door off its hinges, and cart it off to the chemist. His establishment was too small for the barn door, so it was propped up on the pavement while he read the formula, which he entered with particular care in his book, lest, should the medicine require repetition, he need not have to refer to the original prescription.

A deputation from the Pharmaceutical Society again waited on the Minister of Lands on the 26th May in reference to the piece of land promised some time since. Messrs. Zox and Murray Smith, introduced the deputation. The plans of the proposed building were again laid before the Minister, and, after some discussion, Mr. Duffy said it would be well to see the Commissioner of Public Works (Mr. Bent), and if no opposition was offered by him to the site applied for, he would favourably consider the matter. The deputation then interviewed Mr. Bent, and he promised to personally inspect the land applied for, and give his decision as soon as possible.

Mr. Arthur Cooper Lewis has been admitted as a partner in the well-known and old-established firm of Messrs. George Lewis and Son, chemists and druggists, Collins-street, Melbourne. The firm will, from the 1st May, be "George Lewis and Sons."

Meetings.

THE PHARMACY BOARD OF VICTORIA.

THE ordinary monthly meeting was held on the 12th May; present—Messrs. Brind, Bowen, Holdsworth, Lewis, and Kruse. Mr. Henry Brind was in the chair.

The minutes of the previous meeting were read and confirmed.

Permission to carry on business under the 23rd section of the Act was granted to Mrs. Jane Summers, Nagambie; Mrs. Page, Violet Town, and Mrs. Stillings, Taradale, were informed that the Board have no power to allow them to carry on, unless the business was conducted by a registered chemist.

Applications for Registration.—The following applications were passed:—Charles Finch, Collingwood; William W. Caught, Taradale; Francis George Chamberlin, Sandridge, and Alfred Dickinson, Fitzroy. The applications of T. M. Cryer, Kyneton, Robert Soppet, St. Kilda, and Charles A. Kerans being postponed, and that of Edwin Hall, Smith-street, Collingwood, refused.

Name Erased from the Register.—A certificate of the death of Mr. E. Perkins, of Kyneton, having been received, his name was erased from the register.

Apprentices' Indentures Registered.—The following were registered in accordance with the provisions of the 43rd section of the regulations:—R. M'Mullen, Stawell; C. A. Graves, Deniliquin; Thos. J. Woodfull, Prahran; Edward Towl, Benalla (transferred); and John G. Wilson, Hotham.

The registrar was instructed to write to the Adelaide University in reference to the nature of the lectures on chemistry and botany at that University.

A communication was received from the Pharmaceutical Society, accepting the terms for use of offices.

Correspondence.—Letters were received and dealt with from the following persons:—A. Power, Mrs. Page, Mrs. Stillings; the Police, Brunswick, Melbourne, Nathalia, Yarrawonga, Cowes, Cranbourne, Yandoit; F. G. Chamberlin, J. P. H. Tanner; School of Mines, Ballarat; John Davis, Henry Francis, G. J. Newton, deputy-registrar, Ballarat; D. Robertson, J. M. Paul, J. J. Cunningham, H. A. Geyar, the Adelaide University.

The meeting then adjourned.

THE PHARMACEUTICAL SOCIETY OF VICTORIA.

THE ordinary meeting of the council was held at the rooms, Collins-street, Melbourne, on Friday evening, the 4th June; present—Messrs. Bowen, Gamble, Baker, Norris, Jones, Huntsman, Macgowan, and Shillinglaw. The vice-president (Mr. Wm. Bowen), in the absence of the president (Mr. C. R. Blackett), who was unable to be present, took the chair.

The minutes of the previous meeting were read and confirmed.

Election of New Member.—Mr. C. Bock, of 50 Rundle-street, Adelaide, was duly elected a member. The following were also nominated:—Messrs. J. Porter, 152 Rundle-street, Adelaide; J. Davidson Stanthorpe, Queensland; Alfred

Bradley, Melbourne (major certificate from Pharmaceutical Society, Great Britain); Wm. J. Main, 9 Hindlay-street, Adelaide.

Deputation to Minister of Lands.—The honorary secretary reported the result of the interview with the Minister of Lands, and stated that the application now rested with the Commissioner of Public Works, who was in the occupation of the ground applied for. Should the Public Works Department offer no objection, the site asked for would be granted.

Correspondence.—A letter was read from Mr. Holdsworth, of Sandhurst, suggesting the idea of enlarging the number of members of the council by the appointment of a member thereat from each of the large towns of the colony, such members to be honorary members. After some discussion, the hon. secretary was instructed to write to Mr. Holdsworth, and recommend that the chemists of Sandhurst and other large towns should do as Ballarat had done, and form themselves into associations, and seek representation on the council by election instead of hon. membership.

Alteration of the Time of Meeting.—The motion on this subject standing in Mr. Macgowan's name was withdrawn.

Members of Council Absent.—The honorary secretary was instructed to call the attention of those members of council who did not attend to Rule XI.

POISONING BY SUBCUTANEOUS INJECTION OF MORPHIA.

The following paper was read by Mr. W. Bowen:—"I beg to submit for the information of the Pharmaceutical Society the following epitome of a remarkable case of poisoning by subcutaneous injection of morphia, which I have gleaned from *The Times of India*, resulting in the death of the Italian Consul in Bombay, Chevalier Charles Grondona. The deceased gentleman, while on a visit at a friend's house, complained of a pain in his knee. A physician, Dr. Lorigiola, who was a personal friend of the deceased, was likewise on a visit at the same house, applied a liniment containing arnica and chloroform. This application not proving effectual, the physician determined to apply a subcutaneous injection, and accordingly wrote a prescription for a solution of morphia, which was forwarded to the establishment of Messrs. D. S. Kemp and Co., and dispensed by the assistant, Mr. Bristed. A portion of this solution—10 minims—was injected into the skin of the inner side of the deceased's right knee, in the presence of another physician, Dr. Barbavara. Immediately afterwards, on examining the phial containing the solution, a white deposit was observed around the stopper, which aroused the suspicion of the medical men, who then proceeded to make inquiry from the dispenser as to the cause of such deposit. The prescription, as intended by the physician was written thus :—

> Morphiæ hydrochlor., grana ij
> Aq. destillat, scrupula x
> Solve.

But instead of this, the word grana, illegibly written, was misread for gramme ij, or 30 grains, being fifteen times the intended strength. The ten minims injected, supposing the whole quantity of the morphia had been in solution, would contain one grain and a half; but as a portion remained undissolved, it was estimated that a grain and one-third had been administered. In justice to the dispenser it should be stated that he had previously dispensed the prescriptions of Dr. Lorigiola, and it is well known that European-Continental practitioners frequently adopt the French system of weights and measures, and likewise that out of several skilled witnesses examined at the inquest, one only could he found who would read the word for *grana*, others read it as gramme, the remaining number could not decipher the word at all. But I cannot exonerate the dispenser from all blame, as I consider it is the duty of every one having the responsibility of dispensing medicines, not only to be careful and precise as regards weights and measures, but likewise to examine the doses ordered of any important drug, and to satisfy himself that they are in accordance with usual practice. Besides, he should know that the solubility of hydrochlorate of morphia, in accordance with the estimate of one of the highest authorities—Mr. Squire—is 1 grain in 20 of cold water, hot water will dissolve a larger quantity, but that excess would be deposited on cooling; accordingly, 200 minims would only dissolve 10 grains, and that a hypodermic injection should always be a complete solution. In bringing this case before the notice of the Pharmaceutical Society, I trust the importance of its character will he deemed a sufficient apology."

Communications have been received from the following persons—F. W. Reay, J. Brinsmead, H. C. M'Burney, W. H. Eager, F. H. Newth.

MODIFIED EXAMINATION.

THE twelfth modified examination of candidates eligible to pass and be registered under the Pharmacy Act was held on the 7th of June, at the Mutual Provident Buildings, 100 Collins-street, before the board of examiners, Messrs. Bosisto *(materia medica)*, Blackett (pharmacy and Latin), and Johnson (chemistry, of the pharmacopœia). The following were the candidates who passed :—

Frederick J. Bartlett, Hotham.
Edward Tunnercliffe, Melbourne.
Alexander A. Morison, East Melbourne.
Hugh Marwick, Collingwood.
Alfred Reeve, Carlton.
Samuel Park, Sandhurst.

PRELIMINARY EXAMINATION.

THE ninth preliminary examination was held on the 3rd of June. The following are the candidates who passed :—

Robert M'Mullen, Stawell.
Cuthbert R. Blackett, jun., Williamstown.
Joseph Barnes, jun., Queensberry-street, Hotham.

VETERINARY MEDICAL ASSOCIATION.

A MEETING of veterinary surgeons took place on the 1st June at Menzie's Hotel for the purpose of forming a veterinary association for Australia ; Mr. Graham Mitchell, F.R.C.V.S., presided. The chairman stated that this movement had been started by Mr. Kendall, and read a letter written by that gentleman, which appeared in the *Leader* a few weeks ago, pointing out the unsatisfactory state of veterinary science in these colonies. He then went on to show that the profession had met with so little encouragement either from the Government or the public that many good scientific men had left the ranks of the profession to follow occupations of a more thankful nature. The prevailing diseases of stock were then briefly alluded to, and it was stated that the regulations of the stock department, as at present existing, were totally unfit to cope with the spread of disease. Mr. Mitchell also observed that tuberculosis (consumption) was a very serious disease in cattle, as instances had been known of the disease being produced in children by drinking the milk from affected cattle. The hydatid disease in sheep is now very prevalent, and as numbers of sheep are pasturing on the watersheds supplying the Yan Yean, the water may possibly become impregnated with the larvæ of these entozana, which in the adult form become developed into tape worms in the human subject and the dog. Many other diseases were mentioned, which it will be the duty of the association to inquire into. The chief objects will be to promote veterinary science by encouraging the united action of members of the profession throughout these colonies in the investigation of diseases of animals and the important effects they have upon the health of the community ; to draw the attention of stockowners to the necessity of rendering all the assistance they can in these investigations by describing outbreaks of disease and noting their progress, and by forwarding whenever opportunities occur, morbid specimens for examination, &c.; to watch the general interests of the profession, and to protect it against the frauds and impositions of unqualified persons. To facilitate these objects it is intended to hold monthly or quarterly meetings, at which papers will be read, pathological specimens exhibited, and subjects brought forward for discussion. Several letters were then read from members of the profession in different parts of the country, regretting their inability to attend, and expressing their sympathy with and approval of the movement. It was then proposed by Mr. Kendall, and seconded by Mr. T. C. Dobson, that a Veterinary Medical Association for Australia be formed, which was carried unanimously. Mr. Kendall was then elected hon. sec. *pro tem.*, and the following gentlemen appointed as a provisional committee to draw up rules for the working of the association, to be submitted at the next meeting to be held at Menzie's Hotel on the 1st July next:—Messrs. J. P. Vincent, G. Mitchell, T. C. Dobson and W. T. Kendall.

Legal and Magisterial.

BALLARAT ASSIZE COURT.

MONDAY, 25TH MAY.

(Before His Honour Mr. Justice Stephen.)

MANSLAUGHTER.

EDWARD MORTENSEN, on bail, pleaded not guilty to the charge of having, on 9th October last, feloniously killed one Ellen Harrington. Mr. Finlayson, who held the brief for the Crown, prosecuted; and Mr. Molesworth, instructed by Mr. Watson, appeared for the defence.

Catherine Harrington, a little girl aged thirteen years, and daughter of the deceased, gave evidence showing that on 9th October last, after she came home from school, her mamma sent her to Mr. Mortensen's shop between six and seven o'clock, and when she got there she saw the boy, and subsequently Mr. Mortensen. The latter asked her what she wanted, and she said two worm powders for an adult. Prisoner said, "All right," and got a mortar, and put in it some brown stuff and some white stuff like sugar, and mixed them up, and, after putting a little more white stuff into the mortar, put the stuff into two pieces of paper, which he then put into an envelope and labelled. Witness took the powders home, and gave them to her mother, who was sitting in the kitchen, in the presence of Mr. Ewins and the other children, who were in the house. Witness shortly afterwards went out of the house, and returned in five or ten minutes. Nobody but witness herself handled the packet from the time the prisoner gave it to her till she gave it to her mother. About five or ten minutes after witness returned her mother "took bad." Her mother put her hands to her head, and, saying she was giddy, lay down on the sofa. She turned quite yellow, and in a short time was unable to move. Witness then went and called a neighbour, Mrs. Savage. Cross-examined—Her mother was never very well; generally had headaches.

Adolphus Mortensen, son of the prisoner, gave evidence showing that he knew of an accident in his father's shop, some time in May, he thought. It was caused by an inside door slamming, three or four bottles being thereby knocked off the shelf. One bottle was broken, but he did not know whether the stoppers came out of other bottles. Witness collected the contents that were spilled, and put them in a bottle, and wrote "santonine" on it. That word had been written on the broken bottle. Witness placed the newly-labelled bottle on the shelf. His father was away at the time, but returned in half an hour. Witness did not tell his father of the accident till several days afterwards; then said that the slamming of the door had knocked down the "santonine" bottle, and that he had replaced it. After Mrs. Harrington's death being asked witness whether any other bottle had been thrown down; and on his replying in the affirmative, prisoner asked him to point out the bottles; but so long a time had then elapsed that witness had not a distinct recollection of the bottles in question. Witness did not remember if a bottle labelled "Strychnine" was amongst those which fell down. Cross-examined—Did not know the difference between strychnine and santonine. There were some bottles marked "Poison" in his father's shop. These bottles were kept in a shelf behind larger bottles. Witness fancied that the santonine was put on the same shelf as the bottles labelled "Poison." Witness replaced all the bottles that fell, but did not recollect whether any of them were marked "Poison." The bottle in which he placed the santonine was quite clear, and was like the bottle two inches by one inch produced. All the poison bottles he had seen in his father's shop were sealed.

The court here adjourned for an hour.

On the court resuming, Thomas Ewins, miner, gave evidence showing that at the time of the death of Mrs. Harrington he was boarding with the deceased. Remembered the little girl bringing in the papers of powders referred to. Witness saw the deceased take a powder out of the paper the little girl brought in, and mix it in an eggcup with a knitting-pin, and sip a little of it, saying it was bitter. She handed the eggcup to witness and the two children. Witness refused to take it, and the deceased then offered it to the children, who tasted it.

The deceased then drank it off. Witness went away and returned in about three-quarters of an hour, and the deceased was then dead. He gave the packet to Senior-constable Crowley.

Edward Stubbs, a boy twelve years of age, who was living at the house of the deceased at the time of her death, deposed that the deceased gave him the mixture in question to taste, and it was bitter.

A Mrs. Savage, who had been called to see the deceased, described the condition in which witness found her. The deceased was apparently in great pain, and her face was distorted. The deceased lived only for half an hour afterwards. She was dead before the doctor arrived.

Ellen Gartside, Errard-street, deposed that when she went to the deceased's place she saw a powder on the table; gave it to Mr. Ewins.

Senior-constable Crowley gave evidence showing that when he went to the deceased's house on the night in question the deceased was dead. He received the packet and envelope now produced from Mr. Ewins. Showed the packet to Dr. Bunce, who took one-fourth of the powder. Witness gave the rest of the powder to the Government analytical chemist. At the post-mortem examination witness received the stomach of the deceased from Dr. Radcliffe, and took it to the Government analytical chemist.

Dr. Radcliffe gave evidence showing that when he arrived at the residence of the deceased on the evening of her death he found the body warm. He tasted the powder given to him; it was very bitter. Witness here gave a description of the appearance of the deceased at the time the post-mortem examination was made, showing that all the indications denoted that the deceased had died from poisoning by strychnine. He also said that he put the stomach of the deceased into a prepared jar, and gave it to Senior-constable Crowley. His opinion was that death was caused through poisoning by strychnine. The ordinary dose of santonine for an adult was from 2 to 5 or 6 grains; 8 grains should not be given in less than two days. After the death of the deceased the prisoner came to witness to consult him as to the proper quantity of santonine to be given for a dose. Witness referred him to the authorities on the subject. Prisoner said he had taken a drachm of santonine and mixed it with jalap, and gave it in two powders. Witness thought the prisoner said a drachm, not half a drachm. Witness said it was a large dose. Subsequently to this witness saw the prisoner at his own house. Asked the prisoner how the occurrence could have taken place, and he said he had given santonine. Asked the prisoner if he had strychnine at the shop, and he showed witness a small bottle which was sealed with red sealing-wax. Asked where the santonine was, and the prisoner brought from the same shelf a paper with santonine, and broken glass in it. Witness said that could not be what was in the powder shown to him. Prisoner accounted for the appearance of the santonine by an accident which had occurred in the shop when he was away. Half a grain of strychnine taken at once had been known to kill. Cross-examined—The prisoner might have said half a drachm of santonine; at this distance of time witness could not be certain.

Dr. Bunce, who assisted at the post-mortem examination, gave corroborating evidence as to the appearance of the deceased's body, and went on to say that the prisoner had called at his place and asked to be allowed to be present at the post-mortem examination, and witness said it was not usual for a person to be present under such circumstances. The cause of death was obviously poisoning from strychnine. Cross-examined—Never used santonine.

Wm. Johnson, Government analytical chemist, gave evidence as to his receiving the powder and the jar referred to. Examined the powder first with a microscope, and detected a number of crystals, and tested them chemically, and they proved to be strychnine. He proceeded to weigh the entire powder; it weighed nearly 15 grains. Witness weighed out 10 grains, and separated the strychnine and weighed it. The result was 7½ grains of strychnine. The 2½ grains not accounted for had the general appearance of jalap. Santonine, when pure, was white. The brown powder could not have been santonine. Next examined the stomach by Stas's process, and extracted the strychnine now produced in the glass. Estimated roughly the weight at 2 grains. Half a grain would generally produce death. The twentieth part of a grain was a dose for an adult. Santonine was an old remedy. It was not considered a poison in the ordinary sense by Taylor. Santonine had the appearance of strychnine.

The statement of the prisoner at the inquest was then read over.

Mr. Johnson, recalled by His Honour, said if there had been any santonine in the powder it must have been a very minute quantity.

Adolphus Mortensen, recalled, said he brushed up the medicine on the floor with a feather, and put it in a paper, and put paper and all in the bottle.

His Honour pointed out that the prisoner, in his account of the matter, said that he found the paper on the shelf, and put all into the bottle.

Mr. Finlayson then addressed the jury on behalf of the Crown, putting all the points of the case very lucidly.

Mr. Molesworth then addressed the jury for the defence in an eloquent and able speech of forty minutes' duration. He quoted the cases of Regina v. Webb, v. Noakes, v. Spencer, to show that the death of Mrs. Harrington was a misadventure only, and the prisoner was entitled to an acquittal, as had been got in the cases referred to.

His Honour then summed up, pointing out that it was necessary, in the interests of the community, for the jury to take a firm view of the case. There was no doubt that this poor woman was poisoned by strychnine. She took one of the powders, and the other remained. The only defence was misadventure. It was not a question of admixture; it was a question of substitution. There was no doubt, however it happened, this dose was made up half jalap, half strychnine, instead of half jalap and half santonine. How was it that such a thing could happen as a chemist sending out a poison for a drug? Who of us could be sure that he would not be poisoned if we had chemists amongst us who substituted one drug for another. His Honour proceeded to condemn the unclean way in which the drugs had been gathered off the floor, and said that in a chemist's shop it was reasonably expected that everything should be in good order, and the drugs kept separate. He also deprecatingly adverted to the circumstance of a person ¦being allowed to mix up drugs without having had a prescription. He further said that he did not see how the jury could acquit the prisoner of unpardonable negligence. He did not wish to appear to press the case against the prisoner ; but for the safety of the public it was necessary that if it was proved that the deceased was killed by want of ordinary care the prisoner should be punished. If they considered that this death was caused by the want of reasonable skill, they could not acquit the prisoner. In this community, where medical skill and advice could not be always obtained, it was necessary, in the interest of the safety of the public, that all reasonable precaution should be used by those to whom the people looked for treatment.

The jury then retired, and after an absence of about an hour and a half returned with a verdict of guilty, with a strong recommendation to mercy, on the ground that no previous charge had been brought against him, and also on account of his age.

The prisoner, in answer to the usual question as to whether he had anything to say, replied that he had two things to say. Referring to the proportion of chemicals, he said that it was very difficult to decide in analysis the respective quantities of two alkaloids such as strychnine and santonine. He could not feel himself that he had done any harm through carelessness, and he could not explain how it occurred. He could not explain how the strychnine got into the hottle, but it was through no mistake of his. He was satisfied His Honour would deal fairly with him.

His Honour, addressing the prisoner, said he was very sorry to see him in that position. He had had the advantage of a temperate trial. He had been ably defended by superior counsel. The case had been mercifully put by the gentleman who prosecuted on behalf of the Crown ; the medical gentlemen and the Government analytical chemist had given their evidence with great clearness ; and the jury had given great consideration to the case. It seemed to him that the prisoner had substituted one drug for another, or one poison for another drug. The prisoner had been many years in business, and, perhaps, his eyes were not so good as they had been. Nobody thought the prisoner did it wilfully ; but the law held negligence to be criminal. The jury were justified in assuming that this was his first offence. There was no evidence that the prisoner had made any mistakes before. But he (His Honour) must mark his sense of the gravity of the offence. We might all he poisoned unless special care were exercised. After a most careful consideration of the whole case he (His Honour) sentenced him to one year's imprisonment.

The prisoner on hearing his sentence fell down on the floor of the dock. He was lifted by the police and removed. The court then adjourned *sine die*.

BALLARAT.

THE BALLARAT DISTRICT CHEMISTS' ASSOCIATION.

THE monthly meeting of the association was held on Wednesday evening, 21st May, at Lester's Hotel. There was a fair attendance of members. Mr. T. P. Palmer, president, took the chair at twenty minutes past nine p.m. The minutes of the previous meeting were read and confirmed.

A letter was read from Mr. D. M. A. Gray, manager of the Melbourne Friendly Societies' Dispensary, in reply to one to him from the hon. secretary, relative to the cost of maintaining the dispensaries. It was resolved that the minimum price for all future tenders for dispensing for friendly societies be 7s. 6d. per member per annum.

The President referred in feeling terms to the death of the late Mr. Joseph Longstaff, whom all had known so long and so agreeably. It was resolved that a letter of condolence, signed by the officers of the association, be sent to Mrs. Longstaff.

The hon. secretary stated that he had attended the meeting of the Pharmaceutical Council, on 7th May, as also the adjourned general meeting that was held afterwards ; had voted for the new offices, considering that they were much needed, were central, suitable, and commodious ; had endeavoured to re-introduce the motion of Mr. Whittle with respect to voting for members of council by ballot instead of proxy ; but the subject was considered as having been finally closed at the last meeting. The adjourned general meeting was not largely attended, the sitting of the council being rather long, and several members of the society who had come early went away before the meeting commenced. The association endorsed the hon. secretary's action in voting for the new offices.

Addition of articles, with prices agreed upon, for new list as follows :—Glass syringes, 3 ij oz., 1s. ; 1 oz., 1s. 6d. ; 2 ozs., 2s. Pancreatic emulsion, 4s. and 7s. ; Walton's cake annatto, 1s. 6d. ; Fulwood's do.—1 oz., 6d. ; 2 ozs., 1s. 6d. ; 4 ozs., 1s. 6d. (two for 2s. 6d.). Walton's liquid—4 ozs., 1s. ; 6 ozs., 1s. 6d. ; 8 ozs., 2s. 6d. ; pint, 3s. 6d. ; quart, 6s. Revalenta—½ oz., 2s. 6d. ; 1 oz., 4s. 6d. Extract of meat, 2s. and 3s. 6d.

The president stated that he and the hon. secretary had waited upon one of the members of the association with respect to the infringement of the price-list, and that the matter had been explained.

Some accounts were passed for payment, and the meeting closed, as usual, with a vote of thanks to the chair.

The remains of the late Dr. Nicholson were conveyed to the New Cemetery on the 7th June, the funeral *cortége* leaving the deceased's late residence, Albert-street, at two o'clock. Although in accordance with the wishes of immediate friends the funeral was a private one, still the late doctor was held in such general estimation that a very large number of persons were anxious to pay the last tribute of respect to his memory, and the consequence was that the funeral procession was a long one. The pall-bearers were Drs. Owen, Radcliffe, Jakins, and Hudson, and Messrs. A. Anderson and W. Little. The funeral was conducted in strict accordance with the rules of the Ballarat Funeral Reform Association, and was divested of all the " trappings of woe" which usually characterises such sad ceremonials. The Rev. H. E. Cooper officiated at the grave.

MODIFIED EXAMINATIONS.

IN order to afford intending candidates some idea of the character of the examination before the Pharmacy Board, we publish the last examination papers :—

THE TWELFTH MODIFIED EXAMINATION.—7th June, 1880.

Questions in Materia Medica.

Time allowed, one hour.—Examiner, J. Bosisto.

1. Name the tree from which mastich is obtained, and state in what way the characters of mastich differ from those of sandarach.

2. Name the active principles of the following plants :—Belladonna, gentian, ipecacuanha, nux vomica.

3. Give some of the constituents of plants under the following heads :—(1.) Organic matter. (2.) Inorganic matter.

4. How would you distinguish the stigmas of *Croci sativus* from the florets of *Carthamus tinctorius*, the latter being often employed as an adulterant of the former ?

5. *Linum usitatissimum:*—What part is officinal? State the preparations.

6. Give the natural order of matico.

Note.—3 and 4 well answered will receive special marks.

Questions in Practical Pharmacy.

Time allowed, one hour.—Examiner, C. R. Blackett.

1. What is specific gravity? What is the use of the hydrometer ? Name the principal scales in use.

2. What is the actual value in avoirdupois weight of the gramme ?

3. Give the official names of the liquid preparations of opium, and the dose of each.

4. State the official process for preparing morphia.

5. How is hydrocyanic acid prepared? State the official test for its strength.

6. How is official belladonna plaster prepared ?

MY FIRST AQUARIUM.—(By Mr. C. A. Atkin.)

(Continued from page 95.)

My first afternoon's haul consisted of small Yarra trout, perch, or, in more vulgar parlance, mud-fish (who, by-the-way, is a very inquisitive, interesting little fellow), shrimps, water scorpions, large aquatic beetles, singing beetles, dyticus marginalis, caddis worms, &c. Indeed, I now thought I was getting on swimmingly, and the daily increasing curiosity of my friends went far to confirm me in that opinion.

About this time, my esteemed fellow-townsman, the late Dr. Howitt, called. He was, like myself, an amateur naturalist, and probably possessed the largest collection of land and water beetles in the colony. The worthy doctor at once took a lively interest in my collection, told me the scientific names of each specimen, their habits, &c.; and on the occasion of his next visit brought me a valuable aquatic plant.

Another friend, the late Rev. J—— D——, was scarcely less useful to me in this particular aquarium, and I cannot help relating an incident which goes far to support such a statement. One week-night, rather late, he dropped in, and almost his first inquiry was, "Well, how is the aquarium getting on !" My reply was satisfactory, and without more ado he said—"I have brought you an interesting contribution. While on my way to preach at Footscray I passed a man who, whilst digging a post-hole, had come upon a lot of small eels, which he showed me. I at once thought of you, but the difficulty was, how could I convey them? After searching for some time, we managed to find a jam tin, and putting them in my coat-pocket, I continued my journey, and conducted the service with the eels in my pocket. Here they are, and I trust you will find them all right." Sure enough there were. The ball-shape in which they were coiled up contained about two dozen of them, from 2 in. to 4 in. long, and after a week's stay in the aquarium they became the objects of unflagging interest, not only to my reverend friend but to many others.

My next addition to the aquarium was an inverted propagating glass, placed on a wooden stand. This receptacle only held about a gallon of water, but it was amply large enough for the experiment I intended it for—viz., to ascertain how long I could keep the fish alive without changing the water. The result of this case showed about eighteen months, during which time very few of the fish died.

The whole theory may be explained in a few words. Living animals absorb oxygen gas, and exhale or throw off carbonic acid gas. By a like continuous process plants separate the carbonic acid gas into its constituent elements, carbon and oxygen. The plants absorb the carbon, which is converted into their vegetable tissue, and in their turn throw off the free oxygen for the animals to breathe. In this way animal and vegetable life are balanced, and so long as this equilibrium is preserved the two can be kept together in clear colourless water for any length of time.

My next grade in the aquarium line was a more elaborate affair altogether. I wished to have a fountain in the centre of a tank, as well as the vegetation and fish already described. For this purpose I had a small tank made with plate-glass sides, and ends bedded into brass pillars, and a slate bottom.

In this I put 4 in. deep of washed sand and several aquatic plants, including the white and blue flag, small bulbs of the white arum lily, and some of the finest specimens of the graceful Vallisneria spiralis I ever saw, presented to me by my friend, Mr. J. Bosisto, who obtained them, I believe, in Gippsland, where, he informed me, it grows in abundance. Notwithstanding the distance it had been brought, the plant had still the graceful spirals and elegant flowers attached. I may mention that this, of all others, is esteemed the best aquatic plant for the purposes of a fresh-water aquarium, and in Europe it is extensively used by chemists and those who deal in leeches to oxygenate the water in which those bloodthirsty creatures are kept. It is indigenous to the south of Europe.

My next requirement was a framework of wood, which I covered over when made with a coating of Portland cement. This I left in water—frequently cleaning it—for weeks, so that when put into the tank the lime in the cement would not destroy the fish. Soon after its completion I was cheered by the sight of my first goldfish. In the year of the great flood, 1864, a large number of the fish that had accumulated at Mr. Coppin's Cremorne-gardens was washed out into the Yarra, and from thence found their way into the North Melbourne swamp. A youth came to me one day with, I think, the first specimen of the kind that had been seen out of Cremorne. Who sent him I know not, but I presume that some kind friend who had heard of my icthyological vagaries or eccentricities considered that it was the right thing to do, and I have not heard since that any one regretted the proceeding. My hobby (and every one has, or ought to have, a hobby, provided it is an interesting and instructive one, and interferes with no one else's comfort) cost me 7s. 6d. on that occasion.

I now added to my large aquarium some fresh-water turtle, about the size of a five-shilling piece, from the Murray River ; a few crayfish from the quarryholes at Brunswick ; and, in fact, I had quite the nucleus of an amateur's aquarium. There was, however, a daily increasing desire for more wonders of nature, as distinguished from those which art can display. My next ambition was to breed goldfish, and I ultimately succeeded in bringing them to perfection in a tank I had made in my back garden. The spawning season for them commences about December. On closely watching the fish I saw them frequently brush quickly past any aquatic vegetation that came in their way, and on clipping some of those plants off with a pair of scissors I discovered several small jelly bags about the size of a pin's head deposited upon them. These I carefully lodged in a large glass vase, in which some vegetation had previously been growing, and after a few days I was able to distinguish two little black spots (the eyes) in each jelly bag ; on the sixth day they were liberated, and adhering to the sides of the glass vase, just like the small mosquitoes without wings. A few days later, they commenced to dart about in the water, a distance of about two or three inches at a time ; then, after a few weeks, the fins were developed, they were of age, and away on their own account.

I kept some of them for a length of time; but owing to their confinement in such a limited space they remained very small. Subsequent experience proved to me that the carp, although brown at first, assumes a golden colour, and grow much quicker in a stream of dirty, muddy water, to which circumstance they are probably indebted for their appellation of a mud-fish.

I think I have said enough to encourage any amateur who, like myself, is inclined to give this interesting study a fair trial.

Many, if not all, of the doubts and uncertainties I had to contend with have been cleared away by the creation of such monster establishments as that of the Trocadéro Aquarium, at Paris, an account of which appeared in the last number of the *Victorian Review*. Besides, the very "difficulties" of such a pursuit are, to most minds, the best "incentives" to further diligence, and, in this case, I guarantee that the reward of such perseverance will be ample.

It was my intention to have added a *résumé* of my experience with marine aquaria. Space alone prevents me, for the material at my command is much more extensive than that already employed, and the interest it awakens is, to my mind, proportionately greater.

I will, therefore, await the result of this first instalment, and, should opportunity afford, will do my best to save those who have followed me thus far a disappointment in the future article.

Correspondence.

PILL COATING.

To the Editor of The Australasian Supplement to the Chemist and Druggist.

DEAR SIR—I have to thank your correspondent for the information contained in last issue in reference to coating pills, and hope to at last succeed.—Yours, &c.,   AMBITION.

DRUGGISTS AND THEIR POISONS.

THE following letter appeared in the *Ballarat Star :—* "To the Editor of the *Star.*—Sir—On behalf of the Ballarat District Chemists' Association, I am directed respectfully to request the insertion of this letter in your valuable columns on the above subject, for the information and security of the public—viz., that in all well-ordered chemists' shops the bottles are classified upon the shelves, with regard to colour, contents, &c., and poisons of a virulent nature—such as strychnine, morphia, arsenic, prussic acid, &c.—are invariably kept in a cupboard as far distant as possible from the dispensing department. These rules are observed in all the chemists' shops in Ballarat. Moreover, the chemists here consider they have good cause for self-congratulation, seeing that the unfortunate case just concluded is the only one that has ever occurred in this district through carelessness or mistake on the part of a druggist.—Yours, &c.,
"28th May.   "J. T. MACGOWAN, Hon. Sec. B.D.C.A."

STOREKEEPERS AND DRUGS.

To the Editor of The Australasian Supplement to the Chemist and Druggist.

DEAR SIR—I think it is quite time some action was taken to protect chemists from intrusion on their business by storekeepers, &c. The Pharmacy Act has done a great deal of good for the trade, but it does not apply to storekeepers dealing in drugs, &c., unless they call themselves chemists and druggists. They have long dealt in patent medicines, and cut them as fine as it is possible to do, and now the evil of their selling drugs is growing greater every year.

I will confine my remarks to the action of the storekeeper in my own township; and perhaps some of my country brethren will follow suit.

Some have said that patent medicines are a curse to our business, and so they are ; but the public will have Holloway's, Cockle's, &c., and if the chemist persuades them to take his own article, they will at times be offended, and go for the future to the storekeeper, where sometimes they will get them cheaper and at longer credit.

Leaving patents alone, I will direct the attention of my brethren to the fact that in this township the storekeeper retails liq. ammon. fort., ext. tarax. aaci., acs : sulph., nitric, and muriatic, ammon : mur : sodæ, bibor., pot. bitart., and others too numerous to mention. Could not an Act be brought before Parliament to suppress this evil?

Coming to patents again, the storekeeper here is not satisfied with dealing merely in Holloway's, Cockle's, Steedman's, salts and senna, &c., but goes in for Churchill's syrup, Jayne's preparation, Row's embrocation, &c.—in fact, one corner of the shop is stocked larger than my own with such articles as I have mentioned.—I have the honour to be, yours, &c.,
COUNTRY CHEMIST.

PRESERVATION OF MUCILAGE OF GUM ARABIC.

To the Editor of The Australasian Supplement to the Chemist and Druggist.

SIR—There are few pharmacists, I think, who have not experienced considerable annoyance in consequence of the difficulty of keeping a supply of *sweet* mucilage of gum arabic, and various have been the methods proposed for attaining this end, most of them aiming at the complete exclusion of air from the vessels containing the mucilage. "Squire" recommends filling six-ounce bottles with mucilage as soon as made, and corking them. My own experience has led me to an exactly opposite opinion. I have frequently noticed that mucilage when kept in open-mouthed vessels has invariably kept longer than when closed up in bottles so as to partially or entirely exclude the air. Three weeks ago I made ten pints of mucilage. About three pints of this were unused, and of this about a pint was put into a bottle, and closely covered with paper ; the remainder was allowed to remain in the jar in which it was made (which, by the way, has a diameter internally of $8\frac{1}{4}$ inches, with perfectly straight sides); it was loosely covered with a piece of paper, thrown over it to exclude dust, &c. That which had been kept in the bottle was quite sour, and effervesced briskly on the addition of some solution of bicarbonate of potash ; that which had remained in the jar smelt and tasted perfectly sweet, and, although litmus paper distinctly indicated acidity, still on the addition of some solution of bicarbonate of potash not the slightest perceptible effervescence took place ; it was, in fact, practically unaltered. Thinking the acidity indicated in the *sweet* mucilage might be due to the presence of a small quantity of acetic acid, I applied the usual tests, but failed to find any.

I then powdered some of the same sample of gum, and dissolved it in distilled water, and again applied the litmus paper, and again obtained the indication of the presence of an acid, which confirmed an opinion I had already entertained, that the acid reaction might be due to the presence of some free gummic acid, or that gummate of calcium might be an acid-salt.

I enclose for your inspection the respective pieces of test paper used, and although there is a decidedly more apparent indication in favour of the older mucilage, there is still undeniable evidence of the existence of an acid in the perfectly fresh.

I then thought that probably the acid present might be sulphurous acid, thinking that some of the gum might have been bleached by this agent; but upon applying the tests therefor I failed to find even a trace.

I think that these facts are most decidedly in favour of keeping mucilage in open vessels, and, I think, proves, or tends to, that air is not the cause of mucilage becoming sour. As to what may be the reason of this singular phenomenon I will not even venture an opinion ; but these facts have led me to the belief that the best method of preserving mucilage of gum arabic is to keep it in vessels in which it is as much exposed to the air as is consistent with the exclusion of dust and other extraneous matter.

I shall be glad to see this matter taken up by some one more capable of throwing some light upon this apparent anomaly.—
Yours faithfully,   S. M. DALTON.
Sandhurst, 7th June, 1880.

THE PHARMACY ACT IN NEW ZEALAND.

To the Editor of The Australasian Supplement to the Chemist and Druggist.

SIR—Our New Zealand *confrères* deserve much commendation for their activity in attempting to assimilate the educational standard of the trade there to that legalised by the Government here ; and I am sure that we all heartily hope their endeavours to get a bill passed through the Legislative Houses for this purpose may be crowned by the most complete and speedy success. If, as I see by editorial note in our *Supplement* (folio 83), and in the *Chemist and Druggist Journal* (folio 15), they have already drafted a bill on the model of our Victorian Act, I would like, through your journal, to offer a suggestion to the pharmacists of New Zealand, ere it be too late—that instead of accepting our Act in its entirety as a perfect one, they should go further than ours, adding to it an additional grafting, that ours much requires, and one that I take to be a future necessity, and one which, ere many years have flown away, I trust may be carried out. Those gentlemen in New Zealand familiar with our Act will know that it is administered and carried out by a board of seven members ; that the Pharmaceutical Society is governed by another board or council of twelve members ; the one not necessarily connected with the other in any way, excepting in having the one qualification of being "registered pharmacists." Now, my impression is that there is in this mode of conducting our affairs a great deal of superfluous and supererogatory work, and the machinery, so to speak, unnecessarily large and unwieldly ; but considering the time, circumstances, and anxieties attendant on the introduction and consummation of passing the Act to the few zealous pharmacists on whose shoulders the whole responsibilities rested (many must have said, "'Tis greatly to their credit"), the Act has worked hitherto remarkably well ; and, though in some points it is not quite as perfect as its framers desired it to be, it was, I believe, by them accepted on the law of expediency, as being as near perfection as at that time it could he made. The supererogatory work and heavy machinery to which I have alluded should be, if possible, avoided. I would, therefore, most strongly advise that the new Act for New Zealand should more closely follow the English than the Victorian in its constitution, for there the council have the power and undertake the triplicate duties of legislative, educational, and commercial; here, the board directs the two former, and the council the latter; so that if the Pharmacy Board, in the course of their duties, are desirous of initiating anything commercially to the advantage of the trade, it has to he relegated to the council, and the same see-saw work has to he done hy it to the hoard in like circum-stances; and as both have the one and self-same object in view, such a fault shonld, if possible, he remedied. Again, in order to make the Act a benefit and success to the puhlic as well as to pharmacists, its governing hody must be provided with the necessary sinews of war. Now, the Victorian Act has made provision only for the board's receipt of registration and examination fees, and any penalties obtained from the infringe-ment of the Act. Clearly, therefore, as soon as the registration fees, which are its real and only positive income, hccome expended, so soon must the Board, without an appeal he made for a grant of money from the Government, be eleemosynary on the proverbially poor druggist, or cease to he effective. The English Act, being made a self-supporting one, should, there-fore, in this direction, I think, he most decidedly followed. I cannot see any hardship in compelling pharmacists to suh-scribe, say, nearly fivepence (! ! !) per week towards the expenses incurred in self-protection, seeing that, in addition to it, a journal worth the annual guinea subscribed can be obtained by them; though I very much regret that there are still in Victoria registered pharmacists who think differently, and hold aloof from the Pharmaceutical Society altogether. I think our register shows there are over six hundred registered pharmacists, and not half of this number are members of the Pharmaceutical Society. "Tis true, 'tis pity," &c. But it only shows the usual reticence of druggists in all matters which may—nay, they—vitally affect their individual and collective interests. If the New Zealand pharmacists get their Act passed, I have no doubt, sir, hut that arrangements could he made with our society for the transmission of the journal to their members as to ours, reserving a certain number of folios for their exclusive use, which could also he done for the New South Welshmen, South Australians, Qucenslanders, &c. Our *Supplement* would then be highly interesting—a fair reflex of pharmacy south of the line—and well repay pharmacists for their modicum of financial assistance in advancing trade and intellectual interests for the present and future generations.—I am, &c.,   HENRICUS.

ANSWERS TO CORRESPONDENTS.

" INQUIRER."—Bauncheit's oil is composed of croton oil and olive oil.

PRUSSIAN BLUE PHOTOGRAPHS.

MR. C. L. LOCHMAN, of Bethlehem, Pa., describes in the *Druggists' Circular* the following simple process for obtaining beautiful photographic impressions in Prussian blue:—

Dissolve 210 grains of double citrate of iron and ammonia in 3 fluid ounces of pure water, and add 10 grains of citric acid to the solution; then, separately, dissolve 180 grains of ferri-cyanide of potassium (red prussiate of potash) in 3 fluid ounces of water; mix the solutions, and filter through paper. Float a good quality of unruled white ledger paper on this liquid for three or four minutes, or wash one side of it with the liquid by means of a pellet of cotton, and hang it up to dry in a dark place. This liquid or the paper can he kept in a good condition for a considerable time in a dark place. The paper is exposed under a negative or other media to sunlight, until the parts which are to receive the darkest impression have assumed a bronze-like appearance and the lighter parts a pale blue colour. The print is then developed to a brilliant blue, simply by washing it in water, until the water runs off clear. If the exposure is merely carried so far as to produce a blue impression, and the darker parts are not bronzed, it leaves the print too pale after washing. This method produces prints of a splendid blue, with fine half tones, from a negative.

Impressions of ferns, leaves, small plants, tracings made in black on tracing paper or muslin can be readily copied with-out a camera. In these cases the ground, of course, will he blue, and the object or tracing light. A thin, flat piece of board of the requisite size is employed, a piece of cloth spread over it, and then the paper, with the sensitised side upwards, laid on the leaves or tracings, super-imposed and pressed in contact by covering it with a flat piece of glass, which is held in place by means of spring cloth clips. For negatives, a regular printing frame is better, or the hoard may be hinged in the middle, so that one half can be turned back for inspec-tion of the print. The leaves of plants should be pressed and dried, and fastened on the glass with mucilage.

In printing from natural specimens the paper must be ex-posed to a strong sunlight until it has passed the bronzed stage and assumed a metallic gray colour in the hody, in order to let the light penetrate sufficiently through the dark green leaves and show the veins. The process is exceedingly simple, and the results are beautiful.

DETECTION OF AMMONIA IN WATER.—Ammonia is usually present in water as carbonate, but frequently in such small quantities that it cannot be detected by the ordinary tests. In such cases Hager ascertains its presence by mixing 2 to 3 litres of the water with 20 drops hydrochloric acid, evaporat-ing to dryness, dissolving the residue in 10 or 15 cc. distilled water, filtering, and applying Bohlig's test, which consists in adding, first, 5 drops of solution of corrosive sublimate (1 part in 30 parts of water), and then 5 drops of solution of potassium carbonate (1 part in 50 parts of water), when a cloudiness indicates the presence of ammonia.—*Pharm. Centralb.*, 25th December, 1879.

TO PULVERISE SHELLAC.—Any one who has tried to pound up shellac in a mortar knows that the attempt is more favour-able to perspiration and profanity than to the pulverisation of the slippery stuff. A correspondent of the *Druggists' Circular* has devised the following method :—" Enclose the shellac in a strong, closely woven piece of cloth, at first compressing the folds rather tightly, hut gradually relaxing them. Then, after placing the hunch, which must be held in position with the hand, upon a solid block or smooth counter, the strokes of a heavy iron pestle are applied, gently at first, while the hunch is kept moving from side to side, so as to expose every part to the strokes of the pestle. After the large, sharp pieces are hroken, the strokes are increased in velocity and power, with wonderful effect upon the resin, and but little injury to the cloth. In this way shellac may be reduced to a granular form sufficiently fine for pyrotechnic purposes at very short notice, and to an almost impalpable powder in a comparatively short space of time. To produce this result, however, it is neces-sary to wield the pestle forcibly, and then from time to time separate the finer particles from the coarser by sifting."

Pharmacy Board of Victoria Notices.

THE TENTH PRELIMINARY EXAMINATION of Apprentices will be held at this office on THURS-DAY, the 2nd day of SEPTEMBER, 1880, at Eleven a.m. The attention of apprentices is directed to Clause 43 of the Regulations to the Act, which obliges indentures to be registered within twelve months of their being executed.

HARRY SHILLINGLAW, Secretary and Registrar.

Office of the Pharmacy Board, Mutual Provident Buildings, Collins-street West, Melbourne.

THE THIRTEENTH MODIFIED EXAMINATION of Candidates for Registration under the Pharmacy Act will be held at this office on MONDAY, the 6th SEPTEMBER, 1880, at Ten o'clock a.m. Candidates must give to the Secretary notice of their intention to present themselves for examination, together with their indentures of apprenticeship and the fee of three guineas, ten days prior to the day.

HARRY SHILLINGLAW, Secretary and Registrar.

Office of the Pharmacy Board, Mutual Provident Buildings, Collins-street West, Melbourne.

MARTIN & CO.,

WHOLESALE

Homœopathic Chemists,

85 COLLINS STREET EAST,

MELBOURNE.

HOMŒOPATHIC GOODS of EVERY DESCRIPTION SUPPLIED AT ENGLISH QUOTATIONS.

MARTIN & CO.'S Homœopathic Preparations can be obtained from any of the Melbourne Wholesale Drug Houses.

Price List, Show Cards, Illustrated List of Chests, Order Sheets, &c., forwarded free on application.

FELTON, GRIMWADE & CO.,

WHOLESALE DRUGGISTS AND MANUFACTURING CHEMISTS,

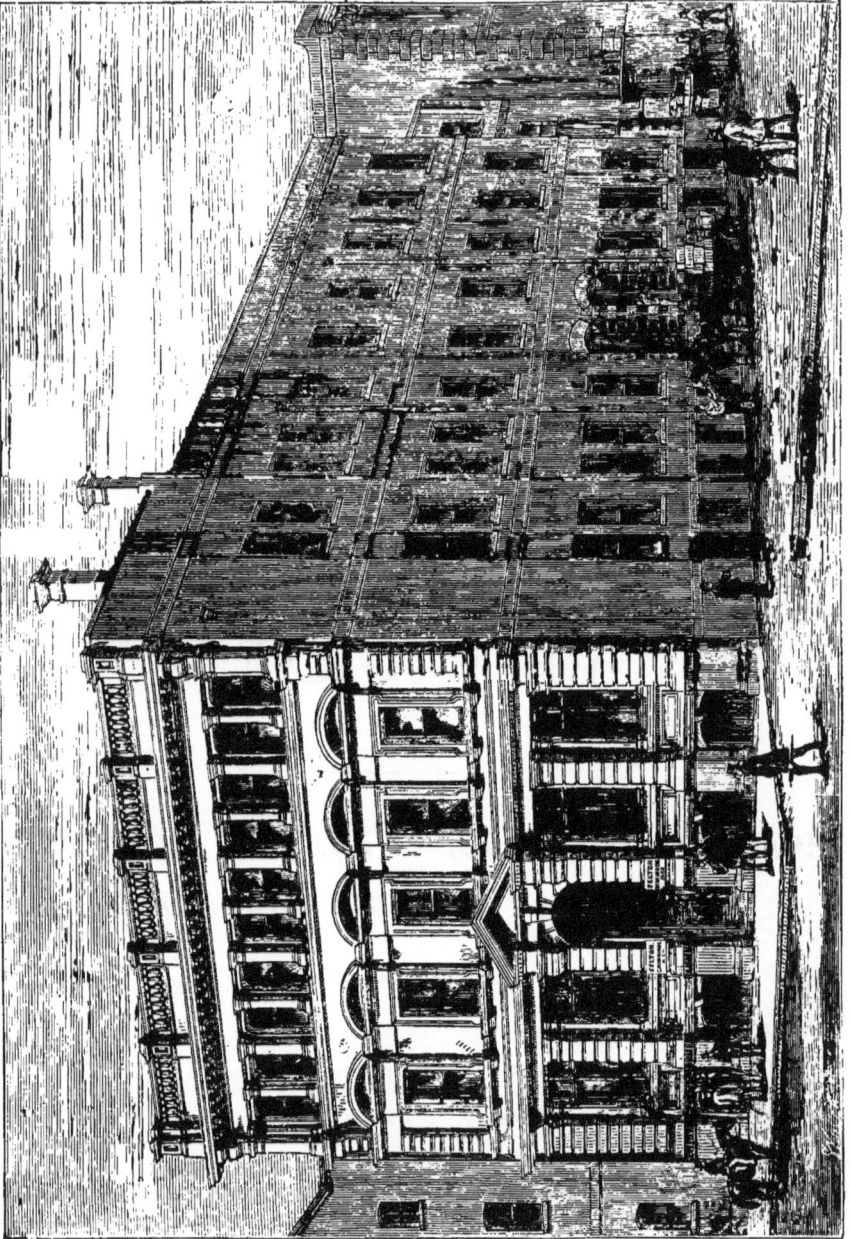

31 & 33 FLINDERS LANE WEST,

Chemist & Druggist.

WITH AUSTRALASIAN SUPPLEMENT.

(Published under direction of the Pharmaceutical Society of Victoria.)

No. 27. { PUBLISHED ON THE 15TH OF EVERY MONTH. }
Registered for Transmission as a Newspaper.

JULY, 1880.

{ SUBSCRIPTION, 15s. PER ANNUM, INCLUDING DIARY, POST FREE.

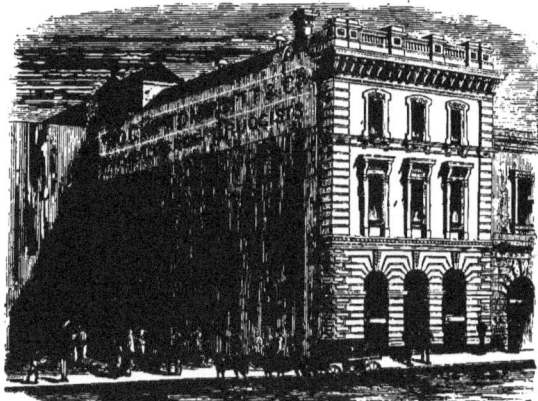

HEMMONS, LAWS & CO.

WHOLESALE DRUGGISTS,

55 & 57

RUSSELL STREET,

MELBOURNE.

FLINDERS LANE
MELBOURNE.

The Chemist and Druggist.

WITH AUSTRALASIAN SUPPLEMENT.

OFFICE: MUTUAL PROVIDENT BUILDINGS, COLLINS STREET WEST.

Published on the 15th of each Month.

THIS Journal is issued gratis to all paid-up Members of the PHARMACEUTICAL SOCIETY OF VICTORIA, and to non-members at Fifteen Shillings per annum, payable in advance. A copy of *The Chemists and Druggists' Diary*, published annually, is forwarded post free to every subscriber.

Advertisements, remittances, and all business communications to be addressed to THE HONORARY SECRETARY OF THE PHARMACEUTICAL SOCIETY, MELBOURNE.

SCALE OF CHARGES FOR ADVERTISEMENTS:

	Per annum.		Per annum.
One Page	..£8 0 0	Quarter Page	..£3 0 0
Half do.	.. 5 0 0	Business Cards	.. 2 0 0

Special rates for wrapper and pages preceding and following literary matter. Advertisements of Assistants Wanting Situations, 2s. 6d. each.

Advertisements for insertion in the current month should be sent to the office before the 10th.

COMMUNICATIONS for the EDITORIAL department of this journal should be addressed to THE EDITOR, MUTUAL PROVIDENT BUILDINGS, COLLINS STREET WEST, MELBOURNE.

No notice can be taken of anonymous communications. Whatever is intended for insertion must be authenticated by the name and address of the writer—not necessarily for publication, but as a guarantee of good faith.

NOTICE.

Subscriptions for the year 1880 are now due, and members are respectfully requested to remit the same.

APPRENTICES AND THE PRELIMINARY EXAMINATION.

IT is now nearly four years since the Pharmacy Act became law, and yet a great many of those who have been apprenticed have not passed the preliminary examination, which is the first step to be taken before proceeding to the studies and examination demanded by the law of the land, as a *sine qua non* before any person can commence business on his own account—indeed, to speak strictly, before a young man can hold the position of a qualified assistant to a pharmaceutical chemist, as without the full qualification required by law no one has the right to sell or dispense any of the drugs enumerated in schedule A of the Poisons Act ; and as it is the intention of the authorities to now enforce more stringently the application of the law, it behoves all principals to seriously consider the anomalous and dangerous position in which they are placed in disregarding the clearly defined conditions sanctioned by Parliament. The law *cannot*, and certainly *will not*, be allowed to be disobeyed with impunity. There is no longer the smallest excuse for masters to go on any longer in a selfish and lazy indifference ; it is the duty of all those who take apprentices and assistants to insist upon a prompt conformity to the wise provisions of the Pharmacy Act—an Act which was passed most fortunately at a time when useful legislation *was* possible, and which was enacted to protect the public against ignorance and incompetency. It is a matter of surprise that the followers of so important and responsible a calling as that of pharmacy should in so many instances show themselves so careless of their own interest and reputation, for surely it is, even on the low ground of self-interest, culpable for any one to neglect to urge upon their pupils—who have in most instances paid good premiums—the duty of preparing themselves for so easy an examination as the "preliminary." Any youth who has had a fairly liberal education ought to pass this examination as soon as his indentures are signed, so that he may have more time to give to those studies and practical lessons which are to prepare him for the higher examinations in chemistry, *materia medica*, botany, &c. We feel sure that it rests mainly with the master whether an apprentice realises or not his true position ; if the principal is regardless of the future success of the youth confided to his charge, we may rest assured that the "parents and guardians," and the pupil himself, will have cause to regret and feel aggrieved at the non-performance of a *contract !* It ought to be the pleasure and pride of all pharmaceutical chemists to spare no effort, whether by example or precept, to instil into the minds of their apprentices a spirit of emulation, for without some energetic moral stimulus, how can we expect the often thoughtless youth to "burn the midnight oil," and take a delight in study, especially when we consider how many and enticing are the temptations to profitless pleasure abounding in our large cities ?

The anxiety of those earnest men, who, at much sacrifice of their time and energy, were the promoters of an improved education for pharmacists in Victoria, is great, and the ultimate success of their labour depends in no small degree upon a dutiful and cordial co-operation on the part of the pharmacists. We feel confident that all conscientious persons will feel the force of our appeal, and do all they can to support the Pharmacy Board in their efforts to enforce the provisions of the Pharmacy Act. We trust that those young men who have masters indifferent to their obvious duties will come forward, and without fear or delay pass the "preliminary."

The Month.

THE Victorian branch of the British Medical Association gave a supper at Clement's Café. About forty gentlemen were present. Mr. W. Gillbee, the president of the Victorian branch, presided. The guests present were—Mr. Gray, president of the Medical Society; Mr. Ellery, president of the Royal Society; Mr. Blackett, president of the Pharmaceutical Society; Mr. Ralph, president of the Microscopical Society; Dr. Lucas, president of the Naturalists' Society; Dr. Brownless, vice-chancellor of the Melbourne University; and Baron von Müeller, Government botanist.

"Through the exertions of the *Public Record*, a newspaper of Philadelphia, the operations there in selling bogus medical diplomas have probably been broken up. The proprietor of the *Record* has been for several weeks gathering evidence, his city editor, under assumed names, getting eight medical diplomas from the American University of Philadelphia, the

Eclectic Medical College of Pennsylvania, and the Livingstone University. This work was done in connection with the Government authorities. · Everything being ready, Dr. John Buchanan, the chief dealer in bogus diplomas, with three others of his faculty, were arrested on Wednesday, and charged with using the mails for improper purposes, also with fraud. Buchanan was to-day held in bail for 10,000 dol. to answer the charge in the United States Court, and the others will be examined to-night. The papers captured in Buchanan's office showed a sale of 3000 spurious diplomas, while there was a large quantity on hand. Buchanan's trade was chiefly with Germany, but some diplomas were sent to England. His prices varied from 65 dol. to 110 dol. each. Nearly all the diplomas issued were ante-dated. Buchanan's colleges are legally incorporated by the Pennsylvania Legislature, but this exposure will be made the basis of forfeiting the charters."— *Telegraph.*

Mr. Joseph Bosisto, M.L.A., whose exhibits of essential oils and pharmaceutical preparations, obtained from the indigenous vegetation of Victoria, have formed a conspicuous feature in the collections forwarded to all the great exhibitions of the last fifteen or twenty years, has just been awarded the handsome gold medal of the Sydney International Exhibition. This is the highest award made by the Sydney commissioners, and as very few gold medals have been awarded the distinction must be regarded as a very valuable one.

Amongst other passengers who left by the "Wotonga," on the 17th July, was Mr. Duncan Carson, who goes on a botanical mission to the South Pacific with H.M.S.S. "Wolverine." Mr. Carson studied practical botany at Edinburgh, and scientific botany under Sir William Hooker, at Kew. Mr. D. Carson is a son of Mr. John Carson of this city, and although young in years, is well grounded in botanical science.

In accordance with a resolution carried some time since by the council of the Pharmaceutical Society, that proceedings should be taken against a number of persons who were known to be illegally selling poisons, the first two cases were heard in the District Court on the 2nd August. The evidence was perfectly clear, and showed that the defendants had sold poisons mentioned in part 1 of the Poisons Act, not being qualified, and without taking any precaution as to registering or labelling. In the face of this evidence, Mr. Call, the P.M., fined each of the defendants 1s., and £3 3s. costs. The decision of the Bench took every one by surprise, and is certainly a miscarriage of justice. The society, acting in the interest of its members and the public, had gone to considerable expense in getting evidence in these and several other cases, fully expecting that the bench would recognise the importance of such illegal practices being stopped. This does not, however, appear to have weight with the magistrates, who, by their decision, rather protected than punished the offenders.

It is contemplated to hold the annual dinner of the Pharmaceutical Society about the middle of November next; the date will be fixed at the next meeting of council.

The *Licensed Victuallers' Advocate*, in a leading article on the late prosecutions under the Poisons Act by the Pharmaceutical Society, says :—"We consider the penalty inflicted utterly inadequate. Here were two unlicensed men deliberately selling arsenic and tartar emetic—deadly poisons—in unlabelled bottles ! The lives of a dozen people might have been jeopardised by such conduct, if our brewers did not resort to chemical purification of bottles, yet the offenders get

off with a fine of 1s. each. Mr. Call is an admirable magistrate, but in this instance we think he tempered justice with a little too much mercy—drowned the miller, in fact. However, future offenders may have an opposite experience to that of Leith and Miscamble."

Meetings.

THE PHARMACEUTICAL SOCIETY OF VICTORIA.
THE meeting of the council was held at the rooms, 100 Collins-street West, on Friday, 6th August ; present—Messrs. Bowen, Huntsman, Gamble, MacGowan, Jones, Baker, Hooper, and Shillinglaw ; the vice-president, Mr. Wm. Bowen, in the chair. An apology was received from the president, who was unable to attend.

The minutes of the previous meeting were read and adopted.

New Members.—The following were elected :—Fergus J. Heeney, Ipswich, Queensland; John T. Barker, Gawler, South Australia; Albert Andrews, Beaufort ; Frederick J. Bartlett, Hotham ; John Davidson, Springthorpe, Queensland. Alfred Dickinson, of Nicholson-street, Fitzroy, was also nominated.

Prosecutions under the Poisons Act.—The hon. secretary reported that, in accordance with a resolution passed some time since, a number of prosecutions had been instituted ; the first two cases had resulted in convictions. The council decided to go on with the other cases.

The Annual Dinner.—It is contemplated to hold the annual dinner in the month of November ; the date will be fixed at the next meeting.

Correspondence and financial business brought the meeting to a close.

THE PHARMACY BOARD OF VICTORIA.
THE ordinary monthly meeting was held at the office of the board on the 21st July ; the president (Mr. J. Bosisto, M.P.) in the chair.

The minutes of the previous meeting were read and confirmed.

Applications for Registration.—The following were approved :—Arthur Power, Narracoorte (South Australia); Rawson Parke Francis, 31 Bourke-street, Melbourne (examination certificate, Pharmaceutical Society, Great Britain); Walter Thomas Siddall, Footscray ; and Frederick Wm. Reeve Wilcannia. A provisional certificate was also granted to James Anderson, Moonee Ponds.

Apprentices' Indentures Registered.—F. A. Groening, Sandhurst ; E. C. Longson, Narracoorte (South Australia) ; Albert E. Pilley, Windsor ; J. A. Davy, Melbourne.

Names Erased from the Register.—Certificates were received from the deputy-registrar of births and deaths of the death of Joseph Jelfs (Hotham) and James Edward Bryant (Collingwood), and their names erased from the register.

Correspondence.—Letters from the following were read and dealt with :—A. H. Florance, John Lay, T. M. Cryer, A. C. Dunn, the Adelaide University, deputy-registrars of Hotham and Collingwood, Mrs. Jelfs, the police of Cowes, Melbourne, and Ballarat, J. C. O'Keaney, W. H. Frost, E. H. Hall, W. E. Matthews, the secretary Pharmaceutical Society, Great Britain, J. T. Poock, R. Soppet, the secretary Pharmaceutical Society of South Wales.

Financial and general routine business brought the meeting to a close.

PHARMACEUTICAL SOCIETY OF NEW SOUTH WALES.
FOURTH ANNUAL REPORT.
THE annual meeting of the members and associates of the Pharmaceutical Society of New South Wales was held in the

board-room of the institution, Phillip-street, yesterday afternoon. Mr. F. Senior, J.P., president of the society, occupied the chair. There was a good attendance of members.

Mr. W. T. Pinhey, the secretary, submitted the annual report, which was as follows :—

"Your council, in presenting this, their fourth annual report, have considerable gratification in being enabled to state that the past year has been one of prosperity, and that the money placed at their disposal has enabled them to form a reserve fund to meet emergencies, or to make purchases as opportunities offer advantageous to the interests of the society.

"Your council are of opinion that the time has arrived when the chemists ought to possess the power of self-government ; in other words, power to admit into their ranks only those who have acquired sufficient knowledge in the leading branches appertaining to and inseparable from the legitimate carrying out the practice of pharmacy with comfort to the chemist and security to the public.

"Your council trust the ensuing year of the society's operations will form an era in the history of pharmacy, for the long-required and ardently desired Pharmaceutical Bill will in all probability soon be laid before Parliament. Its object will be to raise the status of the chemist, and give assurance to the public that in future none but those qualified to deal in or dispense medicines will be permitted to do so. The Pharmaceutical Bill will have, *inter alia*, this beneficial effect ; for it contains a clause bearing upon the necessity of those who may be desirous of commencing business undergoing an examination in chemistry, pharmacy, and *materia medica*, which, if carried out, will meet one of the grand objects the founders of this society had in view, and the education and qualification of the chemist will be clearly defined.

"The Medical Bill, brought before Parliament for the second time by Dr. Bowker, is for the present shelved ; but your council felt constrained to petition against the last clause of section three of that measure, because it had a tendency to interfere with the rights and privileges secured to the chemist and druggist under the Apothecaries Act of 1815.

"Your council are of opinion that it would be well if an arrangement were entered into with the University for special lectures to be given there on chemistry, pharmacy, and toxicology. This subject will be brought up for discussion at an early date.

"Your council have to acknowledge with gratitude the gifts of valuable books from Messrs. W. H. H. Lane, A. J. Watt, L. B. Bush, T. Humphreys, your secretary, and others ; which have enabled your council to invest a sum which would otherwise have been expended in adding to the collection of standard works now in your library.

"Your council have instituted a minor examination for associates, and a major examination for members. Every candidate will be expected to be able to translate medical prescriptions, to be acquainted with a certain amount of practical pharmacy, as well as conversant with toxicology.

"The following have been selected as texts-books for examination :—Proctor's or Redwood's *Pharmacy*, Pereira's *Selecta è Prescriptis*, *British Pharmacopœia*, Squire's *Companion to the British Pharmacopœia*, Attfield's or Bowman's *Chemistry*, and Bentley's *Botany*.

"Your council would impress upon all chemists and druggists that the Pharmaceutical Society is for the protection of the chemist, and to study his interest ; they, therefore, trust that by and through your continued support your society may be further benefited, and its usefulness extended, involving as it does the welfare of the public, upon whose patronage and confidence all are dependent upon for success.

"During the year four vacancies in the council have occurred. These were filled by the appointment of Messrs. Wm. Larmer, Wm. Pratt, Edward Row, and John C. Burrell, but their seats becoming vacant at the expiration of the year, notification to that effect was made by advertisement, and the following gentlemen have given the required notice to fill the vacancies, viz.:—Messrs. Wm. Larmer, Wm. Pratt, Edward Row, and John W. Guise.

"The honorary treasurer will now lay before you the balance-sheet, duly audited, which your council trust will be gratifying to all concerned."

The report and balance-sheet were unanimously adopted.

The treasurer's financial statement showed that the receipts for the past year amounted to £269 10s. 11d., which included a balance of £75 11s. 7d. brought forward from the previous year. The sum received during the past twelve months in subscriptions was £163 10s. The expenditure for the year was £82 1s. 2d., leaving a credit balance of £187 9s. 9d.

Messrs. Wm. Hume and J. Henry were elected auditors for the current year.

A vote of thanks was most cordially accorded to the council for their services during the year. Messrs. W. Larmer, W. Pratt, Edward Row, and J. W. Guise were declared members of the council, being the only members who had given the required notice.

The chairman returned thanks on behalf of the council, and bore special testimony to the exertions of Mr. W. T. Pinhey on behalf of the society. In alluding to the various matters touched upon in the annual report the chairman said he could not help thinking that some of their brethren, who, from various causes, had withdrawn from the council, would be rather astonished to find the society at its fourth general meeting in such a prosperous state, considering the lukewarmness the society had met with until the last twelve months. In proof of this prosperity he drew attention to the following facts :—They would see by the audited account-sheet that the income from fees was doubled, and that the sum of the invested funds, though small, was increasing. They had purchased, and had now on order many of the latest works, both English, American, and foreign, on subjects pertaining to pharmacy. They had had several valuable gifts of books from kind well-wishers, and had now ordered from America a large quantity of specimen bottles, with which to commence the formation of a Pharmaceutical Museum. He thought they would allow these were all marks of progress in their young society. And the time had now arrived to make another progressive step, as their *confrères* in other parts of the world had done. By the kind assistance of the Government they were taking measures for the introduction of a new Pharmacy Bill, which would no doubt raise their status, and benefit their fellow-colonists by educating a more scientific body of dispensing chemists ; and already they have evidence of a better class of youths seeking admission into the society. As there seemed in the minds of some of their brethren a doubt as to what effect on their business Dr. Bowker's Bill would have, they thought proper to petition against it, and for the present that Bill seemed to have dropped out, though he should hope before long the Government would be induced to introduce one, when he trusted no undue interference would be made with their privileges. He would advise all those who had not yet joined the society to do so at once, as it must be evident to every intelligent pharmacist that each year would necessitate their examinations being of a more stringent character, and he felt sure that all those who really felt an interest in pharmacy would have no difficulty in going through the curriculum laid down, and to which they were determined to adhere. He could not conclude without taking the opportunity of thanking the older society of Victoria for the interest they took in the society by regularly sending to them their examination papers and periodicals, and he hoped this kindly sympathetic feeling would always exist.

The meeting then closed.

Notes and Abstracts.

WICKERSHEIMER'S preservative fluid for animal and vegetable tissues is composed as follows :—

Alum	...	...	...	100 parts
Common salt ...	...	...	...	25 „
Saltpetre	...	...	...	12 „
Potash ...	...	...	...	60 „
Arsenious acid...	...	...	...	10 „

Dissolve in 3000 parts of boiling water. After cooling and filtering, add to every 10 pints of this solution 4 pints of glycerine and 1 pint of methyl alcohol.

According to the *American Journal of Microscopy*, silver-wire, in which the most delicate test could detect no difference of diameter, has been run through plates of rubies to the length of 170 miles.

The new Royal Irish University does not promise to become of great importance in science. The senate consists of ecclesiastics, politicians, and lawyers—classes of men seldom favourable to the investigation of nature.

NOTE ON UNGUENTUM HYDRARGYRI AMMONIATI.

(By C. R. Blackett, President of the Pharmaceutical Society.)

Pharmaceutical chemists have alway found a difficulty in the keeping of the ointment of ammonio-chloride of mercury, notwithstanding the most scrupulous care in seeing to the purity of the various ingredients officially ordered for the preparation of this compound. In seeking for an improved method to remedy the defective formula in use, various fatty substances suggested themselves as desirable substitutes for the simple ointment recommended by the *British Pharmacopœia*. As lard is so prone to undergo rapid change, it is the very worst material that can be used in any preparations in which there are any chemical substances liable to decompose with great facility; and as ammonio-chloride of mercury is of this character, it is not to be wondered at that the ointment, as usually prepared, will not keep for any length of time. It is not necessary to go into any detailed account of the chemical changes which take place in this ointment when kept, as the true constitution of white precipitate has been the subject of much discussion. Hitherto it has been the practice of pharmacists to prepare this ointment as required, or in small quantities at a time. By adopting the improvement which I now suggest, this need no longer be the case. Paraffine oil and wax were at first thought of as a desirable basis for the ointment, as it would resist rancidity longer than the ordinary ointments containing animal or vegetable fats. Vaseline, cosmoline, &c., are probably merely paraffine oil and wax in varying proportions, and are excellent bases for such ointments as ung. hyd. am.-chlor., or ung. hyd. ox. rubri, &c., and will keep their condition for a very long time; but it was found objectionable to use these patented compounds on account of their colour, and the B.P. formula was altered by substituting pure castor oil for the lard and almond oil with the most perfect success. Some ung. hyd. ammonio-chloridi, made many months since, has been found not to have undergone any, even the slightest, decomposition. As the substitution of castor oil cannot possibly cause any difference in the action of this preparation, there need be no hesitation in adopting this change in the formula as suggested.

CHLORIDE OF METHYL FOR EXTRACTING PERFUMES.

Professor Vincent, of the Ecole des Arts et Metiers, Paris has communicated to the Société d'Encouragement a process for the extraction of perfumes by chloride of methyl, which seems to yield greater results and finer perfumes than are obtained by the ordinary methods.

The idea was suggested by M. Massignon, a manufacturing perfumer, who is now constructing a laboratory at Cannes, which will be able to exhaust on this principle 1000 kilogrammes of flowers daily.

The experiments were first made with odorous woods. The perfume was extracted, but it was tainted with a very persistent disagreeable odour, derived from the chloride of methyl itself. Professor Vincent set himself to remove this, and succeeded in doing so perfectly by treating the chloride of methyl in a gaseous state with concentrated sulphuric acid.

Orange flowers were then experimented on, and the perfume obtained was pronounced by several practical men superior to *neroli* obtained by distillation of the flowers with water.

An apparatus was then set up which has been regularly worked for some months. Its working is thus described :—A digester is filled with the flowers to be treated. On these a sufficient quantity of chloride of methyl is poured, from a reservoir in connection, to cover the flowers; after being left in contact for two minutes, the liquid is drawn off into a third air-tight vessel. Further charges of chloride of methyl are passed through the flowers until the latter are believed to be exhausted. The chloride retained by the flowers is extracted by means of an air-pump, and a steam jet forces that which has combined with the moisture of the flowers into a gasometer, from whence all the chloride is obtained by means of the air-pump.

The chloride charged with perfume is evaporated *in vacuo* by passing round the vessel a stream of water at about 30° C., the air-pump meanwhile withdrawing the chloride in vapour. A manometer is attached to the apparatus, and this, which at first indicates a pressure of three to four atmospheres, is allowed to show a vacuum of half an atmosphere, when the operation is considered complete. The vessel is then opened

and the perfume is found in combination with fatty and waxy matters. This compound treated with alcohol yields the perfume, possessing all the sweetness of the fresh plant.

The process is applicable not only to those plants which are usually obtained by distillation with water, but also to those like jasmine and violet, which can only be extracted by *enfleurage*.

Flowers, seeds, barks, and roots have all been tested, and in each case an increased yield of 25 per cent. has been obtained over the old method.

PROSECUTIONS UNDER THE "SALE OF POISONS ACT."

At the District Police Court, on the 2nd August, before Mr. Call, P.M., James Leith and John R. Miscamble, described as veterinary surgeons, were summoned for that, not being duly qualified medical practitioners or registered pharmaceutical chemists, they did sell certain poisons, to wit, a solution of arsenic and tartar emetic, contrary to the provisions of the "Sale and Use of Poisons Act."

Mr. D. Wilkie appeared to prosecute on behalf of the Pharmaceutical Society, and Mr. Frank Stephen appeared for the defendants.

In opening the cases, Mr. Wilkie stated that, in consequence of the great increase of the number of deaths by poison, public attention had been directed to general evasions of the provisions of the "Sale and Use of Poisons Act." It was also well known that numbers of unqualified persons were selling poison without complying with the requirements of the Act in registering and labelling. Under these circumstances the society felt that, in the public interest, some steps should be taken; and these cases were the first of a number that would be brought before the court. The evidence would show that no precautions had been taken, that the defendants had sold the articles to a person who was a perfect stranger to them, and that there was no label "poison" on them. The following evidence was taken :—

William Lee deposed that, acting under instructions from the secretary of the Pharmaceutical Society he called at the defendant's place of business and asked to be supplied with 4 oz. of Fowler's solution of arsenic, four doses of tartar emetic, and a horse-ball; that these articles were supplied to him, for which he paid the sum of 7s. The witness stated that he was not asked to sign any book, neither was there any witness to the sale. Upon receiving the poisons he took them to the office of the Pharmaceutical Society, and initialled each package, sealing them up, and then, by order of Mr. Shillinglaw, he took them to Mr. Blackett for analysis. He identified the packages now before the court, as those he had received from the defendants.

In cross-examination by Mr. Stephen, the witness stated that he informed the defendants that the medicines were for a friend up the country.

Mr. C. R. Blackett was then examined, and said :—" I am an analytical chemist ; I received the articles produced from the last witness for analysis. Upon examination I found arsenic in one bottle and tartar emetic in all the packets. Arsenic and tartar emetic are both in part 1 of the schedule to the Poisons Act. This closed the case for the prosecution.

No evidence was tendered by the defendants that they were legally qualified veterinary surgeons, and it was admitted by Mr. Stephen that his clients had practically no defence.

Mr. Call said that, as this was the first case of the sort that had been brought forward in Melbourne, he thought a nominal fine would meet the case. He might, however, remark that any future cases would be severely dealt with. The defendants would be fined 1s. and £3 3s. costs.

Mr. Wilkie drew the attention of the Bench to the small amount of costs allowed. As the prosecutions were for the public good, he thought it scarcely fair that the society should be put to expense in bringing the cases forward, and the verdict was not one to induce the society to continue the good work they had commenced.

According to M. Des Cloiseaux the crystalline form of magnesium is a regular hexagonal prism.

Dr. Huggins most truly declares that one of the great charms of the study of nature lies in the circumstance that no new advance, however small, is ever final. There are no blind alleys in scientific investigation. Every new fact is the opening of a new path.

Notice of Book.

Eucalyptographia: A descriptive Atlas of the Eucalypts of Australia and the adjoining Islands. By Baron Ferd. von Müeller, K.C.M.G., &c. Sixth decade.

WE have received from the Government Botanist the sixth decade of the important work of Baron von Müeller, on the Eucalypts of Australia. The present number is the most valuable of those hitherto issued, and containing as it does a full botanical description of the Eucalyptus globulus, is especially interesting. The learned and accomplished botanist, with his usual laboriousness, gives us also a complete bibliography on the subject, which will be found very useful to scientific botanists. The lithographic illustrations of this, as of the preceding decades, are exceedingly well done, giving in life-like exactness all the parts of those remarkable plants. As Baron von Müeller was the first to draw attention to the peculiar characteristics of the Eucalypts, and more particularly the Eucalyptus globulus, his historical references will be read with interest by botanists in Europe. It would appear that we owe to the enlightened foresight of Baron von Müeller, (when Director of the Botanic Gardens), and Mons. Prosper Ramel, the transmission of the seeds of the Eucalyptus globulus to France, Algeria, and Italy; in the two latter countries this tree so important for *reboisement* purposes, and in a sanitary point of view has been extensively cultivated with the best results. In the Campagna the planting of the Eucalyptus globulus, from seeds supplied by Baron von Müeller, has produced the most wholesome effects upon the poisonous air of the Pontinian swamps, thus solving a problem in sanitation that has baffled the ablest rulers from the days of Appius Claudius to our own times !

We do not intend to write a review of these contributions to botanical science, as it would be, perhaps, beyond the scope of our journal, and therefore, must conclude by referring to a few points which are more particularly interesting, and to which, in justice to our eminent but insufficiently appreciated author, we feel it our duty to draw attention. The careful and exhaustive experiments made, under the direction of Baron von Müeller, upon the quality, strength, and durability of this timber, are worthy of close examination by builders and others. Upon the yield of Potash from the Eucalyptus globulus some valuable data are given, the result of experiments made by the author. Upon the febrifuge properties of the Eucalyptus some details will be found, which will interest those who believe in the therapeutical value of the Eucalypts. We cannot speak too highly of this work, the publication of which does credit to the Government of Victoria.—C. R. B.

BALLARAT.

WE are in receipt of the annual report of the School of Mines, Ballarat, which deals exhaustively with the progress and work of the school during the past year, which seems to have merged from the uncertain babyhood of existence, and to have developed into a robust youthfulness. Its finances appear to be on a more satisfactory, reliable, and permanent basis, and the superstructure, so to speak, of intellectuality, which will, we think, be endeavoured to raise on it, will be both *utile et dulce*, and alike creditable to the council, registrar, lecturers, and the country at large. With much pleasure we note the appointment of permanent professors and lecturers as a great advancement in the school's history, and having the honour of knowing some of the scientific capabilities of the appointees, we have every confidence that the prestige of the school will be greatly advanced and benefited thereby. It seems a pity that as yet no gentleman has answered the appeal of the council to lead the way in forming a microscopical society, but the absence of special scientists in a provincial city is unfortunately by no means rare. Nearly thirty certificates have been granted by the council to those attendants of the school who have successfully passed their examinations. The number of pupils during the year has been 266 for the four terms, and Government subsidy received, only £862 3s. 5d. Classes have been held in Euclid, algebra, logarithms, trigonometry mining and land surveying, mechanical engineering, elementary, organic, inorganic and pharmaceutical chemistry, botany and *materia medica*, animal physiology and telegraphy. In addition to the above subjects the council intend securing lecturers for geology, mineralogy, electricity, and magnetism. Since last report

1220 assays and analyses have been made, and upwards of 22,000 ozs. of gold and 500 ozs. of silver melted for the public. We have before alluded to the council's great desire to increase the facilities for the introduction of free students, and with this view arrangements have been completed whereby a donor of £50 can always have one free student at the school, or an annual subscriber of £6 6s., after the second year, the right of retaining three students on the school-roll.

It appears to us that the school offers grand facilities to our rising young men for acquiring scientific knowledge cheaply and profitably, and the only apparent difficulty in the way is how to popularise it more. To say that the two Ballarats, with their large populations, has only some seventy of their youths attending the classes at the School of Mines is at present, perhaps, an unjust reflection on their scientific aspirations. Time, the great magician, will, however, we hope, soon alter this; and now that the council's endeavours to thoroughly establish the schools having been to a certain extent consummated, we hope to see their energy directed into popularising it, and in educating parents to see the many and great advantages the school offers our children over, above, and beyond the ordinary amusements now followed by them. We cannot do better than cull from the *addendum* to the report a clause which we think merits general attention :— "The council take the opportunity of again inviting inventors and manufacturers to exhibit at the school any kind of appliance for the more effective carrying on of operations in connection with the great industry of mining, or with any other industry. Beside the direct advantage to the class of persons indicated, a positive benefit to the community at large is likely to arise from the adoption of such a scheme. But the council are the more anxious to obtain this co-operation, in order to render the school as useful as possible ; for although instruction and examinations in the art of mining, and in the sciences pertaining thereto, are doubtless of primary importance, it cannot be denied that the public naturally look to this institution for a solution of difficulties met with in the practice of the art, and the practical application of those sciences, the teaching of which is generally considered peculiarly within the province of a school of mines and industries."

BALLARAT DISTRICT CHEMISTS' ASSOCIATION.

THE usual monthly meeting of the association was held at Lester's Hotel, Sturt-street, on Wednesday evening 21st July. There was a fair attendance of members.

The president, Mr. Palmer, occupied the chair. The minutes of previous meeting were read and confirmed.

The hon. secretary read a letter from Mr. Joseph Bradbury, of Sandhurst, asking for a copy of the rules of the association, and seeking information relative thereto, with the intention of initiating a similar association in that city. The hon. secretary said he had forwarded a copy of the rules as requested, and had written to Mr. Bradbury, stating the pleasure the members of the association here would derive from the knowledge that their hands would probably be strengthened by the formation of a kindred association at Sandhurst, and hoping that no obstacles would prevent its immediate formation, and that the association here would be most happy to render all the aid in its power to help them forward. The action of the secretary was endorsed by the meeting.

The hon. secretary stated that there were several reasons which prompted him to resign his position as member of the Pharmaceutical Council, and wished the association to allow him to do so. All the members present regarded such an action as highly undesirable, as they considered it very important that the association should be represented on the council, and unanimously passed a resolution urging upon the secretary not to resign, and adopting measures to remove some of the obstacles that had arisen. Several additions and alterations were made to the price-list, and a hundred copies ordered to be printed. A vote of thanks to the chair closed the meeting.

Personalities.

MR. JOHN REED, formerly of St. Arnaud, and Mr. O. M Davies have both opened very pretty new shops at St. Kilda Pharmacy is exceedingly well represented in this suburb now

Mr. J. K. Blogg, for some time well known as town traveller for one of the principal wholesale drug-houses, has retired from that position, and has taken charge of the manufacturing department for the same firm. Mr. M. Brown succeeds Mr. Blogg as traveller.

We notice, with pleasure, the return to Melbourne of Mr. Geo. Swift, so well known as a member of the firm of Francis and Swift, Bourke-street. On his retiring from that firm Mr. Swift entered into business in Sale, Gippsland, where he has been for the past year, and he returns to the metropolis as the proprietor of the old-established and well-known business of Wm. Ford and Co., Swanston-street, Melbourne. So esteemed a pharmacist as Mr. Swift will, we trust, meet with that measure of business success he so well deserves.

We are glad to hear that Mr. Alfred Brady, whose registration we lately recorded, has been engaged as town traveller by one of our leading wholesale drug houses. Mr. Brady is a brother of the well-known English pharmacist of that name, whose researches on *Foraminifera* are known to all microscopists, and, though a new comer, his knowledge of the drug trade ought to well qualify him for the post he has obtained.

We learn that the business in Elizabeth-street North, carried on for many years by the late Mr. Jelfs, has been sold to Mr. Alfred E. Hughes, for some time past assistant to Mr. Henry Francis, of Bourke-street. Another change has also to be recorded in the purchase of Mr. Swift's business, at Sale, by Mr. George Wilson. Mr. Wilson was apprenticed several years ago to Mr. Bosisto, and has been since in business at Beaufort, and subsequently at Deniliquin.

THE ACCIDENTAL POISONING CASE AT COLAC.

THE inquest on the death of Joseph Joshua Clark was held on the 30th July, at the courthouse, Colac, before Mr. Heron, P.M., coroner.

The jury having answered to their names, the first witness called was

George Farmer Turner, who deposed — I am a chemist residing in Colac. I remember Mrs. Clark coming to my shop on the evening of 14th July. She had a child in her arms. She asked me to give her something for a tightness at the child's chest. I put up a mixture of almond oil and syrup of squills, and my apprentice, John Moir, put up some hartshorn and sweet oil and some soothing powders. I mentioned what I had given her, and labelled the bottles. I recollect being called to see Miss Moore between eight and nine o'clock that same evening. I was called by my apprentice. I did not see the prescription. I saw it first about nine the next morning. The lad did not ask me for any directions as to making it up. I first found out that a mistake had been made with Dr. Dobie's prescription the next morning between nine and ten. I went to look over the previous day's prescriptions, as I usually do. The thing that drew my attention to the prescription was that it was very badly written. It was signed by Dr. Dobie. This is the prescription. Noticing the top line written in a very bad style, I called my apprentice, who has been with me two years and two months, and pointed out that line to him, and asked him how he read it. He answered, "L'aqua morphia acet." I knew from the nature of the prescription more than from the reading of that line that it was "L'aqua ammonia acet." intended. I felt very much stunned by the blow. I immediately said, "Whatever comes, the child must not take another dose." I immediately made up the prescription correctly, and sent it down to Mrs. Clark by the apprentice. I told him to give them the bottle, and tell them that a mistake had been made. I told him to ask for the first bottle in exchange. I did not see any directions that may have been given the night before. The prescription directs a teaspoonful to be taken every four hours. The boy has been with me two years and two months. He has been very careful and intelligent.

Mr. Heron — Does it not strike you that, to put the mildest face upon it, you were very lax in not looking at this prescription before the lad made it up. Was that not a neglect of duty ?

Witness — No thought occurred to my mind.

Mr. Heron — I ask you again why you did not, on the 14th of July, when this prescription was brought to you by Miss Moore to make up, look at it before the boy made it up. Your feeling that it might not be right because Mr. Dobie had left Dr. Foster's service ought to have made you more careful.

Witness — I never entertained any suspicion of the prescription. I did not know it was badly written. The next

morning I found out that the prescription had been wrongly made up. I did not apply to Dr. Foster or Dr. Dobie to do anything to save the child. I knew the child must have taken some of it, but it did not occur to my mind to do more than acquaint the parents. I did not think of it. I saw Dr. Foster that morning before discovering the mistake. He told me the child was dying. He said I had prescribed for a child named Clark. It was between nine and ten. I told him I had not prescribed, and never did. Selling medicines and labelling them as such is a very different thing from prescribing. Mrs. Clark did not ask for the particular medicine I gave her. She paid for it. Dr. Foster said there would be some difficulty in the matter ; that he should not give a certificate as to the cause of death. I did not take any other steps to save the child's life.

The Foreman — Has your apprentice passed any examination qualifying him to dispense prescriptions ?

Witness — No.

To Mr. Hebb — Have you allowed your apprentice to make up prescriptions before ?

Witness — Occasionally, when I have been busy.

Mr. Hebb — Did you warn your apprentice that the prescriptions were badly written ?

Witness — All his previous prescriptions have been well written.

To Mr. Hebb — Have you ever had any previous mistake ?

Witness — No. This is the first I have ever had in the place.

To Mr. Hancock — The lad has been with me two years and two months. He has been very careful. He has assisted me in putting medicines up. I have given my assistant the necessary instructions to qualify him for dispensing, and he has studied the necessary books.

John Moir — I am an apprentice to Mr. Turner, chemist, of Colac. I remember Mrs. Clark coming to the shop with the baby on the 14th of July. She spoke to Mr. Turner. She said, "My baby has a little tightness on the chest ; will you give me something for it ?" He said, "I will give you some syrup of squills and oil of almonds." He went and looked at the baby ; he did not examine it. I do not know what he said. He gave some syrup of squills and oil of almonds. I do not know whether she paid for it. She gave the baby a dose of it in the shop. He told her to rub its chest and back with hartshorn and oil, and give it the mixture every four hours. About eight that night Miss Moore came to the shop. She said she brought a prescription from Dr. Dobie. She told me to make it up. I said I would not till Mr. Turner came. Mr. Turner was out then at Mr. Robertson's committee rooms. I went up and found him. I took the prescription with me. I asked Mr. Turner whether "L'aqua morphia acet." was the same as that in the bottle labelled "L'aqua morphia." He said it was. I did not show the prescription to Mr. Turner. I had it in my hand. I thought they were the same, but was not sure. I did not then know the difference between the two names. Mr. Turner told me they were the same thing. I put up the medicine when I had found out the dose. Mr. Turner did not ask me anything about the prescription. I mean by finding out the dose consulting some medical authority. I was not competent enough to make it up from my own experience or training as a chemist. When he discovered that a mistake had been made, Mr. Turner said they must not, on any account, have an opportunity of giving another dose. Mr. Turner put up another bottle himself. He sent me down with it to Mrs. Moore's. I asked for Mrs. Clark, and told her a mistake had been made in the medicine. I asked her to give me the other bottle and I would give her the right one. She said, "It was no use, the child was dying." I came back and told Mr. Turner. This would be about eleven o'clock. Nothing was done to acquaint Dr. Foster, or to try and save the child. I said nothing about it.

To the Foreman — I went to Mr. Turner twice. It was at the first time that he told me that "L'aqua morphia acet." was the same as "L'aqua morphia." The second time I told him I had a prescription from Dr. Dobie for Mrs. Clark. Then he came to the shop, and said to Miss Moore, "You have been to Dr. Dobie ; you can please yourself."

To the Coroner — Mr. Turner's evidence was quite correct on that point.

To Mr. Forbes — I did not think to show Mr. Turner the prescription.

To Mr. Hebb — I understand the nature of poisons. I thought the quantity ordered enormous till I looked at the book and found the dose to be from ten to sixty minims.

To the Foreman—I thought the word "ammonia" on the prescription was "morphia." I think it looks like it now. I should take it for morphia now.

To Mr. Mitchell—The mistake occurred entirely in the reading of the prescription.

To Mr. Hancock—I have received instructions from Mr. Turner, and I have had the necessary books to inform myself. I took the word on the prescription to be morphia. I felt sure it was written morphia. I referred to Squire's *Companion to the Pharmacopœia*. I found the dose to be from ten to sixty minims. The prescription I made up would allow fifteen minims to each dose. I thought this a simple prescription. I have previously put up such prescriptions with morphia as an ingredient. I had no doubt about the prescription or I would not have put it up. I had been instructed by Mr. Turner not to put up a prescription where I had any doubt about it.

To Mr. Forbes—I only went a second time to Mr. Turner because I doubted Dr. Dobie's right to give a prescription. The first time I went was to ascertain whether the "L'aqua morphia acet." was the same as "L'aqua morphia ;" and the second time was to inquire if Dr. Dobie had a right to prescribe, and to fetch Mr. Turner.

To Mr. Hebb—I do not usually refer to books instead of to Mr. Turner.

The Coroner—I would be quite right in referring to any recognised and proper authority.

To Mr. Hancock—I never put up any prescription with the same quantity of morphia in it. This is why I referred to the book, from which I found, as I thought, that it was a proper quantity.

William Johnson—I am the Government Analytical Chemist, residing at St. Kilda. On the 20th instant I received from Constable Williams one jar containing some viscera, one box of powders (produced), two four-ounce medicine bottles (one quite full, the other nearly so). The one nearly full is marked E.H., No. 1 ; the other is marked No. 2. I examined No. 1, and found the presence of morphia immediately. I made an estimate of the amount of morphia the bottle No. 1 would have contained when full. It was equal to three grains of acetate or muriate of morphia. A teaspoonful of such a mixture, which is the dose ordered to be given every four hours, would be equivalent to one-tenth part of a grain of either of the morphia salts I have mentioned. The bottle No. 2 is free from morphia. There is nothing remarkable about the powders. They consist of James's powder and a little calomel. They are ordinary fever powders. I examined the viscera, and there I failed to find any trace of morphia whatever.

To the Senior-constable—The dose given would contain the tenth part of a grain. Children of a few months old might be killed by the fifteenth part of a grain. There is a case on record where one-nineteenth part of a grain has proved fatal. The prescription produced could be read by an experienced hand. The word might have been read morphia, but the context would have enabled an experienced man to know that it could not be morphia.

To the Foreman—Morphia is very seldom found in the stomach after death. It is only the portion left over after causing death that could be found. The portion that had caused death would be absorbed into the system, and never found at all.

To Mr. Hancock—I cannot say how much had been taken out of the bottle when I got it. Supposing it to have been full to a certain mark on the label when I got it, then half an ounce must have been taken out. That is, about four doses. If that quantity were given by carelessness, the mischief would have been greater. In that case there would be four-tenths of a grain taken ; that would be a full dose for you or me.

Rupert Pincott, medical practitioner—I have heard the evidence of Mr. Johnson. There is no doubt that the dose of morphia given would cause death. At the same time I am bound to inform the jury that the appearances left by morphia or opium are quite negative. In point of fact there are none. Having made the *post-mortem*, I say that had the child been brought to me by the police I should have said that it died from inflammation of the lungs, but now having heard the evidence of Mr. Johnson, I think it died from an overdose of morphia.

To Mr. Mitchell—The child might have recovered from the inflammation of the lungs. The morphia would accelerate its death. I have seen the prescription given by Dr. Dobie. I read it thus—" L'aqua ammonia acet." I must say, and I regret to say it, as it is a reflection on my own profession, that it is shamefully written. Prescriptions are often illegible, but this is very shamefully written. Still, even a mere tyro should not take it for morphia, considering the size of the dose. I do not consider it fairly written as it stands, and I do not think any physician should send such a prescription to a dispenser.

This concluded the evidence. Mr. Heron recapitulated the circumstances attendant upon Mrs. Clark's consulting Mr. Dobie and the preparation of the prescription. He said—" I tell you fairly and distinctly that when the boy Moir came to Mr. Turner with those questions it was his duty to look carefully at the prescription, and to see it properly made up. It was culpable neglect not to do so. Mrs. Clark has told you that the child was better before she gave it the physic, and Dr. Pincott has given his opinion that the death resulted from an overdose of morphia. You have to consider whether the lad Moir has been negligent or careless, and whether his carelessness amounts to criminality. You must not imply manslaughter, but if you consider this lad committed manslaughter, you must find a direct verdict ; and he must have the fullest benefit of any doubt in your mind. I ask you to dismiss from your minds everything that you have heard outside these walls, and give your verdict solely on the evidence."

The court was cleared, and at one o'clock the jury gave the following verdict :—" This jury find that the deceased, Joseph Joshua Clark, died by an overdose of morphia, the same being accidentally dispensed as medicine ; the said morphia being mixed in a prescription prepared by John Moir, apprentice to G. F. Turner, chemist, he making a mistake in reading morphia for ammonia in the first line of the prescription, which was illegibly written." They added the following rider :—" We consider that the said G. F. Turner is guilty of gross carelessness in not reading the prescription, and seeing the same properly dispensed."

Correspondence.

To the Editor of The Australasian Supplement to the Chemist and Druggist.

DEAR SIR—Will you kindly allow me to say a few words on a subject broached by your correspondent "Princeps" in your last issue?

As one of those who were present at the meeting held at the Clarence Hotel on the 17th of October last, to fix prices for patents and arrange other matters, I assented to the various proposals, with a full determination to carry them faithfully out ; and have done so up to the present time, so far as patent and proprietary medicines are concerned, and adhered, as near as I could, to the scale fixed for dispensing prescriptions.

I thought the suggestion of a particular mark, to place over our stamp, to indicate the price charged for compounding a prescription a very good one, as it would enable us to see what had been charged elsewhere, and thus put us in a position to confute the too ready fib of parties, who, seeking only to get their medicine on the cheap, are not particular as to the means they use to do so. Well, Mr. Editor, for some time I acted as I thought others were doing, and duly marked, or caused to be marked, with the symbol agreed upon, every recipe dispensed at my establishment. But I, like "Princeps," soon found that this practice was not carried on by my compeers ; for of all the prescriptions which have passed through my hands, from the date of the meeting until now, which had been dispensed at other places, only two bore the mark which had been agreed upon ; and now I own to having dropped the practice too, partly because I do not care to appear singular, and partly because it has been intimated to me by a brother chemist that there were some in the business mean enough to take advantage of the knowledge the mark gave them, to charge something under the price of the first dispenser, with a view of securing the future custom to themselves.

I do not say that there are any members of our honourable calling so low down in the scale of rectitude as to do this, but it has certainly been intimated to me that there are ; and as other chemists would be sorry to give them the chance, neither does your humble servant,

· MEL. BORACIS.

IS THERE AN ANTIDOTE AGAINST STRYCHNINE?

To the Editor of The Australasian Supplement to the Chemist and Druggist.

SIR—It appears to me singular that in this age of discovery that no antidote against the above dangerous poison has yet been discovered! Persons who are desirous of ending their career in this life chiefly resort to it, knowing that under no circumstances can they recover from its effects; instances I know have been recorded where chloroform, properly administered, has succeeded; but the action of the poison is so quick that before a medical man arrives he generally finds it too late to use the means at his disposal.

Some time ago a bank manager, residing in an Australian bush township, informed me that he thought prussic acid was an antidote for it, and gave me his reasons. He stated that in riding through a sheep run accompanied by a greyhound, the dog must have picked up some poisoned meat, probably laid there for that purpose, for as soon as he arrived at home the dog was seized with tetanus, and continued in such dreadful agony that he determined to destroy it by administering to it some prussic acid. Soon after doing so he was surprised to see the dog completely recover, although he administered enough acid to kill two or three dogs. Knowing this gentleman very well, I communicated the fact to a learned professor in Melbourne with a view to inquiry, but, as yet, without effect.

I trust, however, that as your valuable supplement is read by most of the pharmacists and chemists in Victoria the above facts may tend to elucidate further inquiry.—In the meantime, I remain, your obedient servant,

Sandhurst, 23rd July, 1880.   J. HOLDSWORTH.

[We on one occasion administered a large dose of prussic acid to a dog, which had been poisoned with carbolic acid, for the purpose of speedily putting an end to his sufferings, and, strange to say, instead of causing death, it acted as an apparent antidote.—EDITOR.]

MY FIRST AQUARIUM.

(BY C. A. ATKIN.)

(Concluded.)

THEN I collected some lovely rose-coloured anemones from the Black Rock or Rickard's Point, below Brighton. I obtained a few small flounders from the back beach at Williamstown, renewed my researches along the shore at St. Kilda, where those useful scavengers—periwinkles—may also be found at low tides, and everything went on prosperously for the next twelve months.

By a strange fatality, which a friend, in true prosodical style, attributed to *tempus edax rerum*, I was dismayed one day to find that the chord by which a bird-cage hung over this aquarium had suddenly snapped, and in its downfall involved the total destruction of so much pains and pride.

Once more the right hand of fellowship which such studies engender was held out to me, in the shape of an invitation from the Microscopical Society to join in one of their very enjoyable marine excursions. I accepted with some misgivings as to the prudence of such a course, seeing that I possessed none of the appliances required on such an occasion. However, all doubts on that head were speedily removed by the indulgence of my new-found friends, and I gratefully refer to the incident as having served as a fresh starting-point to my subsequent experiences in this matter. To those who keep aquaria, not merely for the sake of being amused, but of learning the higher lessons which animated nature is ever so ready to teach us, both fresh-water and marine parlour aquaria may easily be converted into nurseries for microscopic research. In them may be reared myriads of minute forms of life, whose ephemeral history and various conditions may be positively seen enacted upon the stage of the microscope. Human eyes can thus look down upon and witness the evolutions of these lower forms of life, just as, it is possible, other eyes look down upon our own terrestrial career.

Stimulated by the commendable zeal and rivalry for the *place d'honneur* I had witnessed amongst the members of the Microscopical Society, I determined once more to have a marine aquarium, or, more properly speaking, an artificial sea-water collection of *curios*. The necessary ingredients for the former were ready to my hand, and

can easily be procured in bottles containing sufficient for an aquarium of any reasonable size. Twenty-four hours after being mixed, all impurities are thrown down in the shape of a deposit, and the top water must then be carefully removed by means of a lead tube bent as a syphon. Having thrown away the deposit, the clear water may then be returned to the aquarium, after which, or even before, a few pieces of rock, with patches of seaweed adhering to them, should be carefully arranged to suit the taste of the proprietor, and to prevent, as far as possible, any damage to the glass front. Now, place your aquarium in a strong light, not too much exposed to the sun, and let it remain there quietly for some six or eight weeks. At or about the expiration of that time you will frequently notice a number of beautiful pearl-like beadlets rising quickly to the surface. This is a good indication that the vegetation on your rockery is thriving, and you may then commence to stock the aquarium with animal life, such as anemones, periwinkles, an oyster or two, and a few live shrimps or prawns. I am not quite sure whether they are procurable here, but a gentleman who has had large experience in this matter at home was telling me the other day of the endless diversion which may be procured by watching the evolutions of the hermit-crab, one of the most pugnacious creatures, he asserts, in the animal kingdom. As is well known, the huge whelk shell this gentleman usually appropriates to himself as a domicile is not his natural covering; but, given a certain number of unprotected hermit-crabs, and drop a couple of empty whelk shells, or even a thimble, between them, the *fracas* indulged in to obtain possession of the huts, and the assaults and batteries to which the *locum tenens* is subjected after he is there, until he finds suitable shelter amongst the rocks, surpasses comprehension. I think I have now said all that is necessary to enable any one to make a start with a small marine aquarium; perhaps a supplementary word of caution as to overstocking will not be altogether needless, and I will therefore add that the water should be well aërated, at first, by the aid of a glass syringe, failing which a teacupful may be taken out and poured back again for a few minutes each day. Notwithstanding these precautions, some of the specimens may not live, probably owing to carelessness in their capture, or injuries received *en route* to their destination. So long as the anemones thrive after the ninth or tenth day of their arrival, it may be concluded, however, that the aquarium is in proper working order, and if it contained no other specimens than those mentioned, I maintain that they would well repay all the trouble. In support of such a statement I quote the opinion of one of our most eminent naturalists:—"If sea anemones were all of one kind and form, however exquisite that one form or colour might be, its constant repetition would tire the senses, and having seen one or two specimens, we should soon cease to admire the rest. It is so with flowers, it is so with beauty of every kind. If our ladies were uniformly fashioned after the strict model of beauty, as set forth in the statues of Venus, it is doubtful whether they would find so many admirers as they do now, with their charming variety of feature, complexion, and expression. No tiresome sameness marks our sea-flowers, but every one presents some variation from others of its class. Each individual varies in itself, assuming now one shape, then another, now displaying one tint, then setting forth another in a different part of the body. Each specimen shows some slight peculiarity by which it may be known from others of the same variety. Each species has a distinct range of variation, clustered in crowded colonies, on sea rocks, and in pools on the beach, enriching the sands and pebbles with strange flowers as bright and variable as any terrestrial flowers that can be ranged out for prizes on a gala day. Such are the 'anemones.' The more we know of them the more we shall admire their structure, economy, and transcendent loveliness."

It would serve no immediate public purpose that I am aware of to inquire why the few terse remarks offered in my last letter on the fresh-water aquarium have elicited such a large amount of inquiry. I dwell on the fact for the encouragement of others who have greater facilities than myself for promoting researches in the vast field of subaqueous zoology we have at our very feet. Viewed in every direction, that field is manifestly capable of producing grand additions to our knowledge of nature. Problems that are suggested by the facts already discovered await a satisfactory answer, and I trust the time is approaching when such studies will enjoy a far larger share of public attention than they have hitherto done in Victoria.

J. BOSISTO

Desires to direct the Medical Profession and Pharmaceutical Chemists to his

Special Chemical and Pharmaceutical Preparations from Australian Vegetation.

OL. EUCALYPTI ESS.

Obtained from the Amygdalina Odorata species : the Eucalyptus Oil of Commerce. This Essential Oil of the Eucalyptus family is now recognised in the Hospitals of Europe as an antiseptic of great power. A few drops sprinkled on a cloth and suspended in a sick room renders the air refreshing ; and for disinfecting and deodorising, a tablespoonful of the Oil added to two or three pounds' weight of sawdust, well mixed and distributed, will speedily produce a purifying effect. It is also employed as a valuable Rubefacient in all Rheumatic Affections, as a Basic Odour in aromatising Soaps, and as a Solvent of Resins difficult of solution.

☞ NOTE.—To ensure the certainty of obtaining this Oil is by purchasing it from the Wholesale Houses in packages or bottles, bearing the certificate and signed "J. Bosisto and Co.," together with the trade mark—Parrot Brand, yellow ground.

SYRUPUS ROSTRATI.

Prepared from the Inspissated Juice of the Red Gum Tree. A delicate mucilaginous astringent, employed in all affections of the mucous membrane, particularly in Diarrhœa and Chronic Dysentery. In bottles of 1 lb. each.

OL. EUCALYPTI GLOBULI ESS. C_{12}, H_{40}, O.

Anthelmintic—By Enema 30 to 60 minims in mucilage of starch. Internally—Dose 3 to 5 minims in gum mucilage, syrup, or glycerine. Tonic, Stimulant, and Antiseptic. A small dose promotes appetite ; a large one destroys it. In stronger doses of 10 to 20 minims it first accelerates the pulse, produces pleasant general excitement (shown by irresistible desire for moving about) and a feeling of buoyancy and strength. Intoxicating in very large doses, but, unlike alcohol or opium, the effects are not followed by torpor, but produce a general calmness and soothing sleep. A strong cup of Coffee will at once remove any unpleasantness arising from an over-dose.

EUCALYPTOL. C_{12}, H_{20}, O.

From Eucalyptus Globulus. Therapeutic use. For Inhalation in Bronchial Affection. Quantity employed —From half to one teaspoonful with half a pint of hot water in the Inhaler.

TINCT. EUCALYPTI GLOBULI.

Stimulant, Tonic, Antiperiodic, and Antiseptic. Employed in purulent Catarrhal Affections of the Urethra and Vagina in dilution ; and for Disinfecting the Dressings of wounds.

CIGARETTES OF EUCALYPTUS GLOBULUS.

Recommended for Bronchial and Asthmatic Affections, and also for the Disinfecting and Antiseptic Properties. NOTE.—The Cigarettes are numbered 1 and 2. No. 1 are without Tobacco : No. 2 contain a small quantity, and are recommended for general smokers.

EUCALYPTENE : from Eucalyptus Globulus:

The Tonic or bitter principle in an amorphous condition ; employed in Low Fevers in doses of one to three grains.

LIQUOR EUCALYPTI GLOBULI.

The Fever and Ague Remedy. Dose—For Ague and Dengue Fever 30 to 60 minims in half a wineglassful of mucilage and water, or glycerine and water, with the occasional addition of two minims of Eucalyptol every two or three hours during the paroxysms of Ague. Incompatibles—The Mineral Salts.

UNG. EUCALYPTI VIRIDIS.

Antiseptic Emollient ; rapidly sets up a healthy action. In 1lb. jars.

OL. ATHEROSPERMA MOSCHATA ESS.

The physiological effects of this Oil, in small doses, are Diaphoretic, Diuretic, and Sedative, and it appears to exert a specific lowering influence upon the heart's action. As a medicine it has been introduced into the Colonial Hospitals, and employed successfully in cases of Heart Disease. Administered in one or two drop doses at intervals of six or eight hours.

LIQUOR ATHEROSPERMA MOSCH.

Employed in Asthma and all affections of the respiratory organs.

The following Articles are prepared ready for the Counter Trade :—

EUCALYPTUS OIL, in Bottles 1s., 2s. each.
———————— OINTMENT, in Pots 1s. each.
———————— PILLS, in Bottles 2s. each.
———————— CIGARETTES, in Boxes 2s. each.
———————— LOZENGES, RED GUM, in Boxes 1s., 2s. each.
———————— SYRUP, RED GUM, in Bottles 1s. 6d., 2s. 6d. each.
ATHEROSPERMA, in Bottles 1s. 6d., 2s. 6d. each.

Each bears the Trade Mark—Parrot Brand.

J. BOSISTO,

MANUFACTURING PHARMACEUTICAL CHEMIST

(LABORATORY : RICHMOND, MELBOURNE),

By whom the Eucalyptus Preparations were first introduced, both in Australia and in Europe, and to whom has been awarded the Silver Medal of the Society of Arts, London, and Special Medals of Merit from the various European and Australian Exhibitions, dating from the first of his investigations in 1853, and published in the Transactions of the Royal Society of Victoria, and other publications, European and Colonial.

NOTE.—The Medical Profession and Pharmaceutical Chemists are requested when ordering through Wholesale Houses to state distinctly that Bosisto's Preparations are wanted.

FELTON, GRIMWADE & CO.,

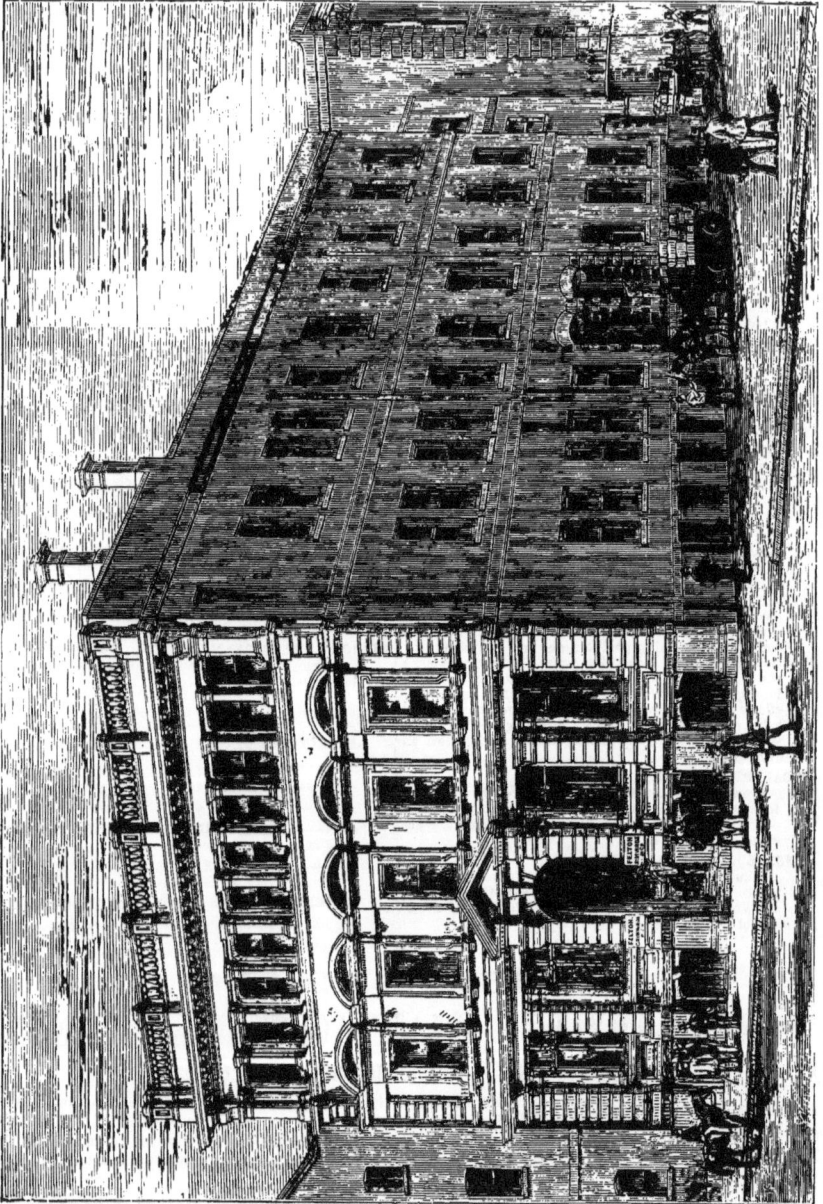

31 & 33 FLINDERS LANE WEST,
MELBOURNE.

[SUPPLEMENT ONLY.]

Chem. & Drugg. Aust. Suppl.
V. 3, no. 30, 41-48, (Oct., 1880).

THE
Chemist & Druggist.

WITH AUSTRALASIAN SUPPLEMENT.

. (Published under direction of the Pharmaceutical Society of Victoria.)

No. 30. { PUBLISHED ON THE 15TH OF EVERY MONTH. }
Registered for Transmission as a Newspaper.
OCTOBER, 1880.
{ SUBSCRIPTION, 15s. PER ANNUM, INCLUDING DIARY, POST FREE.

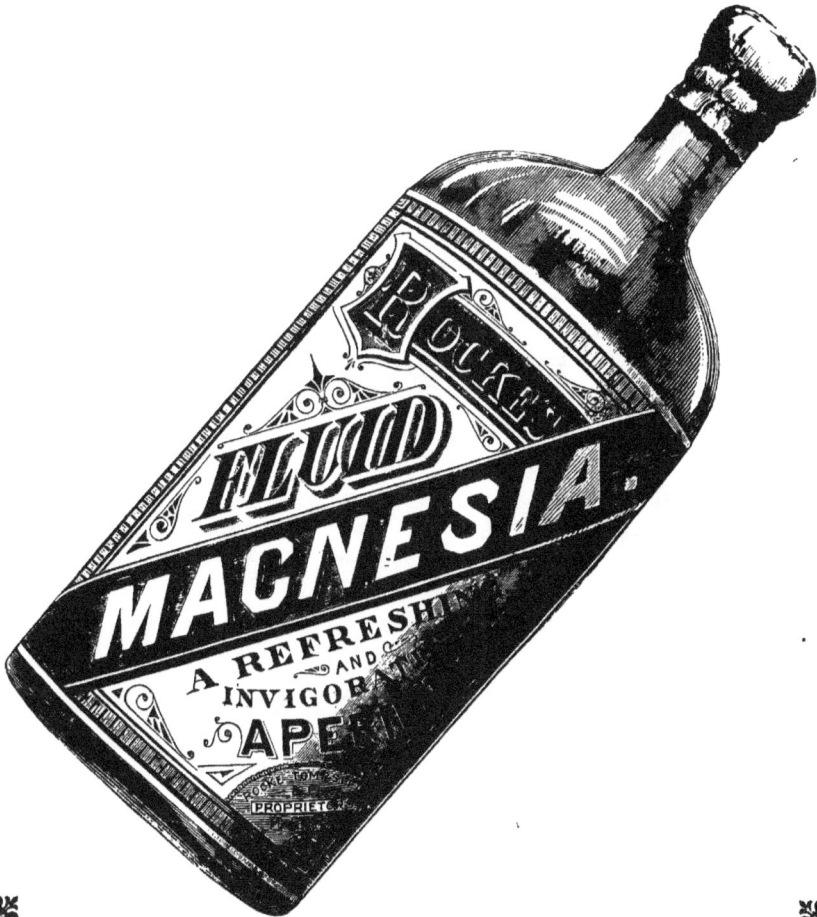

V. 3. no. 30 : 41-48, (Oct., 1880).

INDEX TO LITERARY CONTENTS.

The Chemist and Druggist.
WITH AUSTRALASIAN SUPPLEMENT.

OFFICE: MUTUAL PROVIDENT BUILDINGS, COLLINS STREET WEST.
Published on the 15th of each Month.

THIS Journal is issued gratis to all paid-up Members of the PHARMA-CEUTICAL SOCIETY OF VICTORIA, and to non-members at Fifteen Shillings per annum, payable in advance. A copy of *The Chemists and Druggists' Diary*, published annually, is forwarded post free to every subscriber.

Advertisements, remittances, and all business communications to be addressed to THE HONORARY SECRETARY OF THE PHARMACEUTICAL SOCIETY, MELBOURNE.

SCALE OF CHARGES FOR ADVERTISEMENTS:

	Per annum.		Per annum.
One Page	.. £3 0 0	Quarter Page	.. £3 0 0
Half do.	.. 5 0 0	Business Cards	.. 2 0 0

Special rates for wrapper and pages preceding and following literary matter. Advertisements of Assistants Wanting Situations, 2s. 6d. each.

Advertisements for insertion in the current month should be sent to the office before the 10th.

COMMUNICATIONS for the EDITORIAL department of this journal should be addressed to THE EDITOR, MUTUAL PROVIDENT BUILDINGS, COLLINS STREET WEST, MELBOURNE.

No notice can be taken of anonymous communications. Whatever is intended for insertion must be authenticated by the name and address of the writer—not necessarily for publication, but as a guarantee of good faith.

NOTICE.

Subscriptions for the year 1880 *are now due, and members are respectfully requested to remit the same.*

BIRTH.

FRANCIS.—On the 3rd November, at 48 St. Vincent-place South, the wife of Henry Francis of a son.

M'FARLANE.—On the 28th October, at 72 Smith-street, Collingwood, the wife of R. J. M'Farlane, chemist, of a son.

MARRIAGE.

GRACE—MACKENNAL.—On the 20th October, at St. Peter's, Melbourne, by the Rev. Canon Handfield, J. F. F. Grace, only son of J. F. Grace, M.D., M.R.S.E., West Melbourne, to Henrietta, only daughter of J. S. Mackennal, sculptor, 108 Collins-street East and Jolimont.

AMERICAN BOGUS DIPLOMAS.

IT has long been a matter of surprise to observers as to how certain uneducated or imperfectly educated people contrived to get their credentials as medical practitioners. It has been generally understood that at some second-rate and obscure universities in Europe diplomas were granted *in absentiâ* on payment of certain fees; but that demoralising practice has ceased. It would seem, however, that in some of the States of the great republic of America "bogus diploma manufacture" has, under the sanction of the Legislature (State charter!), been carried on to a disgraceful extent. Pennsylvania, which in former years obtained a world-wide and unenviable notoriety for having been guilty of "repudiation," has, according to the editor of the *Philadelphia Record*, been the seat of this manufactory of swindling quacks. The *Pharmaceutical Journal* gives the following account of the way in which this impudent business is or was until very recently carried on :—

"The *Philadelphia Record* is carrying on the work of exposure with great zeal, and is evidently determined to spare no effort to tread the swindle out of existence. Column after column is filled with lists of persons who are alleged to have countenanced these 'universities' and those who have obtained diplomas from them. It appears, however, that the charters of Buchanan's colleges are still valid, and have been distributed gratuitously among coloured voters to influence local elections—that at length a committee was appointed by the Senate to investigate the scandal, the result being a resolution to repeal the charter. But the power of the Senate to repeal it was disputed in the law courts by Buchanan, and eventually successfully, and in the meanwhile he fell back upon another charter that he had obtained for the 'American University,' which had been overlooked. This *contretemps* seems to have given an impetus and additional audacity to the movement, so that when recently the proprietors of the *Philadelphia Record* entered into a compact with the legal authorities to find the funds necessary for an attempt to break up the system, the agent employed, it is said, obtained for a sum equal to about £45 sterling no less than eight diplomas from seven 'universities' and 'colleges,' five being for the degree of M.D., and one each for those of D.D., LL.D., and D.C.L.

"The story of the schemes by which several diplomas were obtained by the same person under different names is very amusing, but cannot be recapitulated here. One of the most expensive—having cost twenty-five hours in time and £26 in cash—was for the curious degree of 'Master in Electro-Therapeutics,' and was declared to be granted to one 'qui bene curriculo studiorum praescripto perfunctus est, et quem justo et rigido examine prius habito, hoc gradu dignissimum censuimus.' The result was that Dr. Buchanan and some of his colleagues were arrested, he being charged with devising a scheme to defraud by means of the post-office of the United States. A few days afterwards proceedings were commenced against the trustees and officers of the 'Philadelphia University of Medicine and Surgery,' concerning whom it is in evidence that, in conferring degrees upon a person of whom they knew nothing except the name, they had made an infant two years old an M.D. and LL.D.

"Some idea may be formed of the extent to which this traffic extended from the statement that when Buchanan was arrested the officers discovered on the premises nearly half a ton weight of blank diplomas, some of them signed by the 'faculty' and prepared for the insertion of the names of buyers. Receipts were also found showing that fully three thousand diplomas have been sold during the past six years, and it is estimated that during the last twenty-two years Buchanan has sold at least eleven thousand diplomas."

Unless a diploma is granted by Harvard, or some such old established and reputed seat of learning, we should imagine that American certificates will in future be received with little respect.

The Month.

THE following additional names have been added to the list of legally qualified medical practitioners in Victoria :—James de Burgh Griffith, South Yarra; Edward George Keighly Marks, Mornington.

In the last number of the *Australian Medical Journal* Dr. Maloney contributes an interesting paper on the therapeutics of tea-drinking.

The annual dinner of the Pharmaceutical Society, to be held at Clement's Hotel on the 18th November, promises to be well attended by both town and country members ; there are, also, several visitors from England and the neighbouring colonies who are likely to be present.

Apropos of Dr. Embling's paper, read before the Social Science Congress, we may quote the following suggestions of Dr. Beyrauds. He says that a practical test by which real death may be recognised is the application of the cautery to the supposed corpse. If the eschar does not show itself, the subject is dead ; if it be yellow and transparent, the subject is dead ; if it be black or reddish-brown, the subject is living.

A vacancy has occurred in the Pharmacy Board of Victoria by the resignation of Mr. R. F. Kennedy. The announcement of the returning officer in reference to the election to fill the vacancy appears in the advertising portion of this issue. We are, at the same time, requested to draw special attention to the time when the ballot-papers must be returned. At the last election a number of votes were informal in consequence of the papers not being received *before* four o'clock on the *afternoon of the day preceding the election.*

We have received from Messrs. C. H. Grondona and Co. a sample of Schlobach's eucalyptus tobacco. This is a new preparation, and it is stated that instead of being injurious to smokers it is beneficial, besides which, it emits a fragrance altogether unknown to ordinary tobacco, and is of great value as a disinfectant, especially where such epidemics as measles, fevers, &c., are prevalent, and in sick-rooms and all unhealthy localities. It also affords relief in cases of asthma, and all diseases of the chest. It is prepared solely in Melbourne.

The circumlocution office and the Tite Barnacle family are admirably represented at our Melbourne University, where it is quite a crime " to want to know, you know." During the examination of the registrar of the University before the select committee at present sitting on the bill it came out in evidence that some three years ago the faculty of medicine had decided that it was _ desirable pharmaceutical education should be recognised and taught at the Melbourne University, and that an examiner in pharmacy should be appointed. This determination of the faculty of medicine to introduce persons connected with trade into the Melbourne University appears to have quite upset the Tite Barnacle mind, and, in consequence, we find every opposition and obstruction offered to the recommendation of the faculty of medicine. After the lapse of a year the matter was referred to the senate, and from thence to the council, who referred it back to the faculty of medicine, who referred it to the council, who reversed the decision previously arrived at, and after two years' departmental routine it was finally wiped out from the business paper. The greatest joke of all this appears in the fact that the Pharmacy Board, who were the persons most interested, were kept quite in the dark as to what was going on, and are not, as Sir Joseph Porter, K.C.B., remarks, even now " officially " informed of the fact.

We are very much gratified to read that Dr. Attfield, F.R.S., so long the able and respected Professor of Chemistry to the Pharmaceutical Society, has received an address and a handsome present of books (about five hundred volumes). No one who knows the Professor but will endorse every word said by Mr. Schact, upon whom devolved the duty of making the presentation on behalf of the Pharmaceutical Conference. From the remarks made by the President we cannot forbear quoting the following :—"For many years I have had the pleasure of an intimate acquaintance with our friend, and charging my memory to strict accuracy, I can trace throughout all my knowledge of him nothing but one steady, constant effort to lead a good and useful life. As to its goodness, this is not, perhaps, the place to speak, and I will not dilate upon it further than to say that I believe that side of his character to be the mainspring of the other. It may not be inappropriate, perhaps, to say just a word or two on the point of Professor Attfield's usefulness in his public life, which is, indeed, the cause of what we are now doing, and explains the enthusiasm with which the project has been received. Broadly speaking, it occurs to me that the usefulness of our friend's life has consisted in this, that he first of all achieved a high and distinguished position for himself, and from that moment he has endeavoured to hold up both for our admiration and achievement that higher life of mental culture which is so plainly open to us in the very nature of our calling, but which we are very prone to forget in the experiences of business. It seems to me it has been in that constant protest against pharmacists sinking into anything like perfunctory drudges, and in his recommendation of the only genuine remedy for that, viz., that each man should do something, or at least try to do something, for the general good, that the main influence of Professor Attfield has rested."

Meeting.

THE PHARMACY BOARD OF VICTORIA.

THE monthly meeting of the board was held on the 13th October. Present—Messrs. Bosisto, Brind, Power, Lewis, Holdsworth, and Kruse.

The President (Mr. J. Bosisto, M.P.) in the chair.

The minutes of the previous meeting were read and confirmed.

Applications for Registration.—The following persons were registered :—Henry James Massey, Emerald Hill ; James Edward Gribble, Castlemaine, and William Gray, East Melbourne. These three passed the modified examination. Robert Soppet, St. Kilda, certificate Pharmaceutical Society of Great Britain ; John Davidson, Stanthorpe, Queensland, in business before passing of Act ; William Paul Green, Geelong ; and Robert Dalziell Murray, Sandhurst Hospital, were restored to the Register.

Apprentices Indentures Registered.—John Kennedy Peterson and William Alexander Taylor, both of Stawell.

Name Erased from the Register.—A certificate of death of Theodore W. Jones, late of Warrnambool, was received, and his name erased from the Register.

School of Pharmacy.—Mr. Bowen's motion on this subject was postponed until the next meeting, when the nature of the report of the Select Committee on the University Bill will be known.

The Major Examination.—The first practical pharmacy examination under the major examination was fixed to be held in the presence of the whole Board on the 3rd December, 1880.

Resignation of Mr. R. F. Kennedy.—Mr. Kennedy forwarded his resignation as a member of the Board, which, on the motion of Mr. Lewis, was accepted with regret.

The registrar was instructed to notify to the returning-officer that an extraordinary vacancy had occurred, and to request him to take the necessary steps to fill the vacancy.

Correspondence.—Communications were received from the registrar, School of Mines, Ballarat, intimating that the Governor in Council had appointed the President of the Pharmacy Board a member of the Council of the School.

From A. J. Allan, Wellington, New Zealand, forwarding a copy of the Pharmacy Act of New Zealand. From the Secretary Pharmaceutical Society, Great Britain, enclosing copy of the Register for 1880. A number of other letters of no special interest were also dealt with.

Financial business brought the meeting to a close.

BOOKS, &c., RECEIVED.—*American Journal of Pharmacy, Boston Journal of Chemistry, Pharmaceutical Journal, Australian Medical Journal, New York Druggists' Circular, The First Annual Report of the Pharmaceutical Society of New Zealand.*

BALLARAT.

THE SCHOOL OF MINES, BALLARAT.

THE ordinary quarterly meeting of the council was held on the 20th instant. Present—Councillors H. R. Caselli, J.P. (in the chair,) J. M. Bickett, A. Hoelscher, T. Mann, B.A., J. F. Usher, M.D., and W. H. Barnard, F.G.S. A telegram from his lordship the Bishop of Ballarat, and a letter from Mr. James Campbell, apologising for unavoidable absence, were read and received. Minutes of meeting held 21st July last were read and confirmed. On the report and recommendation of the examiners, the council granted certificates of proficiency in the art of telegraphy to the following students, all having passed satisfactory examinations, the first six with credit:—David Richard Davies, James Robert Bradshaw, Emily Ann Radley, Thomas Williams, Peter Alroe, Catherine Mary Wilmer Howe, Elizabeth Lee, Ruth Miller, Alice June Ryan, Isabella Reardon, and William Arthur Goode. Professor F. M'Coy, J.P., F.G.S., and R. L. J. Ellery, Esq., F.R.S., were appointed examiners—the former in natural philosophy and geology, and the latter in electricity. H. B. de la Poer Wall, M.A., C.E., was appointed the fifth delegate from this institution to the Social Science Congress. The recommendation of the administrative council *re* fees—viz., £12 12s. for a three-year's course by students going up for examination as pharmaceutical chemists, and £20 for attendance at all classes by perpetual students—was approved of and adopted. As the architect was not prepared with the plans for the tower erection, required for the apparatus for testing vacuum and steam pressure gauges, this matter was postponed. It was deemed desirable that reports of lecturers as to the students attending, and other matters connected with their respective classes, be submitted at meetings of the administrative council in the future. The registrar submitted the following report, which was received and adopted:—"That the site of The School had been gazetted, and that since the Council last met there had been a change of Ministry, but it was not thought that the new estimates would vary from those previously prepared in the matter of grants in aid of mining schools. That it might be advisable to obtain dies for the striking of medals as prizes to be given to students. That the additions of store-room and office to the laboratories, at a cost of £95, and a new class-room, 33 ft. by 23 ft., at a cost of £177, as approved by the administrative council, were being proceeded with expeditiously. That a large number of exhibits at the Melbourne International Exhibition might be obtained by the school if proper and immediate steps were taken. That arrangements had been made for the treatment and testing of samples of quartz sent to The School for that purpose, the following charges being fixed:—From one lode only, 1 ton, £5; 2 tons, £9; 5 tons, £15; 10 tons, £20; 20 tons, £35—inclusive of all costs for crushing, grinding, amalgamating, assays, reports, and advice as to modes of treatment." The resignation of Mr. Newman as a member of the administrative council was accepted with regret, and Mr. J. M. Bickett appointed in his stead. The council then adjourned.

THE FIRST ANNUAL REPORT OF THE PHARMACEUTICAL SOCIETY OF NEW ZEALAND.

THE PRESIDENT'S ADDRESS.

GENTLEMEN—It gives me great pleasure, and I am sure it does also those who have been working with me here, to welcome the representatives from the other large centres to take part in the work of building up "The Pharmaceutical Society of New Zealand." Before going into the business which we have met to consider, I will say a few words as to the origin and progress of the Society so far, though I fear what I have to say will not be very new to any of you.

As most of you are aware, it originated in a meeting of the chemists in this city, called by me two years since, to consider what steps could be taken to put the profession generally throughout the colony in a better position with the public, and, also, for self-protection.

This met with cordial support here, and was very generally approved by those in other parts of the colony, as is evidenced by the number of members, associates, and apprentices who have enrolled their names, the former numbering 128, associates 60, and apprentices 27, previous to 1st July. In fact, a large proportion of those connected with the business have joined the Society. In Otago this is especially the case, there being scarcely an exception, and I feel confident we shall yet see it universally supported, as it deserves to be. And, although the movement commenced here, it must not be thought that we wished to make it centre in Wellington, or have the entire management of it. It might be fairly said to be a happy thought of ours.

It seemed to us that the time had come when something should be done to raise the standard of education for those who wished to qualify themselves for the business; and by doing this, more thoroughly to secure the public safety, and at the same time insure a certain amount of protection for ourselves, and that it was better that a movement in this direction should emanate from ourselves. That we should show the public we wished that, for the future, those who were desirous of entering into business, and engaging in the responsible work of dispensing medicines, should by a proper course of education become more thoroughly fitted for it—following, in fact, the example set by the pharmaceutical chemists of Great Britain and some of her dependencies.

I think we all felt this was most desirable, and that such a course would meet with the approval of the public generally; and I believe in this we were not mistaken, judging from remarks that have reached us.

And it certainly should be so, as at present there is nothing to prevent a person, however uneducated he may be, from keeping open shop for dispensing and dealing in medicines, the nature and use of which he may be entirely ignorant of. However, the Pharmacy Act is now an accomplished fact, and all this will be changed. And although we have been charged by some persons with trying to create a monopoly, by asking the Government to introduce a Pharmacy Bill, we fully believe the public are thoroughly on our side, and that it is universally considered a step in the right direction.

How it could be looked upon as an attempt at a monopoly by any sensible person I fail to see. It is clearly no more so than the making a course of education necessary to qualify a surgeon or a solicitor for their professions. The opposition shown to the measure appeared to be chiefly from those who were ignorant of its object and did not trouble themselves to understand it. And had it not been for the support given by those who made themselves thoroughly acquainted with it, and with English and colonial legislation on the subject, there is little doubt it would have been thrown out.

We may, I think, congratulate ourselves that a Society so recently established has been enabled in so short a time to accomplish so much; and though the Pharmacy Act now passed may not be all that could be desired, I think it is generally admitted that it is a great point gained, giving us a standing which we had not before, and it rests with ourselves now to make the most of it.

It is to be hoped that now we have met to consider matters of general interest we shall make a fresh start from this point, and by vigorous and united action set in motion plans which in future will raise the profession in the eyes of the public, and that the Pharmaceutical Society of New Zealand will follow in the steps of the Pharmaceutical Society of Great Britain, and be a credit to the colony and to those who have taken part in its promotion.

The minute-book of the Society and the Treasurer's balance-sheet will be laid before you, and by reference to them I think you will find that in all we have done our aim has been, as far as possible, to consult our members throughout the colony, to exercise the greatest economy consistent with working the Society, and to make it as popular as possible; and we have been pleased to receive their suggestions, and very generally their confirmation of our action.

So much for what has been done. It may to some extent be considered of a preliminary character. We have been feeling our way, and it now remains for us thoroughly to organise our work for the future, which can be much more effectually done by our all meeting to discuss. The revision of our rules and many other matters will engage our attention.

In conclusion, I would say that the fact of our being brought together, as we have been, to consider matters of general interest, has already had a good effect, and made us know one another better. And the establishment of the Society bringing the chemists of all parts of the colony into frequent communication with each other, by meetings held in connection with it, should have a tendency to do away with local jealousies. If we can only bear in mind the old motto that "union is strength," and act upon it, we may accomplish a great deal.

CHARLES D. BARRAUD, President.
Wellington, September 27, 1880.

MELBOURNE INTERNATIONAL EXHIBITION.

VISITORS to the Exhibition will have noticed that chemical and pharmaceutical products have been assigned a prominent place. All the most important exhibits under this class are to be found in the main avenue, on the right-hand side on leaving the main building. Our wholesale and manufacturing chemists make a creditable display. As most of our readers have inspected the various exhibits for themselves, it is unnecessary for us to describe them in detail, especially as on some future occasion—after the jurors have made their examinations—we shall be called upon to return to the subject. The following list includes the names and exhibits of the Victorian and foreign manufacturers. There are in the official catalogues 435 chemical and pharmaceutical exhibits. Great Britain furnishes 64; France, 56; Germany, 51; Victoria, 63; New South Wales, 18; United States, America, 22; Italy, 43; Japan, 6. There are 76 exhibits of perfumery. Under the classification of chemical and pharmaceutical products are included many articles which have little, or at least only a remote, relation to pharmacy, and are, consequently, in many instances omitted from enumeration in our list. The Philadelphia College of Pharmacy has, in a letter addressed to Mr. Bosisto, very courteously given the exhibits No. 190 in catalogue to the Pharmaceutical Society of Victoria—which offer has been accepted and acknowledged. At the close of the Exhibition the specimens will be added to the museum of the Society, and carefully preserved. We may take this opportunity of expressing a hope that some of the other exhibitors will follow the laudable example of our American friends, and so enrich our collection; the necessity for a more complete repository of materia medica and chemical specimens being increasingly felt by the Society.

VICTORIA.—G. Adams, Latrobe-terrace, Ashley, Geelong, eye lotion. L. C. Andreson and Co., 9 Market-buildings, William-street, Melbourne, chemicals, chemical and pharmaceutical preparations, varnishes, &c. Apollo Stearine Candle Co. Limited, Footscray, Melbourne, candles in variety, oils, chemicals, glycerine (medicinal and crude), &c. C. A. Atkin, 43 Errol-street, Hotham, Melbourne, quinine tonic made with colonial wine. Australian Lithofracteur Co., 29 Little Collins-street East, Melbourne, nitric, sulphuric, and other acids. W. Beckwith, 43 Little Collins-street East, Melbourne, medicines for horses and cattle. J. Bosisto, Bridge-road, Richmond, Melbourne, essential oils from eucalyptus, others from indigenous trees, &c., chemical products from same. Bull and Owen, 9 Malop-street, Geelong, chemicals, pharmaceutical preparations. S. Capper and Co., 97 Webb-street, Fitzroy, Melbourne, blue, blacking, washing-powder, knife-polish, epsom salts, senna leaves, &c. Cumming, Smith and Co., 47 William-street, Melbourne, chemicals. T. O. Dunstone, High-street, St. Kilda, Melbourne, medicines. Felton, Grimwade and Co., 31 and 33 Little Flinders-street West, Melbourne, chemicals, dugs, &c. R. J. Fullwood, Barkly and Canning streets, Carlton, Melbourne, drugs, chemicals, proprietary preparations. A. Hall, 48 Douglas-parade, Williamstown, Melbourne, aërated

waters. Hemmons, Laws and Co., 55 Russell-street, Melbourne, pharmaceutical chemicals. Hepburn Spring Water Co., 142 Collins-street East, Melbourne, aërated waters. L. Hesse, Argyle-street, St. Kilda, Melbourne, disinfectants (liquid and in powder). Hood and Co., 147 Elizabeth-street, Melbourne, sheep-dipping composition, Hood and Co.'s proprietary medicine. G. Kingsland, 259 King-street, West Melbourne, chemical and pharmaceutical preparations. J. Kitchen and Sons, 28 Little Flinders-street West, Melbourne, stearine candles, soda crystals. F. Longmore, Flinders and King streets, Melbourne, beeswax (bleached and prepared), insecticide, pharmaceutical chemicals and medicines. R. M'Call, Swan-street, Richmond, Melbourne, cough mixture. N. S. Marks, 108 Collins-street West, Melbourne, pharmaceutical products, ointments, tonic syrup, chlorodyne. T. W. Norris, 68 and 70 Chapel-street, Prahran, Melbourne, medicines for domestic animals. Rocke, Tompsitt and Co., 3 Flinders-street, Melbourne, insectibane. Sander and Sons, Bridge-street, Sandhurst, Eucalyptus globulus extract. W. H. Slater, Mitcham Grove, Box Hill Distillery, Nunawading, essential oils and extracts from medicinal herbs. J. Sullivan, 15 King William-street, Fitzroy, Melbourne, Sullivan's disinfecting preparations.

NEW SOUTH WALES.—L. J. Altman, 277 Pitt-street, Sydney, cement for glass and china. Barratt and Co., Buckingham-street, Sydney, aërated waters, cordials, &c.; balsam of aniseed. G. Bogerly and Co., Botany, gelatine and glue. W. Davies, Goulburn, Dr. Waugh's baking-powder. G. W. Gibson, Forcaux-street, Surrey Hills, odontalgic essence. Grogan and Co., 497 George-street, Sydney, pure india-rubber stamps, seals, signatures, crests. B. O. Holterman, 674 George-street, Sydney, furniture polish, Holterman's life drops, Hudson Brothers, Botany-road, Redfern, non-poisonous paint. C. Icke, Wickham, Newcastle, pure soldering liquid, invented and produced by exhibitor. E. Kerr 508 George-street, Sydney, cement for veneers, cabinet work, household purposes. J. and J. Mulcahy, Regent-street, Redfern, toilet and other soaps, candles. A. Orchard, 145 Cleveland-street, Redfern, exhibition cement and marking ink. L. Peate, George-street, Bathurst, baking-powder. J. Pottie, 215 Elizabeth-street, Sydney, patent medicines. M. Saunderson, 55 Point-street, Pyrmont, bonanza (a cleansing cream). J. Schweppe and Co., 62 Margaret-street, Sydney, mineral waters (non-competitive). J. Starkey, 156 Phillip-street, Sydney, aërated waters. Watson and Young, Albury, aërated waters.

SOUTH AUSTRALIA.—A. M. Bickford and Son, wholesale druggists, Adelaide, aërated waters—viz., soda-water, lemonade, ginger ale, ginger beer, sarsaparilla. W. H. Burford and Sons, soap and candle makers, Adelaide, superior yellow soap. A. Centauri, veterinary surgeon, Adelaide, "Time" metal polish. B. M. and H. Conigrave, manufacturers, Macclesfield, aërated waters, assorted. W. Evans, valet, Government House, Adelaide, boot varnish. G. Hall and Sons, aërated water manufacturers, Norwood, aërated waters—viz., soda, seltzer, tonic, lemonade, ginger ale, sarsaparilla. W. H. Malpas, Adelaide, patent anti-ant compound. J. Tidmarsh, soap and candle maker, Adelaide, (1) stearine, (2) stearine candles, (3) soap.

NEW ZEALAND.—Kelly and Frazer, Puriri Mineral Springs, Thames, aërated and medicinal waters. Kitchen and Sons, Wellington, candles and soaps. M'Leod Brothers, crown soap and candle works, Dunedin, stearine candles, soaps. J. Neil, herbalist, Dunedin, selection of botanic medicines. F. Bennett, Thames, raw and calcined hematite, and specimen board showing tint effects. F. Bennett, Thames, specimens of raw and manufactured hematite. J. Gomez, Bulls, Rangitikei, soda-water, lemonade, and sarsaparilla. H. A. H. Hitchens, Auckland, vegetable compound for purifying the blood. Hokitika Local Committe, Hokitika, dozen mineral waters, from Waihoauri, Westland. W. Innis, Port Chalmers, five pint bottles cod liver oil, warranted pure.

QUEENSLAND.—Berkley, Taylor and Co., dugong oil (unrefined). Botanic gardens, Brisbane, essential oils, tinctures, &c., prepared by L. Carmichael, chemist. D. Clarke, Warwick, collection of essences, perfumes, and tooth-powders. K. T. Staiger, F.L.S., samples of pyroligueous acid, acetic acid, methylated alcohol, wood tar, acetate of soda, kerosene, paraffine. K. T. Staiger, F.L.S., essential oil, made from the leaves of the Eucalyptus citriodora, found near Gladstone. K. T. Staiger, F.L.S., essential oil, from leaves of ironbark-tree on the Palmer River (not yet named); samples of the leaves therewith. K. T. Staiger, F.L.S., essence made from the leaves of the ironbark-tree on the Palmer River (not yet named);

samples of the leaves therewith. K. T. Staiger, F.L.S., essence made from the leaves of the Eucalyptus citriodora, found near Gladstone. K. T. Staiger, F.L.S., duboisine, extract from duboisa leaves. K. T. Staiger, F.L.S., crystalline alkaloid, alstonine crystals, like quinine. Stiller and Co., Amity Point, Moreton Bay, dugong oil. C. H. F. Yeo, Brisbane, collection of essences and perfumes.

AMERICA.—Barclay and Co., 7 Burling Slip, New York, toilet articles. J. Burnett and Co., Boston, Massachusetts, extracts, cologne, &c. Eastman and Brother, 1011 Marble-street, Philadelphia, toilet soap and perfumery. Fell and Co., Philadelphia, toilet soaps. H. S. Fox and Co., Philadelphia, Oriental balm, &c. Greenfelder Brothers, St. Louis, extracts, A. Pirz, New York City, chemicals. H. Tetlow Brothers. Philadelphia, perfumery, &c. A. J. Vaught and Co., Washington-street, Buffalo, New York, tooth-powder, perfumery, &c. Barclay and Co., medical specialties. F. K. Brown, Philadelphia, extract of Jamaica ginger. J. Burnett and Co., Boston, Massachusetts, flavouring extracts, florimel, essence of ginger. The superiority of Burnett's flavouring extracts consists in their perfect purity and great strength. They are warranted free from the poisonous oils and acids which enter into the composition of many of the factitious fruit flavours now in the market. Burnett's essence of Jamaica ginger, a household remedy for colic, cholera morbus, colds, chills, and diarrhœa, warming and stimulating the whole system. Carniola Chemical Works, Anthony Pirz, Long Island, City of New York, U.S.A., Cosmoroma (toilet vinegar), various chemical products, premium white sugar of lead, orange acetic acid, C.P. premium acetic acid, and photo-acetic acid. All of the preparations manufactured by Professor Pirz are of the highest standard, and have invariably secured the first prizes in State, National, and International Exhibitions. His manufactures of sugar of lead, acetic acid, vinegar, and litharge are known as chemically pure ; the sulphuric acid full standard and renowned for purity. The Pirz fertilizer, or his super-phosphate of lime, is acknowledged as the best fertilizer now known, not exhausting soil, but acting as a permanent stimulant. Over 50,000 tons have been sold the past year. The Pirz cosmoroma is now recognised as a toilet article of great value for bathing purposes, headache, &c., greatly invigorating the body. The Pirzil anti-congestion powders are largely used by physicians in the relief of constipation, piles, and apoplexy. All these articles can be ordered direct from Professor Pirz, or through Newell and Co., Melbourne. Cherry and Myrick, Boston, Massachusetts, botanic medicines. T. Gill, New York City, soap (borax). A. S. Hale, Lyons, Wayne, New York, oil of peppermint, ("Hale and Parshall" brand). E. Lilley and Co., Indianapolis, drugs and medicines. Philadelphia College of Pharmacy, Philadelphia, drugs. W. H. Schieffeln and Co., 170 and 172 William-street, New York, pharmaceutical preparations, fluid extracts, elixirs, syrups, &c. W. H. Schieffeln and Co., 170 and 172 William-street, New York, soluble pills and granules. Seabury and Johnson, New York, pharmaceutical plasters. W. R. Warner and Co., Philadelphia, drugs and pills.

MADRAS.—Dr. G. King, cinchona febrifuge. Rai Kanny Loll Dey Bahadur, Calcutta, collection of indigenous drugs.

JAPAN.—Government Mint, Osaka, nitric acid, sulphuric acid, &c. Government Printing Office, Tokio, blacking, soaps, and colours. Kaitakushi, Department for the Colonisation of the Island of Yesso, Tokio, sulphur. Kogio Shokuwai, Tokio, sulphur, camphor, and wax. Kiritsu Kosho Kuwaisha and T. Akiyama, Tokio, Japanese candles. S. Wooyesugi, Osaka, gum.

GERMANY.—Van Baerle and Sponnagel (proprietor, F. G. Sponnagel), Berlin, water-glass, its raw materials, and articles made from it. Dr. F. V. Heyden, Dresden, salicylic acid and preparations. E. Merck, Darmstadt, chemical preparations. Dr. T. Schuchardt, Görlitz, chemical technical products. Associated Stassfurt, Leopoldshall, Douglashall Salt Industry, Stassfurt, raw salt and products; explanations, both written and pictured, of every kind—twenty exhibitors, viz.:—Andrae and Gruneberg, Leopoldshall. Askania Act Co., Leopoldshall. Royal Mine Inspection, Stassfurt. Chemical Factory, Harburg-Stassfurt (late Thörl and Heydtmann Co., Stassfurt). Concordia Chemical Factory Co., Leopoldshall. Douglashall, Westeregeln. Hell and Sthamer, Schönebeck. Kali and Stein Salt Mine, Douglashall, near Westeregeln. Friedrich's Smelting-house, Leopoldshall. Lindemann and Co., Stassfurt. N. F. Locfasz, Stassfurt. Maigatter, Green and Co., Leopoldshall. Muller and Allihn, Leopoldshall. F. Muller, Leopoldshall. C. Nette, Faulwasser and Co., Leopoldshall. Salt Mines, Neu-

Stassfurt, near Stassfurt. Stassfurt Chemical Factory (formerly Vorster and Grüneberg), Stassfurt. Associated Chemical Works, Leopoldshall. Wustenhagen and Co., Hecklingen, near Stassfurt. Zimmer and Co., Stassfurt.—Baden Aniline and Soda Factory, Stuttgart, aniline colours. J. E. Devrient, Zwickau, chemicals and artists' colours. Gademann and Co., Schweinfurt, ehemical colours. Pfannenschmidt and Kruger, Danzig, amber, lac, &c. J. Bernhardi, Leipsig, drugs. Bruckner, Lampe and Co., Leipzig, drugs, cut and in powder. J. B. Feilner and Grienwaldt, Bremen, collodium, gelatine for photographic purposes. Dr. F. Witte, Rostock, in Mecklenberg, dry rennet for whey (sole agents : Schmedes, Erbslöh and Co., Melbourne). L. Ziffer, Berlin, butter and cheese colouring and preserving powder, cheese rennet extract. Brunswick Quinine Works, Brunswick, quinine, quinine compounds. Haarmann and Reimer, Holzminden, vanilin, heliotropin, &c. E. Sachsse and Co., Leipzig, etherised oils and essences. J. Gautsch, Munich, wax goods (sole agents : Schmedes, Erbslöh and Co., Melbourne). American India-rubber and Celluloid Factory, Mannheim, articles in strong india-rubber. E. Cuntze, Cologne, Ehrenfeld, eau-de-Cologne (sole agents : Schmedes, Erbslöh and Co., Melbourne). F. M. Farina, opposite the Alten Market, Cologne, eau-de-Cologne and perfumes (sole agents : Schmedes, Erbslöh and Co., Melbourne). F. M. Farina, 4711 Glockengasse, Cologne, eau-de-Cologne and perfumes. J. M. Farina, 4 Jülichsplatz, Cologne, eau-de-Cologne. J. A. Farina, Zur Stadt Mailand, Cologne, eau-de-Cologne. J. M. Farina, opposite the Neumarkt, Cologne, eau-de-Cologne. K. Fievet, Cologne, eau-de-Cologne and perfumes (sole agents : Schmedes, Erbslöh and Co., Melbourne). M. C. Martin, Nun, Cologne, eau-de-Cologne and "Carmeliter-Geist." G. Bohm, Offenbach, perfumes and soaps. Junger and Gebhardt, Berlin, essences, scented and washing waters, soaps, pomades, &c. L. Leichner, Berlin, powder and rouge.

(To be continued.)

SOCIAL SCIENCE CONGRESS.

THE first of a series of horticultural shows will be held in the great hall about the middle of November. At a recent meeting Mr. Bosisto, chairman of the Vegetable Products Committee, was requested to undertake the details.

At a meeting of the agricultural section of the Social Science Congress papers on the following subjects were laid on the table :—" The Cultivation of the Olive in Victoria," by C. May, Sunbury ; " The Clearing of Land," by C. H. Lyon, Ballan ; " Manufacture of Beetroot Sugar," by W. Murray Ross ; " Scientific Agricultural Education," by D. B. Smith, Buln Buln ; " Sylvian Streets," by W. R. Guilfoyle ; " Insect Pests on Fruit-bearing Trees," by C. May ; " Rust in Wheat " and "An Economical Scheme of Experimental Farming," by R. W. E. MacIvor.

The health section of the Social Science Congress commenced its sitting on 18th October, when Dr. M'Crae delivered his presidential address ; and the following papers were read : —By Mr. H. K. Rusden, on "The Prevention of Lunacy ;" by Dr. M'Carthy, on "The Use and Abuse of Stimulants as Articles of Diet." An interesting discussion followed upon the two subjects of lunacy and drunkenness. In the evening Dr. Louis Henry read a paper on "The Comparative Immunity from Disease among the Jews," and Dr. Jamieson another on "Infant Mortality." He pointed out that the Melbourne rate was disproportionately high, being 168 per 1000, and greater than that of London. He attributed this to the result of artificial feeding.

On the 20th October Mr. A. Sutherland, M.A., read a paper on "Health Insurance."

On the 21st October Mr. Bosisto, M.L.A., read a valuable paper on "The Forests and Timber Growth of Victoria in Relation to Health, Conservation, and Culture." He pointed out the disastrous effects likely to result from a diminution of our forests, and suggested the appointment of a forest trust, independent of Government control. An interesting discussion followed, in which the importance of the subject was fully recognised. Dr. Day, of Geelong, read a paper on "The Application of Spontaneously Generated Peroxide of Hydrogen to Purifying and Disinfecting Purposes." In the evening Mr. H. K. Rusden contributed a paper on "Contagious Diseases," in which he urged the rigid enforcement of quarantine in the case of every contagious disease. Dr. Paterson, of Adelaide, read a paper on "Quarantine."

The health section of the Social Science Congress concluded

its proceedings on the 22nd October. In the afternoon three papers were read and discussed, the first being "Notes on Ventilation," by Mr. Le Capelain; the second on "Hospital Architecture," by Dr. Henry; and the third by Mr. T. R. Wilson, on "The Prevention of the Spread of Infectious Diseases." In the evening Mr. T. Embling contributed a paper on "Premature Interments." He urged that the State should exercise a vigilant scrutiny to prevent the possibility of any one being buried alive; and he thought that no burials should take place until indubitable evidences of decay had set in. The remaining papers were by Dr. Cleland, of Adelaide, on "The Committal and Care of Insane Paying Patients," and by Dr. Ginders, of New Zealand, on "School Hygiene."

Mr. E. L. Marks, lecturer on chemistry at the Sandhurst School of Mines, in his paper, read before the Education Section, on "Technical Education," made some excellent remarks on the chemistry of many bodies, such as iodine, tartaric acid, fibrous plants, artists' pigments, &c. He also particularly drew attention to pharmacy in the following words:—"In the matter of drugs and chemicals, how infinitely more genuine are they now than was the case formerly. The change has been brought about by the higher technical education required from those practising pharmacy—a change inducing emulation, a change that has intensely impressed the line that distinguishes the chemist from the mere druggist, a change beneficial to society by assuring to it every possible care in every detail of the business, a change beneficial to the individual by expanding the mind and investing mere drudgery with elegance. To a scientific pharmacist no wholesale druggist, no traveller in druggists' wares, would venture to offer, much less to supply, an inferior or a spurious drug; hence in every way technical training has here been a success." Again, he said—"By an extended education we raise the quality of articles of food and clothing, since the knowledge of how simply to detect adulterations is the best way to stamp them out. How easy is it to teach the means of recognising admixtures of cotton with linen, of those with wool or silk, both by chemical means or by the microscope. The intrinsic peculiarities existing in potato starch, maizena, and genuine arrowroot, by which each is at once verified, the genuine tea-leaf from leaves used as adulterants; how the recognition of chalk, iron oxides, Prussian blue, logwood, &c., said to be more or less used to deceive the purchaser, may easily be taught." "Take, again, the question of sweetmeats. Who does not recollect the agonies that children formerly suffered; the pains in the stomach so distracting as to their causes, so difficult to allay? We see the causes in the plaster-of-Paris, the vermilion, the chrome yellow, the arsenical pigments formerly used. Happily, now, thanks to technical training, sugar alone and vegetable colours only are used in the manufacture." It is gratifying to find that, although actively engaged in teaching and lecturing, Mr. Marks has found time and opportunity to bring these important matters prominently forward.

Personalities.

Mr. T. Lakeman, Messrs. Burgoyne, Burbridges and Co.'s representative, has opened an extensive show-room at 24 O'Connell-street, Sydney.

Mr. Edwin Plummer, who for the last four years was in business in Wellington, New Zealand, has returned to Victoria, with a view, it is reported, of again settling here.

Mr. Henry Trumble, late of Eaglehawk, has purchased the business of Mr. Nielson, Lonsdale-street. A man of Mr. Trumble's energy will be an acquisition to our city pharmacists.

The business for some time past conducted by Mr. J. Churchus, at Mount Egerton, has changed hands, and is now being conducted by Mr. Archibald M'Gowan. Mr. Churchus is, we believe, in search of "fresh woods and pastures new."

The business of Mr. Henry Trumble, pharmaceutical chemist, Eaglehawk, changed hands during the past fortnight, Mr. Berriman, a former apprentice of Mr. Trumble, and lately dispenser to the late Dr. Cheyne, being the purchaser. We wish the young man every success.

The races, Exhibition, and other attractions have caused many of our friends in the other colonies to visit us. Mr. Wm. Jas. Main, of Adelaide, being in Melbourne, has paid several visits to the rooms of the society. Mr. Main hopes that South

Australia will shortly follow the example of the other colonies in the matter of a Pharmacy Act.

Mr. James W. Henton, of Auckland, New Zealand, the local secretary of the Pharmaceutical Society at that place, is in Melbourne, and has taken advantage of his visit to make himself acquainted with details of the working of the Pharmacy Act in Victoria. Mr. Henton expresses himself as greatly pleased with the highly effective manner in which the Act is carried out.

THE PHARMACY BOARD ELECTION.

The election for a member of this board, in the place of Mr. R. F. Kennedy, resigned, will be held on the 17th November next. The nomination closed on the 4th November, at four p.m. The following are the candididates nominated:—

Clemes, A. B., Stawell,
Owen, A. J., Geelong,
MacGowan, J. T., Ballarat.

Correspondence.

ELECTION OF THE PHARMACY BOARD.

To the Editor of The Australasian Supplement to the Chemist and Druggist.

Sir—The retirement of Mr. Kennedy from the Pharmacy Board allows the original equilibrium of representation to be restored thereto, if our Melbourne Pharmacists will but kindly lend their assistance in this direction. At the inception of the Pharmacy Act it was deemed as advisable as it was judicious that the principal centres of population should be represented at the Board. This was done by nominating one gentleman each from Geelong, Sandhurst, Ballarat, and four for Melbourne and all its suburbs; and, though at the late election, the *personnel* of the board was considerably altered, through the unfortunate retirements of Messrs. Johnstone and Blackett, yet still the original idea was fairly consummated, except in the case of Geelong, which was left out in the cold through, I think, the casting vote of the returning officer. An opportunity now offers which should, I think, be embraced, of restoring things to the military dictum—"As you were." With this view, I would suggest that Geelong should nominate a gentleman, and then work for his return, calling upon us in Melbourne, to assist them. Why not elect Mr. Green, who is already familiar with the duties required, and proved himself, while there (as far as I can learn), a fair representative man. I think it behoves all Pharmacists to take an interest in these elections, though how they are to arrive at the qualifications of new aspirants, except from hearsay, or, perhaps, the interested motives of drug houses or their travellers, or modest trumpeting by aspirants of their own virtues, I admit, puzzles me, though I suppose Old Time, like it does to everything else, will unravel even this difficulty.

Senes Pilulæ.

DARNEL.

To the Editor of The Australasian Supplement to the Chemist and Druggist.

Sir—I forward you the following, which no doubt will be interesting to your readers:—A cow-keeper consulted me a few days ago in reference to the illness of some of his cows and death of one as yet, and no doubt others may have suffered likewise.

I suspected poison, and on inquiry found the "mash" or grain obtained from a distillery contained a large proportion of "darnel." I therefore had no hesitation in declaring the cause of the cows illness. The question is, should mash of this description be used or sold as cattle food, and what is the effect on the milk? The use of this seed in distillation is also questionable, although it is supposed none of the deleterous principle is retained by the spirit. With brewing it is very different, and may the stupefying effect of some of the trashy ales not owe their injurious effect to "darnel" either accidentally or otherwise mixed with the malt. I draw attention to this subject entirely on public grounds, and warn unfortunate dairymen of the danger of mash such as the samples I have on hand, a portion of which I have placed in the Exhibition. Perhaps some of your readers may think the subject worthy of remark with the view of an investigation being instituted, and the use of this poison for any purposes of food made punishable by law. The quantity supplied appears to be annually on the increase, and is in fact a recognised marketable commodity. You kindly published extracts on the poisonous action of Lolium temulentum when used in flour, &c., from some of the best authorities of the day. The subject is one peculiarly suited to your columns, and on that account request your insertion of these remarks. In conclusion I have to ask your able assistance in throwing all the fresh light possible to prevent the evil increasing as it has been, and undoubtedly is at present.

GRAHAM MITCHELL, F.R.C.V.S.
Melbourne, 1st November, 1880.

P.S.—I herewith forward a sample of the "mash" referred to, which you might place on view.   G. M.

THE APOLLO CANDLE COMPANY.

AMONGST the principal Victorian exhibits at the International Exhibition, that of the Apollo Stearine Candle Co. (Lmtd.) may fairly claim a place in the foremost rank. Their trophies are two in number—one representing the stearine industry, and the other one of the various soaps made by this firm. The more important of their two trophies is naturally that devoted to stearine candles of every description, glycerine, and various oils produced in their process of manufacture. The form is octagon, with an octagon dome, and here we may draw attention to the fact that this exhibit is unique in kind. The whole of the case containing the candle exhibit is made of stearine. This case is sixteen feet in diameter, and twenty-three feet high. The dome is surmounted by a large bust of Apollo, on a pedestal also of stearine, and on the columns stand eight stearine figures representing the four quarters of the globe and the four seasons. The whole case has the appearance of a marble temple, and contains nearly four hundred separate castings. Within is an octagon pyramid with carved sides, on which are arranged, according to size and colour, candles of every possible description and material, amongst which may be mentioned—stearine, paraffine, spermaceti, wax, ozokerit, composite, &c., in sizes varying from the large 2-lb. altar candle, to the tiny taper of eighty to the pound. Every kind of fancy candle is here shown—cable, spiral, fluted, star-shaped, painted ; various patent ends, to fit any candlestick ; aërated candles, with internal channels to prevent guttering and wash ; tulip candles, holly candles, and candles in the shape of Cleopatra's needle—hieroglyphics and all—besides the more ordinary candles for household and mining purposes, for cabs, omnibusses, coaches, ship-lanterns, &c. Within the case appear, also, various bottles containing crude glycerine-oleine for lubricating, saponified and oleic acid, and the various products of the stearine industry.

The second trophy is hexagon in form, and is made entirely of household and wool-washing soap. This soap is manufactured from oleic acid, a by-product of the stearine industry, which, until lately, was virtually useless here, and had to be shipped hence to find a market. The company, however, after repeated and costly trials, have succeeded in working it up into various soaps, of which they are the first and only successful makers in Australia from this article. The company's soft soap, specially made from pure oil and potash for wool-scouring, is also here shown. In addition to the ordinary soaps, they also exhibit transparent glycerine soaps in many varieties, as eucalyptus, carbolic, camphor, rose, honey, Oxford, and Cambridge, which appear in every size and shape of tablet, bar, and ball. These soaps are made by a process, peculiar to the company, from the very finest glycerine and other materials ; and their eucalyptus soap has a very wide reputation as a pleasant and healthy detergent.

The company has branch factories in Sydney and Brisbane, and an agency in Adelaide. Its candles have almost entirely superseded the foreign article. In fact, the company produces and sells more candles throughout Australia than all foreign and colonial makers combined. Its consumption of tallow is about eighty tons weekly, and its machinery is of the most modern and powerful description. Its yearly production is about thirty million candles, which, if placed end to end, would extend about five thousand miles, and if burned consecutively would last for twenty-eight thousand years.

ſlotes and Abstracts.

A NOVEL SUTURE.—The Rev. J. G. Wood, the well-known writer on entomology, says the Medical Times, is responsible for the statement that in some parts of Brazil ants are used for sewing up wounds. He says—"They simply pinch the edges of the wound together and hold the ant to it. The creature immediately bites at the obstacle, making its jaws meet. The native surgeon pulls away the body, leaving the head still adhering. Seven or eight ants' heads are sometimes employed for a single wound."

SANTONIN CONTAMINATED WITH STRYCHNIA.—Strychnia is stated to be a common impurity in commercial samples of santonin. Forquate Gigli recommends for its detection, in preference to Flückiger's method, the following process :—1 gram of the sample is placed in a small beaker, covered with a little distilled water and acidulated with a few drops of sulphuric acid. On agitating with a glass rod, the strychnia dissolves while the santonin remains insoluble. The liquid is filtered, the residue washed with a little water and the washing added to the filtrate, which is then distributed in several test-glasses and examined for strychnia by means of the usual reagents.—Chem. News, 18th June, 1880, p. 283.

De Vrij's improved method of preparing fluid Extract of Cinchona is as follows : 100 grams of the powdered bark of the trunk of East India Cinchona succirubra, containing at least 6 per cent. alkaloids, are mixed with 38 grams normal hydrochloric acid and 362 grams water, and are macerated for 12 hours, at the expiration of which, 20 grams glycerin are added and the whole mixture is transferred to a percolator. When the clear percolate ceases to pass, clear water is passed through the percolator until the percolate is only coloured, but no longer rendered cloudy by soda lye, which usually is the case before 800 grams percolate are obtained. The latter is then evaporated to 100 grams, the obtained fluid extract thus corresponding in strength to the fluid extracts of the U. S. Pharmacopœia.—Pharm. Ztg., 27th March, 1880, p. 187.

BUTTERMILK AS SUMMER FOOD, DRINK, AND MEDICINE. —A Detroit physician asserts that, for a hot weather drink, nothing equals buttermilk. It is, he says, "both drink and food, and for the labourer is the best known. It supports the system, and even in fever will cool the stomach admirably. It is also a most valuable domestic remedy. It will cure dysentery as well and more quickly than any other remedy known. Dysentery is really a constipation, and is the opposite of diarrhœa. It is inflammation of the bowels with congestion of the 'portal circulation'—the circulation of blood through the bowels and liver. It is a disease always prevalent in the summer and autumn. From considerable observation I feel warranted in saying that buttermilk, drunk moderately, will cure every case of it—certainly when taken in the early stages."

NEW WAY OF PRESERVING HOPS.—The principal feature in this new system consists in sprinkling the hops with alcohol prior to packing, and then pressing them tightly into air-tight vessels. In course of time the alcohol combines with some of the constituents of the hop, and certain volatile ethers are thus formed ; these possess a strong and peculiar fruity smell, but being very volatile they are all dissipated during the boiling. Dr. Lintner has experimented on these preserved hops at Weihenstephan, and speaks well of them ; he says the fine colour is retained, and there is a full development of aroma ; the fermentation of worts made with these hops worked well, and the resulting beer possessed a fine bitter flavour. If this method of sprinkling with alcohol will stop the development of valerianic acid, which takes place in hops when stored in the usual manner, it ought to come into general use.—Journal of Chemistry.

PHOSPHATE OF LIME FOR CLARIFYING MUDDY WATER.— Philadelphia appears at present to be supplied with muddy water extremely difficult to clarify even by filtration through paper. Mr. R. F. Fairthorne offers, in the Am. Jour. of Pharm., a simple method for remedying the evil. He says—"After many fruitless or only partially successful efforts, I found the following plan to succeed admirably, namely, to agitate each quart of water with an ounce of phosphate of lime, and allow it to settle. This only requires a few minutes, and it will be found that most of the impurities are carried down to the bottom. The supernatant water is now filtered without any trouble through absorbent cotton. Ordinary cotton will answer as well if previously moistened with alcohol and then washed with water. Of course, either of them must be pressed tightly into the neck of a funnel. By this means perfectly clear water can be obtained in about five minutes.

CHEMICALLY PURE HYDRIODIC ACID.—Winkler proposes, in the *Chem. Centralblatt*, the following improvement on the usual method with sulphuretted hydrogen. Iodine is dissolved in bisulphide of carbon almost to saturation. The solution being poured into a tall glass jar, some water is added on top, in a proportion corresponding to the degree of concentration desired. The tube of the sulphuretted hydrogen generator is conducted to nearly the bottom of the glass jar. As soon as the sulphuretted hydrogen gas acts on the solution of iodine in the bisulphide, hydriodic acid is formed, which is immediately taken up by the water. The free sulphur, which in the ordinary method of making the above acid would separate, remains here dissolved in the bisulphide. As soon as the dark violet colour of the iodine solution has been replaced by a colour like sherry wine, the reaction is completed, and the glass jar contains a heavy, oily solution of sulphur in bisulphide of carbon and an aqueous solution of hydriodic acid. It will, of course, be necessary to heat the acid to the boiling point for a short time, in order to free it from sulphuretted hydrogen gas.—*Journal of Chemistry.*

At Greenwich, Henry Morton, chemist, Broadway, Deptford, appeared to an adjourned summons, at the instance of the Greenwich Board of Works, under Section 4 of the Adulteration of Food and Drugs Act, for having mixed a drug, to wit, tincture of quinine, with ingredients or materials so as to affect injuriously the quality or potency of such drug, by which he had rendered himself liable to a penalty of £50. Mr. Corden, inspector under the Board, said on 16th June he went to the defendant's shop and asked for 3 ozs. of tincture of quinine, for which he paid 1s. 8d. He divided it into three parts, and told the defendant it would be analysed by the public analyst. While he was getting the sealing-wax from his pocket the defendant took two of the bottles containing the samples and threw them away. He offered to mix him up some more, as he said he had made a mistake and put six grains instead of eight to the ounce; but the witness took the remaining sample, and told him he should report the matter. The magistrate was handed the certificate of the public analyst, Mr. Wigner, showing that the sample was more than 60 per cent. deficient, some other comparatively worthless alkaloids being added. Mr. Marsham fined the defendant £5, with £1 costs.

At the British Pharmaceutical Conference, after the reading of a paper on the "Supply of Cinchona Bark," the *Pharmaceutical Journal* reports as follows upon an exhibit of a peculiar kind of bark by Dr. Paul :—" Closely connected with the subject of the foregoing paper was the exhibition, by Dr. Paul, of a peculiar kind of cinchona bark, with the object of showing that it is now no longer possible to arrive even at an approximate conclusion as to the value of a sample of bark from mere visual examination. Leaving out of account the fact that the officinalis, or crown bark, now coming from India contains a large amount of quinine, while that hitherto known as 'crown bark,' or 'Loxa bark,' from South America seldom contains much, if any, it is also to be noted that amongst the bark derived from South America it is equally impossible to judge of the value of a sample from its outward appearance alone. The old landmarks are no longer sufficient for indicating whether a bark is worth only a few pence a pound or the same number of shillings. Thus, for instance, the official 'yellow bark,' or 'flat calisaya,' of the present day is rarely what it used to be, but, on the contrary, seldom contains much or any quinine at all, and only a little cinchonine. On the contrary it often happens that bark of unusual or novel characters comes into the market containing an amount of quinine and other alkaloids that renders it intrinsically very valuable. In the case of the specimen exhibited this fact was well shown, for to all appearance it was of little or no value. It represented a somewhat considerable parcel of bark that was imported in June, 1879. It did not recommend itself for making pharmaceutical preparations, and quinine manufacturers were disinclined to buy it at any price. However, the analysis of the bark gave it a different character, showing that in addition to mere traces of quinidine, cinchonidine, and cinchonine it yielded nearly 2½ per cent. of sulphate of quinine, so that for either or both of the purposes above referred to it was an excellent bark, notwithstanding its unfavourable appearance."

Election Notices.

FELTON, GRIMWADE & CO.,

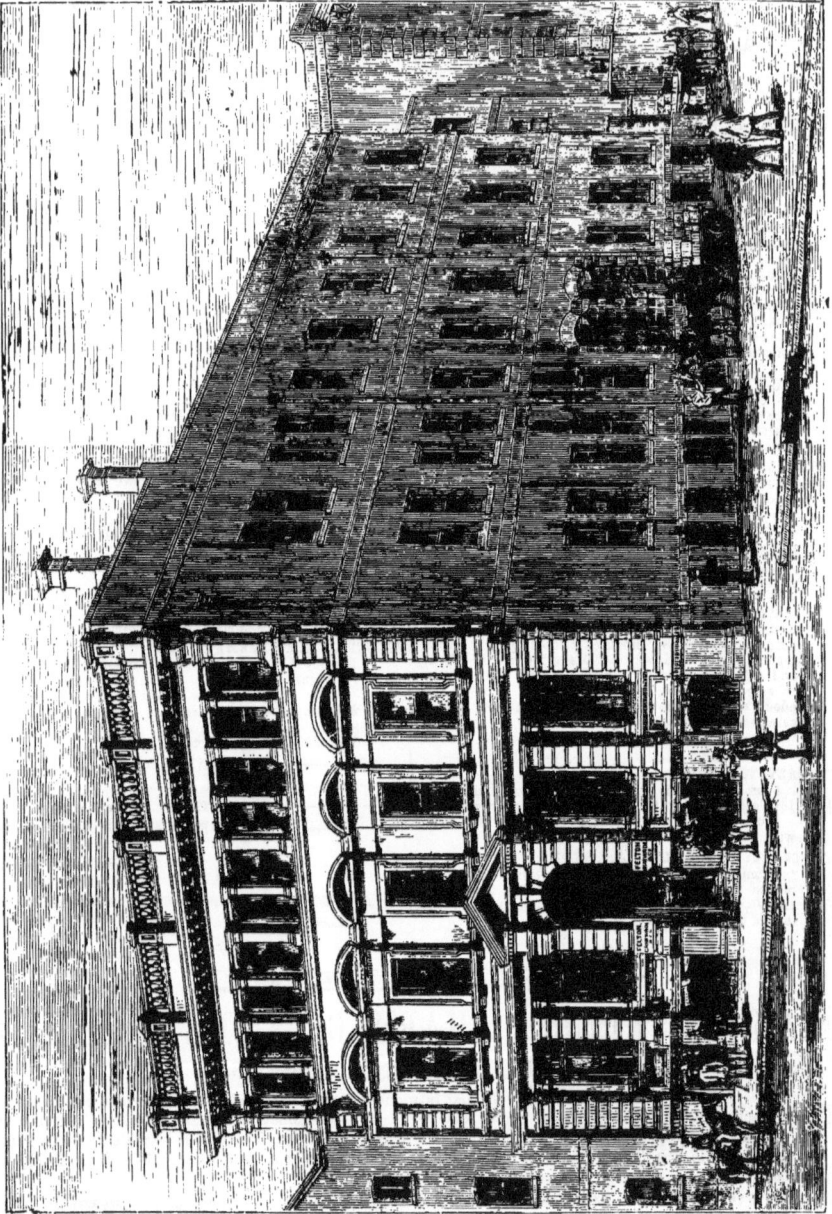

31 & 33 FLINDERS LANE WEST,
MELBOURNE.

[SUPPLEMENT ONLY.]

Chem. & Drugg. Aust. Suppl.
Vol. 3, no. 31 : 49-56, (Nov, 1880)

THE

Chemist & Druggist.

WITH AUSTRALASIAN SUPPLEMENT.

(Published under direction of the Pharmaceutical Society of Victoria.)

No. 31. { Published on the 15th } { of every month. }
Registered for Transmission as a Newspaper.

NOVEMBER, 1880.

{ Subscription, 15s. per Annum, { including Diary, Post Free.

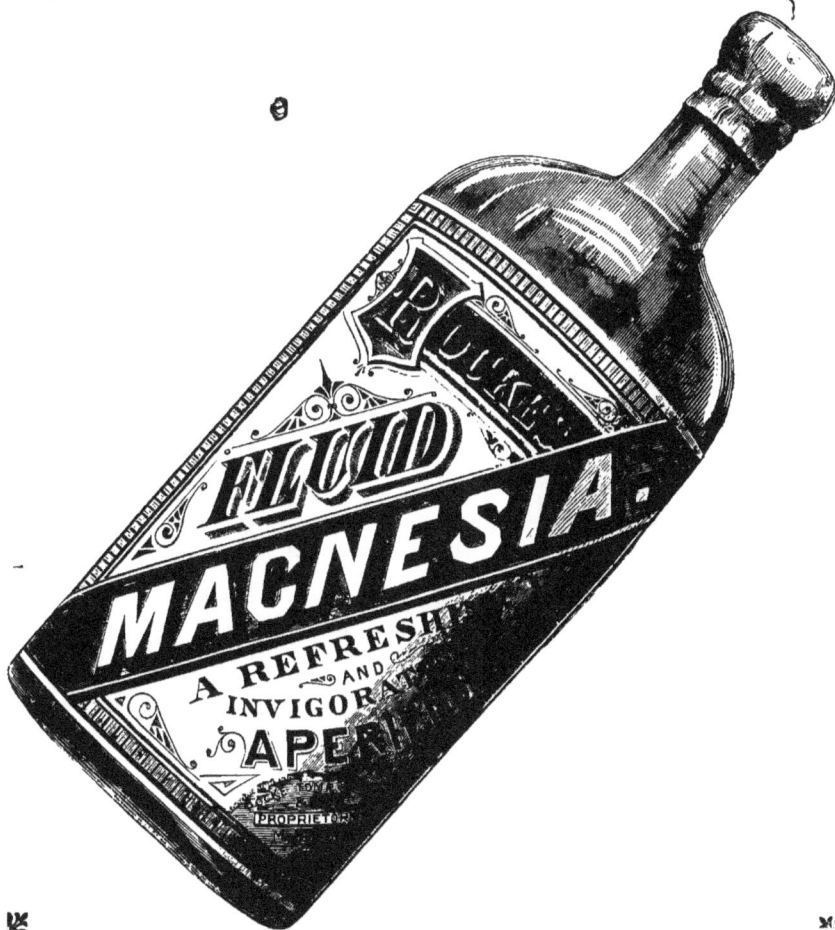

The Chemist and Druggist.
WITH AUSTRALASIAN SUPPLEMENT.

OFFICE: MUTUAL PROVIDENT BUILDINGS, COLLINS STREET WEST.
Published on the 15th of each Month.

THIS Journal is issued gratis to all paid-up Members of the PHARMA-CEUTICAL SOCIETY OF VICTORIA, and to non-members at Fifteen Shillings per annum, payable in advance. A copy of *The Chemists and Druggists' Diary*, published annually, is forwarded post free to every subscriber.

Advertisements, remittances, and all business communications to be addressed to THE HONORARY SECRETARY OF THE PHARMACEUTICAL SOCIETY, MELBOURNE.

SCALE OF CHARGES FOR ADVERTISEMENTS:

	Per annum.		Per annum.
One Page	..£8 0 0	Quarter Page	..£3 0 0
Half do.	.. 5 0 0	Business Cards	.. 2 0 0

Special rates for wrapper and pages preceding and following literary matter. Advertisements of Assistants Wanting Situations, 2s. 6d. each.

Advertisements for insertion in the current month should be sent to the office before the 10th.

COMMUNICATIONS for the EDITORIAL department of this journal should be addressed to THE EDITOR, MUTUAL PROVIDENT BUILDINGS, COLLINS STREET WEST, MELBOURNE.

No notice can be taken of anonymous communications. Whatever is intended for insertion must be authenticated by the name and address of the writer—not necessarily for publication, but as a guarantee of good faith.

SPECIAL NOTICE.

Members are informed that, unless their subscriptions for the current year are paid on or before the 31st December, 1880, they cease to be members, and, in accordance with Rule 14, their names are omitted from the list.

BIRTHS.

FULLWOOD.—On the 19th November, at Barkly and Canning streets, Carlton, the wife of R. Jackson Fullwood, chemist, of a daughter.

THOMPSON.—On the 25th November, at 122 Bourke-street East, the wife of J. D. Thompson of a daughter.

MARRIAGES.

SIMPSON—JAMES.—On the 24th November, at the residence of the bride's parents, Gore-street, Fitzroy, by the Rev. W. L. Binks, David Arthur, youngest son of John Simpson, of Carlton, to Sara, only daughter of Joseph James, of Fitzroy.

HOGARTH—DON.—On the 25th November, at the residence of the bride's parents, by the Rev. Andrew Hardie, William Peel, eldest son of the late Mr. William Hogarth, of Connell, Hogarth and Co., merchants, Melbourne, to Marion Katarine (Minnie), eldest daughter of Mr. J. W. Don, Richmond.

ROWLEY—PYNE.—On the 25th November, by special licence, at St. John's Church, Latrobe-street West, Melbourne, by the Rev. Canon Chase, assisted by the Rev. Walter W. Mantell, of Essendon, Walter M. Rowley, chemist, of 8 Bourke-street East, Melbourne, second son of the late George William Rowley, Cheltenham, Gloucestershire, England, to Florence Ada Pyne, eldest daughter of Mr. Charles Pyne, of West Melbourne, granddaughter of the late George Pyne, Esq., Bristol, Gloucestershire, England.

DEATH.

HACKETT.—On the 1st December, at 203 Bourke-street East, Thomas Masters, second son of Thomas Hackett, aged sixteen years.

ADDRESS TO STUDENTS.

THE *Chemical News* of 17th September has the following excellent address to students. The observations, both to those who are about to commence their studies and also to examiners, are so admirable that we feel confident that the article will be read with profit and pleasure. As the writer says, "Examinations are only a means, real or supposed, to a certain end, and not the end itself." Our youths must be taught and impressed with the idea that they must study "to know" as well as "pass," or the result will be disastrous, and end in intellectual debase-ment and futility. We therefore venture to think that this timely and judicious advice may have a salutary effect:—

"The duty or the policy—and the two are here identical—of a man entering upon any course of serious study is not as simple as was the case in former days. We refer not merely to the vastly increased extent of every science, to the enhanced accuracy now expected in all investigations, or to the rapid progress made in every department, which frequently compels us to revise before the end of the year views which we had adopted at its beginning. There is another and a more perplexing difficulty. Formerly, and even at present in some countries, the student had to keep in view one paramount object only. To whatever science he had devoted himself he had to make himself thoroughly master of its principles and its methods. The purpose of study was not so much to acquire a mere summary of what had already been discovered by others, as to become capable of continuing their work and of adding to the stores of truth which they had accumulated. The power of effecting such continuations and of making such additions is surely the best, the all-sufficient proof that the student's time has not been misspent.

"But in higher education, as conducted in modern England, this unity of purpose no longer exists, and this test of proficiency is no longer accepted. The student is required not merely to make himself, if possible, thoroughly acquainted with his subject, but to satisfy certain official persons that he has obtained such an acquaintance. If he does not succeed in the latter object his actual proficiency in the science in question will be of no avail. And if a due knowledge of such science be a part of the preparation required for some professional career, his time will have been in one sense wasted. Hence this latter object assumes the preponderance—the shadow outweighs the substance—and, in the never-to-be-forgotten words of Professor Huxley, we study in these days not to know but to 'pass,' the consequence being that we pass and don't know. The difficulty, then, placed before the British student is how to combine the two purposes; how, whilst qualifying himself to take a good position at an examination, he may at the same time become fitted for a career of research hereafter. We cannot, unfortunately, give any neat formula or recipe for compassing this object, but there are some considerations which may profitably be kept in mind. Let it be remembered that examinations are only a means, real or supposed, towards a certain end—not the end itself. When a man has got so far as to define, even in his secret thoughts, science as a mere something to be examined in, he is intellectually dead. In conjunction with this caution we must make a demand upon the moral nature of the student. We must exhort him, at whatever cost of time and labour, to eschew cram, including under the term all the tricks and dodges by which a really undisciplined mind is made to put on a false appearance of mastership. It is not safe to argue that the English system of examinations being essentially a sham, it may be legitimately evaded. He who wins degrees and diplomas by deceit will have acquired habits of dishonesty which will cling to him in after-life, and which will manifest themselves in a propensity for trimming and cooking results, for suppressing inconvenient facts, and forging evidences for a tottering theory. He who cheats examiners in his youth will in after-life be apt to cheat scientific societies and the learned world at large for his own glorification, and may, perhaps, for a time succeed.

"If we might presume to address a word of advice to examiners, we would recommend them, in place of reading up recondite matter in order to puzzle a student, to devise means for distinguishing true knowledge from mere cram, and intelligent comprehension of principles from the results of verbal memory."

The Month.

AT the termination of the meeting of the council of the Pharmaceutical Society an adjournment was made to the Union Club, where the health of our visitors—Messrs. Aicken and Langton—was drunk. In responding, Mr. Aicken said he felt very much the very kind and hospitable manner in which he had been treated in Victoria, and he trusted at no distant time to have the pleasure of seeing some of those present in New Zealand.

The Chemists and Druggists' Diary for 1881 will be issued to members and subscribers as early in the year as possible. They are expected to arrive the first week in January.

Mr. Rivers Langton (Messrs. Langton, Edden, Hicks and Clark, Thames-street, London), in response to the toast of his health, which was proposed at the conclusion of the Pharmaceutical Society's meeting at the Union Club, said that he had some experience in essential oils, and the truly magnificent Eucalyptus oil exhibit of Mr. Bosisto's at the International Exhibition reflected the greatest credit on that gentleman. The samples shown would successfully compare with the best makes of the world. Mr. Langton also spoke of the very great kindness and attention that had been shown him during his visit to the colonies.

The election of a member of the Pharmacy Board in the place of Mr. R. F. Kennedy, resigned, took place on the 18th November. There were three candidates—Messrs. Owen, Clemes, and Macgowan. The polling was not heavy, 320 only voting out of a possible 570. As usual, there were a great many informal and unsigned papers. The following are the numbers for each candidate :—Owen, 125 ; Clemes, 112 ; Macgowan, 83.

At the last council meeting of the Pharmaceutical Society a communication was read from Mr. Edward Mortensen, Ballarat, expressing his thanks for the assistance given to him in bringing his case before the Executive Council, which has resulted in his liberation.

Professor Halford, who is about to leave the colony on a visit to the medical schools of Europe, after eighteen years' labour in connection with the Melbourne University, was entertained at dinner at Gunsler's Café on the 11th November.

The gathering was a most successful one ; there were about sixty-five gentlemen present.

We are desired to state that the Pharmaceutical Register will not, as heretofore, be published in *The Chemist and Druggist.* The council of the Pharmaceutical Society have decided, in consequence of the expense attendant on its re-publication, to discontinue it. The official copy can be obtained—price one shilling—at the offices of the Pharmacy Board, 100 Collins-street West.

The following have been added to the legally qualified medical practitioners registered under the provisions of the Medical Practitioners Statute, 1865 :—Joseph Higham Hill, Fitzroy; Arthur Alma Johnston, Moonee Ponds; Richard Henry Symes, Melbourne.

Meetings.

THE PHARMACEUTICAL SOCIETY OF VICTORIA.

THE monthly meeting of the council was held at the rooms on the 5th November, 1880 ; present—Messrs. Blackett, Baker, Bowen, Jones, Francis, Hooper, Huntsman, Norris, and Shillinglaw ; the president, Mr. Blackett, in the chair.

The minutes of the previous meeting were read and confirmed.

An apology was read from Mr. Macgowan for his absence.

New Members.—John Nathaniel Bird, of Carlton, was elected, and Frederick C. Cook, Prahan ; Henry W. Potts, Brisbane ; George Fox Ward, Semaphore, Port Adelaide ; David Jones, Ballarat, and Charles Ross, Chapel-street, Windsor, were nominated as members.

School of Pharmacy.—A copy of a resolution passed by the Pharmacy Board on this subject was received and discussed, and, on the motion of Mr. Bowen, a committee appointed to deal with the matter.

Finance and other Committees.—Mr. J. C. Jones's motion in reference to the appointment of a number of committees to manage the affairs of the society was after some discussion rejected, a motion being proposed by Mr. Francis, and carried, that the business be conducted as at present.

The Dinner Committee.— On the motion of Mr. J. C. Jones, a vote of thanks was carried to Messrs. Bowen, Thomas, and Shillinglaw for the very satisfactory manner in which the dinner was carried out.

The President of the Pharmaceutical Society of New Zealand was elected an honorary member.

During the evening Mr. Graves Aicken and Mr. Rivers Langton were present as visitors.

Correspondence.—Letters were received and dealt with from the following persons :—G. A. Prichard, A. Kibblewhite, W. C. Bohn, H. W. Potts, J. M. Murphy, James Tipping, J. G. Bloore, G. Gammon, R. W. Fairthorne, J. B. Hudson, D. Tomlinson, G. B. Fairbourne, John Barker, G. P. Philpots, the Secretary Pharmaceutical Society, New South Wales.

Financial and routine business brought the meeting to a close.

BOOKS, &c., RECEIVED.—*American Journal of Pharmacy, Boston Journal of Chemistry, Pharmaceutical Journal, Australian Medical Journal, New York Druggists' Circular, The Seventh Decade of the Eucalyptus of Australia.*

THE PHARMACY BOARD OF VICTORIA.

THE monthly meeting was held on the 10th November ; present—Messrs. Bowen, Brind, Holdsworth, Lewis, and Kruse. On the motion of Mr. Lewis, Mr. Brind took the chair.

A telegram was received from the president, who was unable, from business engagements, to attend.

Applications for Registration as Pharmaceutical Chemists. —The following were passed :—Daniel C. O'Connor, Beechworth ; Charles Ross, Chapel-street, Windsor ; Augustus F. Sapsford, Maryborough, Queensland ; and James Anderson Moonee Ponds. The indentures of S. V. Say were transferred from J. Jelfs, deceased, to A. E. Hughes.

School of Pharmacy.—The notice of motion given by Mr. Bowen on this subject was further discussed, and the following resolution agreed to :—Moved by Mr. Bowen, and seconded by Mr. Lewis, and carried—"That in consequence of the unsatisfactory nature of the reply from the Melbourne University, this board is of opinion that it would be desirable to establish, and is prepared to recognise any efficient School of Pharmacy where the instruction required by part 4, clause 18, of the Pharmacy Act could be obtained ; and that a copy of this resolution be forwarded to the council of the Pharmaceutical Society."

Names Erased from the Register.—In accordance with the provisions of the 13th section of the Pharmacy Act, letters were sent to the last known address of the following persons, asking if they had changed their residence. The letters having been returned unclaimed, their names were removed from the register :—J. M. Ryan, Warrnambool ; A. Bekkevold, Stawell ; J. L. Anderson, Castlemaine ; J. E. Williams, St. Kilda ; F. J. Searle, Fitzroy ; G. S. Allingham, Peel-street, Windsor ; L. Meyring, Melbourne ; R. Hustwick, Geelong ; T. D. Rutter, Buln Buln ; F. J. Negus, Williamstown ; A. S. Beaven, Romsey ; J. C. Hallam, Melbourne.

Correspondence.—Letters were received and dealt with from the following persons :—Mrs. Summers, F. H. Smith, F. Longmore, R. D. Murray, the police (Clunes and Sandhurst), the Registrar Melbourne University.

The Pharmaceutical Register for 1881.—The registrar was authorised to take the necessary steps to print and circulate the register for the year.

Financial and general business brought the meeting to a close.

THE ANNUAL DINNER.

THE annual dinner of the Pharmaceutical Society of Victoria was held at Clement's Café on Thursday, the 18th November, when there was a good attendance. The president, Mr. C. R. Blackett, occupied the chair, and on his right was seated Mr. Cosmo Newbery, and on his left Dr. Moloney and Mr. Gillbee, Messrs. Bosisto and Bowen occupying the vice-chairs. The country districts were represented by Mr. Holdsworth, Sandhurst ; Messrs. Wheeler and Macgowan, Ballarat ; and Mr. A. J. Owen, Geelong. Letters of apology were received from Messrs. H. Brind, Ballarat ; R. Ellery, F. S. Grimwade, A. E. Pulling, T. M. Blackett, S. S. Strutt, W. J. Branscombe, and Drs. Day, Nield, Girdlestone, and Henry. The catering, as might be expected, was served in Mr. Clement's best style, and afforded satisfaction. The president proposed the usual loyal toasts in suitable terms, and they were drunk with musical honours.

Dr. Moloney then proposed the health of the Pharmaceutical Society of Victoria, coupling with it the name of the president, Mr. Blackett. The society had started in 1857, and but very few of the originators of it were now present. It was to the founders that the Pharmaceutical Society owed the fact that it was now a powerful and influential body. (Cheers.) If there were proportionately as many such downright earnest men in his profession, he felt sure that the status of medical men would vastly improve. (Applause.) It was strange, though true, that the medical profession was not represented in Parliament, when the Pharmaceutical Society had a representative of whom they might be justly proud—(applause)—and he regretted that another gentleman, their respected president, had failed to obtain his seat in the Legislative Assembly ; but if that gentleman desired to be still honest and a patriot, he must content himself with remaining a little longer out of Parliament. (Laughter and cheers.) He was glad to observe that the pharmacists were at last obtaining that which they had so long been foreign to—fair play. (Cheers.) It was a strange fact that amateurs in every other sphere of life, except in pharmacy and medicine, were treated with contempt, but even in regard to this matter, the prospects of the Pharmaceutical Society were vastly improving. (Applause.) He had to say that the medical man received a great amount of assistance from the chemist and druggist which often proved valuable to him. It was true there were instances where medical men had to complain of their chemists and druggists, but every one expected to find black sheep in every flock ; and the same had to be said of the profession of which he was a representative. But these remarks of his did not refer to the members of the Pharmaceutical Society, but to the impertinent outsider who foists himself on the public, and will, he was sure, die out by "effluxion of time." (Laughter and applause.) He would very much like to see fairer play given to the society and medical men as well, and a chair of pharmacy established, the beneficial results of which he would not attempt to estimate. (Applause.) This could not be done, but by united action. The Government, he was sure, would afford no help ; and from the University but little assistance could be expected. The only way would be to establish a School of Pharmacy, and then they could boast of having such men as their president and other worthy representatives of the society as "professors" of it. (Cheers.) This proposition, if carried out, would remove all difficulties in the way of examinations, &c., for he had only the other day learnt with great regret from the worthy secretary of the society that there were several students awaiting examination, and unable to undertake what they desired. The establishment of the school would foster *reunions* and establish an *esprit de corps* necessary to the welfare of the society, besides stimulating young and promising men to spend time in the discovery of new and useful drugs. (Hear, hear.) Mr. Bosisto had done much towards the consummation of this latter object, and had given Australia a prominent position in the pharmaceutical world. In conclusion, he had only to say again, that from his personal experience the greatest care and vigilance was practised by pharmacists in the preparation of prescriptions. The manner in which this was carried out was unique ; and in the suburbs just as well as in town a medical man could depend on having his prescriptions prepared with the greatest care. He proposed the health of the Pharmaceutical Society coupled with the name of Mr. Blackett. (Applause.)

The toast was drunk enthusiastically.

Mr. Blackett, in responding, thanked the proposer for the kind terms in which he had couched the language of his toast. He regretted the absence of Dr. Gray, the president of the Medical Society, who was unavoidably absent. The Pharmaceutical Society of Victoria was the first of its kind in the southern hemisphere, and it was a matter for congratulation to the members of the society that they had first led the way to the opening of so many other similar institutions in the other colonies. The founders of the society had undoubtedly done much good ; and he trusted that those who would follow would strive to emulate the example of their predecessors—(cheers)—and that the future might be more glorious than the past. (Applause.) He was one of the few left who started the society in 1857 ; and then there was Mr. Bosisto, whose name had already become so much respected, and Mr. Johnson, who had held the position of Government analyst for so long a period, and discharged his duties in such a manner that he had gained a reputation for himself, and reflected honour on the Pharmaceutical Society, and some others who were happily still with us. He would like to see those coming after them treading in the footsteps of these men. The establishment of the Victorian society stimulated the pharmacists of New Zealand to originate one themselves. New South Wales followed, and now Queensland, and there was a prospect of South Australia adopting the good example of the sister colonies. (Cheers.) He trusted the laws of the Pharmaceutical Societies would not diverge, but be more in unison. They had wished for a Pharmacy Act, and now had the pleasure of seeing their desire fulfilled. He remembered the time when that Act was under debate in the House, and how Mr. Bosisto had to answer the criticisms of Messrs. Gaunson, Longmore, and other members who were opposed to it. He had only to say that their representative stood the attacks like a martyr, and his replies silenced the opponents of the

Act. (Applause.) Of course that Act was not perfect, but it was the best they could get at the time. By the light of experience they found in it flaws, which at the time were not detected. These mistakes, he trusted, would be rectified as soon as the Assembly settled down to useful legislation, and peace was restored to this politically afflicted country. (Laughter and cheers.) The new Pharmacy Act would give larger powers than those possessed at present, and limit the sale of patent medicines. It was monstrous to suppose that ignorant men should be allowed to dispense poisonous medicines simply because the bottle or packet had a stamp and a seal on it. It was also, in his opinion, a dangerous practice to allow grocers to sell unchecked such large quantities of patent medicines, and he considered that any wise Government would remedy this defect. In regard to the suggestion to establish a school of pharmacy, he was convinced that there was abundance of talent in the members of the society to carry out the undertaking, but what seemed to stand in the way was the want of cash. (Laughter.) He would, however, in the event of the suggestion being carried out, like to see the school taken under the wing of the University. If, however, this could not be effected, he would be satisfied to see pharmacy added to the curriculum of studies in the University for medicine. (Cheers.) Why, he (the speaker) knew of an instance where an M.B. did not know the difference between opium and asafœtida. (Laughter.) To his mind it was incumbent for medical men to study *materia medica* more than they did. (Cheers.) And now he had to say a word about the journal representing the society. He admitted that it was an imperfect one, but he was quite certain that it was better than nothing, and that efforts were made to make it interesting and valuable. (Cheers.) What the paper wanted was fresh writing. He did what he could, and was ably assisted by Mr. Shillinglaw, but much could be done by young pharmacists contributing original papers. He hoped that this matter would be attended to, and his appeal receive a ready response. The journal, he was sure, had done much good, not only here, but in the neighbouring colonies; and, with support, was sure it would become a valuable property; and he hoped that it would ultimately be able to run alone, and become, like the *Medical Journal*, the independent organ of pharmacy in Australasia.

Mr. Best, in a few well-chosen remarks, couched in eulogistic terms, proposed the health of the members of the Pharmacy Board, coupled with the name of Mr. Bosisto.

Mr. Bosisto, in thanking the company for the hearty manner in which the toast of the Pharmacy Board had been drunk, said the object of the Board was to seek to educate the young pharmacists in this colony to a standpoint equal to those in other countries of the old world. He was astonished at the progress made by the Board, and at the beneficial results that had accrued from its establishment. He felt sure that what had been done would prove an incentive to the rising generation. He regretted to find that the University did not recognise pharmacy as it ought to, as, in his opinion, it ought to be included in the curriculum of medical studies. (Hear, hear.) He trusted that in the alteration of the University Amendment Bill the medical faculty would recognise this fact, and endeavour to have the study of *materia medica* enforced on a broader basis than the present. And not only did he desire to see this object attained, but that medical botany would be taught as well. (Hear, hear.) He trusted that the day was not far distant when the University would see its way to establish a school of pharmacy, which would meet all the difficulties that they had at present to encounter. (Cheers.) He did not think that it was the duty of a chemist to merely learn the art of coating pills, but to obtain knowledge regarding the different plants and other vegetation which so vast a field lay open for them in Australia. By so doing they would thereby be handing down to posterity knowledge which would be at once useful to generations to come and make to themselves great names. The Pharmacy Board were willing to help, and he hoped that young men would take advantage of the opportunities.

Mr. Francis proposed the health of the Pharmaceutical Society of Great Britain and kindred societies.

Mr. Bowen, in responding, referred to the names of Jacob Bell, William Allen, Thomas Nurson, Dr. Pereira, Theophilus Redwood, and others, who had so readily come forward to establish the Pharmaceutical Society of Great Britain, and otherwise to promote the cause of pharmacy. The names of these gentlemen were still fresh in the memory of some around us, and associated with many great and good deeds,

especially so, the exposure of the frauds perpetrated by some of the English and Continental manufacturers of chemical and pharmaceutical products. It was a singular circumstance that Great Britain, which usually takes the lead in art, science, and literature, should be the last to recognise the necessity of establishing a school of pharmacy. Norway, a country possessing at that period a population of about 350,000 souls—less than half that of the colony of Victoria—was the first to do so in the year 1673. France followed in 1803; the United States next; Germany in 1823; Russia in 1839; and, last of all, Great Britain, in 1841. The establishment of these schools, to his mind, was an imperative necessity, for however skilful the physician or general practitioner might be, unless the prescription was uniformly and honestly dispensed that skill would be thrown away. (Cheers.)

Mr. Johnson proposed the medical societies of Victoria, coupled with the name of Mr. Gillbee. He was nothing of a speaker, and had only experience in that line when badgered by counsel in the witness-box.

Mr. Gillbee, in responding, said he had need scarcely to mention that, as a rule, physicians endeavoured to keep up as friendly an association with their chemists as practicable. The medical man depended entirely in them for the proper preparation of his prescriptions, and he had to say, from his own experience and that of other members of his profession, that their directions were attended to with the greatest care and precision. (Hear, hear.) He trusted that the Pharmaceutical Society would soon rise above a trade, and establish itself into a profession—(cheers)—so that no one would be allowed to tamper with the lives of the general public without having a State certificate of competency to dispense medicines. (Applause.)

The president said that the next toast he had to propose was one he knew they would all drink with great pleasure. The toast was the health of Mr. Shillinglaw, the honorary secretary of the society. (Applause.) As the president of the society, perhaps no one was better acquainted with the large amount of work annually performed by the honorary secretary, and he felt certain all would agree with him when he said that the present prosperous condition of the society was in a great degree owing to the admirable manner in which the business was conducted; no matter what information was required, you had but to apply to Mr. Shillinglaw for it, and it was at once forthcoming. They were not, perhaps, aware of the very large amount of additional work the publication of *The Chemist and Druggist* had entailed. In the official position held by Mr. Shillinglaw as registrar to the Pharmacy Board, he had earned the respect and esteem of all with whom he had been brought in contact. The toast was drunk amidst great cheering.

Mr. Shillinglaw, in replying, said that he felt very much pleased at the kind and hearty manner in which his health had been drunk. His duties had been very much lightened by uniform kindness and courtesy shown to him by the members of the council. He had endeavoured to extend the members' roll outside Victoria, he was glad to find, with some success, and a number of leading pharmacists in the neighbouring colonies were now members of the society; and the circulation of the journal had trebled itself during the last three years; not a little of the success of the journal was due to Mr. Blackett, who gave a deal of valuable time to it. There could be no doubt that the journal had done much good, and induced the other colonies to form societies. He again begged to thank them for the kind manner in which the toast had been received.

"The Ballarat District Chemists' Association," coupled with the names of Messrs. Wheeler and Macgowan, was the next toast proposed by Mr. Blackett, who said it was highly gratifying to find this district society so well represented. He hoped to see the other districts follow in the footsteps of Ballarat, and form local societies.

Mr. Macgowan returned thanks, and remarked that it was owing to the troubles and difficulties of the tariff some twelve months ago that had called their society into existence. He was glad to say the formation of the association had done great good in promoting general unanimity and good feeling. He hoped to see the other large centres of population follow their example; and he thanked them very much for the kind manner in which they had drunk the toast.

The health of Mr. Holdsworth, as the representative of Sandhurst, was also proposed.

In responding, Mr. Holdsworth remarked that he was gratified to take part in so successful a gathering. He had attended the first meeting of the society, which consisted of Messrs. Ford, Croad, Plummer, Glover, Drewry, and himself. That was just twenty-four years ago. He had always taken a great interest in the society, and was pleased to see it attain the importance it had.

Mr. Rocke, in a humorous speech, proposed " The Press," which was responded to hy Dr. Moloney.

" The Ladies" was proposed by the chairman, and responded to by Mr. Ross, who remarked that he thought that it was a pity that the annual ball had been discontinued, and ladies excluded from taking part in the festive gatherings.

During the evening Messrs. Plunket, Atkin, Rocke, and Blogg sang several songs, which added greatly to the enjoyment of the evening. The music was by Plock's band.

SOCIAL SCIENCE CONGRESS.

THE Agricultural and Horticultural Section of the Social Science Congress was opened on the 29th November, when Baron von Mueller, president of the section, delivered the opening address. On the following day Mr. Abraham Lincolne read a paper on ' The Milk Supply of Towns," and in the discussion which followed the necessity was urged for the appointment of an official to inspect the dairies which now supply milk to Melbourne and its suburbs. Mr. J. C. Cole also read a paper on " Pomology." In the evening Mr. W. Murray Ross contributed a paper showing the advantages to be gained by encouraging the manufacture of beet-root sugar in Victoria. Mr. C. May, of Sunbury, read two papers—one upon " The Olive and its Cultivation in Victoria," and the other upon " Insect Pests of Fruit-bearing Trees." The following papers were also read :—By Mr. C. H. Lyon, of Ballan, on the " Clearing of Land ;" by Mr. E. Hulme, of Oxley, on the " Comparative Merits of Large and Small Farms;" by Mr. R. W. E. Macfvor, on " Experimental Farming." Two interesting subjects were dealt with on the 1st December. Mr. D. Howitz read a paper upon the " Climate Influence and Preservation of Forests ;" and Mr. W. R. Guilfoyle, F.L.S., another upon " Sylvan Streets," in which he gave some useful information with respect to the best mode of planting trees in the streets and the best trees to be selected. In the evening Mr. W. Kendall contributed a paper upon "Veterinary Education," and Mr. Graham Mitchell one upon " Diseases of Stock." The following papers were read at the afternoon meeting :—By Mr. D. Howitz, on " The Relative Timber Producing Capabilities of Exotic and Indigenous Trees ;" by Mr. J. Hall, of Hastings, on " Some Exotic Trees ;" by Mr. A. D. Hunter, on " The Utilisation of Sewage." In the evening Mr. B. D. Smith, of Buln Buln, and Mr. R. W. F. Macfvor contributed papers upon " Scientific Agricultural Education."

Personalities.

MR. CHARLES ROSS, who was for some time at Malden Island, has returned to Victoria, and purchased a business in Prahran. The premises and stock of Mr. J. F. F. Grace, of St. Arnaud, have been destroyed by fire. Mr. Grace announces hy circular that he will re-open with a new stock, &c., on the 29th inst.

We regret to state that Mr. Jackson, manufacturing chemist for Messrs. Felton, Grimwade, met with an accident by the bursting of a bottle at the Exhibition. We are glad to say it is, however, not of so serious a nature as was at first expected.

Amongst the visitors attracted by the Exhibition from the other colonies, we have pleasure in noticing the arrival of Mr. Graves Aicken from Auckland. Mr. Aicken, who is a member of the Pharmacy Board of New Zealand, and one of the vice-presidents of the Pharmaceutical Society, was entertained at dinner by Mr. Johnson, the Government analyst, on the 26th instant. On the 29th, by invitation of Mr. Bosisto, he met the members of the Pharmacy Board at dinner. Mr. Aicken was entertained at lunch by Mr. Blackett on the 3rd December. In response to his health, which was drunk at the various festivities, he expressed himself as much gratified at the hospitality and courtesy shown him. We feel certain Mr. Aicken's visit will do a great deal of good in promoting that good feeling which should exist between the kindred societies.

UNIVERSITY OF MELBOURNE.

ORDINARY EXAMINATIONS.—OCTOBER TERM, 1880.

Practical Chemistry.—R. Aitchison, H. R. Maclean, F. A. Nyulasy, C. H. Flack, P. Wisewould.

Materia Medica.—F. H. Cole, G. J. Scantlebury, P. Wisewould.

PHARMACY BOARD EXAMINATIONS.

PRELIMINARY.—2ND DECEMBER, 1880.

THE following passed in the order of merit in which their names appear :—
Charles Alfred Graves, Sale.
George Clark, Sandhurst.
A. E. Pilley, Windsor.
T. S. Woodfull, Melbourne.
Thomas Gardiner, Sandhurst.

FOURTEENTH MODIFIED EXAMINATION.—6TH DECEMBER.

The following passed, and are now eligible for registration as pharmaceutical chemists :—
Joseph Thomas Poock, 183 Bourke-street, Melbourne.
Thomas Shanassy, Mount Gambier.
Walter Fisher, Sandhurst.

BALLARAT.

THE School of Mines, at the late Horticultural Society's Show, made a splendid exhibit of about seventy specimens of medicinal plants, nicely arranged, and labelled with its botanical and vulgar name, class, natural order, genus, species, country, the portion of plant used, and its therapeutic properties ; and when we mention that the whole of these were grown in the small botanical garden attached to the school especially for the use of students studying *materia medica*, &c., it must be taken as another illustration of the school's efficiency and earnestness in imparting a practical and perfect pharmaceutical education to our young men, and is well deserving the liberal support of our local pharmacists.

Either the serious illness of Mr. Mortensen, or the powerful and influential petition presented to His Excellency on his behalf, or both combined, have had the effect of restoring him once more to his family circle, from which he had been estranged. To this change, care of his medical attendants, and the comforts of his home must be attributed for producing a favourable reaction on his system ; and though his trials must have undermined a rather weekly constitution, the sympathy evinced by his brother pharmacists and other gentlemen have acted most favourably on him. We are requested, on his behalf, to acknowledge, with much gratitude, his indebtedness to those who lent their influence for his release, as it will enable him once more to battle hopefully with the world, and to maintain himself and family independently.

The dispensary of our district hospital has lately, at the hands of Mr. G. Bailey, a recent arrival from London, undergone a thorough renovation—walls repainted, fixtures French polished, bottles re-lettered, and it now looks speck, span, and new ; this was a work much needed, and we congratulate the committee on getting it done in such a neat and appropriate style.

An example of the carelessness and ignorance that still unhappily prevails with some regarding medicines was aptly illustrated by one John Hellyer (aged eighteen years), of Mount Clear, who, instead of taking, as he intended, a dose of Eno's Fruit Salt, made a mistake, and took half a powder containing antim. nig., which had been prepared and intended for one of his master's horses ; his feelings, however, soon warned him that something was wrong, and the cause being found, he was then taken to the district hospital, promptly treated, and is now, we hope, a wiser, if sadder young man.

BALLARAT DISTRICT CHEMISTS' ASSOCIATION.

THE usual monthly meeting was held at Lester's Hotel, Sturt-street, on Wednesday evening, 17th November. There was a fair attendance of members ; Mr. Palmer, president, in the chair.

A letter was read from Mr. H. W. Potts, of the firm of Potts and Berkley, chemists, Brisbane, Queensland, asking for a copy of the rules and regulations of the association, and for any further information that could be given, as they were desirous of forming a similar association in Brisbane. The honorary secretary said that he had forwarded a copy of the rules, and written to Mr. Potts, offering some suggestions upon the initiation of the society.

The president remarked upon the influence the association was exercising, even in the other colonies.

The honorary secretary reported that the Governor-in-Council had released Mortensen from gaol before the expiration of his sentence.

The committee of the friendly societies had determined upon opening a dispensary, and expected to be ready to commence on 1st January, 1881. They were about to advertise for a dispenser.

A telegram was received from Mr. Shillinglaw, stating that Mr. Owen, of Geelong, had been elected to a seat on the Pharmacy Board, vice Mr. Kennedy, resigned.

Some matters of business routine having been transacted, the meeting closed with a vote of thanks to the chair.

COSTLESS VENTILATION.

Mr. Holdsworth sends us clippings from Sleeman's *Export Drug Circular*, and directs attention to a process of "costless ventilation," which he says has been used with great success in his own house for the last three years, and recommends others to try the experiment. Mr. H. says that a room or nursery so ventilated have none of the unpleasant smells (when entering them from the fresh air) that bedrooms usually have, which clearly proves the efficacy of the method. Attention is also drawn to an excellent method of disinfecting rooms after and during sickness by the means of carbolic acid (No. 5 will answer) ; and its efficacy at the present time may be clearly proved, in cases of sickness from measles and whooping cough—in the latter case especially, as by the inhalation of the vapour it produces the same effect that is supposed to be produced by taking children to a gas house during that malady, which is no uncommon thing on Sandhurst. The simplicity of the process recommends itself as much superior to only placing deodorants or disinfectants on the floors or furniture of the apartments, as by burning the acid on hot coals or embers the vapour reaches the ceiling, and every nook and corner of the room. Directions : Take a small pan of red hot embers from the fire, and drop upon them about a teaspoonful of No. 5 carbolic acid, moving about the room during the process. If this is done at night, it can be repeated in the morning with excellent effect. Be careful of the fingers during the process.

A constant supply of fresh air is so important to our well-being, and in the prevention and cure of disease, that the subject needs no comment ; an attendance, however, at any public meeting is only necessary to convince how much this axiom is ignored—or, if admitted, how unsuccessfully met— "crowded to suffocation," indeed, being the conventional term used to express a full assemblage.

For some time, says Dr. Hinckes-Bird, I recommended to my patients the plan of opening the window-sash at the top, and stretching out on a frame a corresponding depth of tarlatan to intercept blacks and prevent draughts ; but the principle is wrong, and the results unsatisfactory, as the draught is directed downwards on the sitter, and not upwards towards the ceiling ; the screen, too, is anything but ornamental, and becomes clogged with blacks, so as to require removal and repair.

The method I now use is simple, economical, quite free from draught, can be regulated to a nicety, and does not get out of order. Raise the lower sash of the window, and place in front of the opening at the bottom rail a piece of wood of any approved depth—from two to three inches is sufficient ; this leaves a corresponding space between the meeting rails in the middle of the window through which the current of air is directed upwards towards the ceiling ; heavy blacks cannot ascend with the air, which is driven so high as to be warm before it descends ; light blacks are not admitted in ordinary conditions of the atmosphere, though doubtless they are in cases of violent commotion caused by very high wind—the more the lower sash is raised the more the difficulty of blacks entering between the meeting rails is increased. The principle may be modified in various ways, making the lower bending of wire blinds supersede the strip of wood, or if this be placed above and the top sash drawn down, to a corresponding depth, the same result will obtain ; in a word, open the lower sash of the window two or three inches, and block it up anyhow, and the air enters the space

in the middle and is carried to the ceiling. In the *Sanitary Hints* I have circulated in the district to which I am medical officer of health, it is more tersely described thus :—" Raise the lower sash of the window two or three inches, and fill the opening underneath the bottom rail with a piece of wood— this leaves a corresponding space between the meeting rails in the middle of the window, through which a current of air enters, and is directed towards the ceiling, whence it should escape by a valvular opening." The sand-bag, so frequently placed over the meeting-rails to prevent fresh air coming in, should, the greater part of the year, be placed under the lower sash, so as to allow air to enter at the meeting rails.

Correspondence.

THE CASE OF THE QUEEN V. TURNER.
To the Editor of The Australasian Supplement to the Chemist and Druggist.

Sir—When a person seeks the advice of an attorney or doctor-at-law, or as in the case of the Pharmaceutical Society of Victoria did in the above case, you are generally bound to accept his advice ; but it appears to me that the privileges enjoyed by the druggists of Victoria were not properly understood by the magistrates who heard the case at Colac. Even the Medical Practitioners Statute does not infringe upon those privileges, but rather upholds them, in that it provides a clause for that purpose. Part 2 section 14 of that Act provides that " Nothing in this part of the Act shall be *construed* to infringe on the rights and privileges hitherto enjoyed by chemists and druggists and dentists." Now, I uphold that Mr. Turner did nothing at all wrong in prescribing the simple remedies he did, and if any one was to be blamed or prosecuted it was the person who employed Mr. Turner, for if a child dies without medical attendance a certificate of death is refused, hence an inquest ; and if neglect can be proved, a committal of the parents or guardians follows. Again, even a properly qualified medical man is always open for damages if mal-treatment can be proved ; but this, even, was not proved against Turner ! I for one am not satisfied ; for if a chemist can be fined through a clause in the Pharmacy Act, it is like being condemned out of the mouth of babes and sucklings.
J. HOLDSWORTH.

"DARNEL."
To the Editor of The Australasian Supplement to the Chemist and Druggist.

Sir—Mr. Mitchell's inferential deduction regarding the seed of Lolium temulentum causing the death of one and illness of other cows because of its having been found in the mash or grains obtained from a distillery, and on which the cows were fed, has, I think, been drawn a little too precipitately, inasmuch as the poisonous properties of this grass seed has, I think, on the whole, been rather disproved than supported. I have heard of its having been given to pigs with impunity ; and though this may be no proof it would not kill cows, yet the researches which, some time since, were made on the Continent, completely established its perfect harmlessness and to this view I incline.

The contamination of malt with this seed, ergo, affecting the beer produced therefrom, I cannot think in any way can be supported, doubting whether a hundred grains of it could be found in a hundred thousand bushels of any malt used by any brewers either in town or country ; for when the barley is steeped any light grain such as the darnel (or drake) will always float, even if the barley is of such an even quality as not to require screening (the first and usual preparatory step to malting). Now, either of these processes should, and I think does, effectually remove it from the grain to be malted ; and having seen a good deal of malt, I cannot recall one instance of ever seeing darnel in it, so that I think we must look further afield than to the one in question for the ill effects found in the trashy ales alluded to. Darnel is only grown by tyro farmers and dirty farming, and will ultimately be as scarce in samples of grain here as at the present time it is in those from England or New Zealand ; but even now I do not think it a recognised or marketable commodity, or ever should or will be, but I should very much like to hear of Mr. Mitchell, or other scientist, conducting a few experiments, so that its actual properties may be elicited beyond a doubt.—Yours, HORDEUM.

A WORD FOR THE PHARMACEUTICAL SOCIETY.

To the Editor of The Australasian Supplement to the Chemist and Druggist.

SIR—The present seems an opportune time to say a word to those pharmacists who have not yet joined our society. The senate of the University having declined to institute a chair of pharmacy, the entire responsibility of pharmaceutical education is thrown back upon ourselves. We must establish our own school; this requires money and organisation. In the Pharmaceutical Society we have the latter; to the whole body of chemists we must reasonably look for the former. Hitherto the "sinews of war" have been furnished by a section only, who have voluntarily borne the whole burden. It is not fair that this should continue. Since all are interested, each man should contribute. At home membership of the society is compelled by law; but I hope better things of my brethren here than that an Act of Parliament will be needed to teach them their duty. I know there are those who are not satisfied with the society, but I would urge that the remedy is in their own hands. Let them join its ranks, and it will be what they make it; and I would further suggest that a better acquaintance would remove or modify some of the objections. It is often said—What is the good of all this education? It neither puts money into our pockets, nor makes us more respected. Time will prove this statement to be unfounded. But, even if it were true, we cannot help it. We dare not stand still; we cannot. The rest of the world is moving on, and, if we do not move with it, we shall be left behind. Every schoolboy will know more of chemistry, and botany, and of physical science generally, than did the chemists of a few years ago. When the mechanic calls science to his aid, the chemist dare not neglect it, if he values his reputation or his bread. The public will soon learn to discriminate between the educated pharmacist and the mere seller of drugs, and will bestow their patronage accordingly. I will not, however, further enlarge upon this theme; but, in conclusion, will re-state the facts:—The fiat has gone forth—we must be educated; the Pharmaceutical Society must undertake the work, and money is needed. This the chemists must supply. The question is—Will each man join the society, and so contribute his share, or must the willing horse do all the work. I trust, for our credit's sake, "that every man will do his duty."—I am, yours truly,   ALFRED OWEN.

Notes and Abstracts.

CLOTH, linen, paper, straw, &c., can be rendered fire proof (incombustible) by immersing them into a boiling solution of pure ammonium sulphate eight parts, ammonium carbonate 2½ parts, boracic acid three parts, pure borax 1·7 parts, and starch two parts, in water 100 parts.—*Pharm. Ztschr. f. Russl.,* 15th Feb., 1880, p. 120.

Concentrated tincture of insect powder (tinctura pyrethri florum concentrata) is highly recommended as an insecticide by Finzelberg, who prepares the tincture in the proportion of one part Persian insect powder to ten parts absolute alcohol, and claims that in order to prove efficient, it is necessary to scatter it by means of a perfume atomiser. When thus used in a closed room all flies soon drop dead, while scattering it over linen, &c., acts as a protection against fleas, &c.—*Pharm. Centralh.,* 1st April, 1880, p. 118.

Grimault's Indian hemp cigarettes are highly recommended for asthma, other affections of the breathing organs, and various other diseases, consist almost altogether, as the French manufacturer claims, of Indian hemp and a little saltpetre, and are far superior to the ordinary remedies, which consist of the leaves of belladonna, of nicotina, or of paper—all impregnated with saltpetre, opium, or even arsenic. An analysis, made by Dr. H. Braun, proved, however, that Grimault's cigarettes consist chiefly, in contradiction to the manufacturer's statements, of belladonna leaves, contaminated (we might almost say) with a few fragments of cannabis, and of two other species of leaves, one of which greatly resembles the leaves of epilobium. — *Ztschr. d. Allg. Oest. Apoth. Ver.,* 10th April, 1880, p. 168.

COLD AIR FRUIT CURING.—The California *Mountain Messenger* reports an interesting experiment in fruit curing lately made at a Placerville foundry. About a peck of sliced apples were placed in a sieve and subjected to a cold air blast for three and a-half hours in the cupola furnace of the foundry, and the fruit is reported to have been completely and beauti-

fully cured by the treatment, remaining soft and without the slightest discolouration. The cured fruit showed none of the harsh, stiff dryness which results from hot curing, the cold blast completely freeing the fruit from excess of moisture, with no possibility of burning or shrivelling it. The *Messenger* says:—"Compared with our sun-drying, it effects a great saving of expense, attention, and risk. Anybody who can command or devise a strong blast of cold air, can dry fruit in a superior—we might say perfect—manner, without being dependent on the weather and waiting on the slow process of sun-drying, and without the most expensive resort to fuel and the risk of overheating."

THE GREENING OF PRESERVED VEGETABLES.—It is known that the green colour given to preserved vegetables is generally obtained by means of the salts of copper, the presence of which in preserves is both dangerous and fraudulent. M. Lecourt, a preserve manufacturer of Paris, and Professor Guillemare, of the Lycée of Rheims, have devised a new process for such colouration which is the subject of an interesting report addressed to the Consultative Committee of Public Hygiene of France by MM. Wurtz, Gavarre, and Bussy. This new process consists in adding to the vegetables employed a surcharge of chlorophyll, so that after the inevitable loss caused by boiling at 120 deg. Cent., they still retain sufficient to present the green colour of fresh vegetables. MM. Lecourt and Guillemare obtain all the green colour thus utilised from table vegetables, especially spinach, which contains a great quantity that is easily extracted. By an appropriate manipulation they obtain this green matter in solution in water alkalised by soda. The application of the colour is made thus:—The vegetables being plunged in boiling water, previously acidulated by chlorohydric acid, a suitable quantity of the solution of chlorophyll is turned into the water; by saturation of the soda, by means of chlorohydric acid, sea salt is produced, and the colouring matter is deposited in the organic tissue to increase the intensity of its proper colour. The vegetables thus treated are submitted to several washings before being enclosed in the vessels in which they are to be submitted to the high temperature necessary for their conservation.

PALM OIL.—That portion of the west coast of Africa which lies south of the River Volta furnishes the principal supplies of palm oil. Nearly 1,000,000 cwt. of this oil are annually exported to Great Britain, of the value of 7,500,000 dols., its principal use being in the manufacture of soaps, perfumery, candles, and similar articles. Among the natives it is highly valued, both for food (taking the place of butter), for lighting and cooking purposes, and for anointing the head and body. The so-called oil, which is rather a fatty substance, resembling butter in appearance, is obtained from the fruit of several species of palms, but especially from the one known botanically as *Elais guineensis,* which grows in abundance on the western coast of Africa, and from which it takes its specific name. So thickly do these trees grow, and so regular and rapid are their supplies of fruit, that in some localities where the regular collection of the produce is not practised the ground becomes covered with a thick deposit of the oily, fatty matter produced by the ripe berries. Deposits of palm oil, which may almost be called "mines" of vegetable fat, exist in some parts of the Gold Coast, and which, if not in themselves worth working, at least practically illustrate the natural wealth of the country in such productions, and indicate its undeveloped resources. These "mines" would probably not repay the cost of exploration, as the palm oil is apt to become rancid and valueless for its general uses after long exposure, though for such purposes as candle making these deposits might still be valuable.— *Colonies and India.*

NOTES ON NITRITE OF AMYL.

(BY JAMES MAYNE.)

AMYL nitris, nitrite of amyl, amylo nitrous ether ($C_5 H_{11} No._2$), is an amber-coloured, very volatile liquid, of a penetrating, peculiar odour, resembling that of ripe pears, the sp. gr. of the liquid being 0·877; of the vapour, 4·30; the boiling point is 205° F., but when perfectly dry it boils at 210° F. It is insoluble in water, freely soluble in alcohol. Fused caustic potash converts it into valerianate of potassium. Nitrite of amyl can be prepared by passing a stream of hyponitric acid (nitrous acid) gas through amylic alcohol (purified) at a temperature of 132° C. This process is very long and tedious, taking hours for the amylic alcohol to become saturated, and the resultant contains not only the nitrite, but also valerianate of amyl, also nitrate of ammonium, and a black, non-volatile substance, so that to purify a complicated process is required.

The best process for preparing nitrite of amyl is a modification of Balard's process. Amylic alcohol is first rectified until pure, until its boiling point is about 270° F. This alcohol, with an equal quantity of nitric acid, is introduced into a large glass retort, and moderate heat applied, gradually increasing. When the mixture approaches boiling the fire is removed and reaction allowed to continue. If the application of the heat has been too rapid or too long continued great frothing occurs, and contents of retort may froth over. Moderate and slowly increasing heat must be used, when the reaction is much less violent, the temperature rising gradually after removal of the fire and the beginning of boiling. As soon as the thermometer inserted in the tubulus rises above 212° F. the receiver is changed, the distillate now becoming more and more mixed with ethyl amylic ether, and nitrate of amyl, readily perceived by change in ordour. The distillate obtained below 112° F. is shaken with an aqueous solution of carbonate of potassium to remove free acids, and after separation the oily liquid is introduced into a clean retort and again slowly heated. The first portion coming over is amylic aldehyde. When the very slowly increased heat has risen to 205° F. the receiver is changed, and the distillate now collected is nitrate of amyl, until the thermometer reaches 212° F., when distillation is stopped.

To Dr. Brunton belongs great merit of being one of the first to use this remedy, and of inferring correctly its therapeutic effect from its physiological action; also to the researches of Dr. Richardson is a very great deal due.

In thirty to forty seconds, whether inhaled, subcutaneously injected, or swallowed, it flushes the face and increases the heat and perspiration of the head, face, and neck; sometimes the increased warmth and perspiration affect the whole surface; or while the rest of the surface glows the hands and feet may become very cold, and this condition of the extremities may last for hours. It quickens the pulse in a variable degree, sometimes doubling its pace. This augmented heat of the pulse precedes the flushing by a few seconds.

It causes the heart and carotides to beat strongly, and sometimes produces slight cough and breathlessness.

It often causes slight giddiness, mental confusion, and a dream-like state.

It relaxes the whole arterial system, probably by partially paralysing the sympathetic ganglia and motor nerves. This paralysing effect of the arterial system is well shown by sphygmographic tracings, the flushing of the face, and the increase of the size of visible arteries, like the temporal, which often becomes notably large, sometimes, indeed, being doubled in size, and branches previously invisible become plainly apparent; and by the interesting fact that has been observed by several who, while cupping a patient over the loins, and finding the blood would not flow, administered nitrite of amyl by inhalation when the cuts immediately began to bleed freely. Nitrite of amyl is administered generally by inhalation, doses being two to five drops. If administered internally, should be given in sugar or dissolved in alcohol. It is of extreme value in angina pectoris, and in many spasmodic diseases it has proved valuable.

Relief in asthma is often immediate, and in almost any convulsive disorder much good may be expected from its employment.

MELBOURNE INTERNATIONAL EXHIBITION.
(Continued.)

BELGIUM.—T. X. De Beuklaer, 77 Rue Kipdorp, Antwerp, hygienic liqueur. A. Deelereq, 18 Rue du Convent, Antwerp, elixir. B. Dupuy, 80 Montague de la Cour, Brussels, cressine nasitorine (concentrated juice of watercress and lozenges). Kock and Reis, raffinerie du Noid, Antwerp, sulphur, raw, refined, crystallised, &c. A. J. Laurent, 36 Rue Fousmy, Brussels, pharmaceutical substances. Solvay and Co., Couillet, carbonate of soda and chloride of calcium. C. Vanderbruggen, 13 Rue du Fort, St. Gilles, near Brussels, hygienic liqueurs. L. E. Verbist, pharmaceutical chemist, aessehot, mercurial ointment. G. G. Verzyl, and Co., Chemical Works, Louvain, chemicals used in the manufacture of saltpetre and nitrate of soda, chloride of potassium.

FRANCE.—Candes and Co., 26 Boulevard St. Denis, Paris, antephelic milk for the toilet. — Carcano, 35 Notre Dame de Nazareth, Paris, perfumed satchets. — Cottance, 19 Rue des Lombards, Paris, perfumery. E. Coudray and Sons, 13 Rue

d'Enghien, Paris, perfumery, toilet soap, tooth paste, powders, &c. A. Delettrez, 54 and 56 Rue Richer, Paris, perfumery. — Guerlain, 15 Rue de la Paix, Paris, perfumery. Lyonnet Maison (Gautier and Co.), 28 Rue d'Enghien, Paris, perfumes for the toilet, soaps, pomades, concentrated perfumes and tooth pastes; agents—Paris, Wedeles and Co., and in Melbourne, Schmedes, Erbslöh and Co. Muraour and Co., 25 Rue d'Enghien, Paris, Laferriere water, scents, perfumed oil for the hair, rice powder, &c. Raynaud Maison (L. Legrand), 207 Rue St. Honoré, Paris, perfumery and scented soap. Roger-Gallet, 38 Rue Hauteville, Paris, eau-de-Cologne, soaps, and perfumery. Bertrand Roure, Grasse, Alpes-Maritimes, scents, perfumed oils, pomades. — Viard, Levallois-Perret, Seine, eau-de-Ninon and Velontine Viard toilet vinegar, &c. A. Allenet, Angoulême, Charente, wine king, tonic and aperient wine. Armet de Lisle and Co., 18 Rue Malher, Paris, sulphate of quinine. — Arnaud, 141 Rue Montmartre, Paris, chemical and pharmaceutical products. — Bandon, 11 Rue des Francs-Bourgeois, Paris, Bandon wine, elixir eupeptic of Tissy. D. Belugon, Montpellier, quina curaçoa Belugon. V. Beyer, 32 Rue Delahorde, Paris, elixir water and dentrifrice. Blaquart and Genevoix, 14 Rue des Beaux Arts, Paris, quevenne iron, hydrogene iron. A. Boude and Sons, 52 Rue St. Ferreol, Marseilles, sulphur of every description. A. Catillon, 1 Rue Fontaine and 2 Rue Chaptal, Paris, pepsine Catillon, syrup of Catillon, ferruginous wine of Catillon. Charras and Co., Nyons (Drome), essential oils of different kinds. A. Chevrier, 21 Rue du Faubourg Montmartre, Paris, codliver oil, cocoa wine, codliver wine. Chouet and Co., 8 Place de l'Opéra, Paris, tooth powder and dentrifrice of Dr. Pierre. E. Chouillon, 13 Quai du Havre, Rouen, chemical manures. Coignet, Sons and Co., 131 Rue Lafayette, Paris, gelatine, gelatine gum, and strong gum. Compaigne des Eaux Minerales Naturelles de Vichy (sources, Elizabethand Ste. Marie), 124 Rue St. Lazare, Paris, Vichy water. Desnoix and Co., 17 Rue Vieille du Temple, Paris, blisters, sticking-plasters, &c. E. Duriez, 20 Place des Vosges, Paris, quinordine Duriez, elixir Duero. — Dutant, 26 Rue d'Enghien, Paris, Dutant's food for young children, invalids, and the aged. Favier, Berard and Co., Valence (Drome), Glycirrhizine amonicale, ducime in powder, essential oils. Feil and Son, 56 Rue Lebrun, Paris, artificial reproduction of minerals, crystallisation of alluminium of magnesia. — Freyssinge, 97 Rue de Rennes, Paris, Freyssinge tar, salicale Dusaule, Dartois' pills, &c. Genevoix and Co., 7 Rue de Jouy, Paris, chemical and pharmaceutical products. St. G. Girandeau, 12 Rue Richer, Paris, Rob hoycean laffecteur, vegetable syrup. A. Guislain, Galleries de Valois, 185 Palais Royal, Paris, Peruvian cocoa wine. Homolle and Blaquart, 7 Rue de Belzunce, Paris, Homolle and Quevenne digitaline. A. Hottot and Co., 7 Avenue Victoria, Paris, pure pepsine, pepsine and peptine preparations. Jounet and Serret, 118 Grand Chemin de Toulon, Marseilles, pale blue soap (called "Marseilles soap"), white soap. E. Julien, St. Amand, Nord, anti-asthmatic trochus. — Lefehvre, Illiers, Eure et Loire, green water Lefehvre—a remedy against fever amongst animals. Limousin and Co., 4 Rue des Vieilles, Handriettes, Paris, pharmaceutical products, seals for bottles. Montreuil Bros., A. Vignat and Co., 40 Boulevard National, Clichy, Paris, chemical and pharmaceutical products; agents—Paris, Wedeles and Co., and in Melbourne, Schmedes, Erbslöh and Co. Mothes, Lamouroux and Co., 68 Rue J. J. Rousseau, Paris, capsules, Mothes. La Cie. des Eaux de Pestrin, Perhrin, natural mineral waters of Pestrin (acidulated, ferruginous, arsenical, &c). A. Pontois, Monthard, Cote d'Or, quina pontois, prepared with quinquina calysaya, and the rind of the shaddock, &c. Poulenc and Son, 7 Rue Neuve St. Merri, Paris, chemical products, for photographers, chemists, and for commerce. E. de Ricqles and Co., 41 Rue Richer, Paris, and 9 Cour d'Her Bouville, Lyons, alcohol de Menthe de Ricqles. Roseau & Co., 57 Rue Rambuteau, Paris, insect-destroying powder. Solvay and Co., Varangeville Dombasle, Meurthe et Moselle, carbonate of soda manufactured by E. Solvay's process, soda crystals manufactured from Solvay's soda. (Annual production of this firm equals 50,000,000 kilog. of pure carbonate of soda. Diploma of Honour, Vienna, 1873; Medal, Philadelphia, 1876; Grand Prize, Grand Medal, Paris, 1878. Agents, Arlès, Dufour and Co. — Surun, 378 Rue St. Honoré, Paris, Seguin's quinquina wine. Thessier-Fevre, 398 Rue St. Honoré, Paris, apparatus for making seltzer water at home. C. Torchon, 19 Rue Jacob, Paris, chemical and pharmaceutical products.

(To be continued.)

FELTON, GRIMWADE & CO.,

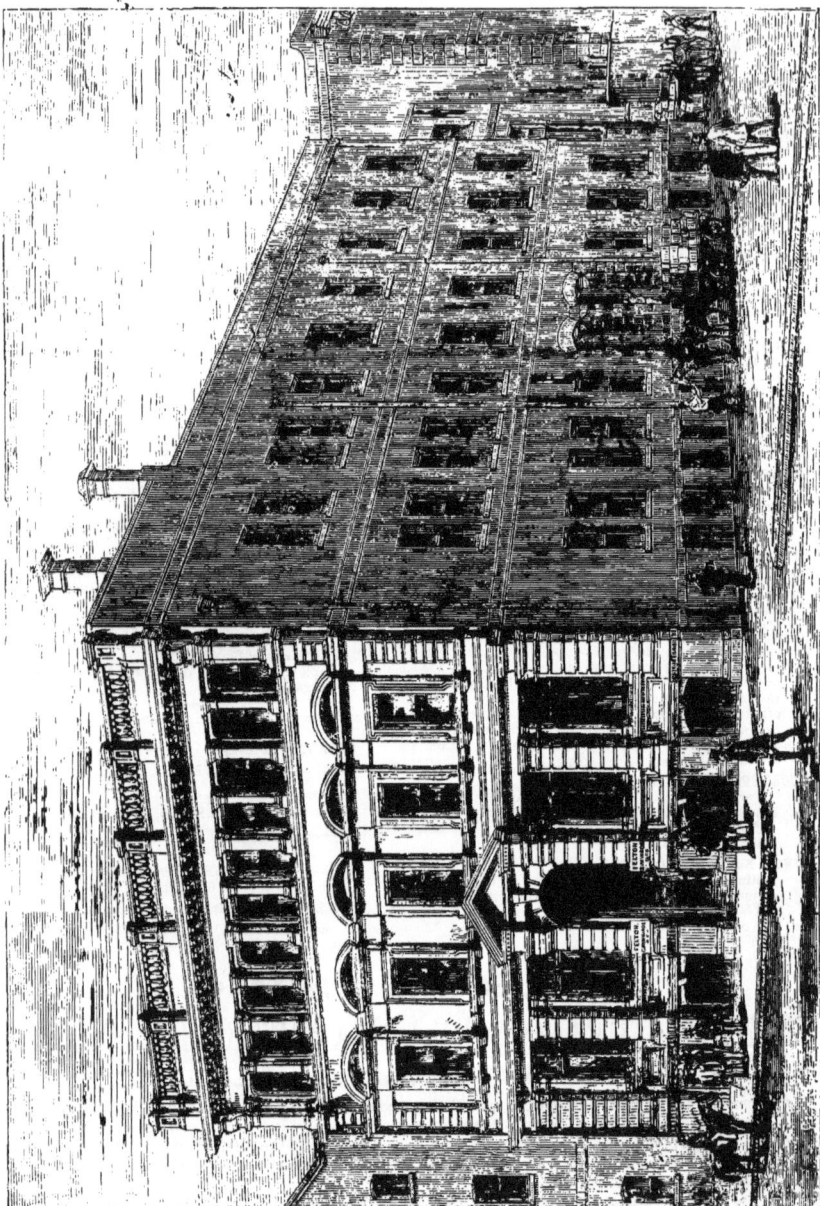

31 & 33 FLINDERS LANE WEST,
MELBOURNE.

INDEX

Australasian Supplement to Chemist and Druggist.

VOL. II.

FROM JUNE, 1879, TO MAY, 1880.

All letters to the Editor will be found arranged under the head of Correspondence.

INDEX—(Continued).

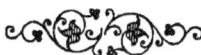

Chem. & Drugg. Aust. Suppl.
Vol. 3, no. 35 : 81-88. (March, 1881)

THE
Chemist & Druggist.

WITH AUSTRALASIAN SUPPLEMENT.

(Published under direction of the Pharmaceutical Society of Victoria.)

No. 35. { PUBLISHED ON THE 15TH } { OF EVERY MONTH. }
Registered for Transmission as a Newspaper.

MARCH, 1881.

{ SUBSCRIPTION, 15s. PER ANNUM, INCLUDING DIARY, POST FREE.

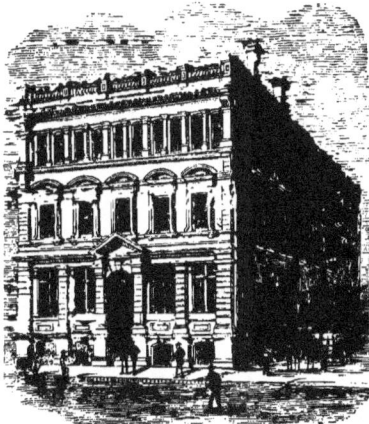

Printed and Published by Mason, Firth & M'Cutcheon, 51 & 53 Flinders Lane West, Melbourne.

The Chemist and Druggist.

WITH AUSTRALASIAN SUPPLEMENT.

OFFICE : MUTUAL PROVIDENT BUILDINGS, COLLINS STREET WEST.

Published on the 15th of each Month.

THIS Journal is issued gratis to all paid-up Members of the PHARMA-CEUTICAL SOCIETY OF VICTORIA, and to non-members at Fifteen Shillings per annum, payable in advance. A copy of *The Chemists and Druggists' Diary*, published annually, is forwarded post free to every subscriber.

Advertisements, remittances, and all business communications to be addressed to THE HONORARY SECRETARY OF THE PHARMACEUTICAL SOCIETY, MELBOURNE.

SCALE OF CHARGES FOR ADVERTISEMENTS :

Per annum.		Per annum.
One Page £8 0 0	Quarter Page .. £3 0 0
Half do. 5 0 0	Business Cards .. 2 0 0

Special rates for wrapper and pages preceding and following literary matter. Advertisements of Assistants Wanting Situations, 2s. 6d. each. Advertisements for insertion in the current month should be sent to the office before the 10th.

COMMUNICATIONS for the EDITORIAL department of this journal should be addressed to THE EDITOR, MUTUAL PROVIDENT BUILDINGS, COLLINS STREET WEST, MELBOURNE.

No notice can be taken of anonymous communications. Whatever is intended for insertion must be authenticated by the name and address of the writer—not necessarily for publication, but as a guarantee of good faith.

MARRIAGES.

BLANCHE—AUGHTIE.—On the 5th March, at the Wesleyan Parsonage, Melbourne, by the Rev. W. L. Binks, Thomas William, eldest son of J. F. Blanche, teacher, Tullamarine, to Elizabeth Laura, eldest daughter of E. S. Aughtie, chemist, Yarrawonga. Home papers please copy.

STODDART—FRITH.—On the 9th March, at Upper Hawthorn, by the Rev. W. H. Fitchett, A. L. Stoddart, chemist, to Jennie, daughter of the late Joseph Frith, formerly of Geelong.

THE SCHOOL OF PHARMACY.

THIS month will be marked in the history of pharmacy in this colony as one of great event—namely, by the establishment of the School of Pharmacy in connection with the Technological Museum. The Pharmaceutical Society not having been successful in obtaining a grant of land for the purpose of erecting thereon a suitable building, with lecture-hall, laboratories, rooms for museums and offices, &c., and the Board of Pharmacy having likewise failed to induce the senate of the Melbourne University to establish a chair for pharmacy, it was proposed by a member of the Pharmacy Board to try to arrange with the trustees of the Technological Museum, who willingly gratified the wishes of the Pharmacy Board. The large lecture-hall, as well as the laboratories and apparatus, are available ; and efficient and experienced lecturers will be nominated by the Pharmacy Board, under whose guidance, in connection with the scientific superintendent of the Industrial and Technological Museum, Mr. J. Cosmo Newbery, the institute will be carried on.

The courses will comprise :—

I. Elementary Chemistry, the introductory lectures of which will include the principal physical forces and chemical philosophy, and then the study of—first, the non-metallic elements and their combinations, *inter se* ; second, the metallic elements and their more important combinations. Organic chemistry will be treated in connection with botany and *materia medica*.

II. Practical Chemistry.—In this division the students will go through a full course of qualitative analysis, the preparation of reagents, &c.

III. Botany.—The lectures on botany will comprise morphology, physiology, the proximate and ultimate constituents of plants ; the systems of Linnæus, Jussieu, and de Candolle ; descriptions of officinal plants, and the diagnoses of the more important natural orders will be illustrated by living and dried specimens.

IV. Materia Medica and Pharmacy will be treated under the following heads :—

1. Organic *materia medica*—vegetable. The study of the officinal substances derived from the vegetable kingdom.

2. Organic *materia medica*—animal. The study of the officinal substances derived from the animal kingdom.

3. Mineral *materia medica*. The study of the chemicals of the *British Pharmacopœia* will include the preparation of them practically, and the testing of their purity and strength volumetrically and otherwise will be carried out.

4. Pharmacy will comprise an explanation of the principles and laws upon which the operations of the *British Pharmacopœia*, dispensing, &c., are based.

A prospectus will at once be issued, with a full synopsis of the course of instruction and a syllabus of subjects for examination, and it is to be hoped that the council of the Pharmaceutical Society and others will offer prizes, and thereby render our new institute in its aspirations and design in every respect identical with that of the School of Pharmacy of the Pharmaceutical Society of Great Britain.

Meetings.

THE PHARMACEUTICAL SOCIETY OF VICTORIA.

THE monthly meeting of the council was held at the rooms, No. 4 Mutual Provident Buildings, Collins-street, on Friday, the 1st April, 1881. Present—Messrs. Blackett, Bowen, Gamble, Thomas, Swift, Huntsman, Francis, Baker, Jones, Hooper, Johnson, and Shillinglaw.

The president, Mr. C. R. Blackett, in the chair.

The minutes of the previous meeting were read and confirmed.

ELECTION OF OFFICE-BEARERS FOR THE YEAR 1881.

President.—Mr. Blackett said the next business to be proceeded with was the election of office-bearers for the year. The first on the list was the office of president, and he felt great pleasure in proposing Mr. William Bowen. The motion was seconded by Mr. William Johnson, and carried unanimously.

Mr. Blackett—" I have great pleasure in informing you that you have been unanimously elected to the honourable position of president of this society."

Mr. Blackett then vacated the chair, which was taken by Mr. Bowen, who then said—" Gentlemen, allow me to thank you very much for the honour you have conferred on me by electing me your president. I must ask you to join me in expressing our most cordial thanks to the gentleman who has just retired from this chair for the manner in which he has filled the position during the last three years." The vote was then put and carried unanimously, and Mr. Blackett briefly replied.

Vice-President.—Mr. William Johnson proposed Mr. John T. Thomas as vice-president; the motion was seconded and carried unanimously, and Mr. Thomas duly returning thanks.

Treasurer.—The office of treasurer was next on the list, and in proposing Mr. H. Gamble for that office, Mr. Blackett said all the members must feel grateful to Mr. Gamble for the very efficient manner in which he had conserved the funds of the society. The motion was seconded by Mr. Bowen. Before the motion was put, Mr. Gamble said he desired to say a few words. He had now been treasurer for three years, and he thought that it might be desirable to allow some one else to take the position.

Mr. Bowen said he believed the office of treasurer was one that should not be shifted from one person to another, Mr. Gamble had filled the position so ably that he trusted he would reconsider the matter and continue to act. Several other members followed Mr. Bowen, and urged Mr. Gamble to reconsider his decision.

Mr. Gamble said he had no wish to complicate the affairs of the society, and as it appeared to be the wish of the council, he would accept the office.

Secretary.—In proposing Mr. H. Shillinglaw as honorary secretary, Mr. Blackett said that it was unnecessary for him to refer to the very good service Mr. Shillinglaw had rendered to the society; it was known to them all.

Mr. Bowen seconded the motion, and in doing so said it gave him pleasure to fully endorse all Mr. Blackett had said of the admirable manner in which the duties had been carried out.

Mr. Shillinglaw said he was in hopes that the council would not have again asked him to accept the position of secretary. There were many young members who, no doubt, would be glad to take the duties, with advantage to the society. He had held the position for three years, and he was pleased to find his efforts had been so highly appreciated. Still he thought a change was desirable; but sooner than see the interests of the society suffer, he would continue the duties for another year.

The motion was then put and carried unanimously.

Correspondence.—A further letter was read from the president of the Pharmaceutical Society of Great Britain in reference to the conference to be held in London in August next. The following letter was also received from Mr. Rivers Langton, resigning his position as one of the representatives of Victoria at the conference :—

"16 Vaughan's Chambers, 48 Queen-street,
"Melbourne, 31st March, 1881.

"Dear Sir—I must ask you to thank, on my behalf, the president and members of the council of the Pharmaceutical Society of Victoria for the great honour they have done me in nominating me as one of their representatives at the Pharmaceutical Conference, to be held in London in August next, and to express to them my high appreciation of the compliment paid me. I am, however, to my great regret, compelled to forego the honour, as I find my business engagements will not permit of so speedy a return to London as I had at first anticipated. Under these circumstances I find it will be impossible for me to take any part in the approaching conference. I am exceedingly sorry I shall not have the opportunity of telling the chemists of Great Britain of the great and boundless resources of your colony, and the large influence on pharmacy they must have in the future; but on my return to London I shall be happy in any way I possibly can to reciprocate the kindness shown me by the chemists of Australia during my visit to the colonies.—Believe me, very faithfully yours,   "RIVERS LANGTON.
"H. Shillinglaw, Esq."

A communication was also read from Mr. R. J. Fulwood, Carlton, in reference to the recent election of the council

complaining that he had received no proxy paper. The secretary was requested to refer Mr. Fulwood to Rule 21.

New Member.—Mr. Edward Gilbert Quorn, South Australia, was nominated.

Donations.—From Graves Aickin, Esq., Auckland, *Transactions and Proceedings of the New Zealand Institute ;* The Government of New South Wales, per Baron Ferd. von Mueller, K.C.M.G., *Select Extra-Tropical Plants* (New South Wales edition), No. 4 and 8, 1858 and 1860 ; *Transactions of the Pharmaceutical Society of Victoria,* from J. C. Jones, Esq.; *The Australian Medical Journal,* The following publications have also been received :—The *Boston Journal of Chemistry,* the *American Journal of Pharmacy,* the *New York Druggists' Circular,* Messrs. Langton, Edden, Hicks and Clark's bi-monthly circular, the *Chicago Pharmacist,* the *Pharmaceutical Journal.*

Financial and general business brought the meeting to a close.

THE PHARMACEUTICAL SOCIETY OF NEW SOUTH WALES.

THE monthly meeting of the Pharmaceutical Council was held on the 1st March, at the society's rooms, Phillip-street; Mr. Senior, president, in the chair. There were also present Messrs. Row, Pratt, Guise, and Watt. The following were duly elected members of the society :—Messrs. H. W. Challinor, A. H. Melville, F. Wright, J. J. O'Reilly, A. Macleod, J. A. Rose, and H. H. Parsons. The secretary reported that the examiners (Messrs. Senior, Larmer, and Watt) had granted a certificate to Mr. A. J. Newling, of Yass, who had passed a very satisfactory examination. The examination of three others was postponed. The indentures of F. J. Thomas (to J. L. Barnett, of Inverell) were registered, and he was admitted as an associate. The usual correspondence was read, several accounts were passed, and the meeting closed.

SANDHURST.

SCHOOL OF MINES, SANDHURST.

UNDER recent regulations of the Education Department examinations were held last Christmas in science subjects, the candidate for the Government certificate of qualification being teachers in State-schools. Amongst the students in chemistry, under Mr. E. L. Mark's tuition, five teachers have most successfully passed, and this is gratifying, seeing that Mr. Marks has for over seven years held the position of lecturer on chemistry in Sandhurst, and that under his guidance such excellent results are possible. The papers set included subjects ranging over all included in *Roscoe's Elements* as far as organic chemistry.

Scientific Summary.

WE cannot present to our readers anything very remarkable. There would seem to be a lull in discovery, but as the International Pharmaceutical Congress will meet in August, in all probability many workers are reserving their results.

Dr. Squibb, at a meeting of the King's County Pharmaceutical Society, drew attention to the varying quality of nux vomica seeds. The manufacturers of strychnia, it appears, buy up the best. Only the large silky seeds should be selected for making tincture and extract. While on this subject it is worth notice that according to some recent experiments by L. J. Morris and others, the active principle colchicia exists only in the skin of the seed, and that it is a waste of time to powder colchicum seeds.

In Dr. Wallace's paper in the *Chemical News* of 11th February he alludes to Dr. Anderson's patent for the precipitation of the solid matter in sewage, in which sulphate of alumnia and lime are employed together with the best possible results.

utical Journal, a valuable
epsine has been contributed
of a large number of com-
rts that, taking fresh pigs'
rgone alteration, and using
:eeded in preparing pepsines
iminose one thousand times
in. Sheep's stomachs yielded
nth as active. It may be
psine, which was vaunted to
>onding to the omnivorons
. preparation from the gizzard
d by the experiments of Mr,
of the power of digestion.
tates that chloral in the solid
toothache in a few minutes,
otton wool is placed in the
o dissolve.
ts upon the dialysis of ferric
of ferric chloride have been
,cademy of Sciences by M, de
r, p. 86). He represents "fer
),.'Fe₂Cl₆, and he states that
a weak solution of this pre-
: chlorine had passed into the
of ferric chloride had been
; of ferric oxide, the chlorine
;o pass through. He is of
tions ferric hydrate *per se* is

ysicians still order lig. ferric
arsentcalis, &c. It cannot be
ferri dialysatic is best given
, All alkaline or acid bodies
decompose iron in this form.
ance prove that oxide of iron
1o stomach.

toriam.

ENT RAMEL.
ill be for ever associated with
eucalyptus in Europe and
was received by the last mail
:nt botanist, who was one of
intimate friends. M. Ramel
It is now many years since
ich he was much attached,
this colony that the writer
i friendship, which has been
>rang up. His last letter was
:ks before his death—a long
he descants with all his old
He was also occupied with
ffle into Australia, and had
n with the late Mr. Edward
s, Planchon, to make experi-
er that this last desire of his
ss._ Mr. E. Wilson's death—
mel, and who entered warmly
realisation of this important
In his last letter M. Ramel
health, "*Bien portant grace*
was, in one form or another,
: used daily. M. Ramel was
that "*La cause de la salubrité*
due to the eucalypts. He it
Mueller, caused these trees to
1, in which latter country he
r the auspices of the late
quote from the Paris corre-
his whole thoughts upon the
;' whole forests of eucalyptus
plains of Algiers." For his
the Cross of the Legion of
:veral scientific societies; and
, among the last sent to him

iished, yet shall rise
n the spark I bore."
C. R. BLACKETT.

JOHN STENHOUSE, F.R.S.

ON the last day of the old year passed away Dr. John Stenhouse, F.R.S., in the seventy-second year of his age. He was
a native of Glasgow, where he received his first education.
Afterwards he was a pupil of Graham and Liebig, and became
an unwearied investigator in the domain of organic chemistry,
his studies being a labour of love to him. In the catalogue of
scientific papers, published by the Royal Society up to the
year 1871, no less than 64 papers are enumerated, written by
him at different periods. He has contributed not a little to
the progress of pharmaceutical knowledge, in recognition of
which he was, in 1856, elected an honorary member of the
Pharmaceutical Society. Aloin, oil of cinnamon leaf, thymol,
from the seeds of *Ptychotis ajowan*, the crystalline deposit in
essential oil of bitter almonds, and myroxocarpine, are a few
of the substances he examined. Of the latter, a crystalline
substance obtained from the white balsam of Peru, a specimen
exists in the museum of the society. Dr. Stenhouse was a
Royal Medallist of the Royal Society, LL.D. of Aberdeen, and
one of the founders of the Chemical Society. On removing
to London he was appointed lecturer on chemistry in St.
Bartholomew's Hospital. In 1865 he succeeded Dr. Hoffmann
as non-resident assayer to the Royal Mint. Though labouring
for many years past under severe physical suffering, yet he
was not deterred from continuing his scientific investigations.
In private life, as a Christian philosopher, as a stern denouncer
of scientific humbug, and as a kind and sympathising friend,
he is said by those who knew him best to have left behind
him but few equals.—*Pharmaceutical Journal.*

FIRE AT ST. ARNAUD.

WE extract from the *St. Arnaud Mercury* of the 30th March
the following :—" The inhabitants were startled from their
slumbers at about half-past one o'clock yesterday morning by
the alarm of fire being given through the medium of the firebell and the shouts of residents in Napier-street, and on proceeding to the scene of the disaster it was discovered that the
lower portion of the premises occupied by Mr. J. F. F. Grace,
chemist, Napier-street, was in flames, in a manner similar to
the fire which broke out in that establishment some three
months ago. From what we can learn of the occurrence, it
appears that a little before the hour named, Mr. F. Fearn, who
had just left a rehearsal of the minstrel troupe held in a private
dwelling, was proceeding down Napier-street on his way home,
and when near the Rose, Shamrock, and Thistle Hotel, observed
the reflection of a peculiar brilliant light in Mr. Grace's
window. On crossing over to see what it was, he observed
that the shop was on fire, the flames appearing to come from
under the window. Mr. Fearn at once gave the alarm, and
with commendable promptitude ran across to the Rose, Shamrock, and Thistle Hotel, knocked up the proprietress, and
obtained a bucket. He then made an aperture in the window,
and with the aid of some water running down the side-channel,
made a desperate attempt to put the fire out, and had nearly
succeeded in doing so, when it caught some explosive, and
was thereby vigorously renewed. In the meantime the firebell was tolled, and Mr. Grace (who was in bed in the upper
story) warned of his perilous position, shortly afterwards
came down scantily dressed to endeavour to save his property.
Meanwhile, the flames had rapidly spread, and the fire brigade
and a crowd of spectators had put in an appearance. The
brigade, though labouring under many difficulties through
being short-handed and being compelled to carry on operations
amidst darkness, rain, and mud, promptly had the hose to
work, and quickly arrested the progress of the flames, the fire
being extinguished in ten minutes after their arrival. The
damage done was confined to the shop and stock, nothing else
being injured. The origin of the fire is a mystery, Mr. Grace
being in bed at the time of the occurrence, and the shop
locked up some time previously apparently all secure. Strange
to relate, although everything was insured, the reverse might
have been the case, as Mr. Grace had only re-insured with the
local agent the afternoon previous."

TO TEST HOUSE DRAINS.—In London house drains are
tested by pouring in at the highest point of the pipes an
emulsion of oil of peppermint and water, following this up
with a couple of buckets of water to wash the emulsion
through the drains. Should there be any leaks they can be
located by the penetrating smell of the peppermint. The
same system is, we believe, used in Boston.

Personalities.

In re O. and A. E. Pulling, of Swanston-street, wholesale druggists, Messrs. Ecroyd, Danby and Gilmour, acting with the committee appointed at the meeting of creditors, invited tenders for the stock, &c., as per statement, in eight lots. The tenders were opened on the 5th April, and that of Messrs. Felton, Grimwade and Co., being the highest, was accepted. There were four tenders sent in.

In re W. Tayler and Co., Sydney, an offer of 6s. 8d. in the pound has been made in this estate, which has been accepted by the creditors.

Mr. W. H. Greeves, after nineteen years' residence in Woodend, has left that district, having disposed of his business to Mr. Geo. Lorimer. Mr. Greeves goes to settle at Hobart, and carries with him the good wishes of a large number of friends.

The business of Mr. W. Stephens, of High-street, St. Kilda, has been purchased by Mr. J. Brinsmead, also of High-street, St. Kilda. We understand that Mr. Brinsmead will remove from his present premises to those lately occupied by Mr. Stephens.

Mr. Edwin Sharpe, 96 Chapel-street, Prahran, has transferred his business to Mr. F. G. Bennett, formerly of Ballarat.

The handsome exhibit of the Crown Perfumery Company at the International Exhibition has been sold to Mr. William Bowen, Collins-street.

Mr. Walter Rowley has just removed into his new premises, No. 10 Bourke-street West; the shop, which is next door to the one formerly occupied by Mr. Rowley, is one of the handsomest in Melbourne, and is most elegantly fitted up.

Mr. Rivers Langton is at present in Melbourne.

At last advice Mr. Thos. Lakeman was in New Zealand (Auckland).

Mr. Forrest (Messrs. Sleeman's, Lime-street, London) is at present in Melbourne.

Messrs. Maw, Son and Thompson advise a representative on the way to the colonies.

Messrs. Jones and Co., surgical instrument makers, 108 Lonsdale-street, have just imported some of the best workmen from their London firm (Mathews Brothers, Carey-street, London), and are now in a position to make instruments of every description in Melbourne.

Mr. Kemptborne (Messrs. Kempthorne, Prossor and Co.), Dunedin, has been in Melbourne; he returned to New Zealand by the last steamer.

We have received from Mr. E. Rowlands, 116 Collins-street, Melbourne, a sample of a new non-alcoholic beverage, "Vigorine." It is an elegant preparation, and will no doubt be much in demand in cases where alcoholic stimulants would be prejudicial.

NOTES ON A HITHERTO UNDEFINED SPECIES OF ENCEPHALARTOS.

(By BARON FERD. VON MUELLER, K.C.M.G., M.D., Ph.D., F.R.S.)

OUR International Exhibition, which is just drawing to a close, has shed on many products of nature, and on numerous works of art from various parts of the world, a "flood of light," which will lead us on to multifarious new commercial and industrial efforts, while, simultaneously, we have gained much additional information on the capabilities and resources of the Australian colonies.

Even among the living plants, which for decorative purposes were displayed, some features of interest occurred in the Exhibition, and thus attention will be drawn in these pages to a cycadeous plant of imposing aspect, which had a place in the Queensland court.

The plant under consideration belongs to the sub-generic group of Macrozamia, which only on geographic considerations can be kept apart from the older South African genus Encephalartos, inasmuch as merely the more or less protruding and pungent summits of the flower and fruit scales offer a distinction of Macrozamia in contrast to Encephalartos; but this characteristic is so variable even in Australian species, that already more than twenty years ago (in the quarterly journal of the Pharmaceutical Society of Victoria II. 90), I combined the two genera. Indeed, it would be no strain on natural arrangement within the order of Cycadeæ to take back both Macrozamia and Encephalartos to the original Linnæan genus Zamia, because the restriction of the latter in modern sense rests solely on a distinct articulation between the leaf-rachis and the leaflets; for even if the entire absence of woody fibres in the medulla of the stem of all American Zamias could be proved, that character alone would not be of generic value, while in the very species of Encephalartos now to be brought under notice the aged leaflets secede on their own accord from the rachis, tardily, it is true, yet at least some of them perfectly as in Zamia proper, leaving a distinct cicatrix at the point of insertion. Nor could a mere geographic limitation of Zamia be maintained when in the order of nearest alliance, that of Coniferæ, we have Araucaria represented as well in South America as in East Australia and the adjoining islands, Libocedrus in West America, South Asia, and New Zealand, and Fitzroya in Chili and Tasmania, not to speak of the occurrence of Cypresses, Taxus, and Juniperus in all the lands around the northern hemisphere, and of Pinus from the Sunda Islands westward to California, nor to mention the dispersion of Podocarpus to all the great divisions of the globe except Europe, and the occurrence of Callitris in North and South Africa as well as Australia.

Alphonse de Candolle's suggestion (*Prodromus* XVI., II., 534) of reducing Bowenia to Encephalartos, as originating, but on other grounds from my own writings (*Fragmenta* V. 171), because the leaf division is as variable in Clematis, Ranunculus, Aralia, Begonia, Manihot, &c., as it would be in Encephalartos if Bowenia were added, is not applicable, inasmuch as comparisons of this kind could only be instituted in orders of close affinity, otherwise the characteristic of invariably opposite leaves in the vast order of Rubiaceæ or the constantly quartering division of the flowers in the large order of Proteaceæ would at once become invalidated.

Whether the new cycadeous plant is placed into Zamia or Encephalartos or Macrozamia will depend on the individual view of any observer, as all genera are mere artificial groups to facilitate classification, and aid memory, while species in their true sense are originally created beings, which when perished, as has already been the case with many of them in St. Helena and some other places on the earth's surface, can by all our human efforts not be restored, but would require the godly might as much for their restoration as they did for their origination.

The species to be defined now is not altogether new, but was much misunderstood, it being mixed from imperfect material in the *Flora Australiensis* (VI. 253) with Macrozamia Miquelii; but the last mentioned plant as originally described from specimens obtained at the Richmond River is very closely akin to M. spiralis, which differs from the stately species exhibited in the Queensland Exhibition court in its very short stem, smaller and twisted leaves, longer leaf-stalks, narrower and above convex rachis, lax and very spreading and less pungent leaflets, which do not regularly approach nor partly overlap each other, in the lower leaflets being nearly as long as the middle ones, in smaller fruit cones on comparatively longer stalks, and in the middle and upper anther-scales being more suddenly contracted into a shorter point. Indeed, the true M. Miquelii is identical with the M. Corallipes, more recently published by Sir Joseph Hooker in his *Botanical Magazine*, t. 5943.

The undescribed species which I wish to name in honour of Mr. Charles Moore, who cultivates it in the Sydney Botanic Garden, and who first drew attention to some of its characteristics, may be recognised by the following diagnosis:—

MACROZAMIA MOOREI.—Tall, *glabrous, leaf-stalks very short, younger leaves but very slightly twisted, older leaves straight,* elongated, rachis very rigid above, almost flat towards the base, dilated, *leaflets but little spreading,* very numerous, all closely approximated, regularly disticbous, very stiff, opaque, flat, very finely nerved, sharply pungent at the apex, *lower leaflets regularly and gradually diminishing in length,* the lowest successively, very short, and ultimately almost toothlike; male cone rather long ellipsoid (cylindric), antheriferous scales rhomboid (wedgeshaped), the lower pointless, those towards the middle of the cone short pointed, the upper antheriferous scales longer and gradually acuminated, fruit-cone very large, elongated, lower fruit-scales pointless, those towards the middle of the cone terminating in an acumen of about half the length of the diameter of the lamina, those towards the summit of the fruit ending in an acumen almost as long as the lamina.

With certainty known from the mountainous regions of Queensland at the verge of the tropics.

It remains to be added that the interest attached to this species rests not merely on its stateliness for scenic purposes in horticulture, its stem (like the trunk of its congeners) containing a peculiar starch, though garden traffic ought to hold this Zamia too valuable to be sacrificed for technical purposes ; but the acrid principle which pervades these plants, and especially the alluring fruits, is so intense that fatal poison cases have actually occurred in these colonies from consuming Zamia fruits without maceration and baking, yet the peculiar principle of acridity has never been chemically ascertained, and thus awaits, perhaps for important therapeutic purposes, careful elucidation.

Correspondence.

To the Editor of The Australasian Supplement to the Chemist and Druggist.

SIR—As there are two sides to every question, so there are two ways of looking at facts. And I am sure your correspondent in last month's issue, "Sensus Communis," will not find fault with a brother pharmacist because he may not have common-sense enough to see things in exactly the same light as he does. No doubt there is enough of the patent medicine trade in the world just now ; so there has been, and ever will be, whilst the orb goes round ; but that we, as a body of reasonable men, have any cause to grumble because certain persons take the trouble to place on the cover of a neatly got up almanac, or on the back of a pretty picture card, our name, without first consulting us, I fail to see. Nor do I think that the mere fact of our names appearing thereon makes us god-fathers to the preparation, whatever it may be ; and if it be intended (as I think it is) to give purchasers some idea of where the genuine article may be procured, instead of allowing them to seek it at the nearest huckster's shop, my opinion is that, so far from complaining, we have reason to be thankful that the transaction was so directed.

Patent medicines will be in demand, and quack pills and powders swallowed, as long as time endures. And if by the use of my humble name the traffic in them can be diverted from the contact of cheese, butter, eggs, and treacle to the counter of the qualified chemist, Drs. Jayne, Ayer, Holloway, and the rest are quite welcome to use it,—I am, sir, your obedient servant, NOSTRUM.

To the Editor of The Australasian Supplement to the Chemist and Druggist.

SIR—As an attendant at the late annual meeting, I was much gratified at not only seeing so influential and numerous an assembly, but also at the tone of thought and unanimity regarding the business of the society. Of course, there was the usual spluttering of a pigmy volcano from simply a misconception of a few details which were effectually illuminated by explanation, and regarding which at future meetings I would like to offer a suggestion to metropolitan members that, if followed, would, I think, to some extent check that carping spirit which is so apt to germinate feelings of an unfavourable character, and with suitable soil make such rapid growth, for

> Small herbs have grace;
> Great weeds do grow apace.

To those desirous of advancing the interests of the society, and who take a vital interest in its concerns, and therefore are its most valued members, being at times placed in a decided disadvantage to other "go-as-you-please," lukewarm members, who are mere subscribing, but otherwise disinterested, adherents, my suggestion is that as the society's office is so centrally situated, and the courtesy of our able honorary secretary so proverbial, that the annual accounts and report being praiseworthily circulated antecedent to the meeting, it would be politic for residents in and near Melbourne feeling a proper interest in its affairs, and desiring further information or details regarding the council's statements than appear in its report, to wait on the honorary secretary, before the meeting, to obtain any explanation that may be deemed necessary, and which, if unexplained or thought unsatisfactory, could then at the meeting be better dealt with, I venture to believe, than by reserving all such inquiries, with all details, till the meeting actually takes place. Such a procedure as I suggest would effectually sift out all but those matters in which the general body of members would feel an interest in hearing discussed, and the introduction and importance of which would be considered by all as desirable and praiseworthy. An honorary council should not, I take it, be questioned at a public meeting on unimportant matters of detail, as it retards progress, and is apt to engender an undesirable and unamiable spirit, ofttimes affecting and lasting during the continuance of the meeting. But where reason and common-sense points to errors or misdirection, I say impugn the ruling authorities in scorn of consequence.

The council should, I think, take into their earliest consideration the advisability of making strenuous exertions for augmenting the number of its members. Surely a direct appeal by circular, enumerating the advantages to be personally derived from joining, and the obligations of every pharmacist to swell the ranks, and thus add to the welfare of the society, would be sure to, on some, have the desired effect ; this, with the creditable and pleasing *esprit de corps* evinced by the heads of our wholesale houses, who, on proper representation, I feel, would allow their representatives to interest themselves in furthering the council's views, who, in turn, would communicate direct to the honorary secretary the views of these gentlemen, to whom they had introduced the question, so that in time the council could state that almost every registered pharmacist had been personally asked "to do his duty" to himself to advance and protect pharmacy throughout the whole of Australasia, and to assist and nourish a young and promising child of science and trade, so that its constitution may be built up a credit to those who nobly father it now and to those who may hereafter take our places in the rank and file of pharmacy.

It is now many years since a determined effort was made to secure to all more freedom from the present unnecessary number of hours (of slavery) to business ; and, as our worthy president alluded to it in his apt address, will our new council again see what may be done in this direction ?—Yours, &c.,
HENRICUS.

ANNUAL CRICKET MATCH.

THE annual match between the wholesale and retail chemists was played on the Melbourne ground on Thursday, 7th April, and resulted, after a very close and exciting finish, in a victory for the retail by two runs. There was a good attendance, and some interest was manifested in the match. Mr. J. Hemmons acted for the wholesale as umpire. The following are the respective scores :—

WHOLESALE.

Treadaway, b Ross	0
Lyons (captain), b Ross	30
Jenkinson, b Ross	21
Coates, st Wade, b Strutt	16
Duff, b Ross	8
Court, b Ross	0
Floyd, b Ross	0
Moss, c Barnard, b Lewis	1
Cherry, b Lewis	0
Anderson, b Ross	0
Fripp, not out	0
Byes	1
Leg-byes	5
Total	82

BOWLING ANALYSIS.—Ross, 66 balls, 31 runs, 7 wickets ; Lewis, 42 balls, 20 runs, 2 wickets ; M'Kie, 18 balls, 10 runs ; Strutt, 18 balls, 15 runs, 1 wicket.

RETAIL.

Hope, b Floyd	13
M'Kie, b Treadaway	1
Lewis, b Floyd	0
Strutt, b Treadaway	11
Ross (captain), b Moss	13
Barnard, run out	7
Cunningham, b Floyd	18
Atkin, c Lyons, b Treadaway	2
Wade, b Treadaway	1
Baker, b Floyd	16
Cunningham, not out	0
Byes	2
Total	84

BOWLING ANALYSIS.—Treadaway, 72 balls, 31 runs, 4 wickets ; Floyd, 54 balls, 20 runs, 4 wickets ; Moss, 18 balls, 9 runs, 1 wicket ; Jenkinson, 12 balls, 18 runs ; Lyons, 12 balls, 6 runs.

In the second innings the wholesale lost eight wickets for 105, Treadaway (60) and Moss (22) being the highest scorers.

A NEW METHOD FOR THE EXAMINATION OF COFFEE.

(By F. M. Rimmington.)

I think it will be generally admitted that the methods in use for estimating the degree of adulteration in coffee are far from satisfactory as regards definiteness and certainty, and that something approaching nearer to chemical accuracy is very desirable. Little has been done in this direction since the days of the Lancet Sanitary Commission.

It may, possibly, not be generally known to analysts that chicory, dandelion, and probably some other substances that are used for mixing with coffee, are readily deprived of colour by a weak solution of chloride of lime (hypochlorite), and that this agent has very little action on the coffee. When this method is adopted a portion of the coffee should be gently boiled a short time in water with a little carbonate of soda, so as to move extractive as much as possible; after subsidence the liquor should be poured off, and the residue washed with distilled water. When this has been sufficiently done, a weak solution of the hypochlorite of lime is to be added and allowed to remain, with occasional stirring, until decoloration has taken place, which will be probably in two or three hours. The coffee will then form a dark stratum at the bottom of the glass, and the chicory a light and almost white stratum floating above it, and showing a clear and sharp line of separation.

The chicory after this operation is in the very best condition for microscopical examination, and it is not difficult to discriminate between chicory, dandelion, or other substances. Although the lower stratum may be dark, and have all the appearance of coffee, other substances may be present and should be sought for. I have recently met with a substance that is entirely new to me, as a coffee substitute, that is not affected by this treatment.—*Pharmaceutical Journal.*

DUST, RAIN, AND FOG.

At a meeting of the Royal Society of Edinburgh, an important paper was read on "Dust, Rain, and Fog," by Mr. John Aitken, of Falkirk. The communication was very interesting, and was illustrated by a number of successful and conclusive experiments. Mr. Aitken's results may be briefly summarised as follows:—A vapour does not condense under ordinary circumstances when cooled below its boiling point, except on a free surface; that is to say, that if steam, for instance, be blown into a receiver filled with ordinary air, a white cloud is immediately formed by the condensation of the vapour on the innumerable particles of dust; but if a jet of steam be blown into a receiver filled with air, which has been filtered through cotton-wool, no cloud is observed. The same fact was demonstrated by means of another experiment. A large inverted flask was fitted with a cork, through which passed a tube, communicating with the air-pump. Over the interior surface of the cork was placed a little water. When the flask was filled with filtered air no effect was produced by exhausting with the pump; while with the flask filled with ordinary air a cloudiness was immediately apparent, which increased in density when the working of the air-pump was continued. By using a flask containing air not perfectly free from dust, an effect resembling a shower of rain in minute drops was produced on rapidly withdrawing a portion of the air. Among other things, it was shown that the fumes of burning sulphur (sulphuric acid will not do) have a powerful effect in producing fog. Into a receiver in which a grain of sulphur had been burned, a jet of steam was blown. This instantly caused a dense fog, through which nothing could be seen, and which continued to fill the receiver for a much longer time than if the atmosphere had simply consisted of unfiltered air.

From these and other observations which Mr. Aitken has made, he concludes that if the air were free from dust we should have no clouds, rain, or fogs; but that the excessive moisture would slowly condense on the surface of the earth, on the trees and houses, keeping them constantly wet. He is also of opinion that the large amount of sulphur which is daily burned in the coal fires in London, is a principal factor in the production of the "pea-soupy" fogs for which that city is famous.—*Pharmaceutical Journal.*

The French Government has allotted to M. Pasteur the sum of 50,000 francs for the purpose of enabling him to carry out his researches on the contagious diseases of animals.

VAPOURS FOR INHALATION.

The following are selected by the *Monthly Magazine of Pharmacy* from the formulæ used at the Hospital for Diseases of the Throat in London:—

VAPOUR CARYOPHYLLI.

Oil of cloves	30 minims.
Light carbonate of magnesia	15 grains.
Water	3 ounces.

VAPOUR CASSIÆ.

Oil of cassia	20 minims.
Light carbonate of magnesia	10 grains.
Water	3 ounces.

VAPOUR CINNAMONI.

Oil of cinnamon	20 minims.
Light carbonate of magnesia	10 grains.
Water	3 ounces.

VAPOUR CREOSOTI.

Beechwood creosote	3 drachms.
Glycerine	3 „
Water	3 ounces.

VAPOUR CUBEBÆ.

Oil of cubebs	2 drachms.
Light carbonate of magnesia	60 grains.
Water	3 ounces.

Useful in laryngorrhœa.

VAPOUR CUBEBÆ C. LIMONE.

Oil of cubebs	1½ drachms.
„ lemon	½ drachm.
Light carbonate of magnesia	60 grains.
Water	3 ounces.

The oil of lemon is added to mask the disagreeable odour of the cubebs.

A teaspoonful to be added to a pint of water at the desired temperature, 150° F., and an additional teaspoonful to be added every five minutes during the time that the inhalation is used. Not more than three teaspoonfuls to be used on any single occasion.

CONTRIBUTIONS TO THE EXAMINATION OF WINE.

(By V. Wartha.)

1. Detection of Magenta in Red Wines.

In all judicial cases the following should be applied in succession:—

a. The Magnesia Test.—20 c.c. of the wine are mixed in a large test-tube with excess of calcined magnesia. After well shaking there is added 1 c.c. of a mixture of equal parts colourless amylic alcohol and ether; the whole is well shaken and allowed to stand for some time. 1 m.grm. magenta in 1 litre of wine may be detected by a rose colouration of the supernatant stratum. In stongly coloured southern wines faint reactions are often masked by a yellowish or light brownish colouring-matter.

b. The Sugar of Lead Test.—20 c.c. of wine are mixed with 10 c.c sub-acetate of lead of officinal strength, and the mixture after being well shaken is filtered into a perfectly dry test-tube. If moderately large quantities of magenta are present they will be detected by the paler or deeper rose colour of the filtrate. But even if it appears perfectly colourless or yellowish, small quantities of magenta or aniline-violet may be present ; 1 c.c. of the above-mentioned mixture of amylic alcohol and ether is therefore added ; the tube shaken up, and then allowed to stand for some time. If held against a white background very small quantities of magenta may be recognised in the upper stratum.

c. The Ether Test.—If the sample has given strong reactions with *a* and *b*, concentration is not necessary. If the reactions were slight, from 150 to 200 c.c. of the wine are evaporated down to one-third to one-fifth of its original volume in a silver capsule, which should have been slightly ignited previously. The concentration is effected over an open flame as rapidly as possible, and the residue while still warm is poured into a stoppered glass cylinder, which should previously be washed with concentrated nitric acid and rinsed with pure water. The wine is mixed with an excess of pure ammonia, 30 to 40 c.c. pure ether are added, the cylinder is stoppered, and shaken carefully to prevent the formation of an emulsion. The clear ethereal stratum is then filtered through a clean dry filter into a perfectly clean porcelain capsule having glazed edges. One or two threads of clean knitting-wool, 3 to 4 c.m. long, which should have been previously washed and dried, are laid in the colourless ether, which is allowed to evaporate in a warm place. The wool takes a colour which may vary, according to the proportion of the magenta, from a faint rose to a red. One of the threads is then reserved in a tube, whilst the other is cut in two, the one half moistened with hydrochloric acid, and the other with ammonia. In both these the red colour should change to a yellowish. If aniline-violet was present the threads will turn to a green. If the wine was pure, however deep the colour, the wool remains white. Particular care must be taken that the ammonia employed contains no traces of organic colouring-matters.

2. *Detection of Sulphurous Acid in Wines.*

About 50 c.c. of the sample are placed in a small distilling flask, the lateral exit-tube of which projects into a test-tube cooled with moistened filter-paper. The wine is kept at a gentle boil till 2 c.c. have distilled over. The test-tube is taken off and a few drops of a neutral solution of silver nitrate are added. If even traces of sulphurous acid were present the liquid becomes opalescent or a white curdy precipitate of silver sulphite is formed, which is distinguished from silver chloride by its solubility in nitric acid. The distillate also reduces mercurous nitrate and decolourises starch iodide and weak solution of potassium permanganate.—*Berichte der Deut. Chem. Gesellschaft zu Berlin,* No. 6, 1880.

MELBOURNE INTERNATIONAL EXHIBITION.

(Continued from page 56.)

ITALY.—A. Aguglione and Co., Turin, elixir. G. Baroni, Modena, mineral waters, &c. N. C. Bosisio, Milan, 12 bottles of elixir. T. H. Bradley, Florence, aquafortis. L. Bronehelli, Pisa, 24 bottles of alimentary pastiles. G. Cantomuso, Vicenza, castor oil. L. Ciosi, Florence, linseed oil and soaps. Annibale Collina, Bologne, elixir "Persiano." G. Controni, Lucca, various bottles of chemical products. G. Curato, Naples, chemical products. F. de Amezaga, Genoa, samples of ceruse. M. de Gioja, Bari, six bottles of tonic, first quality. De Pasquale Brothers and Co., Messina, orange, lemon, and bergamot essences. D. Fiore Franchini, Trani, elixir "Fiore Franchini." G. Guiffrido and Scotta, Catania, almond and castor oils, flour of mustard. Impresa Publici Macelli, Florence, glue, albumen of blood, first and second quality. Prof. P. Leonardi, Venice, medicinal gelatine. Guiseppe Luciano, Turin, essence of mint. G. Malvezzi, Venice, gum made of starch. Ceresina Manufactory, Treviso, samples "Ceresina." Massa, Solari and Co., Genoa, albumen of blood. B. Morelli, Bari, specialty in medicine. A. Mueller, Messina, various essences. G. Oates and Co., Messina, samples of lemon and bergamot essences. G. Parenti, Siena, chemical products. Spadaro Cav. Placido, Catania, samples of chemical products. Itadusa Brothers, Catania, chemical products. C. Rizzuto and Co., Reg. Calabria, orange and lemon essences, &c. Pilade Rossi, Brescia, medicinal waters and chemical products. Cav. Prof. Zinoro Silvestro, Naples, chemical products. G. Tibernacolo, Bari, hair restorer.

GREAT BRITAIN.—Burgoyne, Burbidges, Cyriax and Farries, Coleman-street, London, drugs, chemicals, pharmaceutical preparations. W. J. Bush and Co., Artillery-lane, Bishopsgate (works: Ash Grove, Hackney, London), essential oils, fruit essences, granulated citrate of magnesia, chemical and pharmaceutical preparations, harmless vegetable colours for confectionery purposes, white lead, dry and ground colours, metallic oxide paints, perfumery, toilet soap. F. C. Calvert and Co., Manchester, pure carbolic acid, preparations thereof for disinfecting and agricultural purposes. J. Chambers and Co., 132 Fenchurch-street, London, chemicals, drugs, colours, varnishes. Chassaing, Guenon' and Co., Southwark-street, London, pepsine wine and medicinal preparations. Chippenham Annatto Works, liquid annatto. Corbyn, Stacey, and Company, 300 High Holborn, London, pharmaceutical preparations. Day, Son and Hewitt, 22 Dorset-street, Baker-street, London, horse, cattle, and sheep medicines. E. Grillon, Wool Exchange, Coleman-street, London and Paris, "Tamar Indien" lozenges. Herrings and Co., 40 Aldersgate-street, London, pharmaceutical preparations, essential oils, &c. F. Hitchins, Chippenham, annatto, Hockin, Wilson and Co., 38 Duke-street, Manchester-square, London, seidlitz powders. Home and Colonial Sanitary Co., Dunstable, and Pownall-road, Dalston, London, antozone and carbolic disinfectants. Dr. J. Lelievre, 49 Southwark-street, London, and Paris, Iceland moss poultices, with india-rubber covering. M. Neustadt and Co., 25 Mincing-lane, London, chemicals used in pharmacy and photography, aniline

dyes, &c. W. Nichols and Co., England, third annatto. Maltine Manufacturing Company, 92 and 93 Great Russell-street, and Bloomsbury-mansions, Hart-street, Bloomsbury, London, W.C., maltine food and pharmaceutical preparations. John Richardson and Co., 10 Friar-lane, Leicester, pure chemicals; pharmaceutical preparations; cod liver oil emulsions; colonists medicine chests; pocket pharmacies, &c. Price's Patent Candle Company, Limited, Belmont Works, Battersea, London, stearine, composite, and paraffine candles; night lights, glycerine, toilet soaps, household soap, soap mixture, machinery oils. Wheeler and Co., Southend-on-Sea, and 40 Aldersgate-street, London, Wenham's lime-juice saline, and "chalyheate." Thomas Whiffen, Lombard-road, Battersea, London, pharmaceutical preparations; quinine sulphate and other quinine salts; bark. Rigollot and Co., 49 Southwark-street, London, mustard leaves. T. and H. Smith and Co., 11 Duke-street, Edinburgh, and 12 Worship-street, London, salts of morphia; strychnine, and its salts. Southall Brothers, and Barclay, Birmingham, cod liver oil; drugs and powdered drugs; surgical dressings; the "aquarium" sea salt.

PREPARATION OF OLIVE OIL.

M. PLANCHON has made sundry practical experiments on the yield of olive oil. There is an old custom, followed in all olive-producing countries, of placing the olives in heaps directly after gathering, to induce fermentation. This method is adopted in Spain, Greece, Syria, and in Provence; indeed, it is universal.

The question comes—Is this an ancient prejudice or an empirical rule-of-thumb proceeding; or is it really a method based upon judicious observation of results? We should at once have been inclined to vote for the wisdom of the old practice, for we believe in traditional experience, though a later and more exact chemistry has not guided its handiwork. Whether right or wrong, the fixed theory has been held that olives which have undergone a sort of fermentation give a better yield of oil.

M. Planchon endeavoured to clear up the matter, and to discover whether the increased yield was due to mechanical disintregation, which would afford facility of escape to the fluid, or whether some more potent chemical agency might not be in question. All fermentation depends upon some living being which decomposes and transforms the substances with which it comes in contact; thus some transforms sugar into alcohol, which in turn is seized up by the mycoderma aceti to be changed into vinegar. May not an analogous action be set up in the partial fermentation of the olive?

In order to arrive at a conclusion, M. Planchon collected some olives by his own hand, from the same tree and at the same hour.

These were divided into four lots. The first, reduced to a pulp, dried over the water-bath, and thoroughly washed with sulphuret of carbon. The second was wrapped in paper, separated from each other, and so left without any fear of fermentation. The third and fourth lots were bottled and heated in a stove from 20 deg. to 25 deg. Those exposed to the air never showed a trace of vegetation. After 8, 15, 30, and 40 days the proportion of obtainable oil remained always constant. The bottled olives speedily became covered with green mould, which under the microscope had a close resemblance to a penicillium. In about 15 or 30 days they exhaled an excellent odour of olive oil, and invariably gave 3 or 4 per cent. more oil than the preceding. But the same olives kept in bottle for two months and a half lost from 5 to 6 per cent of their original oil. The odour was disagreeable, and the vegetation on the surface yellow.

Should this augmentation of oil be attributed to the development of vegetable growth, or to the germs of a ferment which many think pre-exist in all fruits? In all the experiments of the author he had never observed any augmentation apart from fermentation; and, when the olives were as usual exposed to stove-heat, previously having been dusted over with borate of soda to prevent the development of the mycoderm, the proportion of oil neither diminished nor increased. No advantage was found to be gained from operating on perfectly ripe olives; they gave no better yield than that obtained from immature fruits.

From all this, M. Planchon was inclined to believe that the heaping of the olives together after gathering, in order to induce fermentation, and thereby to promote the yield of oil, was not a vulgar prejudice. Secondly, that this fermentation should not be continued too long, else the yield will be diminished. Thirdly, that the transformation of part of the pericarp into oil was due to the development of a mycoderm of the germs penicillium on the surface of the olive.

Lastly, the author refrains from giving practical directions about the manner of treating the olives for commercial purposes, assuring the reader that each olive proprietor will be sure to adopt such methods as will best suit his individual wants.—*Sleeman's Circular.*

Notes and Abstracts.

ACCORDING to the Boston *Herald,* an establishment for the manufacture of "bogus diplomas" has been discovered in that city. It is supposed to have manufactured about one hundred doctors, at prices varying from 100 to 145 dollars each.

An eminent physician of Dublin, referring to "those erratic medical hybrids, the lady doctors," very justly remarks— "There are some masculine woman just as there are some effeminate men. Neither are good types of their kind ; and it needs no serious argument to prove the futility of any attempt founded on such exceptional cases, on the part of either sex, to fill the place and assume the functions of the other."—*Journal of Science.*

WHEN SCIENTISTS OUGHT TO BE KILLED.—Professor Huxley says he has long entertained the conviction that any man who has taken an active part in science should be strangled at sixty. In his experience ninety-nine men out of every hundred become simply obstructionists after that age, and not flexible enough to yield to the advance of new ideas. They are, in short, "old fogies," and he thinks the world would be benefited by the operation he suggests. It may be interesting to note, by the way, that the learned professor himself is fifty-five.

CASTOR OIL APPLIED EXTERNALLY.—Mr. M'Nicoll and Dr. Hilliard *(British Medical Journal)* both report that they have found purgative results follow the inunction of castor oil. The latter says—"I have frequently applied castor oil to the abdomen, under spongiopiline, or other waterproof material, in cases where the usual way of administering by the mouth seemed undesirable, and with the happiest results. Within the last few days, in a case of typhoid fever, I applied half-an-ounce of castor oil in this manner, under a hot-water fomentation, which relieved the constipation and tympanitic distention that had been present, without undue purging or irritation of the bowels."

DETECTION OF IODINE IN BROMINE AND METALLIC BROMIDES.—A few drops of the bromine in question are placed in a small porcelain capsule, 30 c.c. of a solution of potassium chlorate, saturated in the cold, are added, and the liquid is boiled till colourless. The solution is then poured into a test-tube, allowed to cool, mixed with a few drops of a solution of morphine sulphate and a little chloroform. If the chloroform takes a violet colour, iodine was present in the sample. The morphine solution is prepared by dissolving 0·5 grm. morphine in an excess of dilute sulphuric acid, and diluting to 50 c.c. In examining potassium bromide the solution is mixed with two or three drops of pure bromine water, and a few c.c. of a cold saturated solution of potassium chlorate, and further treated as above.—*Zeitschrift fur Analytische Chemie.*

WOOD BOOKS AS BOTANICAL SPECIMENS.—In the museum at Hesse Cassel there is a library made from five hundred European trees. The back of each volume is formed of the bark of a tree, the sides of the perfect wood, the top of young wood, and the bottom of old. When opened, the book is found to be a box, containing the flower, seed, fruit, and leaves of the tree, either dried or imitated in wax. At the Melbourne Intercolonial Exhibition of 1866, Col. Clamp exhibited specimens converted into small boxes of book form, according to a design adopted by him at the Victorian Exhibition of 1851, and then suggested by Baron Müeller. Australia alone could furnish a collection of over a thousand such books. At the Paris Exhibition of 1867 Russia showed a similar collection of wooden books, cleverly designed, showing the bark as the binding, and lettered with the popular and scientific names of the wood. Each book contains samples of the leaves and fruit of the tree and a section and shaving or veneer of the same.

ALCOHOL A STIMULANT OR NARCOTIC.—Alcohol, says Dr. Wilks, in the *Monthly Magazine of Pharmacy,* is stated to be a stimulant. If a man is jaded and tired, it affords a tem-

porary support; a little later he is depressed, the stimulant lasting only a short time. It produces dilatation of the vessels and warmth of the surface, but at the expense of internal heat. The fact is, alcohol is not a stimulant at all, *but a depressant and a narcotic.* If the name were changed we should get a proper notion of its character, and Dr. Wilks believes that such a change would tend more than anything else to make people cautious in its imbibition. Alcohol is taken for the same reason as chloral or opium in other countries, and if regarded as a narcotic the consequences of its use would be better understood. It has a sedative effect, and is therefore useful in severe neuralgia when chloral and opium fail. It benumbs the sense of touch as well as that of sight and taste ; but if it were a stimulant, then sense of taste ought under its influence to become more refined.

MANUFACTURE OF QUINIA IN THE UNITED STATES.—An article in the New York *Times* of 13th January, which has evidently been written by one well informed on the subject, refers to the price of quinia, which last year averaged 2 dols. 90 cents, the maximum figure being 3 dols. 25 cents., the minimum 2 dols. 50 cents. This is about equal to the quotations between 1873 and 1876, previous to the removal of duty from quinia. All articles essential for the manufacture of quinia are taxed, such as soda, fusel oil, alcohol; by our navigation laws the valuable barks from the East Indian plantations are diverted to Europe, a discriminating duty of 10 per cent. being imposed upon them here. American manufacturers are thus compelled to use barks very poor in quinia, but richer in cinchondia, which latter alkaloid is protected by a duty of 40 per cent. Prior to 1879, about 900,000 ounces of quinia sulphate was manufactured in the United States ; last year it was not over 500,000 ounces. The largest quinia manufactory is stated to be at Milan, Italy, carried on by a joint stock company, which supplies under contract East India and Russia, and produces annually about 1,200,000 ounces, or about one-third of the entire consumption of the world.—*American Journal of Pharmacy.*

SAL-SODA CRYSTALS BY THE OLD AND THE NEW PROCESS. —The sal-soda, made after the new ammonia process, begins to find its way in commerce. As it is purer than the old product, a ready way to distinguish one from the other from their appearance is of some interest. The sal-soda, made according to the old, or Leblanc, method is in hard, compact, heavy, and lustreless lumps. Unless much efflorosced the crystals show 32 to 33 degrees of the alkalimetric scale, corresponding to 32 or 33 per cent. of caustic soda in combination. The carbonate of soda obtained by the new or Solvay process is in porous, friable, light, and shining lumps. Without any efflorescence they mark 34 to 35 degrees. They are free from chlorides, sulphates, and free alkali. Their very porosity renders them easily freed from mother waters when they are drained. They consist, therefore, of almost chemically pure carbonate of soda. The force of habit, nevertheless, induces buyers to prefer the old kind of sal-soda ; they think that the porosity of the lumps of the new product indicates the presence of sulphate of soda, while, in fact, this salt is never formed at any stage of the process, and an intentional addition of 5 or 10 per cent. of it would suffice to render the crystals as hard as those of the old kind. Others complain that they do not taste sharp to the tongue, while this simply indicates the absence of caustic alkali, another impurity almost always found in the old sal-soda.

𝔑ew and 𝔖tandard 𝔐edical 𝔚orks

ON SALE BY

GEO. ROBERTSON

WHOLESALE AND RETAIL

BOOKSELLER & STATIONER,

33 & 35 Little Collins Street West,

MELBOURNE.

The Cyclopædia of Practical Receipts, Processes, and Collateral Information in the Arts, Manufactures, Professions and Trades, including Pharmacy and Hygiene, by ARNOLD J. COOLEY, 2 volumes ... ... 47s. 6d.

Beasley—The Book of Prescriptions ... ... 7s. 6d.

Beasley—The Druggist's General Receipt Book ... ... 7s.

Beasley—The Pocket Formulary and Synopsis of the British and Foreign Pharmacopœias ... ... 7s. 6d.

Fownes—A Manual of Chemistry, Theoretical and Practical, 2 vols. ... ... 21s.

Mayne—A Medical Vocabulary : being an Explanation of all Terms and Phrases used in the various departments of Medical Science and Practice, giving their Derivation, Meaning, Application, and Pronunciation ... ... 11s. 6d.

Taylor—On Poisons in Relation to Medicine ... ... 18s.

Bloxam—Laboratory Teaching : Progressive Exercises in Practical Chemistry, illustrated ... ... 6s. 6d.

Royle—A Manual of Materia Medica and Therapeutics, illustrated ... ... 17s.

Carpenter —The Microscope and its Revelations, illustrated ... ... 17s.

Dick—Encyclopædia of Practical Receipts and Processes, 6,400 Receipts 25s

Squire—A Companion to the British Pharmacopœia, comparing the strength of its various Preparations with those of the United States and other Foreign Pharmacopœias, &c. ... ... 12s.

Fenwick—The Student's Guide to Medical Diagnosis, illustrated ... ... 7s. 6d.

Savory—A Compendium of Domestic Medicine, and Companion to the Medicine Chest ... ... 6s.

A COMPLETE CATALOGUE OF MEDICAL BOOKS TO BE HAD ON APPLICATION.

GEORGE ROBERTSON,

33 and 35 Little Collins Street West, Melbourne,

AND AT

SYDNEY, BRISBANE, AND ADELAIDE.

INDEX

Australasian Supplement to Chemist and Druggist.

VOL. III.

FROM JUNE, 1880, TO MAY, 1881.

All letters to the Editor will be found arranged under the head of Correspondence.

INDEX

𝔄ustralasian 𝔖upplement to ℭhemist and 𝔇ruggist.

VOL. III.

FROM JUNE, 1880, TO MAY, 1881.

All letters to the Editor will be found arranged under the head of Correspondence.

INDEX

Australasian Supplement to Chemist and Druggist.

VOL. IV.

FROM JUNE, 1881, TO MAY, 1882.

All letters to the Editor will be found arranged under the head of Correspondence.

[SUPPLEMENT ONLY.]

Chem. & Drugg. Aust. Suppl.
Vol 4, no 42. (Oct. 1881). (pp 41–48)

THE

Chemist & Druggist.

WITH AUSTRALASIAN SUPPLEMENT.

(Published under direction of the Pharmaceutical Society of Victoria.)

No. 42. { PUBLISHED ON THE 15TH OF EVERY MONTH. *Registered for Transmission as a Newspaper.* }   OCTOBER, 1881.   { SUBSCRIPTION, 15s. PER ANNUM, INCLUDING DIARY, POST FREE.

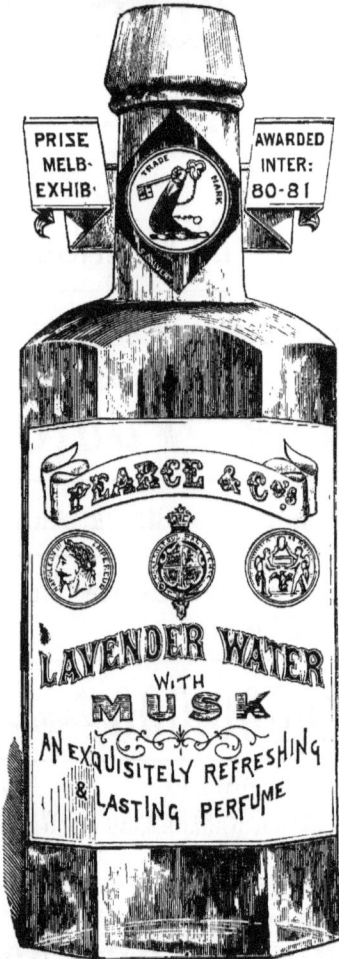

The Chemist and Druggist.

WITH AUSTRALASIAN SUPPLEMENT.

OFFICE: MUTUAL PROVIDENT BUILDINGS, COLLINS STREET WEST.
Published on the 15th of each Month.

THIS Journal is issued gratis to all paid-up Members of the PHARMA-
CEUTICAL SOCIETY OF VICTORIA, and to non-members at Fifteen Shillings
per annum, payable in advance. A copy of *The Chemists and Druggists'
Diary*, published annually, is forwarded post free to every subscriber.

Advertisements, remittances, and all business communications to be
addressed to THE HONORARY SECRETARY OF THE PHARMACEUTICAL SOCIETY,
MELBOURNE.

SCALE OF CHARGES FOR ADVERTISEMENTS:

	Per annum.		Per annum.
One Page ..	..£8 0 0	Quarter Page	..£3 0 0
Half do. ..	..5 0 0	Business Cards	.. 2 0 0

Special rates for wrapper and pages preceding and following literary
matter. Advertisements of Assistants Wanting Situations, 2s. 6d. each.

Advertisements for insertion in the current month should be sent to the
office before the 10th.

COMMUNICATIONS for the EDITORIAL department of this journal should be
addressed to THE EDITOR, MUTUAL PROVIDENT BUILDINGS, COLLINS STREET
WEST, MELBOURNE.

No notice can be taken of anonymous communications. Whatever is
intended for insertion must be authenticated by the name and address of
the writer—not necessarily for publication, but as a guarantee of good faith.

NOTICE TO MEMBERS.

MEMBERS whose subscriptions for the current year
remain unpaid are respectfully requested to forward
the same at their earliest convenience.

LIBRARY NOTICE.

MEMBERS who have books from the library are
respectfully requested to return them at once.
September 28th, 1881.

UNQUALIFIED ASSISTANTS.

IT has for some time been apparent that the employment
of unqualified assistants in pharmacies is too common. It
is in the interest of the public that only examined persons
should dispense prescriptions and sell poisons. The employment of unqualified or imperfectly educated assistants
as juniors under the strict supervision of the principal, or
of a qualified senior-assistant, may not be so objectionable,
although we venture to think that even that is to be
deprecated on many grounds, for it holds out an encouragement to many young men to be lazy; it also is an
injustice to those who have, by commendable effort, qualified themselves and passed the necessary examinations.
In England it has long been felt to be an anomaly that
assistants can in the present state of the law be employed
without having any qualifications whatever. This subject
is now engaging the earnest attention of the leaders of
pharmaceutical education in Great Britain, and there is
no doubt but that a still further amendment of the Pharmacy Act will soon be made in order to bring the education of pharmacists in England as far as possible up to the
high standard of the great continental states. In a
valuable report, very ably drawn up by a special committee appointed by the Pharmaceutical Society, the whole
subject of education and examination is exhaustively
treated, and recommendations are suggested which, if
carried out, will go a long way in this direction. One of

the changes urged by the committee is that the preliminary examination must be passed before apprenticeship. This has, we are happy to say, been done by our
Pharmacy Board, and will, we are sure, be fraught with
the most beneficial results in the immediate future.
During the debate at Bloomsbury-square upon the adoption of the committee's report, Mr. Andrews made the
following observations, with which we agree; and, indeed,
we have frequently expressed ourselves to the same
effect :—" With respect to the second communication,
that the preliminary examination, or its recognised
equivalent, be passed prior to apprenticeship or pupilage, it stated that this could be insured by prohibiting a candidate from presenting himself for the
minor examination until three years after he had
been certified to have passed the preliminary. Now
this could not be insured, as he would show, for a very
painful case had lately come under his notice. A youth
was apprenticed to a pharmaceutical chemist of standing,
and before his indentures were signed—and, by the way,
he might say that the usual form of indentures was, in his
opinion, perfectly unsuited to their business—the chemist
said to his friends that he had great doubt about this
youth passing the preliminary examination. The friends,
however, said they were quite sure he could pass easily,
and he was bound. The result was, he never had passed
the preliminary up to the present time, and he was now a
man of thirty years of age; *he was acting as an assistant,
and was a very good assistant, but he had never passed the
preliminary examination, and never would, and, consequently, he never could come up for the minor examination.*
He did not see how the object the council had in view
could be insured unless there were a provision that the
indentures should be cancelled if the apprentice failed to
pass the preliminary in due time. The chemist in question would have been quite willing to cancel the indentures,
but he could not do so, as the boy's friends held him to his
bargain. There were a large number of young men in the
trade who were in precisely the same position, and unless
some arrangement were made stronger than that proposed
to ensure the preliminary examination being passed before
apprenticeship, this difficulty would always be cropping
up. Mr. Young seemed to think it would be to the
youth's own benefit that he should not be compelled to
pass previously; but he thought it would be very much to
his benefit, and to that of his friends, to know whether he
was fit or unfit for the occupation before he entered upon
it. He had been informed by a member of the council
that there were men throughout the country who took
apprentices and occupied them almost as porters, not
caring one atom as to their future prospects; what they
wanted was cheap labour, and they took these youths on
that account. It was to prevent such a practice as that
that he called particular attention to the second recommendation."

In Germany the young man must pass the "gehülfen-prüfung," corresponding to the English minor examination, before he can act as an assistant.

As the Pharmacy Board has power to permit the widows of pharmacists to carry on the business of her deceased husband under qualified management, it is important that this question should be thoroughly understood, and no injustice or evasion of the law allowed.

The Month.

IN the *Ballarat Evening Post* of 30th September, in an article upon careless dispensing and the sale of poisons, occurs the following :—"Mr. Francis Taylor, a surgeon, was summoned to attend a Mrs. Smyth, at Romsey. He prescribed *salicite (sic) (bark of the willow),* but unfortunately the druggist substituted strychnine." This is a specimen of newspaper scientific knowledge and intelligence. In another part of the same article we find the following remark, *apropos* of chlorodyne :— "No duly qualified medical practitioner would venture to *subscribe (sic)* such a mixture without careful reference to the patient's symptoms and idiosyncracy, and yet any one can purchase it, not only at the druggist's, but at ordinary stores." Surely the State-school has not yet done much for some of our scribes !

In this issue will be found a contribution by Baron F. von Müeller on a new orchid of Victoria. We regret to have to announce the death of Mr. Bentham, the great botanist and co-worker for so many years with Baron F. von Müeller, to whom the news was communicated by the director of the Botanic Gardens, at Florence. This news has not been yet confirmed. As Mr. Bentham is above eighty years of age, his decease would not be unexpected, yet we may cherish the hope that he still lives.

A large audience assembled in the Young Men's Christian Association Hall on the 3rd instant, when the fourth of the present series of health lectures was delivered by Mr. James Smith, who chose as his subject, "The Nervous System ; its Use and Abuse." In clear and incisive language Mr. Smith described the constitution of the brain and the operations of the nervous system. He deprecated the prevalent system of "cramming" in schools as most injurious and detrimental to the healthy development of children, and the imprudence of young ladies of fashion who waste their vital forces in the ballroom was also commented upon. The lecture was followed with close attention by a very appreciative audience.

We have received the first number of the *Australasian Medical Gazette,* the official organ of the combined Australasian branches of the British Medical Association. It is excellently printed, and contains a well-arranged summary of medical intelligence. In the inaugural editorial address, the conductors promise to "follow as near as they can in the footsteps of the *British Medical Journal.*" It is to be issued monthly from Sydney, Drs. Neild and Jamieson being the Melbourne editors.

The arrangements for the annual dinner, to be held on the 16th November, are progressing in a very satisfactory manner, and there is every prospect of a very large attendance. Members of the Society intending to be present will oblige by sending in their names to the hon. secretary at least a week before the date.

We have to acknowledge, with thanks, from Mr. Bosisto, M.L.A., the following donation to the museum :—Specimens of gums and resins, and other products of Australian vegetation.

The second course of lectures at the School of Pharmacy Technological Museum will commence on the 6th February, 1882. It has been resolved that the lectureships shall be annual appointments, and applications will shortly be invited for the positions.

Meetings.

PHARMACEUTICAL SOCIETY OF VICTORIA.

THE monthly meeting of the council was held at the rooms, 100 Collins-street, on Friday, the 7th October, 1881. Present—Messrs. Bowen, Gamble, Blackett, Thomas, Hooper, Huntsman, Swift, Baker, Best, Jones, and Shillinglaw. The president, Mr. William Bowen, in the chair. The minutes of the previous meeting were read and confirmed.

Mr. E. M. Rogers, Emu Bay, Tasmania, was elected a member, and Mr. Charles G. Hill, of Adelaide, was nominated. *Vacancy in the Council.*—Mr. Robert Nicholls, of Emerald Hill, was elected a member of council, *vice* Mr. H. Francis, resigned.

Medal for School of Pharmacy.—Mr. Blackett submitted the design for the gold medal to be given to the student who shall pass the best examination in *materia medica,* botany, and chemistry, which was, after some discussion, agreed to.

Grant of Land from Government.—Some time since, when a deputation waited on the Commissioner of Lands on the above subject, he stated that if no objection was made by the Public Works Department to the occupation of the site applied for on the Eastern Hill, it would be granted. The Commissioner of Public Works having offered no opposition, the Minister of Lands has therefore been asked to carry out his promise.

Correspondence.—A letter was read from Mr. R. J. Poulton, Bourke-street, Melbourne, forwarding his resignation as a member of the society ; the resignation was accepted. A communication was submitted from the secretary of the Pharmaceutical Society of Great Britain, stating that the letter addressed to them in reference to the pharmaceutical journal being supplied to members of the society in Victoria, would be dealt with at the next council meeting, in October.

A number of letters of no special public interest were dealt with, which, with financial business, brought the council meeting to a close.

SPECIAL MEETING.

At the close of the meeting of council a special meeting was held. The meeting was called by requisition, for the purpose of altering and amending certain rules, and more especially to alter the mode of voting for members of council from proxy to ballot.

In addition to the members of council, Messrs. Ross, Dunn, M'Farlane, Brownscombe, Nicholls, and Pendlebury were present.

Mr. Wm. Bowen in the chair.

Mr. J. C. Jones submitted the amendment prepared by Mr. Ross and himself. No important alterations were made until clause 9 was reached, which was altered, making it necessary for persons wishing to become members of council to be nominated by two members of the Pharmaceutical Society.

Upon clause 17 being read—"There shall be a Benevolent Fund, to consist of donations and subscriptions made for the purpose of relieving distressed persons who are or have been members of the society, their widows or orphans, aided by such appropriation of a portion of the general funds as the society at their annual meetings shall think necessary, two trustees for which shall be appointed by the counsel during pleasure"—Mr. Jones said he begged to propose that an addition be made to this clause, giving the council power to grant out of the interest of the Benevolent Fund a sum not exceeding £5, to be applied in the relief of distressed persons, whether they have been members of the society or not. Mr. Nicholls thought the sum so small that he feared that it would be of little use.

Mr. C. R. Blackett said—I desire to offer a few remarks in reference to Mr. Jones's proposition, and, although it may seem very hard not to be able to afford relief to all applicants, I cannot think that the council are acting fairly to apply money subscribed by the members of the society to the relief of persons who have not contributed one shilling towards it. If it became known that the Benevolent Fund was available to any person who applied for assistance, and who was not, and had never been, a member, there would be a number of applications that could not well be refused.

Mr. J. T. Thomas suggested it would be well to establish a special fund to meet cases of this sort. A small contribution of 6d. or 1s. a-week would soon form a sufficient amount to relieve any casual cases that might be found worthy of assistance.

After some remarks from Messrs. Ross, Best, and Brownscombe,

It was moved, as an amendment to Mr. Jones's motion, that clause 17 remain unaltered, and that no money be voted to any persons who are not or have not been members, their widows or orphans. The amendment was put and carried.

Mr. Ross said—The next clause (22) is one that is of the most importance, as it is proposed to substitute voting by ballot instead of by proxy, and I therefore move that clause 22 be rescinded, and the following be substituted :—" If the number of persons nominated to fill the vacancies in the council is greater than the number of persons required to fill such vacancy a poll shall be taken, and the secretary shall cause voting-papers to be printed in the form given in the second schedule hereunto, and shall sign and number each of such papers, and cause one to be enclosed in an envelope, not fastened, with the name and address of the secretary printed thereon, and one of such voting-papers shall be sent by post, under a fastened cover, to the address of each and every member of the Pharmaceutical Society at least seven days before such election. The secretary shall, on the day named, proceed, in the presence of the president and scrutineers appointed at the meeting, to open the envelopes with his printed address thereon, and which have been returned to him, and to take out the voting-papers therein contained, and he shall proceed to ascertain the number of votes for each candidate, and shall declare the candidates that have received the greatest number of votes to be duly elected."

" Clause 23.—If any voter shall suffer to remain upon any voting-paper a greater number of names not struck out than the number of members to be elected, or shall fail to attach his signature thereunto, the vote given on and by such paper shall be void and of no effect. The voter shall enclose such voting-paper in an envelope, furnished to him with the printed address thereon, and shall post the same so that it shall be received by the secretary in course of post before four o'clock p.m. on the day fixed for holding such election. Each candidate shall be entitled to appoint one scrutineer, to be present when the secretary shall open the envelopes containing the voting-papers."

Mr. Blackett : Considering the lateness of the hour and the importance of the alterations, I will move that the meeting adjourn until the 4th November. This will give an opportunity to publish the proposed alterations in the journal, for the information of members.

The meeting then adjourned.

THE PHARMACY BOARD OF VICTORIA.

THE monthly meeting of the board was held at No. 4 Mutual Provident Buildings, on Wednesday, the 12th October ; present—Messrs. Bosisto, Lewis, Holdsworth, Bowen, and Owen. An apology was received from Mr. Brind.

The president, Mr. J. Bosisto, in the chair.

Before the commencement of the business, the registrar stated that he had received a return from Mr. A. T. Best, returning officer under the Act, declaring Mr. C. R. Blackett elected as a member of the board, vice Mr. J. Kruse, resigned. Mr. Blackett then took his seat.

The minutes of the previous meeting were read and confirmed.

Applications for Registration.—The following applications for registration as pharmaceutical chemists were passed :— Millard Johnston, Windsor, passed major examination ; Samuel Breaden, Launceston, an assistant before the passing of the Act ; and Hugh Chalmers Rose, George-street, Sydney, in business in Victoria before the passing of the Act.

Apprentices' Indentures Registered.—George Thos. Whitford and J. A. M. Pearson, Melbourne ; Thos. Edward Turner, Belfast.

Erasure of Names from the Register.—Lane Midworth, Sydney, and James Gerrard, Walhalla, deceased.

Design for certificate major examination was finally agreed to, and the registrar was authorised to have it engraved on copper.

Correspondence.—From Edward Reeve, Rutherglen, forwarding his indentures of apprenticeship for registration, the term being for three years. The indentures were illegal, and could not therefore be registered. From Mr. C. H. Yeo, hon. secretary Pharmaceutical Society of Queensland, forwarding copy of the Queensland Pharmacy Act. From the police, Drouin, Colac, Emerald Hill, and Numurkah. From Mrs. Summers, stating that Dr. M. W. O'Sullivan was now carrying on her business. From the Hon. the Commissioner of Railways, stating that under the new regulations which restrict the issue of passes the Commissioner of Railways is unable to continue the issue of such tickets to the members of the Pharmacy Board.

A case where the widow of a chemist who was granted permission to carry on business came under notice, there being no *bona-fide* registered chemist resident on the premises. It was resolved that unless in one week a qualified resident assistant be placed in charge, the permission to carry on business be cancelled.

A number of reports were received from the police, and after some discussion the following resolution was carried unanimously :—" In consequence of the numerous cases of evasion of the Pharmacy Act by unqualified persons, and of the difficulty of getting the local police to take action upon the same, it was moved that the president and secretary of the Pharmacy Board wait upon the Chief Commissioner of Police, with the view of pointing out to him the necessity of preventing the same."

On the motion of Mr. Bowen, it was resolved that, the next meeting of the board falling on the 9th November (a public holiday), the meeting be postponed until the following Wednesday, the 16th November.

Financial and general business brought the meeting to a close.

PHARMACY IN NEW ZEALAND.

EACH of the four pharmaceutical cities has had, or is about to have, the usual annual meeting of members. Dunedin has led off, and a new vice-president and council have been elected in that energetic southern capital. On Wednesday last, the 7th inst., a well-attended annual meeting was held in Auckland. The retiring vice-president, Mr. Graves Aickin, gave a valedictory address, in which he congratulated the society upon the passing of the new Pharmacy Act. This, however, he considered to be only the precursor of a better one—an amended Act, which should provide for the technical training of apprentices, and a preliminary examination similar to the provisions of the Victorian Act. The ethics of this legislation he took to mean that higher education being made compulsory, higher aims would follow. Scientific inquiry and superior knowledge would render the pharmacist a better man, socially and intellectually. There was a brighter, a better side to our business or profession. The mere " greed of gain," or accumulation of wealth, should not be an only " end and aim." Beyond this is the consciousness that whilst acquiring a competence for ourselves we are also ministering to the necessities of "suffering, sad humanity ; afflicted ones, stooped to the lips in misery," each of us having opportunities of benefiting those around us, and not unfrequently the only requital being the consolation that in our sphere and generation we had had the means of "doing good in the world." The necessity for educating those who may choose pharmacy as a profession was dwelt upon forcibly, and the hope held out that before long the provincial district of Auckland may enjoy the advantages of a local university, with the usual medical school and kindred classes in *matéria medica*, practical pharmacy, &c. The vice-president, who is also a member of the Pharmacy Board, then reported that registration had been nearly completed ; and read a notice from Mr. Allen, the secretary, to the effect that, beyond a certain date, delinquents would be liable to the penalties of the law. The speaker also referred to his visit to the sister colonies, and urged the members to foster friendly feelings, social harmony, and mutual assistance. These excellent qualities had made Victorian pharmacists the model for others to imitate. A ballot for new members was taken, which resulted in the election of the old members. Thanks were voted to the

Pharmaceutical Society of Victoria for their monthly journal; and to the American Pharmaceutical Association for their annual volume of proceedings. At the subsequent meeting of the local council, Mr. James P. King was elected vice-president for the year, and Mr. James W. Henton, hon. secretary. Since last correspondence, Mr. Rivers Langton passed through this colony. In Auckland he succeeded in obtaining large orders—far beyond his anticipation, I fancy; he certainly made a favourable impression. Mr. Lane, who represents the American house of Wm. R. Warner and Co., and Mr. M'Cord, Seabury and Johnson's traveller, were here together, and did a good business. Some of Dr. Lane's clients wonder at his lengthy silence; he was to have opened up a "big trade" here. Mr. C. A. Gosnell and Mrs. Gosnell have been combining business with pleasure. It is quite a brilliant idea of theirs to take a honeymoon trip round the world. They finish their tour in two years or so, and will then have surveyed the chief ethnological features of the globe—ethnological, because the "poor Indian, with his untutored mind" will be taught the civilising influence of "cherry tooth paste" and "trichosayon hair brushes." Mr. Gosnell's chart of travel is a curiosity—a diploma for any *G. T.* Mr. Morgan, the proprietor of the *Chemist and Druggist,* has been the most recent visitor. He is laying up a fund of information in reference to our colonies, with the view to their coming to the front one of these days in the British Parliament. He intends to contest a metropolitan seat at the first general election in the Liberal interest. As the General Council meets next December at Dunedin, I hope to give you an interesting and hopeful account of the future of pharmacy in this colony in my next.

Auckland, 12th September, 1881.

PHARMACY IN FIJI.

WE extract the following from the *Fiji Times* of the 30th July:—

"With reference to the editorial contained in our issue of the 13th instant, we are informed that it was not contemplated by the framer of Ordinance 14, 1881, to subject pharmaceutists holding colonial certificates to an examination before registering them as persons qualified to practise in this colony. It is held that they come within the meaning of the words 'any person holding a diploma or certificate entitling him to practise in any of the capacities aforesaid in the United Kingdom,' occurring in section 3. In accordance with this view, the practice has been to hold them exempt from the necessity of examination, and to register them upon their satisfying the chief medical officer of their identity with the person mentioned in their diploma. Although we thoroughly concur in the good policy and general propriety of the practice adopted, our conviction that it is opposed to the wording of the ordinance remained unchanged; therefore, to determine the matter we have submitted the question to counsel, with the following result:—

"'Question for the opinion of counsel.—Under Ordinance No. 14 of 1881, are pharmaceutists holding colonial diplomas only required to pass the examination as provided for in section 7 before registration, or do they come within the meaning of the words "any person holding a diploma or certificate entitling him to practise in any of the capacities aforesaid in the United Kingdom," occurring in section 3?'

"[OPINION.]

"'Re Ordinance No. 14 of 1881.

"'I have perused the provisions of this ordinance with reference to the question submitted for my opinion—namely, whether pharmaceutists holding colonial diplomas only require to pass an examination under clause 7.

"'Such persons would clearly have to pass such examination; the diplomas of recognised colonial universities are limited to those of doctor or bachelor of medicine or master of surgery, and by omission excludes those of pharmaceutists from recognition. I may also point out that even colonial pharmaceutists' diplomas recognised in the United Kingdom would not enable the holder to practise in the United Kingdom without registration there, a condition extremely difficult to comply with in the majority of cases, and impossible in the residue. "'J. H. GARRICK.

"'Chambers, July 29, 1881.'"

METHOD OF DISTINGUISHING SPURIOUS HONEY.—A solution of twenty pints of honey in sixty of water mixed with alcohol gives a heavy white precipitate of dextrine, if glucose has been added; whilst genuine honey, if treated in the same manner, merely becomes milky.—*Chemical News.*

NOTICE CONCERNING A NEW ORCHID OF VICTORIA.

(BY BARON FERD. VON MUELLER, K.C.M.G., M. AND PH. D., F.R.S.)

AMONG a number of orchideous plants collected this spring by John M'Kibbin, Esq., near the Upper Loddon, occurs a *Thelymitra* which cannot be referred to any described species. That in a colony so much traversed already for botanical purposes still an absolutely unknown plant of conspicuous beauty should hitherto have been overlooked, even in the neighbourhood of a flourishing town, receives its explanation readily enough by the circumstance that this pretty orchid from outward appearance might by a passing collector of flowers readily be taken for a small form of *Thelymitra longifolia,* or *T. ixioides.* Irrespective of this deceptive external resemblance, the new *Thelymitra* may be as rare or local as it is ephemeral, and may thus during the short period of its blooming time—when in spring the ground is gay with flowers —easily escape attention anywhere. In this way also we became aware only during this spring, through Mr. Nancarrow's circumspection, that the lovely *Caladenia coerulea* occurs as a companion of *C. deformis*—in its sisterly resemblance long unnoticed—towards the Lower Murray River, in the whipstick scrub. Facts like these should encourage residents in every district to collect methodically the plants of their vicinity; and this is particularly to be recommended to pharmaceutic gentlemen, settled now in numerous places of Australis, especially as they would thereby raise their scientific standing, and as through their profession they are interested in a flora but scantily as yet investigated as regards the medicinal properties of plants. Of this even the present case is a demonstrative instance, inasmuch as but few of the very many tuberous terrestrial orchids of Australia have been examined for therapeutic purposes. The tubers of any kinds, not having a bitter taste, are likely as valuable for their mucilage as those of several species of orchids, especially the British *O. morio* and *O. mascula,* which yield principally the salep-root, a drug undeservedly sunk into oblivion.

The new tubers soon formed after the flowering time of the plants, are thrown for a moment into boiling water, then briskly and perfectly dried by artificial heat, and finally reduced to powder, which must be preserved in a closed glass vessel. To prepare the salep-mucilage as a very pleasant vehicle for active medicaments in a mixture, one scruple of the powder of salep-root is used for two ounces of boiling water. The mucilage thus instantly obtainable has formerly been used by itself in infantile diarrhoea with very good results. The aborigines were in the habit of utilising the tubers of our terrestrial orchids for food.

The new *Thelymitra,* which with its congeners should also be tested for salep, has been dedicated to its discoverer, and may be characterised as follows:—

Thelymitra M'Kibbini.

Quite glabrous, rather dwarf; basal-leaf very narrow, channelled, stem-leaf bract-like, solitary; flowers two, rarely one; sepals acute, faintly streaked by subtle veins; the outer violet-coloured, the inner as well as the slightly shorter labellum more deeply blue; terminal appendage on each side of the column bright yellow, straight, nearly oblong, almost sessile, minutely papillular-fringed, reaching only as high as the anther; crest between the rather widely disconnected appendages much shorter than the anther, yellow, hardly denticulated; column from below the crest light blue; anther pale yellow, almost smooth, rather blunt.

Among quartz gravel on hills along the Upper Loddon River, near Maryborough; John M'Kibbon, Esq.

This well-marked species belongs to the section Biaurella; from the blue-flowering kinds of that section—namely *T. venosa* and *T. cyanea*—our new congener is at once distinguished by the appendages of the column, neither twisted nor smooth, nor close to each other; furthermore by the anther not acuminated. It verges in some respects to *T. Macmillani,* with which it is associated on the Loddon, as now shown by Mr. M'Kibbin; but the latter plant has the stem more slender and also more flexuous, and provided with two bract-like leaves; its outer sepals, in the earlier state, are brownish purple outside and yellowish at the margin, while the inner sepals and labellum are pale yellow, thus far resembling in colouration those of *T. antennifera,* but all sepals turn finally more or less red; furthermore, the appendages of the column visibly overtop the anther, by which means also the sepals extend not very much beyond the column. *T. Macmillani,* as surmised before, may be a hybrid, perhaps arisen from *T. antennifera* and *T. carnea.* The wide severance, colour, shape and papillar roughness of the column-appendages mark *T. Macmillani* at once as different in all its stages from *T. antennifera*, which at the Loddon is also its companion. In *T. carnea* the column overreaches the anther, the middle space of the summit being nearly at a level with the very short lateral appendages. *T. M'Kibbinii* is in flower towards the end of September and in the beginning of October.

Incidentally it may be here observed that Mr. Bentham has, in one of the very last of his glorious researches, reduced the genus *Ramphidia*, of which one species at least occurs in Queensland, to the older *Etaeria* or *Hetaeria*.

Personalities.

Mr. SAMUEL H. HEALD is about to commence business at Numurkah.

Mr. Edward Thorby Noakes, who was formerly assistant to Messrs. Ford and Co., has purchased the business formerly carried on by Mr Geo. F. Chamberlain, at Rochester.

Mr. Geo. Wm. Francis, son of Mr. H. Francis, has gone to England to finish his pharmaceutical education. Mr. Francis accompanied his son to Adelaide to see him off.

Mr. O. V. Morgan was entertained at dinner by Mr. W. Johnson, at his residence, Windsor, prior to his departure from Victoria. Amongst the gentlemen present were Mr. Bosisto, president of the Pharmacy Board; Mr. Wm. Bowen, president of the Pharmaceutical Society; Mr. C. R. Blackett, Mr. R, Langton, &c. Mr. Morgan spoke very warmly in praise of the hospitality shown to visitors in Melbourne, which he considered the most metropolitan city he had seen since leaving London.

Mr. Wm. Bowen, Toorak, has been appointed to the commission of the peace.

Dr. Cecil Jackson was sued in the Maryborough County Court for medicine supplied by Mr. Ogle, chemist, to lodges of which he was medical attendant. Ogle deposed to a statement by Jackson :—" I have taken all the lodges, and I will take jolly good care I will not prescribe anything expensive for the beggars." Mr. Samuel suggested—" He would give them salts and the scourings of kerosene tins instead of quinine."

POISONING CASES.

A SAD case of poisoning took place on the 10th inst., by which a little girl named Julia Crocker, aged four, living as the adopted daughter of May Anderson, of Sturt-street, Ballarat, lost her life. It appears that the deceased found a bottle containing some caustic potash at the head of an old staircase, the bottle, it is said, being placed there by Richard Waller, the previous occupant of the house, who found it about the premises. The deceased, with the usual curiosity of a child, drank some of it, and shortly afterwards Mrs. Anderson noticed the child lying on the floor. She immediately picked her up and took her to the hospital, where Dr. Owen at once pronounced it to be a hopeless case. Antidotes were, however, administered, but without success, and the little sufferer expired in the greatest agony. From the evidence adduced at the magisterial inquiry held touching the death of the child Julia Crocker, it is palpable that tradesmen and others should exercise great care so that bottles and other vessels containing poisonous substances should not be left carelessly about. It was apparent that the poor child accidentally met her death through drinking poison she had found in a bottle which, presumably, had previously been bestowed there. The evidence also disclosed that a playmate of the deceased, nearly three years old, had partaken of the contents of the bottle to a slight degree, but not dangerously, as it appears she did not like the taste, and spit the substance out. A witness stated that when she heard the deceased screaming after the dose, and perceiving her foaming at the mouth, with her tongue perfectly black, she thought the poor little thing had drunk some ink, but not observing any other bottle about except the one which caused the mischief she took it up and applied it to her lips. She stated the mixture was of "saltish flavour," upon which a premonition came upon her that it was poison, and immediately snatching up the child she carried it to the hospital. If the mixture had been a rank poison instead of an irritant poison, it will at once be seen that three lives would have been sacrificed. It is well known that if a chemist or druggist neglects to label bottles containing deleterious substances with the word "poison" the law takes cognisance of the fact, and the offender is prosecuted. The question naturally arises, why are not other trades or professions using poisonous substances subjected to the same penalties for not labelling the bottles containing them ? It can be plainly seen that poison, when left about, conduces to more danger than when securely kept on a druggist's shelf.

Another fatal case of poisoning occurred on the 14th instant, the victim being a little boy named O'Connor, son of Mr. O'Connor, produce merchant, of Doveton-street North. It seems that about six years ago Mr. O'Connor bought some strychnine, and hid it, as he thought, safely in the stable. About two years ago, when another case of poisoning occurred, he looked for it to put it away in a safer place, but it was not to be found. He gave no further thought to the matter, thinking that it had been got rid of. On Friday, however, the little fellow was playing about in the stables, when his mother came in and told him that she wanted him to go out. He said that he was sick, and could not walk, and that he had eaten something out of a paper he had found. His mother looked at the paper, and recognised it as the one that had contained the strychnine. She immediately sent for Dr. Usher, who set out without delay, but by the time he arrived the child was dead. He had expired in very little pain.

GLYCERINE.

NOTWITHSTANDING the low price which now prevails for almost every description of raw produce and manufactured goods, there are a few articles which form notable exceptions. Perhaps one of the most remarkable of these is refined glycerine, which within the last two years has advanced from about £30 to £130 per ton avoirdupois for 30° B. This enormous advance is due partly to increased consumption, diminished production, and the influence of speculation working on a market devoid of stocks. In view of the present position of the article, and the prospect of a continuance of high prices for a considerable time to come, the attention of soapmakers is now being turned to the utilisation of their waste "leys," and various new processes for recovering the glycerine contained in these liquors have lately been tried with more or less successful results. Apart from minor impurities, waste soap "leys" are generally found to contain glycerine, carbonate of soda or caustic soda, chloride of sodium, gelatin, and albumen. One of the processes for recovering the glycerine which promise to be the most economical and the most successful begins with concentrating the liquor until the salts contained therein begin to crystallise. The liquid is then cooled and filtered to rid it of gelatin and albumen. It is afterwards made to absorb carbonic acid, which precipitates bicarbonate of soda, and first is separated from the liquor in the usual way. After undergoing this process the liquor is then made to absorb gaseous hydrochloric acid until what remains of carbonate of soda has been converted into chloride; and further, until all, or almost all, the chloride of sodium has been precipitated and separated from the liquor in the usual manner. Arrived at this stage, the liquor contains water, glycerine, and hydrochloric acid. The acid is then evaporated entirely and absorbed in water, for using afresh. The dilute glycerine remaining can be purified by filtering it through animal charcoal, or by concentrating and distilling it in the usual way.

THE ONLY AMERICAN LEECH FARM.

IN 1841 Mr. H. Witte established a small leech farm in Kent Avenue, Williamsburg, L.I. In course of time this small establishment was abandoned, and one of thirteen acres was established near Newtown, L.I., and to him the writer is indebted for the following information and description of the only leech farm in America. The breeding ponds consist of oblong squares of one and a-half acres each. The bottoms of these ponds are of clay, the margins of peat. In June the leeches begin forming their cocoons on the peat margins of the pond. The greatest enemies to the young leeches are musk-rats, water-rats, and water-shrews, who dig the cocoons out of the soft peat breeding margins. Next to rats and shrews is overheating of the peat or the water of the pond ; in fact, nothing is so fatal to leeches as a too high temperature. Mr. Witte says he has had leeches frozen in solid ice, but by slowly dissolving the ice and gradually increasing the temperature of the water the leeches sustained no injury. The depth of the water in the ponds during the summer is three feet ; in winter time the depth of water is increased, to avoid freezing.

The leeches are fed every six months on fresh blood placed in thin linen bags, which are suspended in the water. The leeches, as soon as they smell the blood, assemble from all parts of the pond, and attaching themselves to the outside of the bag suck the dissolving coagulated blood through the linen. Digestion proceeds very slowly with the leech, during which time the blood remaining undigested in the stomach of the leech is in a fluid state as if just taken in. The excremental deposits are of a grass-green colour. The best substance for packing leeches in is the peat of their natural ponds made into a stiff mud. Water containing tannin, tanic acid, lime, salt, or brackish water must be guarded against always ; iron is not objectionable, but is an advantage in small quantities.

The demand for leeches in the last few years has somewhat fallen off in the Eastern and Southern States. The Western States and California are now the heaviest buyers. Mr. Witte's sales alone average a thousand a day. The number of leeches imported into the United States amounts to about thirty thousand yearly.

The custom of stripping and salting leeches, to cause them to disgorge after having been applied, has passed away, as many well established cases have occurred of infectious diseases having been communicated on the application of the same leech to a second party. A very popular error exists that a leech when applied takes only the bad blood (whatever that may be) and rejects the good ; this is a mistake. With a leech blood is blood, be it the cold blood of a fish or the warm blood of a human being, no matter how diseased that human being may be. So long as blood is not tainted or putrid the leech will thrive on it. A friend of mine, who was the proprietor of a large leech-breeding establishment at the foot of the Hartz Mountains, when wishing to feed his leeches was in the habit of hiring poor labourers, at six cents per day, to stand in the water for half an hour nearly up to their thighs that the leeches might obtain a full gorging of human blood.

In the marshy lands of Roumania the wild leeches are captured by means of men entering the water and allowing the wild leeches to fasten on to their naked bodies. The leech fisher then strip them off after reaching the shore.

QUACK MEDICINE.

At Warwick recently Henry Norman, called a cheap jack, who travels from town to town, was brought up on remand, charged with having obtained 1s. by false pretences from John Magee, a valet, of Yardley-terrace, Warwick, on the 26th August. The evidence taken at the previous examination was read over. On the day named Inspector Hall visited the prisoner's pavilion, where two or three hundred persons were assembled. Prisoner produced a Chinese tea-chest, which he proceeded to break open. Then he descanted on the wonderful genius of the Chinese, and producing from the chest the bottles, which were carefully packed in sawdust, said—"These have come all the way from China." They contained, he said, "Chinese malachite," a great medicine, which was a specific for rheumatism, shortness of breath, and various other maladies. He said he would give them "a treat for that night only," and would sell it at 1s. a bottle. Then he sold a number of bottles, and Magee, who suffered from tightness in the chest, bought one, which he subsequently handed to the police. He had been unable to test its efficacy, as his wife refused to allow him to take it. Henry Watts, of Coventry, who had been in the prisoner's employ about seven weeks, and, according to his own story, left voluntarily, because he could not stand the prisoner's "swindling," stated the prisoner made the "malachite" himself, and packed it so as to pretend it had just arrived from China, and labelled it up as if it bore the Government stamp. It was made of "Chili pods, aniseed, cloves, cinnamon, cayenne pepper, and black sugar." The cost would be only about a farthing a bottle, and prisoner would sometimes sell 1200 or 1300 bottles. Mr. Hugo Young, Midland Circuit, in addressing the bench for the defence, contended that the accused was entitled to call his medicine Chinese malachite, the same as any concoctor of medicine gave them distinctive names. Magee never heard the alleged statement, but thought the malachite was a patent medicine, and bore the Government stamp, and consequently was not thus deceived. The bench at once dismissed the case without comment. The result was received with immense cheering, repeated outside the court.— *Morning Post.*

PLANTS IN THEIR RELATION TO HEALTH.

(A lecture delivered by Mr. C. R. Blackett before the Australian Health Society.)

One of the most characteristic and satisfactory movements of the present day is that which is so energetically supported by health societies. In former days, in consequence of the general ignorance of all classes of the people of the physical sciences, more particularly chemistry and physiology, little or no attention was paid to the physical laws by which the universe is governed. In the days of our ancestors such questions as drainage, sewage disposal, ventilation, purity of air, tree planting, forest conservation, suitability of clothing and diet, were not thought of much importance ; certainly very little interest was manifested in such subjects, concerning which very imperfect and often extremely erroneous notions were entertained.

It had, however, long been known that residents in the country districts enjoyed better health, and a longer average duration of life, and a greater immunity from many diseases, than inhabitants of cities ; that crowded centres of population were much less salubrious generally. The poet Cowper said—

God made the country, man made the town.

It is now well known that much of the disease which afflicts mankind is preventible ; and although, notwithstanding our greater scientific knowledge, there is much to puzzle us, and often baffle our most earnest and intelligent efforts, yet a great advance has been made in matters relating to the proper methods for preserving health and preventing disease ; and when we consider the importance of the science of sanitation, in its bearing upon the physical and moral well-being of the people, we cannot employ ourselves better than in availing ourselves of every addition to our knowledge, and applying it immediately in active efforts towards the improvement of the health of our population ; for, as Lord Derby observes, "Don't fancy that the mischief done by disease spreading through the community is to be measured by the number of deaths that ensue ; that is the least part of the result. As in battle the killed bear a small proportion to the wounded, it is not merely by the crowded hospitals, the frequent funerals, the destitution of families, or the increased pressure of public burdens that you may test the suffering of a nation over which sickness has passed. The real and lasting injury lies in the deterioration of the race ; in the seeds of disease transmitted to future generations ; in the degeneracy and decay which are never detected till the evil is irreparable, and even then the cause remains often undiscovered." Our national vigour and energy, our social and domestic well-being and happiness, our progress generally, depends upon a wise attention and obedience to those universal, inexorable, and beneficent laws by which the life of the animal is regulated.

The relation which exists between the animal and vegetable world is one of surpassing interest, and a clear conception of the mutual adaptations involved in that relationship is of great utility. We shall see that the two great kingdoms of nature existing upon the earth, living upon the soil, and in the atmosphere, are involved in one ceaseless and mutually dependent revolution. The soil, the animal, the plant, every atom, has its fate determined by fixed and unerring laws.

The visible universe is made up of matter and force, equally indestructible. "The amount of force which is in operation in the earth (and probably in the solar system) is as definite as that of the material elements through which its existence is made known to us."

E.g., a pound of charcoal when burned in air combines with $2\frac{2}{3}$ lbs. of oxygen, and produces $3\frac{2}{3}$ lbs. of anhydrous carbonic acid. This chemical combination is attended with the extrication of a definite amount of heat ; and if it be applied without loss, is sufficient to convert $12\frac{1}{2}$ lbs. of water at 15° C. (59° F.) into steam at 100° C. (212° F.). Associated with each pound of charcoal there must be, therefore, a certain amount of energy or force, which is brought into action when the charcoal is burnt ; in the same way, when phosphorus, sulphur, hydrogen, zinc, and copper, &c., are burnt or oxydised. (The lecturer here conducted several illustrative experiments.) Further, there is no such thing as destruction of force—*ex. gr.*, Joule's *Law of the Mechanical Equivalent of Heat.* The carefully conducted experiments of Dr. Joule show that the actual quantity of heat developed by friction is dependent simply upon the amount of force expended, without regard to the nature of the substances rubbed together. He found, as a mean of forty closely concordant experiments, that when water was agitated by means of a horizontal brass paddle wheel, made to revolve by the descent of a known weight, the temperature of 1 lb. of water was raised 1° F. by the expenditure of an amount of force sufficient to raise 772 lbs. to the height of one foot. The conclusion arrived at was that the quantity of heat capable of raising the temperature of 1 lb. of water (between 55° and 60°) by 1° F. requires for its evolution the expenditure of a mechanical force sufficient to raise 772 lbs. one foot (*Phil. Trans.*, 1859). (Chemical affinity, heat, light, magnetism, and electricity were here briefly touched upon.)

Matter (the various substances of which the universe is composed) is resolvable into simple elementary bodies. Iron, gold, silver, oxygen, &c., are simple bodies; and so on to some 64 undecomposed substances. Water (H_2O) is a compound body. Of these elementary substances only 14 occur in large quantities:—C, H, O, N, P, S, Fe, Ca, Mg, K, Na., Al., Cl., Si. (The lecturer here made remarks on the *soil* and *atmosphere* and the *above constituents* of plants and animals.) Organised beings have been arranged under two heads, two great divisions —animals and plants; and, although the lowest genera in each division approximate so closely that it is almost if not quite impossible to fix where one begins and the other ends, yet in their general relationships they are widely different, and opposed to each other in the functions which they discharge in the order of nature. The operations of vegetable life are complementary to those of animal life in the nicely adjusted balance of organic life, each affording support and nourishment to the other, and mutually dependent. (The contrast between animals and plants was explained by diagrams.)

There are observers of repute who maintain that there are certain organisms which are animals at one period of their lives and plants at another, and *vice versa*. The recent investigation of De Bary have an important bearing upon this question. He describes certain fungi, the spores of which, when germinating, give rise to a body undistinguishable from the *ameba*, one of the lowest forms of animal life. However, we know that plants have a place in nature intermediate between minerals and animals, and derive their nourishment from the earth and atmosphere, and that plants alone have the power of converting the inorganic, or mineral, matter into organic. Animals live on organic matter, and reconvert it into inorganic. Animals cannot produce protoplasm. Professor Huxley, in his work on the *Physical Basis of Life*, says " that a unity of power or faculty, a unity of form, and a unity of substantial composition pervade the whole living world." The attempt to define or explain the phenomena of life in plants or animals has been made, but we are not called upon to detail the various metaphysical and scientific definitions here. Of one thing we are certain—that all the phenomena of life in plants are due to solar radiance. The undulations of the sun's heat penetrate the soil, and set in motion the atoms of the rootlet, and enable them to shake hydrogen atoms out of equilibrium with oxygen atoms, which cluster about them in the compound molecules of water. The swifter undulations are arrested by the leaves, and enable them to dislodge atoms of carbon from the carbonic acid in which they move. These disturbances of equilibrium cause a series of rhythmical motions in the form of the alternately ascending and descending sap. Cells and fibres are then developed. Plants are " the air-woven children of light." As only in special physical conditions can vegetable life exist, so it is also with the animal. In that collection and combination of substance which constitutes an animal there is a perpetual introduction of fresh matter, and a constant departure of the old material. The permanence of the individual depends upon the permanence of external conditions. As they change, so it changes, and a new form is the result. That which we call life is the display of the manner in which the force thus disengaged is expended. As has been said by Draper, a scientific examination of animal life must include two primary facts—it must consider in what manner the stream of material substance has been derived; in what manner and whither it passes away; and since force cannot be created from nothing, and is in its very nature indestructible, it must determine from what source that which is displayed by animals has been obtained, in what manner it has been employed, and what disposal is made of it eventually. As pointed out before, the force expended is originally derived from the sun.

Plants are the intermediate agents for its conveyance. The inorganic saline material of which they are composed is derived from the soil in which they grow, and also the greater part of the water so essential to their existence. The organic matter of plants is derived from the air; and so we may say, to use the words of Mottschut again, " they are the air-woven children of light," condensed from the air.

The chemical explanations of vegetable physiology rest principally upon the discovery of oxygen by the illustrious Priestley, carbonic acid by Lavoiser, and the composition of water by Cavendish and Watt.

When the sun shines the leaves of plants decompose carbonic acid, one of the ingredients of atmospheric air; this substance is composed of the two elements, carbon and oxygen. The carbon is appropriated by the plant, and enters into the composition of the sap, from which organic products, such as starch, sugar, wood-fibre, &c., are made. The oxygen now liberated from the carbon is for the most part refused by the plant, and is *returned to the air*, and as the process goes on, fresh portions of carbonic acid CO_2 are ready to be absorbed and decomposed. The leaves are trembling in an atmosphere warmed by the sun's rays, and over their surface warm currents are continually passing.

The plant's function, then, is to separate the combustible carbon from the air. Carbon is thus obtained from carbonic acid CO_2 and H from water H_2O. Plant life is, chemically speaking, an operation of reduction. Plants decompose in a similar way ammonia into its constituents, nitrogen and hydrogen ; and sulphuric acid and phosphoric acid are made to give up their oxygen, the phosphorus and sulphur being appropriated. The whole vegetable world has thus been and is the result of the solar radiance, formed of matter once united to oxygen. In the wonderful series of decompositions which take place in the plant, force or energy, in the form of light, has disappeared and become incorporated with the organic matter of the vegetal organism. This force is ready to be given up again when oxidation takes place—*e.g.*, coal in our fires. Vegetable products constitute a magazine of force ready for our use ; hence their adaptation to our wants as food, and for the production of warmth. The plant in the secondary geological periods locked up the carbon in its tissues for future ages ! ! Oil, fat, wax, &c., like coal, have all derived their carbon, or force-giving properties, from the sun. " When one takes," says Professor Fiske, "a country ramble on a pleasant summer's day, one may fitly ponder upon the wondrous significance of this law of the transformation of energy. It is wondrous to reflect that all the energy stored up in the timber of the fences and farmhouses which we pass, as well as the grindstone and the axe lying beside it, and in the iron axles and heavy tires of the cart which stands tipped by the roadside ; all the energy from moment to moment given out by the roaring cascade and the busy wheel that rumbles at its foot ; by the undulating stalks of corn in the field, and the swaying branches of the forest beyond ; by the birds that sing in the tree tops, and the butterflies to which anon they give chase ; by the cow standing in the brook, and the water which bathes her lazy feet ; by the sportsman who passes, shooting in the distance, as well as by the dogs and guns ;—that all this multiform energy is nothing but metamorphosed solar radiance, and that all these various objects, giving life and cheerfulness to the landscape, have been built up into their cognisable forms by the agency of sunbeams, such as those by which the scene is now rendered visible. We may well declare with Professor Tyndall that the grandest conceptions of Danté and Milton are dwarfed in comparison with the truths which science discloses. But it seems to me that we can go further than this, and say that we have here reached something deeper than poetry. In the sense of illimitable vastness with which we are oppressed and saddened as we strive to follow out in thought the eternal metamorphosis we may recognise the modern phase of the feeling which led the ancient to fall upon his knees and adore—after his own crude symbolic fashion—the invisible Power, whereof the infinite web of phenomena is but the visible garment."

The lecturer alluded to the sanitary influences produced by plants, the purification of the air, the disintegration of the soil by the roots of trees, the drainage of the soil, the importance of the conservation of forests, the disastrous results which had ensued in many parts of the world through the wanton and ignorant destruction of forests ; and, in conclusion, made the following remarks upon the exhalation of water by leaves and the preservation of forests :—

A common sun-flower, 3½ feet high, with a surface of 5·616 square inches, exhaled 20 ounces a day (Hales). If such a large amount of fluid be thus given off by a single plant, what an enormous quantity must be exhaled by the whole vegetation of the earth. It can easily be understood that the air of a thickly wooded district will be always in a damp condition, while one with a scanty vegetation will be dry ; and hence we conclude that a country to be perfectly healthy should have the proportion of plants carefully preserved. It has also an important bearing upon the fertility of the soil, and thus, indirectly, upon the health of the inhabitants. Many regions, once remarkable for their fertility, now are barren wastes through neglect of these facts.

To quote the forcible language of our eminent botanist, Baron von Mueller—" The existence of many an invalid might be prolonged and rendered more enjoyable, while many a sufferer might be restored to health, were he timely to embrace the patriarchic simplicity of forest life, and were he to seek the pure air, wafted decarbonised in delicious freshness through the forest, ever to invigorate strength and restore exhilaration and buoyancy of mind. Let us regard forests as an inheritance given to us by nature, not to be despoiled or devastated, but to be wisely used, reverently honoured, and carefully maintained. Let us regard the forests as a gift entrusted to us only for transient care, to be surrendered to posterity as an unimpaired property, increased in riches and augmented in blessings ; to pass as a sacred patrimony from generation to generation."

NON-EXPLOSIVE KEROSENE.

VERY frequently of late we have received from correspondents, east and west, samples of "stuff" sold them by peddlers, with the assurance that when a little of these preparations are mixed with the poorest burning oil the latter is rendered *perfectly safe.* Of course one of the chief inducements to use these compositions is the assurance that with them a much cheaper oil of equal illuminating power can be used safely.

This fraud is a very dangerous one, and perhaps the best way to stop it is by the diffusion of a little practical information respecting these oils.

In the first place, there is nothing that can be added to or mixed with poor kerosene oil that will in the least affect its dangerous qualities, or make it any safer to use in lamps. The danger with such oils arises solely from the presence in them of light, easily volatilised, and very inflammable hydro-carbons, such as naphtha, the vapour of which, when mixed with air, explodes on contact with flame.

Kerosene and naphtha, or benzine, are derived by a process of distillation from the same substance—petroleum. The lighter oils—gasoline, naphtha, benzine, &c.—are first volatilised and condensed. As the products distil over they are tested from time to time with a hydrometer, and when it is found that the stream of distilled oil marks about 58 deg. (Baume's hydrometer), what follows is turned into another tank, until it is found that the gravity of the oil coming over has risen to about 40 deg., then the stream is deflected into another tank. The oil distilled between 58 deg. and 38 deg. is called kerosene or burning oil.

In this process about 15 per cent. of the light oils are produced, and, as there is comparatively little demand for them, they are very cheap. Naphtha costs from two to five cents a gallon, while good kerosene costs from twenty to twenty-five cents. As great competition exists among the refiners, there is a strong inducement to turn the heavier portions of the naphtha into the kerosene tank, so as to get for it the price of kerosene, or to cheapen the latter. They change the direction of the stream from the still when it reaches 65 deg. to 60 deg. B., instead of waiting until it reaches 58 deg.; and thus the volatile inflammable naphtha or benzine is allowed to run into the kerosene, rendering the whole of the latter dangerous. It has been shown that one per cent. of naphtha will lower the flashing point of kerosene ten degrees, while with 20 per cent. of naphtha the same oil will flash at 8 deg. (Fahr.) above the freezing point of water. It is, therefore, the cupidity of the refiner that leads him to run as much benzine as possible into the kerosene, regardless of the consequences.

The specific gravity is not a safe guide respecting the character of such oils, as a poor, dangerous oil may be heavier than a safe oil. Astral oil illustrates this. While it does not flash below 125 deg. Fahr., its gravity is 49 deg. B. Poor kerosene flashes at 86 deg. Fahr., but has a gravity of 47 deg. B.

Kerosene when properly refined is nearly colourless by transmitted light and slightly fluorescent by reflected light. Its density should be about 43 deg. B. At ordinary temperatures it should extinguish a match as readily as water, without

becoming inflamed or *flashing,* and when heated it should not evolve an inflammable vapour below 110 deg. Fahr., and should not take fire below 125 deg. to 140 deg. Fahr.

As the temperature in a burning lamp rarely exceeds 100 deg. Fahr., such an oil would be safe. It would produce no vapours to mix with the air in the lamp and make an explosive mixture, and if the lamp were overturned or broken the oil would not take fire.

The standard which has generally been adopted by law as a safe one fixes the flashing point at 100 deg. Fahr., or higher. Professor Chandler, president of the New York city board of health, says :—" Out of 736 samples of kerosene oil tested by me, only 28 were really safe, all the rest evolving inflammable vapour below 100 deg. Fahr." In his paper on the temperature of oil in lamps (*American Chemist,* August, 1872, p. 43), Dr. Chandler has shown that in some cases the temperature of their contents often rises above 100 deg. Fahr. —*Scientific American.*

VARNISH FOR PREVENTING RUST.—A varnish for this purpose may be made of 120 parts resin, 180 sandarac, 50 gum lac. They should be heated gradually until melted, and thoroughly mixed, then 120 parts of turpentine added, and subsequently, after heating, 180 parts rectified alcohol. After careful filtration, it should be put into tightly-corked bottles.

CERTAIN FACTS TOWARDS THE HISTORY OF PHOSPHORESCENCE.—Phosphorus in an atmosphere of pure oxygen is not luminous, but the introduction of a bubble of ozone sets up phosphorescence for a moment. Oil of turpentine prevents phosphorescence, and it possesses the property of destroying ozone. The illumination of phosphorous in oxygen by means of ozone is a means of detecting the presence of the latter.— *J. Chappuis.*

Books, &c., Received.—The *Australian Medical Journal* for October ; the *American Journal of Pharmacy* ; the *Druggists' Circular,* New York ; the *Pharmaceutical Journal* ; the *Australasian Medical Gazette* ; and Messrs. Langton, Edden, Hicks and Clark's " Market Report" of 26th August, which states that the dulness of trade which characterised produce and chemical markets at the date of our last issue has given way to some extent, and a slight activity is noticeable, and more especially in the latter.

THE PHARMACY BOARD OF VICTORIA.

I HEREBY give notice that at an Election of a Member of the Pharmacy Board of Victoria, *vice* John Kruse, resigned, held before me at No. 4 Mutual Provident Buildings, Collins-street, Melbourne, on Monday, the 10th of October, 1881, Cuthbert Robert Blackett, Esq., of Gertrude-street, Fitzroy, was duly elected unopposed ; and I therefore declare the said C. R. Blackett a Member of the Pharmacy Board of Victoria.

ALLAN THOMAS BEST,
Returning Officer.

Dated at Melbourne, the 10th October, 1881.

THE ANNUAL DINNER

Of the

PHARMACEUTICAL SOCIETY OF VICTORIA,

In Aid of the

BENEVOLENT FUND,

Will be held at

CLEMENT'S CAFE, SWANSTON STREET,

On WEDNESDAY, the 16th Nov., 1881,

At Eight o'clock p.m.

Tickets, One Guinea each, can be obtained on application to Mr. Shillinglaw, at the Office, 100 Collins-street, or from any member of the Council.

New and Standard Medical Works

ON SALE BY

GEO. ROBERTSON

WHOLESALE AND RETAIL

BOOKSELLER & STATIONER,

33 & 35 Little Collins Street West,

MELBOURNE.

The Cyclopædia of Practical Receipts, Processes, and Collateral Information in the Arts, Manufactures, Professions and Trades, including Pharmacy and Hygiene, by ARNOLD J. COOLEY, 2 volumes ... ... 47s. 6d.

Beasley—The Book of Prescriptions ... ... 7s. 6d.

Beasley—The Druggist's General Receipt Book ... ... 7s.

Beasley—The Pocket Formulary and Synopsis of the British and Foreign Pharmacopœias ... ... 7s. 6d.

Fownes—A Manual of Chemistry, Theoretical and Practical, 2 vols. ... ... 21s.

Mayne—A Medical Vocabulary: being an Explanation of all Terms and Phrases used in the various departments of Medical Science and Practice, giving their Derivation, Meaning, Application, and Pronunciation ... ... 11s. 6d.

Taylor—On Poisons in Relation to Medicine ... ... 18s.

Bloxam—Laboratory Teaching: Progressive Exercises in Practical Chemistry, illustrated ... ... 6s. 6d.

Royle—A Manual of Materia Medica and Therapeutics, illustrated ... ... 17s.

Carpenter—The Microscope and its Revelations, illustrated ... ... 17s.

Dick—Encyclopædia of Practical Receipts and Processes, 6,400 Receipts ... ... 25s.

Squire—A Companion to the British Pharmacopœia, comparing the strength of its various Preparations with those of the United States and other Foreign Pharmacopœias, &c. ... ... 12s.

Fenwick—The Student's Guide to Medical Diagnosis, illustrated ... ... 7s. 6d.

Savory—A Compendium of Domestic Medicine, and Companion to the Medicine Chest ... ... 6s.

A COMPLETE CATALOGUE OF MEDICAL BOOKS TO BE HAD ON APPLICATION.

GEORGE ROBERTSON,

33 and 35 Little Collins Street West, Melbourne,

· AND AT

SYDNEY, BRISBANE, AND ADELAIDE.

[SUPPLEMENT ONLY.]

Chem. & Drugg. Aust. Suppl.
Vol. 4, no. 43; 49-56 (Nov. 1881).

THE
Chemist & Druggist.

WITH AUSTRALASIAN SUPPLEMENT.

(Published under direction of the Pharmaceutical Society of Victoria.)

No. 43. { PUBLISHED ON THE 15TH }   NOVEMBER, 1881.   { SUBSCRIPTION, 15S. PER ANNUM,
{ OF EVERY MONTH. }   { INCLUDING DIARY, POST FREE.
Registered for Transmission as a Newspaper.

TRADE NOTICE.

REGISTRATION OF MOTHER SEIGEL'S SYRUP IN VICTORIA.

Extract *from* THE GOVERNMENT GAZETTE, *Friday, 9th January,* 1880.

APPLICATION FOR THE REGISTRATION OF ONE TRADE MARK—No. 271.

To the Registrar-General, Melbourne.

I, ANDREW JUDSON WHITE, of 34 and 40 Ludgate Hill, London, patent medicine vendor, apply to be registered as proprietor of a trade mark being an oblong label having the words "Mother Seigel's" on an extended ribbon crossing an American shield surrounding an oval band bearing the words "Curative Syrup" "Operating Pills" and at base another extended ribbon similar to the first bearing the words "Extract of American roots." Within this oval band a sketch of an old woman dressed as a quakeress seated at a table with an open book thereon and (supposed to be) giving directions to a girl standing with a cup and spoon, one in each hand, on the other side of table. Without the oval band the words "A. J. White" and "London," the oval band having on the left but removed thereform a ribbon carried on two supports or rods bearing the words "for impurities of the blood" and on the right but removed from the oval band or ribbon carried similar to the last but bearing the words "for dyspepsia and liver complaints," thus:—

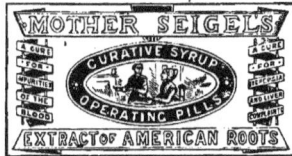

I desire that the said trade mark may be registered in respect of the description of goods following, contained in class 3, that is to say :—Patent Medicines.   A. J. WHITE.
Witness—D. H. McLauchlan, 67 Strand, W.C.
EDWARD WATERS, Agent for Applicant.

Extracted *from* WHITE'S ALMANAC FOR 1882, *now issued throughout the Colonies.*

NOTICE TO CONSUMERS OF MOTHER SEIGEL'S SYRUP.

"I have Registered the Trade Mark Label in all the Colonies, and I shall protect the public from imitations.

"The Wholesale Agents, whose names are printed in this book, receive their supplies direct from me in America, and the public can rely upon the article being genuine."

Melbourne—FELTON, GRIMWADE & CO.; Sydney—ELLIOTT BROS.; Brisbane—ELLIOTT BROS. & CO.;
Adelaide—A. M. BICKFORD & SONS; Hobart—A. P. MILLER; Dunedin, Christchurch, Wellington,
Auckland—KEMPTHORNE, PROSSER & CO.'S NEW ZEALAND DRUG CO. LIMITED;
Launceston—L. FAIRTHORNE & SON.

A. J. WHITE LIMITED,
21 FARRINGDON ROAD, LONDON, E.C.

To guard against Imitations, Note the above facsimile of Label, as printed in
"THE GOVERNMENT GAZETTE."

Printed by Mason, Firth & M'Cutcheon, 51 & 53 Flinders Lane West, Melbourne.

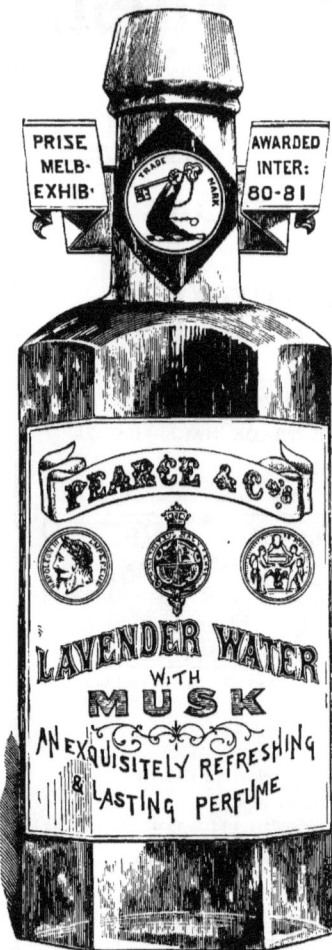

INDEX TO LITERARY CONTENTS.

The Chemist and Druggist.

WITH AUSTRALASIAN SUPPLEMENT.

OFFICE : MUTUAL PROVIDENT BUILDINGS, COLLINS STREET WEST.
Published on the 15th of each Month.

THIS Journal is issued gratis to all paid-up Members of the PHARMA-
CEUTICAL SOCIETY OF VICTORIA, and to non-members at Fifteen Shillings
per annum, payable in advance. A copy of *The Chemists and Druggists'
Diary*, published annually, is forwarded post free to every subscriber.

Advertisements, remittances, and all business communications to be
addressed to THE HONORARY SECRETARY OF THE PHARMACEUTICAL SOCIETY,
MELBOURNE.

SCALE OF CHARGES FOR ADVERTISEMENTS:

Per annum.		Per annum.
One Page £8 0 0	Quarter Page	.. £3 0 0
Half do. 5 0 0	Business Cards	.. 2 0 0

Special rates for wrapper and pages preceding and following literary
matter. Advertisements of Assistants Wanting Situations, 2s. 6d. each.

Advertisements for insertion in the current month should be sent to the
office before the 10th.

COMMUNICATIONS for the EDITORIAL department of this journal should be
addressed to THE EDITOR, MUTUAL PROVIDENT BUILDINGS, COLLINS STREET
WEST, MELBOURNE.

No notice can be taken of anonymous communications. Whatever is
intended for insertion must be authenticated by the name and address of
the writer—not necessarily for publication, but as a guarantee of good faith.

NOTICE TO MEMBERS.

MEMBERS whose subscriptions are unpaid on the 31st
December, 1881, are respectfully informed that in
accordance with Rule 14 their names will be omitted
from the list, and after that date they cease to be
Members of the Society.

THE LIBRARY.

THE Library is open to Members daily, from 9.30 a.m.
to 4.30 p.m.

BIRTH.

MARSHALL.—On the 8th November, at 251 Chapel-street, Windsor, the wife
of W. J. Marshall, pharmacist, of a daughter.

DEATH.

THOMAS.—On the 5th November, at Albert-street, Windsor, Hugh Roberts
Thomas.

A FAILURE OF JUSTICE.

THE horrible tragedy at Sandhurst, which resulted in the
death of an unfortunate young woman, excited throughout
the colony a feeling of disgust and indignation ; and when
it became known that the punishment meted out to the
wretched impostor who perpetrated the foul deed which
ended so fatally, was so absurdly inadequate, every right-
minded person felt that justice had not been done. The
notorious J. E. Wall, who has for years been practising
as a medical man illegally and ignorantly, has escaped
almost "unwhipt of justice." The true story of this
man's life will never be known ; could it be, we have no
doubt but that horrors upon horrors would accumulate.
All the details of the case of the Queen *v.* Wall are so
disgusting that it is most painful to read them, bringing
disgrace upon our common humanity ; and, moreover,
that this convicted quack and murderer is on the roll of
registered pharmaceutical chemists causes us deep regret
and indignation. We trust that the Pharmacy Board
will at once take steps to remove Wall's name from the

register which he has so disgraced. We have no doubt
but that the Board will resolutely do its duty.

The remarks made in a forcible leader in the *Bendigo
Independent* are so thoroughly in accordance with our
feelings upon this case, that we have no hesitation in
quoting them. The italics are our own :—

"Here we have had in our midst for twenty-nine long
years a man, without any legal qualifications to act as a
medical practitioner, has nevertheless usurped the functions conferred by law on men who have, by years of
previous training, fitted themselves to perform the humane,
honourable, and responsible duties of a doctor of medicine,
or of a surgeon. Pursuing his calling—we cannot call it
his profession—for nearly thirty years, how has he
contrived to live ? Holding for many years the *position
of a registrar of births, marriages, and deaths,* the mind
shudders at the thought of this man's life history being
one day laid bare. But the true history of his life will
probably never be written, or, if written, would never find
a publisher. From what little we know as facts, his
unknown deeds can easily be surmised. On several
different occasions he has been called on to answer for
his malpractices. Indeed, it is no exaggeration to say
that he has lived in continual fear of the law, but
until now he has contrived to escape punishment; yet
when conviction at last overtook him, to what did it actually
amount ! Tried *for murder, for one of the fondest crimes
ever perpetrated in the district, the jury returns a merciful
verdict of manslaughter, and the judge sentences the culprit
to a year's imprisonment—less by six months than the
sentence inflicted in the same court only two days before on
a man for stealing a few shillings' worth of sheepskins. It*
is the old story—crimes against the rights of little
regard in the eyes of the law ; it is blasphemy of the
rankest to interfere with the rights of property. With
another judge presiding this—to use the politest language
—excessively mild sentence might, according to recent
precedents, have been expected ; but when in dealing
with the Mitiamo shooting case—rising out of a
drunken quarrel—His Honour Judge Williams, addressing
the prisoner Sugrue, stated that offences against the
person were more heinous than offences against property,
and should be punished accordingly, we scarcely anticipated that Mr. Williams would be found outdoing in
unwarrantable leniency the decision of Judge Holroyd at
the recent sittings of the Central Criminal Court, to which
we referred in last Monday's issue. This time next year
James Egan Wall will again be loose on society, his odious
calling well advertised by the trial throughout the length
and breadth of Victoria and of the neighbouring colonies.
Granting that he possesses some medical skill, will his
twelve months' incarceration change the past character of
the man ? In other words, will he, when he emerges
from the Sandhurst gaol, come out a changed being,
determined to use whatever knowledge he has in a manner

morally, if not legally, right, or will he revert to his old practices, calculating that the danger is counterbalanced by the increased profits? Approaching three-score and ten, can reformation be expected? We think not. And in the sentence recorded, what is there to strike fear into the depraved hearts of others of his calling—who are, there is reason to believe, to be readily found in all centres of population? There is no crime more difficult to prove than the one for which James Egan Wall was convicted; there is no crime more immoral, both in a religious and a physical sense; none more calculated to encourage the meanest, most selfish form of vice to which poor corrupt human nature is susceptible—yet, with all this, the convicted felon—one whose practices were, by a whole generation of Sandhurst residents, regarded as notorious—escapes with punishment such as is every day in ordinary police courts meted out for the most trivial offences."

Our readers will remember that Mr. Mortensen was sentenced to a year's imprisonment for accidentally poisoning a person. A lamentable affair, and, no doubt, the result of carelessness somewhere, but there was no wickedness; it was "death by misadventure." In Wall we have a cold-blooded quack, recklessly causing the death of a human being, and a vile abortionist! and yet the judge thinks twelve months' imprisonment enough.

The Month.

THE annual dinner of the Pharmaceutical Society, held on the 16th of this month, was the most successful gathering of the sort that has ever taken place in the colony. The attendance was very good, and the dinner—an excellent one—reflects great credit on Mr. Clements, the caterer. The company seemed to thoroughly enjoy themselves.

In consequence of the pressure on our space, we are compelled to hold over several reports and letters.

At the next quarterly meeting of the Pharmaceutical Society, which will take place on the 2nd December, Mr. C. R. Blackett will read a paper on "Lolium Temulentum."

We believe that Dr. Bird is a candidate for the appointment of lecturer on medicine in the University, in place of Dr. James Robertson. It is almost needless to add that Dr. Bird's qualifications for the position are of the first order. Dr. Bird's appointment to the chair of medicine would render necessary his resignation of the lectureship on materia medica, which he has held for many years. There are sure to be a good many applications for this position, inasmuch as, financially, it has the advantage of the lectureships of the more advanced years in the Medical School. And as it is proposed to separate the subject into two divisions—namely, materia medica proper and therapeutics and hygiene—it would be necessary to appoint two lecturers to succeed Dr. Bird. The question of a lectureship on pharmacy, which has been several times before the council and the faculty of medicine, may also probably come up again.

Mr. Frank Illingworth (Jones and Co., 108 Lonsdale-street) has been appointed the sole instrument maker to Melbourne Hospital.

Messrs Rocke, Tompsitt and Co. are the successful tenderers for the supply of drugs, &c., to the Melbourne Hospital for the current year.

The next session at the School of Pharmacy will commence on the 6th February, 1882.

The quarterly general meeting of the society will be held at the rooms on Friday, the 2nd December.

Meetings.

THE PHARMACEUTICAL SOCIETY OF VICTORIA.

THE monthly meeting of the Council was held at the rooms, 100 Collins-street, on Friday evening, the 4th November, 1881. Present: Messrs. Bowen, Blackett, Gamble, Huntsman, Nicholls, Baker, Jones, and Shillinglaw. The President (Mr. Wm. Bowen) in the chair. The minutes of the previous meeting were read and confirmed.

New Members.—Mr. Charles G. Hill, of Adelaide, was elected a member, and the President of the Pharmaceutical Society of Queensland, an honorary member.

Gold Medals to Students at the School of Pharmacy.—Mr. Blackett submitted the conditions under which the medals to be given by the Society to the student who shall pass the best examination in materia medica, botany, and elementary and practical chemistry, which were adopted.

The Tariff Commission.—At the suggestion of Mr. George Lewis, it was resolved that action be taken by the Society to ensure some uniformity in the questions to be sent in to the Commission, and the President of the Society (Mr. W. Bowen) was appointed as a delegate to represent the trade before the Commission.

Lectures at the School of Pharmacy.—It was resolved to advertise for lecturers at the school on materia medica, botany, and elementary and practical chemistry for the year 1882.

Amendment of the Sale and Use of Poisons Act.—A communication was received from the Pharmacy Board, asking the Society to consider the advisability of revising the Poisons Act, and a sub-committee, consisting of Messrs. Bowen, Blackett, Johnson, and J. C. Jones, be appointed to deal with the matter, and to report at the next meeting.

Correspondence.—From Mr. Grounds, Levuka, Fiji, stating that the Government had agreed to accept the certificate of the Pharmacy Board as a qualification to carry on business as a pharmaceutical chemist in Fiji. From the Secretary for Lands, in reference to the granting of a piece of land on the Eastern Hill.

At the conclusion of the Council meeting, the adjourned special meeting for the alteration and amendment of the rules, &c., was held. The principal alteration was in the voting for members of the Council by ballot instead of proxy, and the amendments, as published in the last number of the Chemist and Druggist, were passed. The meeting then adjourned.

THE ANNUAL DINNER OF THE PHARMACEUTICAL SOCIETY OF VICTORIA.

THE annual dinner was held at Clements' Café on Wednesday, the 16th November. There was a very good attendance, and the manner in which the dinner was served reflected great credit on Mr. Clements.

The president of the society, Mr. Wm. Bowen, occupied the chair; on his right was seated Dr. J. Robertson, president of the Medical Society of Victoria, and on his left, Dr. Neild, president of the Victorian branch of the British Medical Association. At the same table were also Drs. Gillbee, Thompson, and Henry, Baron F. von Mueller, and Messrs. Grimwade, Brind, Johnson, Harriman, and Blackett. The vice-chairs were occupied by Mr. John T. Thomas, vice-president of the society, and Mr. J. Bosisto, M.L.A., president of the Pharmacy Board. Amongst the visitors present were Messrs. Rivers Langton, W. M. Rogers (Tasmania), J. P. Isaac, W. T. Bowen, Daniel Wilkie, B. C. Harriman, Grimwade (jun.), Goodridge, Bates, Millard Johnson, W. H. H. Lane, Fripp, and D. A. Simpson.

The country districts were represented by Mr. Henry Brind and Mr. J. T. Macgowan (representative of the Ballarat District Chemists' Association), Ballarat; Mr. A. J. Owen, Geelong. Letters of apology were received from Mr. Frank Senior, president of the Pharmaceutical Society, N.S.W.; Drs. Girdlestone, Bird, and Allan; Messrs. Geo. Lewis, H. Wheeler and J. Whittle, Ballarat; Hewlett, Carlton; W. Anderson, Windsor; T. M. Blackett, Williamstown; H. J. Long, Melbourne; J. W. Don, Richmond; C. Marston, Collingwood; John Jackson, West Melbourne; — Walton, Fitzroy; E. Prosser, New Zealand; David Jones, Melbourne; S. S. Strutt, East Melbourne; — Holdsworth, Sandhurst; J. C. Newbery.

The president proposed the usual loyal toasts in suitable terms, and they were drunk with musical honours.

Dr. Robertson proposed "The Pharmaceutical Society of Victoria." He spoke of the close relationship existing between the medical profession and pharmacists, and said that meetings like the present one did much towards fostering and diffusing kindly feelings. It gave him great pleasure to propose the toast entrusted to him, and to couple with it the name of the president of the society, Mr. Wm. Bowen. (Applause.)

Mr. Bowen, who was received with cheers, said :—On behalf of the Pharmaceutical Society of Victoria, I beg to thank you for the cordial manner in which you have been pleased to respond to the last toast ; and in replying thereto I will ask your forbearance for a few moments while I endeavour, in accordance with the usual custom on occasions like the present, to review briefly the principal events which have occurred during the past year, interesting to the pharmaceutical chemist, and to show the systematic progress which pharmacy is making throughout the various countries of Europe and in the United States of America. Without doubt, the most important is that of the International Pharmaceutical Congress, which assembled in London during the month of August last. When I reflect upon the circumstance that it is just thirty years ago since the first International Exhibition was held in London—1851—prior to this date, many present will probably bear me out, that Englishmen knew virtually nothing of the continental countries beyond the number of their standing army and the strength of their naval forces. I well remember at that great world's fair the effect produced upon the minds of my countrymen by the many beautiful works of art, machinery, and other elements of progress brought together by these continental countries to the astonishment and delight of the British public.

I have no hesitation in declaring that I know of no circumstance which marks the progress of civilisation more than this : That within the space of thirty years, socially speaking, from our first acquaintance with the inhabitants of these European nations, that a congress should assemble in the metropolis of the world, of delegates from nearly every country of Europe, the United States of America, and even Victoria—for our little colony had her delegate—a colony not even in existence at the time referred to. I say that nothing marks this progress more than that a congress should be assembled to discuss a subject like that of pharmacy. At this congress one of the principal subjects for discussion was the desirability of establishing an international pharmacopœia ; and when we consider the marvellous rapidity of communication—the telegraphic, postal, and railway systems existing throughout these various countries—when we remember that besides the vast number of persons who avail themselves of such communication for business and pleasure, there is likewise a large proportion who travel for recreative purposes, in search of health—it will at once be apparent the necessity which exists for uniformity in the preparation of medicines which such travellers may require. At this congress many excellent papers were read, among which I observe one by Mr. Peter Squire of a practical character, containing, as it does, a number of tables showing the comparative strength of the various preparations used in these several countries. I have selected a few of the more potent to illustrate my statement :—

Tinct. aconite	...	...	1 and 1 to 1 and 10
Tinct. belladonna	...	...	1 and 1 to 1 and 18
Tinct. colchicum	...	...	1 and 5 to 1 and 10
Tinct. digitalis	...	...	1 and 1 to 1 and 10
Tinct. nuxvomica	...	...	1 and 3 to 1 and 10
Tinct. opium	...	...	1 and 6 to 1 and 20

Although I do not anticipate the immediate success of the movement in establishing an international pharmacopœia, still I have every confidence that some degree of uniformity as regards the more potent of these preparations will be the result. The consideration of these papers will show the importance of another subject brought before this congress— that of pharmaceutical education; and I think you will readily admit the grave responsibility devolving upon pharmaceutical chemists when such difference of strength exists in the pharmacopœias of European countries. But, gentlemen, I contend that the duty of a dispenser is not complete when he simply dispenses accurately the prescription of a medical man with pure and the best of medicines, but consider that another and equally important duty devolves upon him—to read, copy, and carefully examine every prescription brought before him, and to satisfy himself that the doses therein prescribed are in accordance with the latest information. With regard to pharmaceutical education in Victoria, you will probably remember that our late president, Mr. Blackett, informed us that an application had been made to the Melbourne University authorities, requesting them to appoint a lecturer on pharmacy, and that this august body occupied a period of two years in discussing the subject, and at the end of which time sent an acknowledgment of the communication, declining to comply with our request.

I have often endeavoured to satisfy my mind as to the cause of this extraordinary circumstance, and can only arrive at one conclusion. You will probably remember that the late Mr. Buckle, in his book, The History of Civilisation (a book which will be regarded as a standard work so long as the English language may continue), has established the rule "that the climate of a country determines and controls to a very large extent the character of its species ;" and when I remember that the shores of our Australian continental home are washed by the waves of the broad Pacific Ocean, the home of the cephalopoda, a species not remarkable for hasty locomotion, but rather for the tenacity of its grip, I can only arrive at the conclusion that the Melbourne University has become acclimatised. But, gentlemen, however unsatisfactory and discouraging this reply was to the Pharmaceutical Society, I am glad to inform you that it has not proved an unmixed evil ; for there is a remarkable feature in the British character—a determination to overcome difficulties and to remove obstructions in its path—for within a period of two months the Pharmaceutical Society established a school of pharmacy, with a complete staff of lecturers, under the able superintendence of Mr. Cosmo Newbery—a school which, I am proud to anticipate, will occupy no mean position among the educational establishments of Victoria.

At the last meeting of the Pharmaceutical Society it was resolved to offer three gold medals annually to the most proficient among the students, and I have much pleasure in anticipating the results of this incentive to perseverance ; but I would warn the students that it will be an unfortunate circumstance on their part, when passing the board of examiners, should they be unable to define the difference between opium and assafœtida.

There is one feature in the schools of Europe which might well be adopted in our Victorian schools, that of microscopical study ; and I have every confidence that when this subject has been considered by the authorities the same will be recommended. (Applause.)

Dr. Neild next proposed "The Pharmacy Board." He congratulated the society on the success of the Pharmacy Act. Like all useful measures, he said, it was not passed without a great deal of trouble, and much praise was due to Mr. Bosisto for his untiring exertions in connection with it. (Applause.) The Act was the result of the collective deliberations of the two professions, and he was pleased to say it worked admirably. He wished the medical profession had half so good an Act. With reference to the chairman's remarks respecting the refusal of the University authorities to appoint a lecturer on pharmacy, he desired to say something as to how there came to be a failure with respect to the application. Numerous communications on the subject passed between the council and the faculty, and there was some doubt as to what was comprehended by "a lecturer on pharmacy." The medical faculty did not decline to take the question up ; but, somehow or other, he could not exactly tell how, it fell through. (Laughter.) The Pharmacy Board had done a great deal of good, and he was sure it was a source of satisfaction to all concerned. He concluded by asking the company to honour the toast of "The Pharmacy Board," coupled with the name of Mr. J. Bosisto, the president. (Applause.)

Mr. Bosisto, who, on rising to respond, was received with much warmth, returned thanks on behalf of the Board, which, he said, knew its duty and endeavoured to perform it.

Although the members were elected by the pharmaceutical chemists of Victoria, they were responsible to the Chief Secretary of the colony for the working of the "Pharmacy Act;" and so well had it worked, he was pleased to say, that during the five years it had been in force there had not been a single hitch. Some persons had attempted to commence business as chemists without proving their capability; but they had been stopped, and he would take this opportunity of stating that the police of the colony did their duty well in quickly prosecuting for breaches of the Act. The members of the board were the overseers of the rising students in pharmacy, and they felt their responsibility. He would say now, without egotism, that the examination was equal to that in Great Britain. (Hear, hear.) Mr. Johnson, Mr. Blackett, and their humble servant each strove in their respective departments to so rigidly examine, that no certificate should issue from the board unless the applicant had fully proved himself entitled to it. (Applause.) In these days there was a great deal being said about the adulteration of food and everything else, and there was no doubt that the men to deal thoroughly with such subjects must come from pharmaceutical chemists. (Applause.)

Mr. F. S. Grimwade proposed "The Pharmaceutical Society of Great Britain, and Kindred Societies," and said that in May last the Pharmaceutical Society of Great Britain held its fortieth annual dinner. The main object of the society was the promotion of the science of pharmacy. How well it had carried out the intention of its founders could be estimated by comparing the position of pharmacists of the present day with that of forty years ago. Members of the Pharmaceutical Society were connected with the Royal Society, Society of Chemists, the Institute of Chemistry, and in fact more or less were connected with nearly all the scientific societies. Speaking of the Pharmaceutical Society, a whole host of names crowded one's memory—Jacob Bell, Allen, Pareira, Hanbury, Fownes, Sandford, Dean, Burtley, Redwood, Greenish, Schacht, and others who had distinguished themselves. The Pharmaceutical Society of Great Britain should be revered and honoured by pharmacists in all parts of Her Majesty's dominions. (Applause.) The more honour we paid to the Pharmaceutical Society of Great Britain and the names celebrated in connection with it, the more should we appreciate our own society, and as time rolled on, we, too, should have the names of men who had distinguished themselves. We had our Johnson, Bosisto, Blackett, Bowen, and others, who would he held up as examples to our coming pharmacists of men who had laboured hard to promote the best interests of their profession in this country. He called upon the company to honour the toast, coupled with the name of Mr. W. Johnson. (Applause.)

Mr. Johnson briefly returned thanks, and caused some amusement by relating his experiences during the time he was an apprentice, when he had much "dirty work" to perform; work with "good honest dirt," he said, which no man need be ashamed of, but which the apprentices of the present day were not expected to undertake.

Mr. C. R. Blackett proposed "The Medical Society of Victoria, and Kindred Societies." He said the medical profession in Victoria was worthy of its great origin. What profession, he asked, could be more noble? The healing art was the most noble of all. He placed it above divinity. (Hear, hear.) Very soon, he believed, the art of medicine would become a fixed and positive science. It was necessary to constantly bear in mind that the professions must be kept apart, each working in its own line. They were distinct from each other, and the aim of all should be to keep pharmacy to itself and medicine to itself. That there were those who did not endeavour to do this was evident from an advertisement which appeared in the last number of *The Australasian Medical Gazette*, published in Sydney. He would read the advertisement:—"An experienced pharmaceutical and consulting chemist wishes to hear of an opening. A country district preferred, where there is no opposition, and, if possible, no medical practitioner residing in the neighbourhood. Address —'J.G.,' *Australasian Medical Gazette* Office." (Loud laughter.) It was much to be regretted that such an advertisement was allowed to appear. He concluded by coupling with the toast the names of Dr. Robertson and Dr. Neild.

In the absence of the former gentleman, who had been called away,

Dr. Gillbee responded for the Medical Society of Victoria, and said that he and his fellow medical men in the colony placed the utmost confidence in the pharmacists.

Dr. Neild replied for the Victorian branch of the British Medical Association. He referred to the advertisement brought under the notice of the company by Mr. Blackett, and said the only way he could account for its appearance in the *Gazette* was that it had escaped the notice of the editor. The enterprising spirit of the publisher of a newspaper was always in excess of the zeal of the editor. (Laughter.)

Baron von Mueller responded for the Royal Society.

The next toast was "Our Visitors," proposed by Mr. A. T. Best.

Mr. Rivers Langton (Great Britain) replied. He thanked Mr. Best for the flattering reference he had made to him in proposing the toast of the visitors, and begged to assure him that no language he could command would express half the pleasure and astonishment he had felt at what he had seen during his visit to the great Australian colonies. The president in his speech had alluded to the International Exhibition of 1851, which had aroused in Englishmen a desire to travel and become personally acquainted with the continental cities of Europe, and he was sure the splendid exhibition recently held in Melbourne would attract Europeans to visit the colonies. At present at home there was the greatest ignorance as to the boundless resources of Australia, and Englishmen had only to come and experience their delightful climate, and have their eyes opened as to what really was taking place at the antipodes. He was glad to see such a gathering of the medical profession, and to notice the good feeling and unanimity which existed between them and the Pharmaceutical Society; and he had no doubt there was a bright future before the rising pharmacists. It required an educated man well up in his profession to properly dispense drugs, and it was gratifying to observe that in these colonies the medical profession appreciated the labours of the pharmacists. In his younger days he had learned and delighted with the charming tales in the *Arabian Nights*; but no tale of wonder and romance in that entertaining book could compare with the history of this beautiful city of Melbourne. There was a splendid future before the great Australian continent. He had travelled much, and visited the centres of industry in many lands, but the most metropolitan city of all, to his mind, was Melbourne (applause), and he did not know which to admire most, the beauty of the city, or the perseverance and energy which had created it. But perseverance and energy were inherent in the British nature, and always made their way to the front, as exemplified in the career of the great statesman whose life was so recently closed, who, with the disadvantages of birth and prejudice, raised himself to the proud position of Prime Minister of England. The story of this wonderful city of the goldfields would yet form the theme of the poet's song and delight, and enrapture generations yet unborn. It had been a peculiar pleasure to him to be present at this gathering this evening, having experienced so much kindness and courtesy, not only from the pharmacists of Victoria, but throughout the whole of the Australian colonies; nor could he forget the high compliment paid him by the society in electing him as one of their delegates to represent the colony in the congress held so recently in London, and a similar compliment was paid him by the sister colony of New South Wales; and it had been a matter of great regret to him that his business engagements had prevented his being present. He congratulated the society on the able address of their president, and was sure the chemists of Australia would play a part worthy of the glorious future of these great colonies.

Mr. W. H. H. Lane (America) said—Mr. President and gentlemen of the Pharmaceutical Society—I have much pleasure in saying a few words in response to the toast you have so highly honoured; but, after the remarks of my worthy friend, Mr. Langton, and his eulogistic compliments to the United States, I can say but little on our own behalf. There is an old and true saying, that "birds of a feather flock together," and you will find it verified the world over. When I came here this evening I had no idea that I should be called on for any remarks, but it seems that it is to be otherwise. I have the honour of being one of your profession, and I am very proud of it. In the year 1876, at our great exhibition held in the city of Philadelphia, I well remember seeing the exhibits of this colony, and among them those of Mr. Bosisto, and also some of our friend Baron von Mueller's works. I assure you, gentlemen, that Victoria is far better known in the States than you are aware of; but I certainly admit that when I first set out for this country, some three and a-half years ago, I was advised by some of my friends to take my shooting-iron with me and keep a sharp look out for the cannibals, for you know they were at one time here, if not now. No doubt Victoria, as well as her sister colony New South Wales, has come greatly to the front during the past two years; this success, in a great measure, is due to the good effects of your two great International Exhibitions, which have brought you in closer contact with the commercial world. Gentlemen, you have a light in your midst that will take many, many years to obliterate. The one I refer to is my friend on my right, Baron Ferdinand von Müeller. Gentlemen, he has built monuments more enduring than marble or brass, and they will stand for centuries after he has passed away. The people of Victoria will live to do honour to his memory, when too late to acknowledge his sterling worth. Gentlemen you should feel justly proud to have such a valuable adjunct to the profession among you, and I may tell you that we in the United States of America are cognisant of his talents, and have done him the honour to elect him member of some of our leading scientific institutions. Do not for one moment imagine that we are better pharmacists in the United States than in any other part of the world, for, gentlemen, we do not claim that honour. If any one comes over here thinking he can teach you much, he will find himself foiled, for I think, gentlemen, to use an Americanism, "You have cut your eye teeth," and as far as my observations serve me, the chemists of these colonies will compare favourably with any part of the world. I must confess that when leaving San Francisco for this country that tears involuntarily came to my eyes in spite of all I could do to prevent them, for I did not fully know what kind of people I was to cast my lot amongst ; but I have not found you a bad sort after all. I have made many warm friends in these colonies, friends whose friendship I shall cherish to my dying day ; and when I leave these shores I shall always look back with feelings of pleasure and pride, and will no doubt many times long to return to them. Referring to the remarks of your worthy president in regard to an international pharmacopœia, I fully concur in all that has been said this evening. I must say I look forward to its consummation at an early date, and I for one will be glad when there will be no P.B. or U.S.P., &c., or any other of the various pharmacopœias now in existence. Gentlemen, there is also another true saying—"Nature abhors a vacuum," and as I have done my level best for the past three hours to fill that vacuum, will close. Gentlemen, on behalf of the various kindred societies of the United States of America I thank you.

Mr. B. C. Harriman responded on behalf of the Victorian visitors, and expressed the pleasure he experienced at all times in rendering his assistance to societies whose object was the advancement of science.

The toast of " The Press" was proposed by Mr. H. Brind, and responded to by Dr. Neild.

The following donations to the Benevolent Fund have been received :—Dr. Robertson, £1 1s.; Dr. Neild, £1 1s.; R. J. Fullwood, £1 1s.; C. Marston, £1 1s.; T. H. Walton, £1 1s.; H. J. Long, £1 1s.; John Jackson, 10s.

PHARMACEUTICAL SOCIETY'S MEDAL IN GOLD.

School of Pharmacy prizes presented by the Council— Chemistry ("elementary and practical"), botany, *materia medica*, and pharmacy.

At the end of each term a gold medal will be offered for competition. Students who have attended more than one term will be ineligible to compete. The medals can only be taken by students who have worked in the laboratory for not less than 75 per cent. of their period of study, and who are connected with the Society as registered apprentices of the same. On receiving the report of the examiners, the Council will award the prizes.

DEFINITION OF A NEW TREE FROM EAST AUSTRALIA.

By Baron Ferd. von Müeller, Ph.D., M.D., F.R.S., K.C.M.G.

Dysoxylon Schiffneri'—(Section—*Cleisocolyx*).

Leaves and their stalks almost glabrous ; leaflets verging from an oval to a somewhat lanceolar form, opposite or nearly so, thin-chartaceous in texture ; racemous bunches of flowers arising from the stem, short ; stalklets nearly or fully as long as the flowers, silky ; calyx large, before expansion of the

carolla almost egg-shaped, then perfectly entire and closed, without any ruptures or sutural lines, subsequently torn to about the middle into two undivided or once more slightly cleft lobes ; petals four, free, elongated-oblong, about one-third longer than the calyx, and likewise outside silky ; staminal column broadly tubular, seven or oftener eight-toothed, the teeth semilanceolar, about three times shorter than the tube ; anthers seven or oftener eight, sessile between the teeth at the summit of the tube, their connective often minutely pointed ; disk cup-shaped, free, slightly crenulated, as well as the staminal tube glabrous ; style filiform, its lower portion and the ovary densely downy ; stigma depressed-hemispherical ; ovary four-celled, with two super-posed ovules in each cell ; fruit globular, glabrescent, brown outside ; pericarp rather thin, not unless very tardily valvular ; seeds without any arillus.

In the Mount Bellenden-Ker Ranges ; Karsten.

A tree attaining a height of 80 feet. Bark greyish-brown, smooth. Wood yellowish. Leaflets on very short stalklets, in few pairs, so far as the very scanty material admits of judging, 2—5 inches long, somewhat inequilateral, very minutely dotted. Racemes two or more together, 2—4 inches long, fragrant. Petals nearly half an inch long, pure-white, upwards slightly imbricated, downwards valvular. Fruit not seen quite ripe, then not fully an inch long, nor showing any indication of valvular structure, four-celled. Seeds ripening solitary in each cell, turgid, almost longtitudinally adnate ; testa thin, dark-brown, loose. Albumen none. Cotyledons planconvex collateral. Radicle very short, terminal, almost concealed between the minute lobes of the cotyledons.

I have left this remarkable meliaceous tree in the genus Dysoxylon, as constituted at present, although the structure of the calyx is so exceptional in some things, that under the sectional name here adopted, or perhaps under that of Epicharis, this species with its nearest allies might be raised to generic distinction, especially as the fruit does not seem to slit into any valvular divisions, in which anomaly however D. Klanderi coincides (*Vide Fragm. Phytogr. Austr.* IX. 134), thus showing an approach to Sandoricum. The genus Dysoxylon, by admitting into it Hartigshea with arillate seeds, and Didymocheton with sepals overlapping at their margins, has become too artificial, while in Hartigshea spectabilis the anthers are inserted below the merely crenulated summit of the staminal tube, a characteristic on which otherwise much stress has been laid by Casimir de Candolle. The remarkable location of the inflorescence is not without example in the genus, it bursting also in several other species away from the leaves out of the stem or main branches.

This new species is nearest allied to D. caulostachyum from New Guinea, with which and the other species placed by Miquel in the section Epicharis it accords in the peculiar structure of the calyx ; but the leaflets are not coriaceous, the pedicles longer, the calyces twice as long, thus reaching much higher up to the corolla, and the teeth of the column are neither rounded nor retuse-truncate ; the fruits are likely also different.

This noble and singular tree is dedicated to Dr. Rudolph Schiffner, of Vienna, who for many years has been the president of the great and highly scientific Pharmaceutical Society of Austria.

Personalities.

At the suggestion of Mr. Geo. Lewis, united action will be taken to have the trade properly represented before the Tariff Commission now sitting.

Mr. C. J. Plunket, Lonsdale-street, Melbourne, has been appointed to the commission of the peace.

Mr. Rivers Langton desires us to state that he has taken a residence at St. Kilda, and intends remaining in Australia.

Mr. Langton is expecting his wife and family, who will shortly arrive from England.

Mr. J. T. Macgowan has been appointed by the Ballarat District Chemists' Association their represenative at the annual dinner of the Pharmaceutical Society.

At last advices Mr. O. V. Morgan was to leave the colonies about the 6th December.

The secretary of the British Pharmaceutical Conference has forwarded to Mr. W. H. Ford, the representative of Victoria at the Conference, a nicely executed photograph of the picnic as held at Henley-on-Thames during the gathering.

Mr. W. J. Pinhey, the secretary of the Pharmaceutical Society of New South Wales, has courteously forwarded for perusal the drafts of the new Pharmacy Act of New South Wales shortly to be introduced to Parliament.

The Presidents of the Medical and British Medical Societies, Drs. Robertson and Neild, have accepted invitations to the annual dinner of the Pharmaceutical Society.

It is proposed to erase the name of James Egan Wall, who was convicted at the Sandhurst Assizes of manslaughter, from the Pharmaceutical Register.

Mr. Prosser (Messrs. Kempthorne, Prosser and Co.), Dunedin, has returned to New Zealand.

Mr. H. H. Lane (Messrs. Warner and Co.'s representative) has just returned from Tasmania.

At the last meeting of the Council of the Pharmaceutical Society of Victoria the President of the Queensland Pharmaceutical Society was elected an honorary member.

Legal and Magisterial.

CHARGE OF MURDER.

JAMES EGAN WALL GUILTY OF MANSLAUGHTER.

JAMES EGAN WALL surrendered to his bail at the Court of Assize on 28th October, and was placed in the dock, charged with murder, and on a second count of manslaughter. He pleaded "not guilty." Messrs. Casey, Hornbuckle and Quick, instructed by Mr. Rymer, defended the prisoner, and Mr. Chomley prosecuted for the Crown.

All witnesses were ordered out of court, on the application of Mr. Casey, and the prisoner was allowed to take a seat in the dock.

The Crown prosecutor said the prisoner was charged with having feloniously killed and murdered Margaret Smith, a woman twenty-eight years of age, the nature of the charge being that at the time of her death the prisoner was engaged in the commission of an illegal act. According to law, if a person be engaged in the commission of felony, though he may not have the intention to kill, the law regards it as murder. In the present case the prisoner used an instrument to procure abortion of the deceased woman, she being *enciente* at the time. If the jury thought that the purpose of the prisoner was not to procure abortion, or to perform an operation without competent skill to justify such an operation, then he was guilty of manslaughter. The question for the jury was whether the act was a felonious one, or whether the prisoner was guilty of performing an unwarrantable operation. Prisoner had been a resident of Sandhurst for a long time, and the deceased woman was a domestic servant or housekeeper in the employ of Mr. Henry Wrixon, an attorney living at Sandhurst. She had been in his service for some five years, and so far as Mr. Wrixon's evidence went, it would show that the woman was in sound, vigorous health up to the day of her death. On the 1st August she was at her master's house in Sandhurst, and the groom, Thomas Storey, in Mr. Wrixon's employ, last saw her alive about three o'clock in the afternoon, and she was then in good health and spirits, and in the garden watering the flowers. She went from the garden into the house. A little girl named Margaret Beale, came to the place about five o'clock, and went up to the back door of Mr. Wrixon's house. She wanted to see the deceased woman, and called out "Maggy," meaning the deceased woman. A person came to the door, whom the little girl recognised as the prisoner, and asked what was "all this Maggying about," and said that "Margaret was out." The little girl remained about the garden, and saw Wall about six o'clock leave the house. About half-past six, Mr. Wrixon came home, and found the parlour door locked. He went to the groom, and they entered the parlour by the French window, and there found the woman stretched upon the sofa dead, with a sheet thrown over her. She was in good health at half-past three, and at six o'clock she was dead. The deceased, when found, was half undressed, and blood was discovered upon the floor and other things. Drs. MacGillivray and Atkinson made a *post-mortem* examination of the body, and they would tell the jury that death was caused by a wound made by some instrument having been forced against the wall of the vagina behind the abdomen, and, after piercing a number of blood vessels, entered the stomach, inflicting a lacerated wound about a quarter of an inch in diameter. The hemorrhage from the wound flowed into the abdomen, and the doctors concurred in saying that this wound caused death.

Mr. Chomley was going on to state the opinion of the doctors formed upon the appearances, when Mr. Casey took exception to the statement and objected, saying he was going to object when the doctors were being examined, as it was a question for the jury to decide as to the purpose for which the prisoner performed the operation.

Mr. Chomley continued his address, and said the Crown must put this point before the jury, but he would not give Mr. Casey an opportunity of taking exception to his opening address until they had the evidence. Those appearances would be described, and he would offer the evidence, which he thought they would accept. There was nobody about the house except Storey, the groom, until the arrival of the little girl Beale, and the prisoner told the latter that the deceased was out. Prisoner was seen leaving the house, and deceased was found dead shortly afterwards, and with marks of violence upon her body. Those circumstances the prisoner seemed bound to explain, and Wall admitted as a witness at the inquest. The coroner, in most explicit terms, told the prisoner that he was not bound to give evidence unless he chose to do so. That being so, the statement of the prisoner was evidence to go to the jury, and he (Mr. Chomley) intended to put it to them. The prisoner swore then that he had known the deceased for about eight or nine years, and that some seven years ago he treated her while in the employ of Mr. Wrixon's mother in Melbourne for disease of the uterus. As regards that statement, Mr. Wrixon could prove that Mrs. Wrixon never saw the deceased woman, as Mrs. Wrixon had been dead some time before Margaret Smith was engaged by the family. The prisoner had found there was evidence against him, and he floundered in this wild way to make an explanation. Mr. Wrixon would swear that the deceased never went to Melbourne, as sworn by the prisoner at the inquest. The prisoner deposed that he treated her for blood-poisoning, but the evidence would show there was no trace of such. Prisoner also swore that he had been sent for the night before the woman's death, as the deceased had become suddenly enlarged in the abdomen, and that certain discharges had occurred. The medical men would tell the jury that had there been any such discharge of sacs the *post-mortem* appearances would have shown corresponding disease of the organs. It was for the jury to say whether the evidence of Wall was not wholly false. Prisoner swore that he made a diligent examination, and he gave his opinion that the deceased was pregnant; that the deceased denied it, and he told her to see another doctor; that the abdomen was enlarged, and that he told her that he could relieve her if she would consent to take chloroform; that he went into the house, and caused her to partially undress, and put her under chloroform; that he used the catheter, which he found passed the cervix uteri, and on withdrawing the instrument found bloody matter upon it; after he had finished, the deceased woman, according to Wall, said she hoped it would not have to be done again. He told her to put on her clothes, and when about telling her she was pregnant, she asked for brandy, which he gave her. A short time after he heard a gurgling sound in her throat, and Wall put some brandy to her mouth, but she died shortly afterwards. After she was dead he said he put the clothes stained with blood out of sight, so that Mr. Wrixon could not see them, as he did not like to see blood. He locked the door, and put the key in the verandah so as to prevent the little girl going in. Those were the statements of the prisoner; and he was said to have used the instrument most unskilfully. Wall knew the woman was pregnant, as he told her so. There was no trace of those imaginary hydatid sacs referred to by prisoner. What was his object in performing the operation? The evidence of the doctors would form an opinion as to whether he used the instrument to cause a miscarriage. If the jury believed that the prisoner, not having competent knowledge, showed want of skill in handling the instrument, and caused the death of the woman, then it was manslaughter. It was certain that the prisoner had caused the death of the woman, as, according to his own statement, she died before his eyes.

Thomas Storey, groom in the employ of Mr. Wrixon, and the little girl Beale repeated the evidence they gave at the coronial inquiry.

Henry Wrixon, solicitor, deposed to the deceased being in his employ for about five years, and also to finding her dead on the evening of the 1st of August.

Dr. MacGillivray gave similar evidence to that at the inquest. He deposed that, if there were hydatids, they would have found the cysts shrivelled up, or the marks, but there were no such signs. The wound indicated that some person attempted to introduce an instrument to procure abortion, and through unskilfulness in opening the womb, penetrated the vagina behind.

Dr. Atkinson and Mr. R. Strickland, coroner, were next examined.

J. J. Shillinglaw, secretary of the medical board, deposed that the prisoner's name did not appear on the Medical Register.

To Mr. Casey: Had not the pharmaceutical chemist's register.

This closed the case for the Crown, and a certificate of the prisoner being a pharmaceutical chemist was handed in.

Mr. Chomley, in addressing the jury, said the counsel for the prisoner had introduced a new matter, and that was that the prisoner had been in the habit of carrying on the practice of a medical man, and was known as "Dr. Wall." That necessitated him (Mr. Chomley) calling attention to the fact that the prisoner carried on the practice in direct violation of the Medical Practitioners Statute. That statute made it a criminal offence for any person to hold himself forth as a medical practitioner, or to use the title. A certificate, showing that the prisoner was a pharmaceutical chemist, had been put in, and the 25th section of the statute provided that every unqualified person who prescribes or practises as a medical man is liable to a penalty of £10 and six months' imprisonment, so that the very certificate put in the prisoner's favour renders him liable to that penalty. The main facts of the case were undisputed. They had it proved by the witnesses, Storey and Beale, and admitted by the prisoner, that he went to the house, that he was in the house with the unfortunate woman, and when he left she was dead. Drs. MacGillivray and Atkinson, who are well-known and skilled in their profession, and of high repute in the city, had given their evidence fairly, and without the slightest bias towards the prisoner, and they both concurred that death had been caused by the wound, and that it must have been caused by some person trying to force an instrument into the womb. The prisoner knew the woman was pregnant, and the attempt was utterly indefensible and certainly inexcusable, and the effect must have been to procure abortion.

Mr. Casey then addressed the jury. Some of the jury know the prisoner as well as anybody, and he would ask them to divest themselves of all that they had heard outside the four walls of the court. The prisoner had been practising in Bendigo the whole time that he had lived here, and he would ask whether they considered this old grey-haired man unqualified, he having started to practise in the early days of the diggings, and continued ever since. The prisoner had gone through the trying ordeal, and nothing had been said as to whether or not his name was untarnished, and it was for the jury to say whether they would consign him to the public executioner. They would, to find that the prisoner was guilty of murder, have to say that he was guilty of malice aforethought. The prisoner was not wholly unqualified, as he had a certificate as pharmaceutical chemist, but it did not matter whether he was qualified or not in this case. Were the same charges laid against Drs. MacGillivray and Atkinson, the same responsibility would attach to them, according to law, as to Wall. Mr. Casey then cited cases, showing that an unqualified man was not guilty of murder in performing an operation which caused death. Many unqualified persons had practised where people could not afford medical men. Here they had the prisoner poaching upon the doctors, so to speak. There, before Drs. MacGillivray and Atkinson, with their bits of parchment, the prisoner was indicted for murder. Those men came into court by the rules of etiquette, and when they were asked a question they set their ingenuity at work to puzzle counsel. They were inspired with a feeling against the prisoner, and had said they would not consult with him, and certainly had not said anything in favour of the prisoner. The evidence of Mr. Wrixon showed an unnecessarily hostile feeling. The prisoner, in the presence of Sergeant Webb, on the following day after the occurrence, asked Mr. Wrixon whether he remembered prisoner telling him about the woman suffering from hydatids. The fact of the prisoner having asked straight out, satisfied them that there was no triangular connection between the girl and Mr. Wrixon and prisoner. They would have to consider what was in the prisoner's mind when he went there, he being pressed to a certain extent, and as Dr. MacGillivray had said, he had used the proper instrument, if not pushed too far, to relieve the uterus of any collection of serum. He was not going to deny that the wound was made, but they had an entire absence of all intention to kill. Dr. Atkinson had suggested

that he thought the wire had come out of the catheter, which then went the wrong way and caused the wound. If that was so, it was not a crime, but only an accident. It was consistent with his innocence, and the circumstantial evidence was not consistent with his guiltiness.

His Honour summed up, and said that it was a feature worthy of notice that there was no conflict of evidence between the doctors. The only thing, however, that bore out the charge of murder was the statement of the prisoner that he told the girl she was pregnant. He thought that his duty to put the aspect of manslaughter to them, and asked them to consider the prisoner as a medical man, though, for the information of the outside public, he would say that he had no right whatever to the title of doctor. If a man used a well-known medical instrument, and, owing to his unskilfulness, he kills the person in the operation, he is guilty of manslaughter. One of the undisputed facts was that, whether the intention was to remove hydatids from the womb or to procure abortion, he never introduced the instrument into the womb, but forced it up through the vagina. The question shortly was, if they thought he showed gross want of skill it was manslaughter.

The jury retired, and after half an hour's deliberation, returned a verdict of "guilty of manslaughter," and the prisoner was remanded for sentence.

UNEXPECTEDLY LIGHT SENTENCE.

James Egan Wall was placed in the dock to receive sentence for manslaughter.

The prisoner, on being asked whether he had anything to say, remarked that he would like to say something. He hoped there would be no objection to his going into the case diffusely, and he did so with a view to obtaining more justice than he had so far. He would begin by asking to have the uterus brought there, and examined by whom His Honour thought advisable, and he would prove incontestably that it was diseased, notwithstanding that Drs. Atkinson and MacGillivray's evidence was that it was not, but was in a normal state. He had tried "Heaven's hard" at the inquest to have it produced, but he did not know why it was not, unless it was to prevent him from showing the traces of hydatids. (The prisoner here entered into a minute description of the natural disease he alleged the woman was suffering from, but the details are unfitted for general publication. He also at great length endeavoured to refute the evidence of Drs. MacGillivray and Atkinson.)

The prisoner then proceeded: By reference to old works it would be found that such a disease (hydatids) should be treated in the same way that he did, and that some instrument should be used to relieve the water. His Honour having stated—and the fact of the uterus having been kept from him in the most extraordinary manner by the coroner—that he should not have performed the operation, he was willing to wait before his Honour passed sentence, that the examination of the uterus might be made by independent and disinterested authorities. He denied that the blood ever came from use of the stilette touching the veins, and if those medical men came there to give evidence for him, they would have put it down as he had stated. It was impossible for blood to find its way up, and that did not correspond with the medical evidence. There was a pressure of 48 lbs. on the abdomen to bear anything downward, and that alone would have been sufficient to keep the blood down. That was incontestable. He did not think the poor woman knew she was pregnant, but he had written to her telling her she was. He did not perform the operation to take away a child. He could have caught the fœtus with the greatest ease. Nothing could have been easier than for him to do it, but he never went there for the purpose, and he did not think the public would think that his purpose was to procure abortion. Not a man in the colony had more experience in female diseases than he had. "Never since my hair turned grey have I not been called to attend such cases. I was not drunk; my hand was not unsteady, and it was the greatest ease for me to perform such an operation, and I think the public of Sandhurst know that. Mr. Strickland threatened to put me out at the inquest for speaking, and would not allow the uterus to be shown." He (prisoner) had given her medicine to prevent blood-poisoning from the water caused by the disease, and he was was surprised that a new bottle of medicine, which he showed to Sergeant Webb after the occurrence, had not, in justice to himself, been produced. There was no evidence to show it either, and to keep the thing back was not fair, and not justice. He was surprised and astonished to hear Mr. Wrixon say the girl's complexion was of the usual kind. She had a freckled face, and a greasy, miserable look. When it was taken into consideration that Mr. Wrixon contradicted him that the deceased woman was in Melbourne, it was nevertheless true. He also spoke to prisoner about the girl, and he denied she was ever away for three weeks. Mr. Wrixon swore she never lived with his late parents. He (the prisoner) had attended her at the late Mr. Wrixon's place fourteen years ago. He had attended the late Mr. Wrixon in his last hours, and yet his son denied that he ever did so. Moreover, he attended Mr. Wrixon himself up to the woman's death. Probably he had been tedious, and had made to-day an improper application to the court, but, being placed in the position that he was, he required the uterus to be produced to show that he was justified in performing the operation. He was satisfied his Honour would consider the application a just one. He would make an observation, as his Honour appeared in his address to the jury to believe he had no power to practise. He had always maintained that he had a right to practise so long as he never called himself a doctor, and he had the right and the skill to practise. Dr. MacGillivray had tried to convict him three times before. In 1854 he was committed for manslaughter of a man named Roach for doing the most miraculous act ever done ; and when all the others could do nothing, he kept the man for thirty-four days ; and such was the amount of jealousy that a doctor went and sat upon the man's chest, and brought on inflammation, and he died. The case was brought before the late Judge Williams, his Honour's father, and that judge said the case should never have been brought into court.

The prisoner said that twelve years ago a young lady was given up to die, and he saved her life. He said she should be tapped, and a number of medical men, including Dr. Atkinson, consulted as to the performance of the operation. Dr. Rowan said he (prisoner) was perfectly right in going on with the operation, but Dr. Atkinson refused. Prisoner then performed a successful operation, and since the girl had written to Dr. Atkinson, calling him a coward for not assisting her.

His Honour then addressed the prisoner. He said the prisoner had made a request to him to have parts of the unfortunate woman examined in the presence of two medical men who gave evidence yesterday. To that request he had no power then to comply. The case had been dealt with by the proper tribunal—twelve jurymen ; and it was not in his power to review their decision, nor was it in his power to allow the prisoner or any one else to do any act that would have the aspect of reviewing the decision arrived at by the jury. If the request had been made to him by the prisoner's counsel while the case was before the jury, he would have ordered it to be produced. The prisoner began his observations that morning by saying that he was going to make a lengthy address in the hope of getting more justice than in the course of the trial. And having begun his address, he proceeded to reflect upon the course counsel pursued, and the way in which they conducted the case ; upon the finding of the jury, twelve of his fellow-countrymen ; and he had also reflected, not only upon the living witnesses, but on dead persons, and on the dead body of the unfortunate woman. His Honour did not think that the prisoner had done his case any good by his remarks that morning.

The prisoner—" Let me ——"

His Honour to prisoner : I cannot permit you to interrupt me now, sir. I think you have done your cause harm. As far as the verdict of the jury is concerned, I entirely agree with it, and cordially appreciate it. If I did not, it would make no difference, but, as it is, it meets with my thorough concurrence and cordial support, and I do not see how the jury could do otherwise upon the evidence. Prisoner was not guilty of murder, but the verdict of manslaughter did him equal justice. As the prisoner had reflected upon counsel, and the way they had conducted the case, his Honour said he thought counsel exercised a very wise discretion, not only in the line of defence adopted, but also in not making the request for the production of the uterus. Amongst the prisoner's other observations was that he never made the wound in the unfortunate woman. His counsel, who took all the points in the evidence, felt it hopeless to take that point, and he quite agreed with them. It was impossible that the wound could have been done in any other way than by the operation the prisoner had performed, or rather attempted to perform. The prisoner had been addressing the court for the purpose of showing that he did not make use of the instrument to procure abortion. The jury allowed that in his favour, and it seemed that the greater part of the prisoner's address had been made for the purpose of making reflections, and for advertising himself. His Honour noticed that when the prisoner spoke of himself, he was moved to tears, but when he referred to the deed he shed no tears at all. By his gross ignorance the prisoner had caused the woman's death. He might be allowed to tell the prisoner that for some time past he had been violating the provisions of two Acts of Parliament. If he held himself out as a doctor, and called himself as such when not qualified, he was violating the Medical Practitioners Statute ; and when performing the operation, such as in the present case, he violated the Act under which he was registered as a pharmaceutical chemist. Prisoner insisted in violating this Act, and, in consequence, he was liable to six months, in addition to a fine of £10. Therefore, in connection with the crime he had committed, he had criminally and deliberately violated, not only the Medical Practitioners Statute, but also the Pharmacy Act, of which he had taken the benefit. Apart altogether from the Act and the offences he had been committing, his Honour would tell him, and through him would tell others, that he had no right whatever to endeavour to learn the profession by making experiments upon fellow-beings. Prisoner acknowledged that the woman was pregnant, and his Honour should have thought, apart from the medical evidence, that it would commend itself to common sense that such an operation should never have been performed. The evidence showed conclusively that the prisoner never penetrated the uterus, but that by his gross unskilfulness or want of knowledge he ran the instrument into the woman's body, and thereby brought on hemorrhage, causing death. In conclusion, his Honour might be allowed to warn and advise the prisoner that when he had served the sentence he was about to pass he should keep within the bounds of the Act under which he was registered as a pharmaceutical chemist ; because, if he did not, he rendered himself liable to a similar prosecution that he had just undergone, and the sentence would be much heavier. The sentence of the court was that the prisoner should be imprisoned in the Sandhurst gaol for twelve calendar months, and he would order neither hard labour nor any labour, in consequence of his advanced years. In measuring the sentence, his Honour took into due consideration all the circumstances, and all that had been said to him by counsel had weight with him, but the prisoner's statements had no weight. The prisoner, who appeared quite unconcerned on hearing the sentence, was then removed.

Subsequently his Honour told Mr. Gale, the governor of the gaol, that he did not wish any distinction to be made in the prisoner's case than in that of any others.

Mr. Gale said the matter would be attended to.

Notes and Abstracts.

MOSQUITO FUMIGATING PASTILLES.—*Pharm. Zeitung* recommends the following :—

Charcoal	1 pound.	
Saltpetre	2 ounces.	
Carbolic acid	1½ „	
Persian insect powder	8 „	
Tragacanth mucilage, sufficient.		

CLARIFYING SHELLAC SOLUTIONS.—Much trouble is generally experienced in obtaining clear solutions of shellac. If a mixture of 1 part shellac with 7 parts of alcohol of 96 per cent. is heated to a suitable temperature, it quickly clears, but as soon becomes turbid again on cooling. The only practical method of freeing the solution from what some writers call "wax," and others "fatty acid," which is present in shellac in the proportion of 1 to 5 per cent., and is the cause of the turbidity, has hitherto been the tedious process of repeated filtration. M. Peltz recommends the following method :—Shellac, 1 part, is dissolved in alcohol 8 parts, and allowed to stand for a few hours. Powdered chalk is then added in quantity equal to half the weight of shellac in the solution, and the latter is heated to 167°. The greater portion of the solution clears rapidly, and the remainder may be clarified by once filtering. Carbonate of magnesia and sulphate of baryta were tried in the same way, but were not found equally efficacious.—*Design and Work.*

ERRATA.—Page 42, line 5, for *her* read *their ;* line 6, for *husband* read *husbands.* Page 44, line 4 from the bottom, for *pints* read *parts.*

Chem. + Drugg. Aust. Suppl.
Vol. 4, no. 45 : 65-72, (Jan., 1882)

THE
Chemist & Druggist.

WITH AUSTRALASIAN SUPPLEMENT.
(Published under direction of the Pharmaceutical Society of Victoria.)

No. 45. { PUBLISHED ON THE 15TH OF EVERY MONTH. }
Registered for Transmission as a Newspaper.

JANUARY, 1882.

{ SUBSCRIPTION, 15S. PER ANNUM, INCLUDING DIARY, POST FREE. }

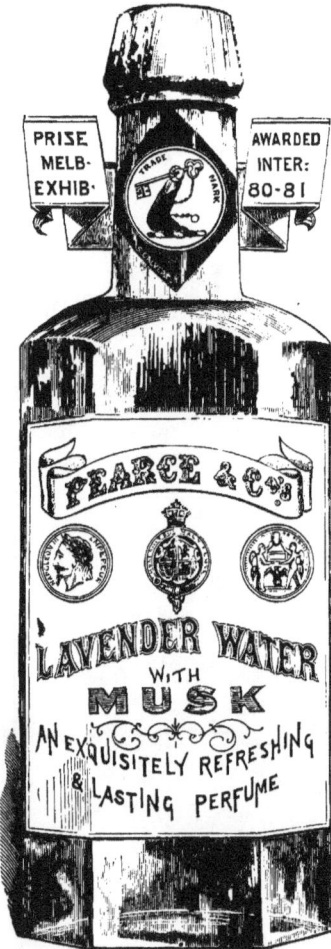

INDEX TO LITERARY CONTENTS.

The Chemist and Druggist.

WITH AUSTRALASIAN SUPPLEMENT.

OFFICE: MUTUAL PROVIDENT BUILDINGS, COLLINS STREET WEST.

Published on the 15th of each Month.

THIS Journal is issued gratis to all paid-up Members of the PHARMACEUTICAL SOCIETY OF VICTORIA, and to non-members at Fifteen Shillings per annum, payable in advance. A copy of *The Chemists and Druggists' Diary*, published annually, is forwarded post free to every subscriber.

Advertisements, remittances, and all business communications to be addressed to THE HONORARY SECRETARY OF THE PHARMACEUTICAL SOCIETY, MELBOURNE.

SCALE OF CHARGES FOR ADVERTISEMENTS:

Per annum.		Per annum.
One Page £8 0 0	Quarter Page .. £3 0 0	
Half do. 5 0 0	Business Cards .. 2 0 0	

Special rates for wrapper and pages preceding and following literary matter. Advertisements of Assistants Wanting Situations, 9s. 6d. each.
Advertisements for insertion in the current month should be sent to the office before the 10th.
COMMUNICATIONS for the EDITORIAL department of this journal should be addressed to THE EDITOR, MUTUAL PROVIDENT BUILDINGS, COLLINS STREET WEST, MELBOURNE.
No notice can be taken of anonymous communications. Whatever is intended for insertion must be authenticated by the name and address of the writer—not necessarily for publication, but as a guarantee of good faith.

NOTICE TO MEMBERS.

MEMBERS whose subscriptions are unpaid on the 31st December, 1881, are respectfully informed that in accordance with Rule 14 their names will be omitted from the list, and after that date they cease to be Members of the Society.

THE LIBRARY.

THE Library is open to Members daily, from 9.30 a.m. to 4.30 p.m.

BIRTH.

BLACKETT.—On the 27th December, at Fitzroy, the wife of C. R. Blackett, M.L.A., of a son.

MARRIAGE.

SHARPE—COOPER.—On the 8th November, at St. Saviour's, Clarborough, by the Rev. L. D. Rowarth, Edwin Sharpe, pharmacist, late of Australia, to Elizabeth, eldest daughter of the late Charles Cooper, Moor-gate, Retford. No Cards.

DEATHS.

GRIFFITHS.—On the 28th December, at 119 High-street, St. Kilda, James William, late of Ballarat, chemist, aged 54 (after a very short illness).

JONES.—On the 31st December, at 308 Bay-street, Sandridge, Walter Llewellyn, infant son of Walter and Adeline Jones, aged four months.

THE SALE OF POISON IN THE FORM OF PATENT MEDICINES.

IN the October number of the *Pharmaceutical Journal* the following observations upon this important subject are so much to the purpose that we feel sure that our readers will fully appreciate them. This question has the same interest for us, and is of as much importance to the public at the antipodes as it is in the mother-country :—

A recent inquest furnishes another instance of the danger attending the inadvertent use of nostrums containing potent drugs; and although the preparation which was the cause of Miss Ashfield's death does not lie under the objection of having its possibly poisonous influence concealed under a fanciful designation, it is, nevertheless, one of a class of preparations which ought not to be sold without the precautionary measures that the Pharmacy Act prescribes in its seventeenth section as proper to be observed for the protection of the public. The

exception allowed in favour of this class of preparations by the sixteenth section of the Pharmacy Act has often been commented upon as unreasonable, and not long ago Dr. Hubbard, of St. Mary's Hospital, justly denounced it as a stultification of the Act, and a fertile source of fatal disaster.
Speaking from his own experience of the conditions under which these preparations can be obtained, and of the consequences attending their indiscreet use, he showed that there were strong reasons for restricting the trade in them, and at least making those who use them more acquainted with the nature and properties of the articles they are taking.

These suggestions of Dr. Hubbard's had a general reference to the "patent medicines" containing potent drugs which are recommended by advertisements as specific remedies; but they appear to have a still more cogent applicability to preparations of such an article as chloral, and the very disclosure of the fact that this substance is an ingredient of the preparation makes it the more evident that the label should bear some impressive caution by the word "Poison."

Dr. Hubbard casts some reproach upon the framers of the Pharmacy Act for the careful and courteous consideration which he thinks they have shown for manufacturers of patent medicines in the sixteenth section of the Act, on the assumption that it was voluntarily inserted by them; but in this respect he has misjudged them, and has failed to take into account the influence and varied interests involved in the patent medicine business. That influence was so strong that it would have been impossible to resist it at the time the Pharmacy Act was passed; and the exemption of patent medicines from the operation of the Act may be looked upon as having been then inevitable, so far as chemists and druggists were concerned. If, however, it can be shown that the sale of patent medicines containing potent drugs, as at present conducted, involves danger to the public, the case would be a very proper one to bring under the notice of the Legislature from a medical point of view, and we have every reason for believing that the application for suitable restrictions upon the sale of such preparations would meet the approval of all qualified pharmacists. We do not hesitate to express our opinion that such a case might well be made out as suggested by Dr. Hubbard.

The need for such a step has not been overlooked by the Council of the Pharmaceutical Society; and quite recently, in drafting a Bill for the Amendment of the Pharmacy Act, the labelling of patent medicines being or containing poison was provided for by a clause which required that on the preparation for sale (whether by wholesale or by retail) of any patent medicine or any article bearing a patent medicine stamp, being or containing a poison within the meaning of the Pharmacy Act, the person so preparing the same shall cause the box, bottle, or vessel containing it to be labelled with his name and address, and the word "Poison." In the same spirit it is provided by another clause of this bill... and without delay will proceed with the erection of suitable premises, fitted with the latest conveniences to facilitate the execution of orders and manufacture of drugs.

Steps are being taken to amalgamate the pharmacy lectures of the Technical College with those of the Pharmaceutical Society. The same lecturer is employed by both institutions, and the same persons attend both courses of lectures. The outcome of the amalgamation will probably be the establishment of a School of Pharmacy in our city.

carry this proposal into effect is an undertaking which is likely to meet with opposition from interested quarters, and it is one in which there is suitable opportunity for the medical profession to support the Society whenever the bill is introduced into Parliament. By such concerted action between the medical profession and the representatives of pharmacy, much good might be effected in the public interest.

The case reported this week serves to show how much restrictions are required in regard to the sale of poisons in the orm of patent medicines, and how thoroughly, under existing conditions, the safeguards provided by the Pharmacy Act are negatived by the sale of such articles by grocers, co-operative stores, or any other unqualified persons. It appears from the evidence in this case that Miss Ashfield's habit of taking chloral was known, not only to her medical attendant—who had expressly warned her to desist from it—but likewise to the chemist with whom she dealt, who had refused to supply her with chloral, except on the order of a medical man. These precautions and the wise intentions of the Act were, however, completely frustrated by the facility with which the obnoxious article was procured from the "stores" upon a wholesale scale, and opportunity afforded for secret indulgence in the practice which led, as in so many other cases, to a fatal result.

In the case we now refer to the jury has given a very emphatic expression of opinion that further precautions should be taken by persons who sell such articles as that which caused Miss Ashfield's death, and that the bottles should be labelled "Poison," notwithstanding the exemptions apparently provided by the sixteenth section of the Pharmacy Act for patent medicines. This is a practical endorsement of the views expressed by Dr. Hubbard, which we hope will speedily bear fruit, by calling attention to the mischief that is being done by the wholly unrestricted and promiscuous sale of poisons in the form of patent medicines. This is an evil that urgently demands a remedy, as being the worst feature of the "patent medicine" trade, alike destructive to medicine and to pharmacy, and pernicious to the public at large.

Whatever reasons there may be for tolerating the sale of patent medicines of a more harmless character, it must be evident that in regard to those of a dangerous nature there can be no question that restrictive measures are requisite. This is felt in other countries as well as our own, and the plausible allurements by which the nostrum traffic is promoted are everywhere attracting the attention of medical men and pharmacists. In America this trade has attained to such dimensions that, as stated in the annual address of the President of the Pennsylvanian Pharmaceutical Association, two-thirds of the total quantity of medicine annually consumed in the United States is sold in the form of secret nostrums. Pharmacists, however, should seek to build up a more legitimate business—that of dispensing to the public such drugs and medicines as are prescribed by the regular medical profession. So long as the public will have quackery in its various forms its sale is safer in the hands of the pharmacists than in any other; but it is not at all desirable that this trade should be promoted by the exhibition of flaming cards, or the distribution of puffing circulars.

The Month.

The examination of students who have attended the School of Pharmacy to obtain the certificates required by the 18th section of the Pharmacy Act will be held on Monday, the 6th March next. The subjects of examination are elementary and practical chemistry, *materia medica*, botany, and pharmacy, and the Pharmaceutical Society have offered three handsome gold medals to the students who pass the best examination in each subject. The conditions under which the medals will be given have already been published, and we refer competitors to them.

The *Pharmaceutical Register of Victoria* for the year 1882 was published early in January, and shows a large addition to the apprentices' list during the year 1881. Copies can be obtained at the office, or from all the wholesale houses.

We are requested to again call attention to the amended regulations to the Pharmacy Act, having reference to apprentices. After 1st January, 1882, all persons *must*, BEFORE entering into apprenticeship indentures, *pass* the preliminary examination, or produce a certificate of having passed the matriculation or civil service examination, Latin being a compulsory subject.

In another column will be found an interesting letter from our Sydney correspondent, who will, for the future, supply the pharmaceutical news of New South Wales to our readers.

The annual report and balance-sheet and the amended rules, and also catalogue of books in the library, will be forwarded to members early next month.

The annual cricket match, Wholesale v. Retail, will be held at the Melbourne Cricket Ground on the 26th January. The wholesale houses have agreed to close at one o'clock ; and the game commencing at noon, an adjournment will be made at two p.m. for lunch, which will be provided on the ground. Two excellent teams have been chosen, whose names, as well as other details of the match, will be found in another column.

The *Chemists and Druggists' Diary* for 1882 have all been issued to members. Should any copies have miscarried, notification may be sent to Mr. Shillinglaw, at the rooms.

The trial of James Egan Wall, of Sandhurst, for a breach of the 23rd section of the Pharmacy Act, will be held on the 23rd instant, at Sandhurst—too late for publication in this issue. It will be remembered that Wall was convicted of manslaughter at the last Sandhurst assizes, and this prosecution arises out of evidence given at the trial. He will be brought up on a writ of *habeas corpus*.

At the last meeting of the council of the Pharmaceutical Society it was stated that there were several persons who attended the annual dinner who had *not yet* paid for their tickets. Surely this is not as it ought to be.

The annual meeting of the Pharmaceutical Society will be held at the rooms on the 8th March next, when the report and balance-sheet for the past year will be presented. The balance-sheet for the year 1881 is an exceedingly satisfactory one.

Meetings.

THE PHARMACY BOARD OF VICTORIA.

THE monthly meeting of the board was held at No. 100 Collins-street, on the 11th January, 1882. Present—Messrs. Bowen, Blackett, Brind, Lewis, Holdsworth, and Owen. An apology was read from Mr. Bosisto.

On the motion of Mr. Lewis, Mr. Brind took the chair.

The minutes of the previous meeting were read and confirmed.

Application for Registration as a Pharmaceutical Chemist. —John Thomas Floyd, Stawell; passed modified examination.

Apprentices' Indentures Registered.—Edward Reeve, Rutherglen; Fred. B. Baker, Richmond; Charles A. Pyne and W. H. Wolfenden, Melbourne; George H. Griffiths and A. S. Edsall, Williamstown; C. L. Henshall, Seymour.

The following renewals of certificates under the "Sale and Use of Poisons Act," were granted:—Nam Shing, Spring Creek; E. Worthington, Avenel; G. R. Berry, Taradale; H. Playford, Dookie South; William Hand, Lilydale; Sun Hi On, Buckland; Ho Lim Sen, Swift's Creek; Ho Ah Yen, Swift's Creek; Samuel Hart, Euroa; C. L. de Buos, Euroa; Hoy Ling, Vaughan.

Amongst the correspondence a number of cases involving breaches of the Pharmacy and Poisons Acts were considered, and most of them were disposed of, a number of prosecutions being ordered; it was also resolved that in all cases where the police prosecute, the registrar be authorised to obtain legal assistance to conduct the cases, so that no technical objection may be taken to the information or summons. A communication was read from the Chief Commissioner of Police, stating that the case against James E. Wall would be heard at the Sandhurst Police-court on the 23rd January.

Annual Balance-sheet.—The annual balance-sheet to 31st December, 1881, duly audited, was submitted and passed.

The Pharmaceutical Register for 1881 was laid on the table.

The Practical Pharmacy Examination.—Mr. Owen submitted a scheme of the manner in which the practical pharmacy examination should be conducted, which, after some discussion, was adopted.

Financial and routine business brought the meeting to a close.

THE PHARMACEUTICAL SOCIETY OF VICTORIA.

THE monthly meeting of the council was held at the rooms, Collins-street, on the 6th January. Present—Messrs. Bowen, Gamble, Huntsman, Thomas, Nicholls, Baker, and Shillinglaw. The president, Mr. Wm. Bowen, in the chair.

The minutes of the previous meeting were read and confirmed.

Election of New Members.—The following new members, nominated at the last meeting, having furnished the necessary declaration, were duly elected:—John C. H. Lilley, Port Pirie, South Australia; Charles Flack, Ballan; J. H. M'Call, Torquay, Tasmania.

New Members Nominated.—W. E. Woods, Napier, New Zealand; P. Fitzsimmons, Brisbane; H. A. Corinaldi, Prahran; H. B. Given, Mount Brown, New South Wales; Jas. R. Laughton, Elizabeth-street, Sydney; Frederick Wright, Pitt-street, Sydney; H. J. Fowles, Glenelg, South Australia; Walter Jones, Sandridge.

The Annual Report and Balance-sheet.—The draft of the annual report and audited balance-sheet for the year 1881 was submitted, and ordered to be printed and distributed to the members.

Appointment of Lecturer, School of Pharmacy.—The application and consideration of all matters relating to the school were postponed, and a special meeting of the whole council called for the 12th January.

Gold Medals.—The dyes and sample of the gold medal to be given to the best student at the school were laid on the table.

Correspondence.—A large amount of correspondence was read, but of no special interest.

The meeting then adjourned.

The following are the retiring members of council for the year 1882:—A. T. Best, R. Nicholls, J. C. Jones, C. Ogg, and H. Gamble, all of whom are eligible for re-election.

A special meeting was held at the rooms on the 12th January. Present—Messrs. Bowen, Blackett, Gamble, Nicholls, Thomas, Huntsman, Best, Hooper, Swift, Baker, and Shillinglaw. The president, Mr. Bowen, in the chair.

The meeting was called to consider the application for the position of lecturer, and for other matters relating to the school.

The President stated that an opinion had been expressed that it would be to the advantage of the school if the classes were removed from the Technological Museum to the rooms of the society, where special advantages existed in the library, museum, &c., and he thought that the first matter to consider was should this be done.

Mr. Swift was of opinion that it would be better to try another term at the Technological Museum before making a change.

Mr. J. T. Thomas: I do not think there can be any doubt of the advantages a school under the immediate supervision of the society would have over the present one.

A general discussion of the subject then took place, in which Messrs. Huntsman, Baker, and Hooper took part.

Mr. Gamble said: To test the question, I will move that the present school of pharmacy at the Technological Museum be discontinued, and that a school be formed, with one lecturer, under the immediate supervision of the Pharmaceutical Society. Seconded by Mr. Best.

Mr. Blackett moved an amendment that the school at the Technological Museum be continued for another session, and that a committee, or board of visitors, be appointed to make any suggestions, &c., that might be found necessary. Seconded by Mr. Swift.

The president put the amemdment, which was lost, and the motion was carried.

Mr. Thomas moved that the arrangement for the school be left to a committee, with power to act, consisting of the president and Messrs. Blacke t, Gamble, and Huntsman.

The appointment of lecturer will therefore stand over until the next meeting of the council on the 3rd February.

NEW SOUTH WALES.
(FROM OUR OWN CORRESPONDENT.)

THE first pharmacy examination of the Technical College was held on the evenings of the 7th and 14th December. Seven candidates presented themselves. The examiners were Mr. James Moore, of Oxford-street, and Mr. Fred. Wright, of Messrs. Elliott Bros. The examination consisted of two papers of ten questions each, and was such as to thoroughly test the candidates' knowledge of the Pharmacopœia. The number of marks gained by the students show, on the whole, very satisfactory results. The lecturer's prize, consisting of a copy of Pareira's *Materia Medica*, was gained by Mr. Fred. Hall. The first prize, consisting of Dr. Carpenter's work on *The Microscope*, Mr. A. Henry; the second prize, four volumes of *Manchester Science Lectures*, Mr. R. Senior. The number of marks stand as follows:—Hall, 147; Henry, 109; Senior, 106; out of a possible 200.

We have to notice the deaths of two persons connected with our profession, one, Mr. C. R. Dowling, who was assistant to Mr. C. F. Turner, Oxford-street. Mr. Dowling is believed to have recently arrived from Melbourne. While in a state of intoxication, he took an overdose of Scheles Acid Hydrocganic. At the inquest it was stated that the deceased was in the habit of taking ten drops of the acid after drinking bouts. The jury returned a verdict of *felo-de-se*. The second case is that of Dr. Hastie, of Lithgow. The deceased gentleman took a large dose of chloroform by mistake, on Monday, 9th January, and died shortly after having swallowed the same. Dr. Hastie was for some time one of the resident medical officers of the Sydney Infirmary, and his death is greatly regretted, his genial manner having rendered him very popular. An inquest has not yet been held.

Mr. E. Prosser (Messrs. Kempthorne, Prosser and Co., Dunedin, New Zealand) has purchased the business lately carried on by H. Beit and Co. Sydney badly needs wholesome competition between the wholesale houses. Messrs. Elliott Bros. have purchased a piece of ground in O'Connell-street, opposite the *Herald* office buildings, and without delay will proceed with the erection of suitable premises, fitted with the latest conveniences to facilitate the execution of orders and manufacture of drugs.

Steps are being taken to amalgamate the pharmacy lectures of the Technical College with those of the Pharmaceutical Society. The same lecturer is employed by both institutions, and the same persons attend both courses of lectures. The outcome of the amalgamation will probably be the establishment of a School of Pharmacy in our city.

NEW ZEALAND.

A SHOCKING occurrence took place at Wellington on 21st December, by which a lady was literally blown to pieces, and a building partially wrecked. The facts are as follow :—At the shop of Mr. Barraud, chemist, Lambton Quay, some blue-fire was in course of preparation for use at the theatre. On testing a small portion of the mixture, it was found dangerously explosive, too much chlorate of potash having been inadvertently used in the composition. Accordingly, Barraud's assistant, named Anthony, formerly of Christchurch, took it out into the back-yard and began to destroy it by slow combustion. He had occasion to leave for an instant, and before he could return, his wife happened to go into the yard, and seeing chemicals on fire, at once threw a bucket of water on the burning mass. A terrific explosion immediately took place, which shook the whole city, and was heard at a distance of some miles. Poor Mrs. Anthony received the full force of the shock, and was frightfully mutilated. Both 'arms were torn off, also one leg, the lower jaw, and the scalp. Wonderful to relate, she lingered for some time. All the windows in the vicinity were smashed, and other damage done. The stone mortar in which the composition had been mixed was hurled many feet into the air, and thrown clear over the tops of the houses into the next street. Fortunately, nobody else was injured. This dreadful occurrence created a profound sensation in the city.

Scientific Summary.

FROM the *Pharmaceutical Journal* and other sources we take the following :—

In an address delivered before the German Pharmaceutical Association at its recent meeting, Dr. Meyer gave an account of the most recent views of the growth and development, as well as the chemical and physical properties of starch. He agreed with Schimper and Musculus *(Bot. Zeit.,* 1880-81), according to whom the starch grains grow, like sphæro-crystals, by apposition of starch molecules. The starch grains are sphærocrystalloids which originate only in the chlorophyll grains of the green parts of plants, whilst in all parts destitute of chlorophyll, as for instance in rhizomes, starch grains are produced by the conversion of other carbohydrates into starch by the so-called starch formers *(Stärkebildner).* To explain the origin of the concentric rings, and the peculiarity of starch grains always being softer in the interior than on the outside, Dr. Meyer made use of a new theory which cannot be here entered upon. Chemically, only the outermost layer of the starch grain consists of anhydride, $(C_6H_{10}O_5)_2$, the inner layers are composed of "*swollen*" anhydride. By the action of acids and ferments water is taken up, and the molecule of anhydride breaks up into several molecules of soluble starch, hydrate of starch $(C_6H_{10}O_5)_2 + H_2O$, which can be obtained in sphærocrystals. By the action of ferments soluble starch is converted into dextrin and maltose, water being again absorbed—

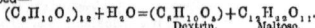

$$(C_6H_{10}O_5)_{12} + H_2O = (C_6H_{10}O_5) + C_{12}H_{22}O_{11}.$$
$$\text{Dextrin.} \qquad \text{Maltose.}$$

This decomposition may be continued ; maltose can then, on absorption of one molecule of water, split up into two molecules of grape sugar. The first step towards the production of starch from grape sugar has been accomplished in the preparation of a dextrin of the formula $(C_6H_{10}O_5)_2$ from chemically pure grape sugar.

In Auckland, New Zealand, an attempt is being made to cultivate liquorice, and if successful it is believed that considerable attention will be devoted to it by farmers, the climate being most suitable. A large quantity of the root has been imported by a local merchant, and has been extensively distributed throughout the country districts.

Professor Hamberg, of Stockholm, has been making a series of experiments as to the relative stability of solutions of different salts of morphia, and has recently brought the subject before the Swedish Medical Association *(Pharm. Zeitung,* xxvi., No. 46). He finds that the sulphate of morphia is more stable than the hydrochlorate, and that the best results are obtained when the solutions are made with boiling distilled water (tested for freedom from ammonia, nitrous, nitric, or phosphoric acids), and filtered directly into small well-filled glass-stoppered bottles, which should afterwards be doubly capped with parchment.

Dr. Lacerda has also discovered that permanganate of potash is an antidote to snake poison. According to a letter to the *Medical Times and Gazette* "repeated successful experiments, positive and negative, have been performed by him in the presence of the Emperor of Brazil," and there is said to be no doubt felt in Rio as to the thorough truth of the discovery.

M. Gautier, in a paper read before the Academy of Medicine, on 26th July last, gives an account of his researches into the nature of snake poisons, more particularly that of the cobra *(Naja tripudians).* He finds that they are not ferments, but chemical bodies of definite composition and considerable stability, whose energy is proportioned to the quantity employed, and but slightly impaired by subjection to a temperature of 125° C. (258° F.) for several hours. Although the poison has the nature of an alkaloid, he found that in its crude state it has an acid reaction, and caustic potash or soda enough to neutralise this acidity, rendered it absolutely inert, and, in fact, decomposed it, since when neutralised with an acid again the energy of the poison was not restored. He, however, failed to prevent death by the subcutaneous injection of alkaline solutions. M. Gautier also verified the fact that the poison may be taken into the digestive canal with impunity.

The existing information as to the solubility under varying conditions of carbonate of magnesia in water charged with carbonic acid gas being contradictory and incomplete, Messrs. Engel and Ville have made a series of determinations, the results of which they have recently laid in a tabular form before the French Academy *(Comptes Rendus,* xciii., 340). It was found that under a pressure of one atmosphere, at a temperature of 19·5 deg. C. one litre of water charged with carbonic acid dissolved 25·79 grams of carbonate of magnesia; under 4·7 atmospheres and a temperature of 19·2 deg., the quantity increased to 43·5 grams ; and under 9 atmospheres and a temperature of 18·7 deg. to 56·69 grams. It was also found that slight variations of temperature—the pressure remaining constant—were sufficient to modify sensibly the solubility of the carbonate of magnesia. Thus with the ordinary atmospheric pressure and a temperature of 13·4 deg. C., a litre of water dissolved 28·45 grams ; at 19·5 deg., 25·79 grams ; at 29·3 deg., 21·945 grams ; at 70 deg., 8·1 grams ; at 90 deg., 2·4 grams.

DEFINITIONS OF SOME NEW AUSTRALIAN PLANTS.

BY BARON FERD. VON MUELLER, K.C.M.G., M. & PH. D., F.R.S.

NOT very long ago I drew attention in the pages of this journal to a new meliaceous tree from Northern Queensland (Dysoxylon Schiffneri) and to a terrestrial orchid, till then unknown, from the Loddon district in our own colony (Thelymitra Mackibbinii) chiefly with an object to interest pharmaceutic gentlemen throughout the Australian colonies more and more in the native vegetation around them. It was hoped, that many pharmacists would be induced to form collections of dried plants, in which it could be shown, that not only the fields of therapeutical and chemical phytology had to be much further investigated, but that even near our own metropolis any assiduous and persevering botanic searches would likely be rewarded with the discovery of quite new species of plants. That this anticipation was well founded, is now again demonstrated by the fact of Mr. D. Sullivan, of Moyston, having added to the three species of the remarkable orchid-genus Caleya a fourth congener, which he obtained in our Grampians. I avail myself of the kind concession of C. R. Blackett, Esq., M.P., of giving in these pages publicity to this new plant and a few others, he sharing my hope that many of his colleagues, especially in remote localities of colonial settlements, may be induced to forward dried specimens also for the further elucidation of the Australian flora, particularly in reference to the *regional* distribution of the species. Researches on the medicinal, industrial or cultural value will follow gradually any systematic descriptive records. Indeed, it would be an immense gain to Australian practical resources also, if in each pharmaceutical establishment gradually a *full* collection of the plants, indigenous in the vicinity, did accumulate, while at the same time the Australian members of the pharmaceutical profession would in botanic inquiries keep thereby pace with their brethren in Europe.

Caleya Sullivanii.—Stem very slender, comparatively short, its lowest portion enclosed in a membranous, narrow, slightly

ir, inserted some distance from
etween the leaf and the floral
small ; inner pair of segments
distant from the outer pair;
from a gradually attenuated
y half the length, pointed at
mply hollow-concave beneath,
dly towards the centre, not
e column terminated on each
fruit oblique egg-shaped.
This evidently rare species
precisely imitates in stature
labellum not in a peltate
nor its apex blunt, nor its
also more dilated towards
margin and apex remaining
I abnormal structure of the
rise from the other congeners,
plesium section of Prasophyl-

ry ; leaves crowded on the
ite, at the margin revolute,
lets, grey-tomentose; flower-
pound corymbs ; involucres
ical, pale yellow, not radia-
irgely pellucid and glabrous,
-stalked, their stipes subtle-
ten to twelve within the
isexual ; fruits very short,
he middle, surrounded at the
s of the pappus sixteen to
towards their summit slightly
r in Central Australia. Rev.
pides, from the coast regions

v. Müeller & Scortechini.—
pinnate ; lateral leaflets in
r or oval-lanceolar, crowded,
at the margin ; rachis some-
e flowers solitary, extremely
ate-lanceolar, nearly half as
i-triangular or quadrangular
mlike nor winglike appen-
distent dissepiments. Near
lland. Rev. B. Scortechini.
ds not yet obtained. The
es pinnate leaves with inap-
, from which this new con-
onspicuous general hairiness,
culated leaflets of only two or
ir fruits, the hairs of which
y and smallness of the leaflets
microzyga (F. v. M. Annual

-

brightest ornaments through
! Hamburg, who, after a brief
ne 21st November last, at the
ars Dr. Sonder conducted, as
cal establishment in the great
for nearly as many years, a
But his zeal, ability, and great
irry on independent progres-
-that of botany—irrespective
gagements. In 1844 he com-
rating for Profess. Lehmann's
Vest Australia the extensive
eæ ; in the year following
lication, the very numerous
once among the masterly
ce. After describing many
r South-African plants, he
escriptive flora of Hamburg,
ions in its surroundings. In
ted Professor Harvey, he ela-
: three large volumes of the
ne his attention was parti-
ions of Australian Algæ, dur-
848, in very frequent com-
ller, and in these researches
aged when death suddenly
ly and large circle of private

and scientific friends. Sixty wreaths from friends adorned his
coffin. So long as the present creation exists Dr. Sonder's
name will be connected honourably with the flora of Australia
and South Africa.

SOME REMARKS UPON MODERN PHARMACEUTICAL STUDY.

(By H. J. MOLLER.)

(From Pharmaceutical Journal.)

ITALY.

THE following facts respecting pharmaceutical education in
Italy I have obtained from Mr. Kernwein, "chimico-far-
macista" in Florence, to which gentleman my friend Mr.
Arthur Meyer (at present an assistant at the pharmaceutical
institute in Strassburg) had the kindness to introduce me.

The most recent law regulating pharmaceutical study is
the royal decree of 12th March, 1876. The course is arranged
in a quite peculiar way which very much resembles the system
employed in Spain and Greece.

There are two classes of pharmacists, viz.:—"farmacista"
and "laureato (or 'dottore') in chimica e farmacia," and
also assistants (called "ministro," "giovane" or "commesso");
these last do not correspond to the German "gehülfen," but
are always examined pharmacists—*i.e.,* have all passed the
"major."

The young man who wishes to commence the study of
pharmacy must first prove that he is qualified to enter the
third class of the "liceo,"* or he must have passed the three
first classes in an "instituto tecnico" (this school corresponds
to the German "höhere Realschule"); in the last case he must
pass a special examination in Latin.

If these demands are fulfilled, the young man does not
begin his *practical* education, but commences immediately to
follow the lectures at the universities, where, according to
Article 2 of the above-mentioned law, special pharmaceutical
schools are to be established. Such a "scuola di farmacia"
already exists in Florence, where it is connected with the
"scuola di medicina." The course occupies from four to five
years, according to the two following plans :—

A. Plan of study, requisite for the degree of *farmacista.*
First year : Inorganic chemistry, botany, mineralogy,
physics. Second year: Organic chemistry, botany, pharmacentical and toxicological chemistry, materia medica ;
practical exercises in pharmaceutical chemistry, toxicology
and qualitative analysis. Third year : Continuation and
termination of the same studies and exercises as in the second
year.

At the end of every year examinations are held in the completed branches. After the last of these examinations, the
student goes to a pharmacy of an hospital, to a military or
other pharmacy, which is authorised by the Government to
this end, and there first he commences his practical education,
which is finished in one year. This last, fourth year of study,
is called the "anno di pratica," and is terminated by a final
examination, which includes qualitative analysis, a chemical
and a "galenical" preparation, medical botany, materia
medica, and the dispensing of prescriptions.

B. Plan of study requisite for the degree of *dottore (or
laureato) in chimica e farmacia.* The studies extend over five
years, and are divided into two periods.

1. The first period (three years) : Inorganic and organic
chemistry, physics, pharmaceutical and toxicological chemistry,
botany, mineralogy, geology, zoology, materia medica, and
toxicology ; practical exercises in physics, botany, mineralogy,
materia medica, qualitative analysis, and chemical preparations.

2. The second period (two years) : In the fourth year the
candidate studies more especially qualitative, toxicological,
and zoochemical analyses ; he must also make some separate
studies in a special branch of natural science, chosen by himself. In the fifth year ("anno di pratica,") he learns practical
pharmacy as above mentioned. Now he passes the final
examination, which consists of three parts ; the first includes
qualitative, quantitative, and toxicological analyses, and an
oral examination in these branches ; the second part embraces
two chemico-pharmaceutical preparations, medical, botany,
and materia medica ; the third consists of a dissertation on a

*The "liceo" is the classical school ; the third class is the highest, and
the final examination of this class is called the "licenza liceale," and thus
corresponds to the German "Maturitätsprüfung," and the French "baccalauréat."

theme, chosen by the candidate himself, and a discussion of this dissertation. It is required of the candidate who wishes to be a "dottore" in pharmacy, that he shall have passed the above-mentioned "licenza liceale."

Legal and Magisterial.

ACCIDENT WITH LIQUOR AMMONIÆ.

AT the Belfast Quarter Sessions, on Tuesday last, before Mr. J. H. Otway, the County Court Judge, a case was heard in which a railway porter, named John Murray, and his wife sought to recover the sum of £50 damages from Mr. John Hogg, druggist, York-street.

Eliza Murray, one of the complainants, deposed that on the 25th ult. she sent her daughter to Mr. Hogg's to buy one pennyworth of "head salts," as she was subjected to headaches. The girl returned with the bottle produced. It was "fizzing" through the cork when she first saw it. It was put on the shelf and not used for a few days. Having a headache she lifted it to apply it, and had it in her hand for a few minutes when it exploded, the contents covering her face. Her eye was destroyed, and her mouth and throat burned, the skins of both having been torn off. It had been put on the mantelpiece previous to the time that she used it. When about to apply it she was sitting near the fire.

John Murray, husband of the injured woman, said that the day after the accident, he went to the defendant to tell him of the occurrence, and Mr. Hogg sympathised with him and gave him 10s. towards paying the expenses of the doctors.

Dr. Gault deposed that on 28th September, he saw Mrs. Murray. Her eyes, mouth, and throat were greatly swollen. The contents of the bottle produced was liquid ammonia. "Smelling" or "head" salts were usually prepared with carbonate of ammonia and a few drops of the liquid ammonia. He did not think that liquid ammonia should be sold by itself for smelling or "head salts." It would be too strong, and the heat of the hand would be sufficient to burst the cork.

Dr. W. A. M'Keown deposed that when Mrs. Murray came to him her eye was completely lost. He knew "head salts" to be the white powder, carbonate of ammonia, with a few drops of the liquid put on. Liquid ammonia was not smelling salts.

John Hogg, the defendant, deposed that he sold the liquid ammonia to the plaintiff's child. The custom of the trade was to give either carbonate of ammonia or the liquid in a diluted form. That given to plaintiff was diluted. He had sent to various druggists in town for the same article that the plaintiff asked for, and in each case the liquid ammonia was given. This liquid would not explode except it were heated.

His Worship granted a decree for £30, with two guineas for expenses.—*Belfast Evening Telegraph.*

SUICIDE OF THE REV. A. F. HARDING.
PROSECUTION FOR SELLING THE POISON.

A CASE arising out of the late suicide of the Rev. A. F. Harding, of St. Kilda, was heard at the St. Kilda Police Court on 9th January, when the chemist, J. W. Thwaites, was prosecuted under the 5th section of the Poisons Statute. It will be remembered that at the inquest Mr. Thwaites was interrogated, and answered as follows:—

Coroner : Are you aware that chloral is one of the articles scheduled in the "Act for Regulating the Sale of Poisons?"

Witness : I never gave it a moment's thought.

Coroner : The Act was passed expressly to prevent suicide by sudden impulse. It provides that no druggist shall sell certain poisons (of which chloral is one) unless a witness is present, and the sale is entered in a book kept for the purpose. Are you in the habit of selling chloral as you did to Mr. Harding yesterday afternoon?

Witness : No. I had no reason to believe that there was anything wrong with the man.

Coroner : It is a very difficult matter even for a medical expert to decide as to a man's mental condition. Why did you not comply with the provisions of the statute? You did not carry out the law, did you ?

Witness : I must admit that, certainly.

Coroner : Had you done your duty, the man, in all probability, would be alive to-day. Was the quantity you gave him poisonous?

Witness : Yes, if taken all at once.

The information laid against the chemist charged him that he "did sell a certain poison specified in the first schedule to the Sale and Use of Poisons Act 1876, to wit the poison called chloral hydrate, to one F. Harding. deceased, without, and before the delivery thereof to the said F. Harding, the purchaser, inquiring his name and place, and occupation, and the place of abode, and occupation, and the purpose for which the said poison was required, or stated to be required, and did not thereupon make a faithful entry of such sale, specifying the said poison and the quantity thereof, together with the day of the month and year of such sale, in a book to be kept by you, such vendor, for the purpose in the form set forth in the second schedule to the said Act, and signed by the said F. Harding as such purchaser, and also by a witness to such sale, the said poison not being made up or compounded by you as a medicine according to the prescription of a legally qualified practitioner, or otherwise being within the exceptions mentioned in the 13th section of the said Act, contrary to the form of the statute."

The magistrates on the bench were the Mayor (Mr. G. Shaw), and Messrs. Keogh, Quinlan, Simpson, Finlay, and Baldwin, J.P.'s.

Mr. Gillott appeared to defend the accused.

On the case being called on, Sub-Inspector Toohey said he had been led to believe that the defendant was going to plead guilty. Seeing, however, that defendant had come prepared with a defence, he would ask their worships to adjourn the case for a week, so that the police might have an opportunity of getting the evidence for the prosecution prepared. The case had been put in his hands only at the last moment.

Mr. Gillott : I scarcely think it is worth while adjourning the case.

Mr. Quinlan : By whom are the proceedings being instituted ?

Sub-Inspector Toohey : By the Chief Commissioner of Police.

Mr. Quinlan : This should guarantee for sufficient time on preparation.

Sub-Inspector Toohey : I had no notice until yesterday that the case was in hand.

Mr. Gillott did not propose to raise many difficulties in the way.

The Bench : Go as far as you can now.

Constable Hoey deposed that on the 3rd inst. he saw the deceased gentleman, Harding, at the Melbourne Hospital, where he had died, death being caused by his having taken inwardly hydrate of chloral. The defendant was present. Witness had shown defendant the bottle in which the poison was contained, and he had acknowledged that it was his bottle.

Mr. Keogh (taking the bottle) : This bottle could not have contained chloral ; it must have been a preparation of chloral ; Chloral is a solid matter.

Cross-examined by Mr. Gillott : Witness said deceased had taken chloral before, when he was attended by a medical man and got over the dose.

Mr. Keogh : Was there any other bottle besides the one produced found on the deceased ?

Witness : Yes ; this one (produced). It was found on deceased, but defendant would not acknowledge it as from his establishment.

Mr. Keogh here interpolated : "It seems by the Act that there is no necessity to enter the sale of a preparation of chloral hydrate in a book. Chloral hydrate is one thing, but a preparation of such a drug is another. The Act does not require the entry of the latter."

Mr. Quinlan : For the purpose of giving a formal aspect to these proceedings they might make the objection suggested, and if a majority of the bench do not think it a valid one they might entertain the request for an adjournment. But there was no use of adjourning if the bench did not think the objection a valid one. He noticed by the Act that there was no interpretation clause to this section.

As further evidence, a deposition of Thwaites was put in by Constable Hoey, to the effect that deceased had been supplied by him with a mixture of 90 of chloral and the rest water. Deceased was in no way excited when he made the purchase. He seemed quiet and rational. He, the chemist, did not carry out the provisions of the Act.

Mr. Quinlan : Was Mr. Thwaites aware that Mr. Harding was a clergyman?

Constable Hoey : He was not so aware. He said he thought he was a German student.

After some further consideration it was decided to remand the case for seven days.

On this decision announced, Mr. Gillott said he and his client would rather plead guilty and throw themselves on the mercy of the bench than be put to the trouble of coming to the court again, which would be a worse punishment than the bench were likely to inflict. He admitted his client had sold the article named. The sale was effected, however, with no intention of fraud, or desire to evade the law. It had been after due inquiry that the preparation had been dispensed. No entry had been made, nor any signature obtained. They had sold the preparation in the usual way.

Mr. Keogh : Yes ; and you have a perfect right to do so.

After some consultation, the Mayor said that although the defendant had admitted the offence a majority of the bench thought there was no case against him, and they had decided to dismiss the case.

SUICIDES BY POISON.

DURING the past month the following cases of suicide by poison have been reported by the police to the Pharmacy Board :—

James Jamieson, aged fifty years, South Preston, died from taking strychnine.

Geo. Smith, Camperdown, attempted to commit suicide by taking strychnine. Recovered.

A recently married woman, aged about twenty, who resides at Dover-road, Williamstown, made a desperate attempt upon her own life on the 27th December. Mrs. Dooley, it would appear, had some altercation with her husband, after which she deliberately went for a bottle of liniment, containing a mixture of aconite and belladonna, in sufficient quantity to poison several persons, and drank off the contents. Mr. Goldie arrived at Dooley's house half an hour afterwards, at half-past five o'clock, and found that some one had prevailed upon the woman to swallow some mustard, by which vomiting had been induced. Mr. Goldie administered another emetic, and had recourse to the stomach-pump. At half-past ten Mr. Goldie, who was continuing the use of restoratives, pronounced the young woman's condition extremely critical.

William A. Black, Little Lonsdale-street, who committed suicide on the 5th January by taking strychnine.

A peculiar poisoning case formed the subject of investigation at the hands of Dr. Youl on the 29th instant. An elderly couple named Benjamin and Mary Anne Morden have been living for some time in Greig-street, Emerald Hill. On Saturday last an acquaintance called in and remained to tea. It would appear from the evidence that the husband, being rather deaf, conceived the idea that his wife was making disparaging remarks about him to their visitor, and, when the latter left, he commenced addressing her in an angry tone of voice. This treatment so influenced the woman's mind that she went to her room, opened a box containing strychnine, mixed a quantity of it in water, and then drank it off. Shortly afterwards she told her husband what she had done. and Dr. Barrett was sent for, but arrived too late to be of any service, as the woman died immediately after his arrival. The jury brought in a verdict of death from strychnine poisoning.

ACCIDENT TO MR. ALFRED FELTON.

WE are glad to be able to state that Mr. Felton, who met with a severe accident while travelling overland from Sydney to Melbourne some time since, is progressing in a satisfactory manner, and, we trust, will soon be convalescent. Mr. Felton is still at Goulburn, and will not be able to be removed for some time.

THE PHARMACEUTICAL SOCIETY OF GREAT BRITAIN.

MEETING OF THE COUNCIL.

WEDNESDAY, 2nd NOVEMBER, 1881.

MR. THOMAS GREENISH, PRESIDENT ; MR. GEORGE FREDERICK SCHACHT, VICE-PRESIDENT.

THE SALE OF CHLORAL HYDRATE.

THE council went into committee to consider a notice of motion given by the president, with regard to the sale of chloral hydrate.

On resuming, the following resolution was passed unanimously :—" That the Law and Parliamentary Committee, in consideration of the frequent deaths occasioned by the use of chloral hydrate, a poison within the meaning of the Pharmacy Act, he requested to consider and report what steps, if any, should be taken with a view to enforce, on the sale of that substance and its preparations, the requirements of the said Act."

DEATH OF MR. A. J. COOLEY.

WE regret to announce the death, on Friday, 28th October, of Mr. A. J. Cooley, the author and compiler of the *Cyclopædia of Practical Receipts*. Although in failing health for two or three years past, he still maintained a lively interest in technical subject with which he was well qualified to deal, and, as a man of integrity, was esteemed by those who had dealings with him.—*Pharmaceutical Journal.*

Correspondence.

To the Editor of The Australasian Supplement to the Chemist and Druggist.

SIR—The " Personalities" column in your last issue leads off, to my astonishment, with the announcement that some one " has succeeded " to my business here. Your informant has been misinformed. I have not disposed of my business ; and, instead of any one having " succeeded " to it, I have to thank my old customers for their not only continued, but increased, support in my new premises. Being a member of the Pharmaceutical Society of many years' standing, I trust you will allow me the *amende honorable* in your next issue.—I am, sir, yours obediently,   ALEXANDER HALL,

Pharmaceutical Chemist, Williamstown.

29th December, 1881.

[The paragraph referred to was taken from the following circular, issued by Mr. Massey :—" H. J. Massey begs to inform the inhabitants of Williamstown that he has commenced business at the above address—in the premises lately occupied by Mr. A. Hall—and trusts, by careful and assiduous attention to business, to merit a share of public patronage."—ED.]

PURSUIT OF KNOWLEDGE UNDER DIFFICULTIES.

ACCORDING to the *Pharmacist*, the members of the American Pharmaceutical Association who attended the recent meeting in Kansas city must have undergone a mild form of martyrdom through their zeal for pharmacy. Kansas city appears to have retained her hottest days for the visitors, and a scorching sun, clay dust, "roily" Missouri water, and mosquitoes, are said to have conspired to make life a burden. All the time that the meeting was in session the thermometer ranged between 104° and 105° F. night and day, and there was no breeze. At the meeting the " comical sight was presented of scientific men sitting in earnest deliberation with coats and vests removed, suspenders down, and shirt sleeves rolled up, all the while manipulating their palmetto fans like so many dames of the ball-room."

THE *AUSTRALASIAN VETERINARY JOURNAL.*

WE have received the first number of the *Australasian Veterinary Journal*, a monthly journal of veterinary science, embracing the breeding, feeding, and management of stock in health and disease ; edited by Graham Mitchell, F.R.C.V.S., Thomas Chalwin, M.R.C.V.S., and William T. Kendall, M.R.C.V.S. The editors in their address say :—" In issuing this our first number of the *Australasian Veterinary Journal*, we have to state that, contrary to our original intention of publishing it quarterly, we have thought it advisable to bring out a monthly number, with the object of having it registered as a newspaper, similar to the medical and pharmaceutical journals. This will not only secure the advantage of the cheap postal rates, and thus bring it within the reach of every veterinary surgeon and stockowner in the colonies, but will also be meeting the views of many of our subscribers who desire to have replies to their communications oftener than once a quarter. " The urgent necessity for a periodical devoted alike to the interests of the veterinary profession and breeders and owners of stock, between whom a greater bond of sympathy ought to exist, is beyond all doubt. Hitherto there has been no publication devoted to the advancement of scientific knowledge in connection with the diseases of animals, or for recording observations on their nature, origin, and distribution, although, from climatic and other influences, many are known to assume forms peculiar to Australia.

"As this country is rapidly becoming one of the greatest stock-raising centres of the world, the health of our animals is of paramount importance. We therefore feel certain that, in publishing the *Australasian Veterinary Journal*—which will provide a ready means of collecting and recording the observations not only of professional men and stock inspectors, but also of many intelligent stock-owners, who have frequently better opportunities of watching the progress of diseases—we shall have the support and assistance of all who have the welfare of the country at heart.

"Australia, probably owing to its isolated position and excellent climate, has so far enjoyed an immunity from many contagious and infectious animal diseases that prevail in other countries ; but the fact that such diseases as pleuro-pneumonia and foot-and-mouth disease in cattle have already made their appearance, proves that our climate and geographical position are not alone sufficient to prevent their introduction.

"The continual importation of foreign stock, and the increased rapidity of transit between this and other countries, renders it highly probable that ere long our shores may be visited by more of these scourges, and it behoves us to be on our guard, so that, if unable to prevent their introduction, we may at least be in possession of information that will enable us to adopt effective measures to arrest their spreading.

"Breeders and owners of stock in this country have, from a combination of circumstances, had to rely almost wholly on their own practical experience in dealing with the diseases of stock. But this experience, which has often been dearly bought, has seldom proved of any avail when any new form of disease has made its appearance, or some unlooked-for mortality, arising from neglect of natural and sanitary laws, has caused serious losses which a general knowledge of veterinary science might have averted.

"One of our most valuable sources of information will be through the Australasian Veterinary Medical Association, which is now represented in all the colonies, and has for one of its main objects the attainment of effective intercolonial legislation for preventing the introduction and spread of contagious and infectious diseases.

"Although aware that some professional men are averse to the circulation of veterinary information amongst owners of animals, we can confidently state, from long experience, that those who are best informed on the breeding, feeding, and management of stock, in health and disease, are invariably our best clients. We therefore feel that, in endeavouring, as far as lies in our power, to diffuse scientific and useful information, we are not only serving the best interests of the veterinary profession, but, by supplying a want that has been long felt, are performing a duty which, as veterinary surgeons, we owe to the country of our adoption.

"Australia presents a field for pathological investigation that, if equalled, is not surpassed by any country in the world. All our domestic animals have been either imported or reared from imported stock; consequently, the opportunities for studying the different modifications of disease from climatic and other causes, as well as of new indigenous forms, are almost unlimited.

"We therefore hope to have the support and assistance of many active workers—lay, as well as professional—who are desirous of promoting the advancement of science and the welfare of the community."

NOTE ON GLYCERINUM ACIDI GALLICI.
(BY T. E. THORPE, F.R.S.)

THIS preparation is made, according to the British Pharmacopœia, by rubbing together one part of gallic acid with four parts of glycerol, and heating the mixture until complete solution is effected. It is advisable to call attention to the fact that unless great care is taken to prevent overheating, the gallic acid may be converted into pyrogallol. I have shown (*Chemical News*, 43, 109 ; *Journal of the Chemical Society, Abstract*, 1881, p. 662) that at a temperature of from 190 deg. to 200 deg. C. this conversion in presence of glycerol takes place very rapidly, the gallic acid being transformed

into the theoretical quantity of pyrogallol, and I have recommended this process as a ready method of preparing pyrogallol for alkaline development in photography. As glycerinum acid gallici is intended for internal use, the possible presence of pyrogallol may be attended by unlooked-for consequences, this body being highly poisonous. According to Personne (*Comptes Rendus*, 69, 749) it acts in the same manner as phosphorus, namely, by abstracting the oxygen of the blood. Two or three fatal cases have been recently reported in the photographic journals from pyrogallol having found its way into wounds or cuts during the processes of dry plate manipulation.

TROCHES OF BORAX.

TROCHES of borax are difficult to prepare by the usual method for preparing troches, because with gum arabic a mass scarcely plastic and difficult to divide is obtained, while tragacanth yields an extremely elastic mass impossible to divide. F. Vigier recommends the following process :—

R Borax ...	...	...	...	...	100 grams.
Powdered Sugar	...	...	...	900	"
Carmine No. 40	...	...	...	0·15	"
Tragacanth in flakes...	...	...	2·50	"
Distilled water	...	...	...	60	"
Tincture of benzoin (Siam)...	...	10	"

Prepare a mucilage from the tragacanth, and one-half each of the water and tincture. Mix the sugar with the carmine, and add one-half of this sugar in small quantities to the mucilage ; then add the remainder of the water and tincture, and with this mixture incorporate the powdered borax and remainder of the sugar, previously thoroughly mixed. Divide the mass into troches, each weighing 1 gram, and containing 0·10 gram of borax.

These troches have been used with good success by M. Poinsot, dentist, in various affections of the mouth, such as aphthæ, &c.

TRANSATLANTIC OFFENCES AGAINST PHARMACY LAWS.

"*Cœlum non animum mutant qui trans mare currunt.*" We regret to notice that the spirit which leads to aggressions and breaches of legislation for the regulation of pharmacy in Great Britain is also represented in her colonies. The Ontario College of Pharmacy has been compelled to consider the subject of breaches of the Pharmacy Act of that province, and it has recently resolved, with a view to protect the public and the members of the College from the sale of drugs by unauthorised vendors, that when such cases of infringement are "credibly reported" to either the registrar or president, those gentlemen shall be authorised in expending a sum not exceeding fifteen dollars in endeavouring to secure the conviction and punishment of the offenders. If the sum of fifteen dollars represents the probable average cost of proceedings in each case, "law" must be a cheaper luxury in Canada than in the old country.—*Pharmaceutical Journal.*

THE ANNUAL CRICKET MATCH.

WHOLESALE CHEMISTS

v.

RETAIL CHEMISTS.

THE match will be played on Melbourne Cricket Ground on Thursday, the 26th January, 1882.

The following are the players from whom the retail team will be selected :—Strutt, Baker, Barnard, Lewis, Gibson, Cooper, M'Kie, Hope, Cattach, Pleasance, Evans, Ross, Gabriel, and Swift.

A practice wicket will be available on Monday next, the 23rd, on Melbourne Cricket Ground, at three o'clock (Richmond end). All the above are requested to be present ; final team to be picked at termination of practice.

Wickets will be pitched on the 26th January, at half-past eleven a.m.; luncheon on the ground at two p.m.

New and Standard Medical Works

ON SALE BY

GEO. ROBERTSON

WHOLESALE AND RETAIL

BOOKSELLER & STATIONER,

33 & 35 Little Collins Street West,

MELBOURNE.

The Cyclopædia of Practical Receipts, Processes, and Collateral Information in the Arts, Manufactures, Professions and Trades, including Pharmacy and Hygiene, by ARNOLD J. COOLEY, 2 volumes ... ... 47s. 6d.

Beasley—The Book of Prescriptions ... ... 7s. 6d.

Beasley—The Druggist's General Receipt Book ... ... 7s.

Beasley—The Pocket Formulary and Synopsis of the British and Foreign Pharmacopœias ... ... 7s. 6d.

Fownes—A Manual of Chemistry, Theoretical and Practical, 2 vols. ... ... 21s.

Mayne—A Medical Vocabulary: being an Explanation of all Terms and Phrases used in the various departments of Medical Science and Practice, giving their Derivation, Meaning, Application, and Pronunciation ... ... 11s. 6d.

Taylor—On Poisons in Relation to Medicine ... ... 18s.

Bloxam—Laboratory Teaching: Progressive Exercises in Practical Chemistry, illustrated ... ... 6s. 6d.

Royle—A Manual of Materia Medica and Therapeutics, illustrated ... ... 17s.

Carpenter—The Microscope and its Revelations, illustrated ... ... 17s.

Dick—Encyclopædia of Practical Receipts and Processes, 6,400 Receipts ... ... 25s.

Squire—A Companion to the British Pharmacopœia, comparing the strength of its various Preparations with those of the United States and other Foreign Pharmacopœias, &c. ... ... 12s.

Fenwick—The Student's Guide to Medical Diagnosis, illustrated ... ... 7s. 6d.

Savory—A Compendium of Domestic Medicine, and Companion to the Medicine Chest ... ... 6s.

A COMPLETE CATALOGUE OF MEDICAL BOOKS TO BE HAD ON APPLICATION.

GEORGE ROBERTSON,

33 and 35 Little Collins Street West, Melbourne,

AND AT

SYDNEY, BRISBANE, AND ADELAIDE.

[SUPPLEMENT ONLY.]

Chem . & Drugg . Aust. Suppl.
Vol. 4, no. 46 : 73-80, (Feb, 1882)

THE
Chemist & Druggist.

WITH AUSTRALASIAN SUPPLEMENT.

(Published under direction of the Pharmaceutical Society of Victoria.)

No. 46. { PUBLISHED ON THE 15TH OF EVERY MONTH. } *Registered for Transmission as a Newspaper.*   **FEBRUARY, 1882.**   { SUBSCRIPTION, 15s. PER ANNUM, INCLUDING DIARY, POST FREE.

Printed by Mason, Firth & M'Cutcheon, 51 & 53 Flinders Lane West, Melbourne.

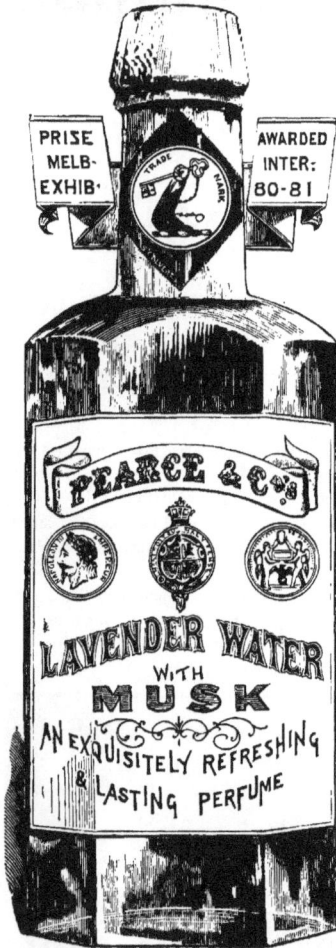

INDEX TO LITERARY CONTENTS.

The Chemist and Druggist.

WITH AUSTRALASIAN SUPPLEMENT.

OFFICE: MUTUAL PROVIDENT BUILDINGS, COLLINS STREET WEST.

Published on the 15th of each Month.

THIS Journal is issued gratis to all paid-up Members of the PHARMACEUTICAL SOCIETY OF VICTORIA, and to non-members at Fifteen Shillings per annum, payable in advance. A copy of *The Chemists and Druggists' Diary*, published annually, is forwarded post free to every subscriber.

Advertisements, remittances, and all business communications to be addressed to THE HONORARY SECRETARY OF THE PHARMACEUTICAL SOCIETY, MELBOURNE.

SCALE OF CHARGES FOR ADVERTISEMENTS:

Per annum.			Per annum.
One Page ..	..£8 0 0	Quarter Page	..£3 0 0
Half do. ..	.. 5 0 0	Business Cards	.. 2 0 0

Special rates for wrapper and pages preceding and following literary matter. Advertisements of Assistants Wanting Situations, 2s. 6d. each.

Advertisements for insertion in the current month should be sent to the office before the 10th.

COMMUNICATIONS for the EDITORIAL department of this journal should be addressed to THE EDITOR, MUTUAL PROVIDENT BUILDINGS, COLLINS STREET WEST, MELBOURNE.

No notice can be taken of anonymous communications. Whatever is intended for insertion must be authenticated by the name and address of the writer—not necessarily for publication, but as a guarantee of good faith.

MELBOURNE SCHOOL OF PHARMACY.

THE Lectures in Materia Medica, Botany, and Elementary and Practical Chemistry commence on Monday, the 6th March next.

For further particulars apply at the office of the Pharmaceutical Society, No. 4 Mutual Provident Buildings, Collins-street.

THE LIBRARY.

THE Library is open to Members daily, from 9.30 a.m. to 4.30 p.m.

DEATH

WHAT IS A PREPARATION?

IN connection with the recent melancholy case of the suicide of the Rev. A. F. Harding the question arose as to what was a poison and a preparation of a poison. No doubt at a first glance the ingenious definition of the word preparation accepted by the justices to some appears conclusive, but we think that very little reflection is required to see that it is quite untenable. The solicitor for the defendant said that he did not intend to raise any unnecessary technical difficulties, but contended that the article sold—chloral and water—was a medical preparation, and not a poison within the meaning of the Act. The magistrates assented to a remand, but decided to hear the evidence available. Thereupon Mr. Gillott advised his client to plead guilty, and throw himself upon the mercy of the court. This course was adopted, and after hearing the case the justices decided that there was no case against the defendant. Although he pleaded guilty, they said he was not. This certainly appears an extraordinary decision. As this case is an important one, as bearing upon the enforcement of an Act

of Parliament passed in the interest of the public to protect human life, we think that a few observations are called for. It is quite evident that the majority of the magistrates were in a confused state of mind on the question submitted to them, and their difficulty turned upon the meaning of the word "preparation." This term has a common and a technical meaning. With the ordinary or dictionary signification we have nothing to do, but have to consider the pharmacopœial use of the word. In the pharmacopœia it will be remembered that under many of the drugs and chemicals a list is given of certain compounds or preparations. *Ex gr.*, under perchloride of mercury, we find preparations, liquor hydrargyri perchloridi, lotio flava. On turning to the first schedule of the Poisons Act we find in part one corrosive sublimate, but no mention of preparations. How is it that there is no mention of "preparations" in this case? Because the so-called preparations are not dangerous, and not likely to be used for felonious purposes. In the same way cantharides and tartar emetic alone are given, and no mention of the preparations. At the time the Poisons Act was drafted there were no "preparations" of chloral. The only preparation—official preparation—now recognised is the syrup which was ordered in the appendix, and was probably then unknown to the framers of the Act. The syrup contains so large a quantity—eighty grains to the ounce—that it is obvious it would not have been overlooked; for it is most absurd to imagine that the framers of the Act intended that a lethal drug could be sold at will simply because it was *dissolved* in sugar and water! If corrosive sublimate, dissolved in, say, spirit, could be sold because there is no such "preparation," the primary intention of the Legislature would be defeated by any ingenious admixture of an official "preparation." Once admit such a postulate as this, and we may as well consign the Poisons Act to the waste-paper basket! According to the dictum of the St. Kilda magistrates, chloral *plus* water, in however small a quantity, is not a poison within the meaning of the Act. By the same reasoning a publican selling brandy mixed with water would not be infringing the Licensed Victuallers Act, if without a license. The sale of poisons by uneducated and irresponsible persons is very properly—or ought to be—restricted, and any failure of justice is to be regretted; and we think that every effort should be made by pharmaceutical chemists to fulfil the letter of the law. There is no doubt that the Act is very defective, and requires immediate amendment; and we hope that as soon as possible the Government will take this matter into consideration. It is, perhaps, impossible by any, however stringent, law to prevent those poor, unhappy persons bent upon self-destruction from "shuffling off this mortal coil" when once possessed with the intention; but the primary object of the Legislature was to prevent the crime of murder, and to render its detection certain.

The Month.

THE quarterly examinations of the Pharmacy Board will be held on the 2nd and 6th of March. The examinations to be held are the preliminary on the 2nd, and the modified and practical pharmacy on the 6th. In addition to these the examination for the certificate of the School of Pharmacy will also take place on the 6th of March.

The annual cricket match, Wholesale v. Retail Chemists, was held on the Melbourne Cricket Ground on the 26th January. There was a much better attendance than on previous occasions, and Mr. J. Hemmons having taken the matter in hand, the wholesale firms agreed to close at one o'clock, so as to allow their *employés* to be present. At the lunch the toast of the wholesale chemists was proposed by Mr. Blackett, M.P., and responded to by Messrs. Grimwade and Hemmons. We hope to see this gathering increase every year in popularity. A full report of the match is given elsewhere.

Messrs. Felton, Grimwade are the successful tenderers to supply the Government with phosphorus.

Mr. James Clezy, M.A., has been appointed by the Pharmacy Board to conduct the preliminary examination required by the Pharmacy Act.

We are glad to be able to state that Mr. A. Felton is slowly recovering from the effects of his late accident, and it is expected that he will be shortly able to be brought to Melbourne.

The council of the Pharmaceutical Society have appointed Mr. John Kruse director and lecturer to the School of Pharmacy. The next session will commence on Monday, the 6th March.

The nominations for members of the council of the Pharmaceutical Society closed on the 15th February. There were five vacancies, and the following are the gentlemen nominated :—Messrs. A. T. Best, Robert Nicholls, Henry Gamble, J. C. Jones, and John Ross. There will not, therefore, be an election.

Members of the Pharmaceutical Society are reminded that the annual meeting takes place at the rooms on Wednesday, the 8th March, at eight p.m., when the President will deliver his annual address.

A small fire occurred at the shop of Mr. W. Bowen, chemist, 43 Collins-street, on the 22nd January. An *employé* of Messrs. Kilpatrick and Co. observed smoke issuing from the rear of the premises, and after throwing a few buckets of water on it gave the alarm at the metropolitan brigade station, the members of which soon extinguished the fire. It is supposed that one of the tins of phosphorus which were stacked in the yard had become ignited by spontaneous combustion.

A young man, fashionably attired and of good address, styling himself Dr. Watson, went into Mr. Rand's chemist shop, Wagga Wagga, on the 4th February, and wrote out a prescription. The medicine was made up, and a cheque for £5 was presented, for which the doctor received the change. After this he hired a buggy and pair and left the town. Suspicion being afterwards aroused a warrant was issued for his

apprehension. He was arrested at Old Junee, and was brought before the local bench and remanded till the 9th inst. It is said that he came from Melbourne.

Shortly after two o'clock on the 26th January a fire broke out in the shop of Messrs. Brown Bros., chemists, at the corner of Clarendon and Raglan streets, Emerald Hill, by which a large portion of the stock was damaged and destroyed. During the day a quantity of benzine was accidentally spilt on the floor, and when lighting the gas the assistant thoughtlessly threw the match on the floor, and the place almost immediately broke out in flames. The local brigades were promptly in attendance, and succeeded after some little trouble in extinguishing the fire. The damage was covered by insurance.

Mr. Kruse, Hanover-street, Fitzroy, requests us to state that he will be glad to supply small quantities of any of the following seeds :—Aconitum Napellus, Aspidium filix mas, Leontodon taraxacum, Actaea spicata, Colchicum officinale, Sorbus aucuparia, Hyorcyamus niger, Angelica archangelica, Helleborus niger, Delphinium staphisagria, Juniperus Sabina, Conium macreatum, Leviationm officinale, and Matricaria chamomilla.

NEW INSOLVENT.—John Frederick Faulkner Grace, of Spencer-street, Melbourne, druggist and chemist. Causes of insolvency—Losses sustained by fire, insufficiency of profits to pay expenses, and want of employment. Liabilities, £366 19s. 10d.; assets, £26 17s. 9d.; deficiency, £340 2s. 1d. Mr. Cohen, assignee.

Meetings.

THE PHARMACY BOARD OF VICTORIA.

THE monthly meeting of the board was held at No. 100 Collins-street, on the 8th February, 1882. Present—Messrs. Bosisto, Bowen, Blackett, Lewis, Holdsworth, and Owen. An apology was read from Mr. Brind.

The President (Mr. Bosisto) was in the chair.

The minutes of the previous meeting were read and confirmed.

Applications for Registration as Pharmaceutical Chemists.—The following were registered :—Sarah Rundle, Wangaratta, Frederick Henry Morris, Drummond-street, Carlton, passed modified examination. The name of John Henry Reed, 67 Swanston-street, was restored to the register. The applications of Thomas Hewson and Abel James were postponed.

Renewals of Certificate under Sale and Use of Poisons Act.—J. T. Player, Mansfield ; Sam Lee On, Omeo.

Examinations.—The following are the arrangements for the next examination :—The preliminary, on 2nd March, at eleven a.m. The modified, on Monday, 6th March, at ten a.m. The examination for the certificate of the School of Pharmacy, on Monday, the 6th March, at noon. The practical pharmacy examination before the board, on Monday, the 6th March, at noon.

The following is the syllabus for the examination :—

PRACTICAL PHARMACY.

Section I.—Dispensing.—Examiners, Messrs. Brind and Lewis.

Reading prescriptions without abbreviations, translating directions literally as well as appropriately, practical dispensing (including the preparation of pills, plasters, emulsions, &c.), writing directions and wrapping packages, incompatabilities and other difficulties, doses, poisons, antidotes, metric system ; general management of dispensing, counter dispensing, conveniences, and whatever will fairly test the candidate's knowledge and fitness for this department of his calling, neatness and care being specially noted.

Section II.—*Materia Medica.*—Examiners, Messrs. Bosisto, Bowen, and Holdsworth.

Recognition of drugs and chemicals by their appearance, taste, smell, form, and other physical characteristics ; use of microscope, estimation of quantity and detection of adulteration by above means; composition of extracts, tinctures, and other preparations not having definite chemical formulæ; the best means of preserving drugs, &c., in a state of efficiency.

Section III.—Chemical and other processes. — Examiners, Messrs. Blackett and Owen.

Operations of pharmacy, such as distillation, sublimation, percolation, evaporation, washing precipitates, taking specific gravities, dialysis, &c.; practical use of quantitive and qualitive tests of the pharmacopœia, chemical formulæ, and decompositions occurring in officinal processes, &c.

PHARMACEUTICAL SOCIETY OF VICTORIA.

THE monthly meeting was held at the rooms, 100 Collins-street, on Friday evening, 3rd February. Present—Messrs. Bowen, Hooper, Johnson, Gamble, Nicholls, Thomas, Best, Baker, Huntsman, Jones, and Shillinglaw; an apology was received from Mr. Swift; the president, Mr. Bowen, in the chair.

The minutes of the previous meeting were read and confirmed.

Election of New Members.—The following new members, nominated at the last meeting, were duly elected :—W. E. Woods, Napier, New Zealand; P. Fitzsimmons, Brisbane; H. A. Corinaldi, Prahran; Jas. R. Laughton, Elizabeth-street, Sydney; Frederick Wright, Pitt-street, Sydney; H. J. Fowles, Glenelg, South Australia; Walter Jones, Sandridge. Harry Jacobs, Canning-street, Carlton, was elected an associate.

New Members Nominated. — H. C. Macaulay, J. Thorby Noakes, J. H. Reed, Frederick Cherry.

Appointment of Lecturer at the School of Pharmacy.— After a personal interview with the candidates for the appointment of lecturer at the School of Pharmacy, a ballot was taken, which resulted in the election of Mr. John Kruse by one vote. It was resolved that the lectures commence on Monday, 6th March, 1882; and a syllabus of the course was agreed to, and is published in another column.

Election of Members of Council.—Wednesday, 15th February is the last day for receiving nominations for the election of Members of Council, to be held at the annual meeting on 8th March next.

The Annual Report.—A printed copy of the report for the year was laid on the table, and the hon. secretary reported that copies had been forwarded to all the members. It is requested that any member who may desire information in reference to any item in the annual report or balance-sheet will apply at the office before the date of the annual meeting.

Correspondence.—A number of letters were dealt with, but of no special interest.

Financial and general business brought the meeting to a close.

Books, &c., Received.—*New Remedies*, June to December, 1880, and *Dental Cosmos*, April to June, 1881, from Mr. W. H. H. Lane; the *Therapeutic Gazette* for December; the *Australian Veterinary Journal* for February; the *Australian Medical Journal*; the *American Journal of Pharmacy*; Report of the proceedings of the Fifth Pharmaceutical Congress of 1881; the *New York Druggist Circular.*

BALLARAT.

IT was "high jinks" with the Ballarat pharmacists on Friday, the 27th January, when at about nine a.m. some forty persons assembled at the shop of the president of the Ballarat Chemists and Druggists' Association (Mr. Wheeler), preparatory to making a start for a picnic to the beautiful Lal Lal Waterfalls, in order to celebrate the second anniversary of their association. One of Cobb and Co.'s very large coaches, splendidly horsed, together with a drag and sundry private buggies, were the vehiculars for conveying the representatives of pharmacy to the trysting ground. The day was simply delightful, Sol's rays being tempered by a beautiful south-westerly breeze. Many were the eulogiums passed while *en route* on the committee of the association for selecting this now somewhat neglected spot in preference to others nearer

and more generally frequented. The drive to and through "ye anciente" village of Buninyong, up to and round the mount, with its expansive and charmingly extensive agricultural and sylvan scenery, then down to Yendon, and so on to Lal Lal Waterfalls, was enough to enchant even those who are ever present with "nature's stores." How much more, then, should this enchantment have been intensified to us, the slaves to pharmacy. Oh, how much we regretted the opportunity was lost to us of witnessing the mind's workings of "one of us," who for the space of twenty-two long but not weary years (for he is still sound in mind and limb, and not at all of that fossiliferous era such a statement would lead one to infer) had not taken such a holiday as this. Shall we *niche* such an one to "pity's" monument, or custom's use and exacting laws? Let us hope such a day with heaven's and nature's bright gifts has made him intoxicated with their delights, and that he will for the remainder of his days behave himself "more seemly," and take such outings much more frequently. Mr. Walker, of Bridge-street, was caterer, and while preparing for an early dinner sundry games were indulged in, the ladies especially distinguishing themselves in rounders, while at quoits and cricket it was easily seen that a good many of the now old boys had not forgotten the cunning of their youth. Awhile after dinner the descent to the basin of the waterfall was undertaken, which was highly difficult, but beautifully picturesque and romantic; and while seated near the water's edge, with wondrously formed walls of basaltic columns towering a hundred and twenty feet above us, immense boulders in wild confusion, and trees and shrubs around us, Mr. Towl, with his well-known amiability and artistic skill, sang several songs, the choruses to which, if lacking in rythm, certainly did not in good will. During tea Messrs. Swifte, Cornell, and Wheeler sang several glees, to the delight of their audience. Before saying good-night, Mr. Wheeler congratulated the pharmacists of Ballarat on initiating and carrying out successfully and pleasantly the picnic of that day. He deemed the wonderful unity now existing amid pharmacy in Ballarat to be a credit and advantage to the entire trade, and was perhaps unparalleled in "the wide, wide world." This state of things was entirely owing to the association of which he had the honour to be the elected president, for its members had learned to know and esteem each other for the good that was in them. It was rather a bold departure from the accustomed celebrations of such an association as this; but the old conventional dinner could not be joined in by those nearest and dearest to them, neither was it in any pleasurable way to be compared to this, which he hoped would be annually repeated. To the hon. secretary, Mr. Macgowan, too much praise could not be given, as he was most untiring in working for the benefit of the association, the success of which he hoped would extend far and wide, permeating even to the metropolitan, Sandhurst, and Geelong districts. He then called upon those present to give three cheers for their hon. secretary, which was responded to most heartily, making the welkin ring again. Mr. Macgowan spoke modestly of his exertions, but was gratified that so much had been done in creating a kindly geniality among the pharmacists of the district, and which, if mutually fostered, must be productive of still greater blessings and advantages in the future. Many apologies had been received from district allies, regretting their unavoidable absence, while that old English gentleman at Carngham (Mr. Hopper) had thoughtfully and liberally contributed to the committee's canteen for the day. Mutual congratulations and good wishes followed, and all were transported back to Ballarat, which was safely reached soon after nine p.m. Much credit must be given to the committee of the association for successfully carrying through what must have been to all a most enjoyable picnic, which to our brother pharmacists in other large centres must seem an extraordinary and uncommon event; to whom we say, "Go and do likewise."

THE BALLARAT CHEMISTS' ASSOCIATION.

THE annual meeting of the Ballarat Chemists' Association was held on Wednesday, the 2nd February. There was a good attendance. The principal items of business were the election of officers, reception of secretary's report for the past year, and reception of report of committee appointed to consider the best means of celebrating the second anniversary of the association. The retiring officers were :—Mr. Towl, president; Mr. Wheeler, vice-president; Mr. King, treasurer; Mr. Macgowan, secretary. Mr. Wheeler was unanimously elected president, and Mr. Whittle vice-president, and Messrs. King and Macgowan re-elected treasurer and secretary. The officers retiring, and those newly elected, duly returned thanks. It was decided to have a picnic at Lal Lal Falls on Friday, 27th January. At the conclusion of the ordinary business, Mr. Wheeler (the newly-elected president) said a very agreeable duty devolved upon him, and one which he accepted with increased pleasure as among the first acts of his presidency, and he felt sure his pleasure would be equally shared by all present, and that was to present their secretary, Mr. Macgowan, with a locket which had been subscribed for by the members as a token of their esteem and approbation of the manner in which Mr. Macgowan had discharged his secretarial duties. Mr. Macgowan expressed his thanks for the honour done him and the gift bestowed. The locket is a handsome gold one, inscribed with monogram, &c.

ANNUAL REPORT OF THE BALLARAT DISTRICT CHEMISTS' ASSOCIATION,

READ AT THE MEETING HELD ON 18TH JANUARY, 1882.

MR. PRESIDENT, Vice-President, and Gentlemen—Time in its ceaseless flight has brought us to the second anniversary of our association; and the year just passed away has not been unmarked by events of interest to us as pharmacists, although no circumstances of special importance have occurred in our own city. During the year throughout the colony there has been an increased number of poisoning cases. In three cases druggists have appeared before the courts. At Sandhurst J. E. Wall was convicted, not of poisoning, but for procuring abortion ; Edward Kilpatrick, of Castlemaine, was acquitted. Coming to ourselves, the year just closed began very auspiciously with our first anniversary dinner, which, as you are aware, passed off with much éclat. Some of the members deeming it would be advisable to have a private room in some public building in which to hold our meetings, it was resolved to engage the room in which we are now met ; but it has not proved so successful as anticipated, and it has been determined to return to Lester's Hotel after the present meeting. During the year, with your concurrence, the hon. secretary resigned his seat at the Pharmaceutical Council. Various alterations have taken place from time to time in the price list. A resolution was carried early in the year altering the rule relating to honorary membership, so that gentlemen in business beyond a radius of twenty miles should have honorary membership at half the annual fee—viz., 5s. per annum. At the election of officers on 19th January last year, Messrs. Towl and Wheeler were elected as president and vice-president respectively, and Messrs. King and Macgowan as treasurer and secretary. These gentlemen retire to-night, and you will be requested to elect their successors. There have been twelve meetings held during the year, the attendances at which have been as follows :—Messrs. Towl, 12 ; Wheeler, 11 ; Whittle, 10 ; Cornell, 11 ; Palmer, 11 ; King, 9 ; Warner, 7 ; Scott, 6 ; Malyon, 8 ; Robertson, 5 ; Bloore, 4 ; Longstaff, 2 ; Wollen, 1 ; Swifte (for Mr. E. Jones), 1 ; Treloar, 0 ; Macgowan, 11 ; no country members attended. The annual dinner of the Pharmaceutical Society was held in Melbourne on 16th November, and your hon. sec. was present, as your representative. The dinner was better attended than that on the previous year, and was a more representative one. The moaning of the *cypress* leaves has been heard in the households of three members of our association—viz., Messrs. King, Longstaff, and Malyon. To the dead, we say, "*Requiescat in pace*," and to the living, "*Viva in spe.*" The "buds" that have sprung up from amongst us have been very numerous, so that in this respect, considering our number, we have been able to hold our own against any other association, as at the close of nearly every meeting a bumper had to be quaffed to some "little stranger." Our worthy past president, Mr. Palmer, has removed into new, commodious, and elegant premises, adjoining his former place of business ; and our worthy president, Mr. Towl, has also made extensive and ornamental alterations to his premises. We trust they may benefit by their enterprise. One more has been added to the list of pharmacists in our city, Mr. Calder having commenced business in Doveton-street North. With regard to medical men, the cry is "Still they come." Dr. Bradford commenced practice here last year, and Dr. Woinarski has commenced this year. The committee appointed to consider the best means of celebrating our second anniversary recommend a picnic, as the ladies will be able to join us in it. The treasurer's balance-sheet shows a small sum

in hand. Members are reminded that the yearly subscriptions are now due. In conclusion, though nothing of an exciting nature has happened during the year to inspire our enthusiasm, yet the meetings have been fairly attended, the price list adhered to ; and those feelings of amity, cordiality, and good fellowship have prevailed which have characterised our association from the beginning.—I am, Mr. President, Vice-President, and gentlemen, yours truly,

J. T. MACGOWAN, Hon. Sec.

SANDHURST.

THE annual meeting of the Bendigo School of Mines was held on the 23rd January. The report was most satisfactory, and shows that the operations of the school are much more extensive than the public generally imagine. It showed that no less than 438 pupils received instruction during the year, of whom 103 attended the chemistry lectures, 22 studied practical chemistry, 30 mathematics, 40 mechanical architectural drawing, 193 freehand drawing, and the remainder were enrolled in the classes for mechanics—practical geometry, surveying, mine management, geology, mineralogy, and metallurgy. The attendance for the past year was greater than during any previous year, and 1881 showed an increase of 100 over 1880, which increase has been more than maintained. Officers for the ensuing year were appointed, ordinary business transacted, and the meeting terminated.

SYDNEY.

(FROM OUR OWN CORRESPONDENT.)

THE annual distribution of prizes of the Technical College took place on Thursday, 2nd February, in the School of Arts Hall. The meeting was presided over by the Hon. F. B. Sutton, Minister for Public Instruction, who in a few appropriate words congratulated the committee upon the remarkable progress of the institution, the number of pupils having increased from a thousand to fourteen hundred during the past twelve months. The chairman then proceeded to distribute the prizes to the students who had excelled in the recent examinations, and the medals and certificates of merit gained by them at the Bathurst Juvenile Exhibition. The Hon. E. Combes, C.M.G., M.L.A., then delivered an instructive address on science and art education ; at the close of which votes of thanks were passed to Mr. Combes and the Hon. F. B. Sutton.

On the platform were the office-bearers of the college and several members of the Legislative Council and Assembly. It has excited some comment that no chemistry prizes were presented.

The annual meeting of the Sydney Mechanics' School of Arts was held on Tuesday, 7th February. The report showed all departments to be in a flourishing condition, and the members showed their confidence in the office-bearers of last year by re-electing nearly all of them to office. There is a general feeling among the members against opening the institution on Sundays.

Three "health lectures" were given last week by Dr. Thos. Dixon, at the Technical College Hall. The subjects touched upon were—"Impure Air and its Effects;" "Dust, and its Action in Spreading Disease;" "Impure Water and Drainage." The lectures were well attended, and highly interesting to the general public, who had again the opportunity of witnessing many well-known experiments.

During the absence of Professor Smith the duties of Experimental Physics Lecturer will be performed by the Rev. Joseph Campbell, B.A., son of Mr. W. B. Campbell, of the Furnishing Arcade, George-street. Mr. Campbell graduated at Sydney University in 1880, gaining the Belmore medal for geology and practical chemistry, and was ordained in December of the same year at St. Andrew's Cathedral. Since that time Mr. Campbell has been curate at St. Michael's Church, Surry Hills.

A meeting of the senate of the University was held on Wednesday, 1st February. Fourteen members were present ; the vice-chancellor, Canon Allwood, presided, and announced the receipt of a petition signed by fifty-four members of the University, urging the senate to invite applications from the

Australian colonies and Great Britain before making the appointments of Professors of Natural History, Physiology, and Anatomy.

Mr. Oliver proposed, and Dr. Badham seconded, a motion to the effect that Mr. W. J. Stephens be invited to the position of Professor of Natural History, which was carried by a majority of three. Dr. Renwick declined to proceed with his motion. Mr. Macleay therefore moved that Dr. MacLaurin be invited to the position of Professor of Anatomy and Physiology, which was also carried.

The lecturerships, of the value of £200 per annum, are being advertised. It is hoped that an efficient staff of lecturers will be thus secured for the medical school.

PHARMACEUTICAL SOCIETY OF NEW SOUTH WALES.

THE monthly meeting of the Pharmaceutical Council was held at the Medical Board Office, Phillip-street, on Tuesday, 14th February, at eleven a.m. Present—the president (in the chair), and Messrs. Abrahams, Guise, Prat, Row, Larmer, and Watt.

The minutes of last meeting were read and confirmed.

Mr. George Woodhouse, M.P.S., Victoria, was admitted a member of the society, and Mr. W. Withers was admitted an associate upon the production of satisfactory credentials.

Mr. J. G. Woods's application for registration of indentures and examination was granted.

Mr. J. S. Abraham was appointed as an extra examiner.

A die was agreed upon for the society's envelopes and papers; and a motion for granting silver medals to all candidates answering seventy-five per cent. of the questions in examinations was postponed until next meeting. The president announced the receipt of valuable works from America as additions to the library.

A NEW PALM FROM QUEENSLAND,
DEFINED BY BARON FERD. VON MUELLER, K.C.M.G., M. & PH. D., F.R.S.

FOR several years it was known through Mr. Eugene Fitzalan, that on Mount Elliott, near Port Denison, a palm occurs, which differs in the structure of its stem as well as in its less elevated habit from Ptychosperma Alexandræ and Pt. Cunninghami. As this seemingly local palm did not yet stand on any phytographic record, I was fortunate to induce Mr. Fitzalan, towards the end of last year, to revisit the locality, with a view of securing flowers and fruits of this species; these he succeeded to obtain, and he placed this new material for elucidation most liberally at my disposal, together with notes on the habit of this palm. Thus, I am enabled to offer now a diagnosis.

Ptychosperma Beatricæ.—Stem robust, moderately high, its basal portion much enlarged, with the annual rings there suddenly and considerably impressed; leaves large, rigid, many of them more erect than divergent; their rachis very straight; their segments numerous, grey underneath, folded back towards the base, gradually narrowed into a pointed apex, not very much spreading, the terminal segments and those nearest to them somewhat convergent at their summit; panicle moderately long, somewhat fascicular, emanating from the stem at no very great height, bearing numerous crowded slender and flexuous spikes; buds rather pointed, hardly oblique; male flowers mostly in pairs, and often a female flower between them; outer sepals from one-third to nearly half the length of the inner sepals; stamens eight to twelve; anthers linear, longer than the filaments; fruits rather small, globular-ovate. On Mount Elliott; Fitzalan. Greatest height of the whole plant 40 ft.; stems solitary from the root; leafstalks channelled; raches of the spikes dark-coloured when dry; flowers evidently smaller than those of Pt. Alexandræ and Pt. Cunninghami, but not available at present in full development; fruits in size, form and structure similar to those of the two above-mentioned species, but rather smaller.

In contrasting such differences, as are best or only observable in native localities, Mr. Fitzalan remarks, that "the stem of Pt. Alexandræ has woody fibres enough to allow of its sometimes being used (I might say sacrilegiously) for fencing and for building bush-huts, while stems of the new palm remain almost as soft as a cabbage-stalk; and while, contrarily again, the stem of Pt. Cunninghami, which is still harder and more durable, than that of Pt. Alexandræ, will sometimes turn the edge of a tomahawk." He further notes, that the basal portion of the stem is "much more massive than that of Pt. Alexandræ," and is remarkable "for the clearly defined steps (at every mark of former yearly foliage) half an inch deep or more, all round up to three to five feet, when these projections cease, and the stem tapers gradually." He adds, that the leaves stand well up, "taper to the point, not having any curvature towards the top," whereas in Pt. Alexandræ and Pt. Cunninghami the upper portion of the leaves is curved downward, and their segments are more spreading. Irrespective of these discrepancies, the Beatrice palm "flowers and fruits already six to eight feet from the ground, when evidently still very young," whereas the two sister species "do not bear fruits at a lesser distance from the base of the stem than about 30 feet." He thinks, that "the hutts of the larger individuals might be fairly called colossal." It does not seem, that the differences between the Alexandra palm and the Beatrice palm, as pointed out by Mr. Fitzalan, arise from mere diversity of places of growth, such as very wet soil and dry ground, or cool valleys and sunny ridges. Pt. Beatricæ shares the paleness of the underside of the leaf-segments with Pt. Alexandræ, agrees likewise with it in the number of stamens, the narrow anthers and short filaments, and is thus more removed from Pt. Cunninghami.

Legal and Magisterial.

BREACH OF THE PHARMACY ACT.
SANDHURST POLICE COURT.

JAMES EGAN WALL, chemist, was brought up at the City Court on 23rd January, before Messrs. Webster, P.M., Wilton and Edwards, Js.P., charged that he, being a registered pharmaceutical chemist, did, at Wattle-street, Sandhurst, practice surgery upon one Margaret Smith (now deceased), otherwise than in accordance with the rights and privileges enjoyed by chemists and druggists in their open shops.

Mr. Kirby, instructed by the police, appeared for the prosecution, and Mr. Hornbuckle, instructed by Mr. Rymer, for the defence.

Mr. Kirby stated that the case was brought under section 25 sub-section 4 of the Pharmacy Act. The evidence against the accused was limited to the evidence given at the inquest on the young woman by Wall himself. There might, however, be an objection to this evidence being admitted. The punishment for the offence with which the accused was charged was £10 and six months' imprisonment. The case was not of a vindictive character. It was purely a Government prosecution. Harry William Shillinglaw, registrar of the Pharmacy Board of Victoria, produced his appointment, and also the original appointment of the board under the hand of the Governor in Council. He deposed that on 1st August, 1881, the prisoner was a registered pharmaceutical chemist, and that he (witness) knew him personally. To Mr. Hornbuckle: The printed pharmaceutical register is a copy of the original document.

Robert Strickland, coroner, deposed, that on the day following the death of Margaret Smith (1st August) witness held an inquest on the body. The prisoner Wall was present, and gave evidence. Witness cautioned him against so doing, as, from the facts of the case, he (witness) thought it probable that the prisoner might stand in the position of an accused person. The depositions (produced) were those taken on the occasion. (Mr. Kirby here put in the depositions as evidence, but this was at once objected to by counsel for the defence, the grounds being that it was not substantially for the same offence as that which was the subject of the enquiry when the depositions were taken; that to make them evidence the charge must be substantially identical, or so connected as to create a reasonable presumption that the prisoner's mind at the time of the first charge was sufficiently directed to the matter which formed the matter of the subsequent charge, and in substantiation the following cases were quoted:—Regina v. Lewis, Regina v. Owen, Regina v. Beeston, in all of which it appeared that, to make the depositions admissible on a subsequent charge, the offences must be identical. On the other side, Mr. Kirby quoted the case of Regina v. Cooke, as heard in 1876 on appeal from the Canadian Court. The Bench, however, decided that the depositions must be rejected.) Dr. H. L. Atkinson gave evidence that he saw the woman Margaret Smith on the day following her death. Made a *post-mortem* examination in conjunction with Dr. M'Gillivray. Prisoner was then present. On the body found a lacerated wound from the vagina to the peritenium, which, by internal and external hemorrhage, was the cause of death. This was probably, as proposed by the prisoner himself, caused by the use of a catheter or stiletto, and was, no doubt, an attempted surgical operation. To Mr. Hornbuckle : The gum catheter can be used with safety by an inexperienced person. Such operations as drawing a tooth, &c., are called minor surgery, and can be performed by a chemist. Dr. P. H. M'Gillivray deposed that on the 2nd of August, in conjunction with the last witness, he made a *post-mortem* examination on the body of Margaret Smith, and found that death had been caused by a lacerated wound, extending from the vagina to the peritenium. It was, no doubt, the result of an attempted surgical operation. Do not remember that anything was said with reference to the matter by the prisoner. To Mr. Hornbuckle : At the *post-mortem* Wall had an opportunity of seeing everything that was done, so that at the inquest he might have cross-examined. During the inquiry the prisoner asked that the uterus might be produced, but this was refused. Mr. Strickland, recalled, in answer to Mr. Kirby, explained that Wall made application to witness, under the 16th section of the medical statute, that he should be allowed to be present at the *post-mortem* examination. Prisoner did not say anything on that occasion, as witness was also present, and prevented him. At the inquest prisoner had an opportunity to cross-examine the witness, which he took advantage of. (Here Mr. Hornbuckle again objected to the depositions being introduced, and was upheld by the Bench.)

John Holdsworth, pharmaceutical chemist, deposed that he had been in business over thirty years. It was not the right and privilege of a chemist to practice surgery. He would not even take a case of diphtheria in hand.

Henry Trumble, pharmaceutical chemist, gave evidence to having been in business for over twenty years. All such operations as drawing a tooth, placing a piece of sticking-plaster over a cut, and drawing the sides together are all minor surgical operations, and witness would consider himself justified in performing such operations.

Richard John Webb, sergeant of police at Sandhurst, deposed to being at Mr. Wrixon's on the 2nd of August. Wall knocked at the door, and asked to see Mr. Wrixon. That gentleman was in the room. Wall then came in and said, "Mr. Wrixon, I am ashamed to meet you." Mr. Wrixon replied that it was a terrible affair. Prisoner then asked Mr. Wrixon whether he remembered his showing him a hydatid cyst which he removed from the woman Smith some three years previously. Mr. Wrixon said he did not. The witness also gave evidence as to a conversation which he had with prisoner with reference to the woman's death.

James Storey, who was a groom employed on the premises at same time, deposed that he last saw the woman Smith alive at half-past three on the 1st of August last. She was found dead at six o'clock, about a quarter of an hour after Wall left the premises.

Margaret Beale, a little girl of thirteen years of age, gave evidence that she was in the house on the 2nd August. The prisoner Wall was there. Witness called out "Maggie," when the prisoner came out of the room and asked "What all this Maggieing meant."

This closed the case for the prosecution.

Mr. Kirby said that once the offence was disclosed on the summons it could be amended by the Bench on the evidence given. An adjournment was here made for lunch.

On resuming at two o'clock, Mr. Kirby resumed his remarks. He argued that section 69 of the Justices Statute said that there was no power to amend where no offence was disclosed on the summons. There had been no occasion to put in the summons what he had about the catheter ; all that need have been said was that the accused had practised surgery. He got those words after reading the depositions, which, however, it had been since stated could not be admitted as evidence. It was plain that surgery had been practised, and they had strong circumstantial evidence that Wall was the man who did it. The act of surgery was performed outside the rights and privileges of chemists. Wall was present at the *post-mortem* examination, and it had been proved that death was caused by an attempt at surgical operation. He thought there was sufficient evidence to find Wall guilty upon. He withdrew his application for an amendment to the summons.

Mr. Hornbuckle said it would be idle for him to ask the magistrates to forget what they had seen in the newspapers of the evidence given at the inquest, for he was sure that their decision would be based merely on what they had heard that day. They were told all that was wanted was to have Wall's name struck off the roll, and this much could be obtained by the infliction of a nominal penalty. But Mr. Kirby asked for more, and he (Mr. Hornbuckle) felt convinced that the whole affair was malicious and vindictive. Sergeant Webb gave evidence as to the death, which was quite in conformity with death from exhaustion, or what Wall stated in his depositions, from chloroform. The doctors did not say that it was a catheter that was used.

The Bench said it did not matter about the catheter, provided it had been clearly shewn that some person attempted to perform an operation.

Mr. Hornbuckle said that there was no evidence of Wall having performed a surgical operation. The only one that could prove he had was dead. The Bench had, no doubt, the whole history of the case in their minds, but they must not think of what they had read.

Mr. Webster : " It so happened that I did not read the depositions at the time."

Mr. Hornbuckle said that it was difficult to decide a matter like this, apart from the previous case. But there had been no evidence to support the charge. There was no direct proof that Wall performed the operation, and a man should not be sent to gaol on a surmise. It had not been proved that Wall was not a surgeon.

The Bench said that he might be a surgeon, but he was not on the medical roll. It was for Mr. Hornbuckle to prove that he was a surgeon.

Mr. Hornbuckle said there was nothing to prevent a man being both a chemist and a surgeon. The offence had not been proved, and even performing an operation was not practising as a surgeon. Practising did not mean a single isolated case. There was no evidence that Wall operated for the purpose of gain. He might even have used the instrument as a friend, just as a farmer might, with a slight knowledge of setting a limb, attend to the broken arm of a friend.

The Bench said that the evidence they had heard was the only evidence that concerned their decision. It had transpired that Wall was the man who performed the operation. There was plenty of evidence to prove that an operation had been attempted. The circumstantial evidence adduced was of a very strong character. It was left to them to decide, and they could not help fixing Wall as the person who did it. They would not inflict a very heavy penalty. They would fine Wall 1s., and three months' imprisonment, which would commence at the expiration of the term he is now serving.

A HOMŒOPATHIC CHEMIST CHARGED WITH LARCENY.

THE St. Kilda Bench—consisting of the Mayor (Mr. Gavan Shaw), and Messrs. Pilley, Simpson, and Balderson, J.P.'s—were engaged on the 6th February in investigating a charge of theft preferred against Mr. Thomas Osmond, homœopathic chemist, High-street, St. Kilda. The facts, as detailed by the prosecutrix, Mrs. Clara Gardner, residing at Leicester-street, St. Kilda, were as follow :— On Monday afternoon she was returning from Melbourne to St. Kilda in an omnibus, in which the prisoner was also a passenger. She placed a small travelling basket on the seat beside her, the prisoner placing her on the opposite side. Her basket contained some small parcels and her purse, in which was a note for £5 and some silver. Mr. J. Mason, a gentleman in the commission of the peace, was also a passenger. In the course of the journey, Mr. Mason remarked the prosecutrix's purse lying on the seat beside her, and before arriving at his destination the prisoner shifted his position to the same side of the omnibus where she was sitting. The prisoner got out at High-street, and then Mr. Mason called the attention of the prosecutrix to the fact that the former had taken up her purse and departed with it in his possession. He had, as he stated in evidence, also watched the movements of the prisoner while in the omnibus, and it appeared to him that in order to possess himself of the purse without detection the prisoner had tried to cover it with the skirt of his coat. By Mr. Mason's advice the prosecutrix obtained the services of a police constable, and they all three went to the prisoner's shop in High-street, and charged him with stealing the purse. He admitted that he had it, but said that it had been his intention to find the owner and restore it. He was then taken into custody. Mr. Weller appeared for the defence, and in a very forcible manner urged the improbability of his client, a man of respectability, seventy-five years of age, and forty-one years resident in the colony, being capable of theft. He said that he had several small parcels of his own, and when leaving the omnibus he took the purse up unknowingly with his own packages. Moreover, it was clear from the fact of Mr. Mason allowing the prisoner to leave the omnibus without challenging him with having Mrs. Gardner's purse, that he must have been actuated by vindictive motives in recommending her to give the prisoner into custody. Mr. Mason corroborated the evidence of the prosecutrix in all essential points, and deprecated the imputation of malice thrown out by Mr. Weller, for which he was sharply rebuked by Mr. Pilley from the bench, who told him he had no right to reply to Mr. Weller's remarks. Cross-examination failed to shake the evidence of either the prosecutrix or Mr. Mason, and on the termination of the case the latter addressed the Bench in justification of the course he had thought it his duty to pursue in the matter. The Bench retired to consider their decision, and after a short deliberation discharged the prisoner, as a majority of the Bench were of opinion there had been no felonious intention in taking the purse. The Mayor dissented from his colleagues in their judgment.

SALES OF ADULTERATED SPIRITS.

At the Richmond Court on Wednesday, the 8th February, Isaac Henry Jones, wine and spirit merchant, corner of Swan and Lennox streets, Richmond, was prosecuted at the instance of the excise authorities, under the 86th section of the Licensing Act, for selling spirits distilled in the colony, mixed with foreign spirits, without causing the bottle containing such spirits to bear upon it the statement that its contents were " a mixture of foreign and colonial spirits." Mr. John O'Connor, senior inspector of excise, appeared to prosecute on behalf of the Customs, and Mr. Gillott represented the defendant.

H. J. Rattray, inspector of excise, stated that on the 27th ult. he inspected the store kept by the defendant, accompanied by Mr. John M'Nee. The defendant said he was the proprietor of the store, and a registered wine and spirit merchant. The witness saw a number of bottles on a shelf labelled "Fine Old Scotch Whisky," and hearing the statement that the contents had been bottled by J. H. Jones, Swan-street, Richmond. On taking down one of the bottles and asking the defendant what whisky it contained, the defendant replied, "Glenlivat Scotch whisky," but that there was some Aikin's colonial whisky mixed with it. Witness purchased a bottle of the spirit, for which he paid 3s. 6d. The defendant then showed the witness over his cellar, and pointed out a cask numbered 3221 of Aikin's colonial whisky, and also a jar of Glenlivat Scotch whisky, which he had purchased from Messrs. Lange and Thoneman, wine and spirit merchants, of Melbourne. He added that the bottle of spirits which had been purchased by the witness was a blended mixture of those spirits. The witness then purchased a bottle of each, paying 2s. 6d. for the Scotch and 1s. 6d. for the colonial spirit. The permit issued for the Aikin's whisky in the cellar was shown to the witness by the defendant; the number upon it was the same as the one upon the cask in the cellar.

For the defence, Mr. Gillott denied that the prosecution had proved their case. The proof rested on the credibility of the witnesses as to whether the defendant had really admitted that the bottle of whisky which had been purchased by Inspector Rattray was a mixture of imported foreign spirits and spirits distilled in the colony. The defendant positively denied having made any such admission. Moreover, there could be no conviction, because it was impossible by any known analysis to prove that the whisky produced in court was a mixture distilled in the colony and an imported foreign spirit. Lastly, as he interpreted the Act, it was not required by law that any statement further than that the bottle contained whisky was necessary to be put on it by the vendor when the spirits were of colonial manufacture.

The Bench recalled Mr. Stubley, who said that in his opinion it was impossible by any analysis to state the constituents of a bottle of whisky, and authoritatively pronounce whether or no it was a mixture of foreign and colonial spirits.

A majority of the Bench were of opinion that the case had been proved, and fined the defendant £10, and £2 2s. costs, the liquor to be forfeited, together with the vessels and kegs in which it was contained.

Mr. Gillott gave notice of appeal.

THE ANNUAL CRICKET MATCH.
WHOLESALE v. RETAIL.

The following report of this match has been furnished by Mr. A. C. Lewis:—The annual cricket match between the wholesale and retail chemists took place on Thursday, the 26th January, on the Melbourne Cricket Ground, and resulted in an easy win for the retail by eighty-six runs. There was a marked improvement upon last year's attendance, and great interest was manifested in the match. This year the retail were the guests of the wholesale, and at two o'clock an adjournment was made to lunch, at which over fifty sat down. Ample justice having been done to the good things provided, before adjourning to resume the game, Mr. Blackett, M.P., rose, and begged to propose a toast — " The Wholesale Chemists." In doing so he said it afforded him great pleasure in being there, and he trusted it would not be the last time he would meet so many under similar circumstances. He was proud to see there were some amongst chemists who could play the grand old English game of cricket, and he was also proud of the position Victorians held in the cricket field, and concluded by hoping the retailers would give the wholesale a good beating. Mr. Grimwade, in responding, said it gave him great pleasure to be present at the match. He had been against these matches before, but now he thought they would help to lead to a better feeling between the wholesale and retail houses. It was through the persuasive powers of Mr. Hemmons that he had given his sanction to a half-holiday, and he hoped now that these matches would become quite an institution. (Loud applause.) He thanked Mr. Blackett for the kind manner he spoke of the wholesale chemists, but did not agree with him in wishing for a victory for the retailers. His sympathy was with the wholesale. Mr. Hemmons, who upon rising was received with much applause, also thanked Mr. Blackett for his kind remarks about the wholesale, and said he was very pleased to see so many present at the lunch. In concluding, he begged to propose the health of the retail chemists, which was drunk with enthusiasm. Mr. Blackett returned thanks in a few words, and the match was then resumed. Mr. Hemmons acted as umpire for the wholesale, and gave great satisfaction, while Mr. Coulthard performed like duties for the retail. It was unanimously agreed by those present to endeavour to make these matches far more popular amongst the trade than they have been. The following are the particulars of the play :—

RETAIL.

F. Baker, c Griffen, b Court	2
F. G. Barnard, b Treadaway	0
Pleasance, b Court	26
Cooper, l b w, b Court	3
Gibson, not out	82
Hope, c Duff, b Jenkinson	10
A. Lewis, b Lyons	0
Cattach, c and b Jenkinson	1
Ross, b Jenkinson	3
Gabriel, b Moss	31
Evans, c Treadaway, b Lyons	15
Sundries	2
Total	175

Bowling Analysis.—Treadaway, 72 balls, 1 maiden, 63 runs, 1 wicket ; Court, 36 balls, 32 runs, 3 wickets ; Jenkinson, 48 balls, 2 maidens, 33 runs, 3 wickets ; Lyons, 37 balls, 14 runs, 2 wickets ; Moss, 42 balls, 31 runs, 1 wicket.

WHOLESALE.

Jenkinson, run out	28
Coates, b Ross	0
Treadaway, c Gabriel, b Baker	3
Lyons, b Ross	18
Moss, b Ross	0
Powell, c and b Ross	4
Rackman, b Gibson	12
Court, b Ross	0
Griffen, b Gibson	4
Duff, not out	10
Whiting, b Ross	1
Sundries	9
Total	89

Bowling Analysis.—Baker, 78 balls, 9 maidens, 25 runs, 1 wicket ; Ross, 97 balls, 6 maidens, 39 runs, 6 wickets ; Gibson, 24 balls, 16 runs, 2 wickets.

Majority for Retail, 86 runs.

PERMANGANATE OF POTASSA AS AN ANTIDOTE FOR SNAKE POISON.

Dr. de Lacerda lately made in Brazil some important experiments on the modification caused by various substances in the effects of the snake poison's inoculation. He found perchloride of iron, borax, acid, nitrate of mercury, tannin, and other chemicals, to be all inert or nearly so, but permanganate of potassa was discovered to afford astonishing results.

The first series of experiments was as follows:—The fresh venom of the bothrops snake, collected on cotton wadding, and corresponding in quantity to that produced by a number of bites, was diluted with eight or ten grammes of water. The liquid being introduced into a Pravaz syringe, about one-half of it was injected into the cellular tissue of the thigh of one of the dogs selected for observation. Then, one or two minutes afterwards, sometimes later, an equal quantity of a one per cent. solution of permanganate of potassa was injected in the same place.

The dogs, on being examined the next day, showed no trace of local lesion, save the usual traces of the puncture. The same poisonous liquid, however, when not followed by the antidote, always produced in other dogs great local tumefaction, and abscesses more or less voluminous accompanied with loss of substance and destruction of tissues.

The next series of experiments was in injecting the poison into the veins, when the antidote failed in only two cases out of thirty. The lack of success in these two instances is explained by the fact that, in order to vary the experiments, some of the dogs operated upon were ill-fed, very young, or weak, and in some cases the introduction of the permanganate was made very late, when the heart's beats were ready to cease.

In a number of cases the injections consisted of half a syringeful of a poisonous solution containing the venom produced by twelve or fifteen snakes' bites, mixed with ten grammes of water. Half-a-minute afterwards two c.c. of the one per cent. permanganate solution were injected. With the exception of a transient agitation and occasional cardiac acceleration scarcely lasting a few minutes, no disturbances were noted. The animals were kept under observation for several days, and their health remained good.

In another series of cases, after injecting the poison, the operator waited for the manifestation of the characteristic troubles. When the animal already exhibited great pupillary dilatation, respiratory and cardiac disturbances, constriction, &c., Dr. de Lacerda injected into the vein two to three cubic centimeters of the permanganate solution. After two or three minutes, five at the utmost, all disturbances ceased; slight general prostration only remained, which never lasted longer than twenty-five minutes. Then the animal, being placed on the ground, could walk and even run. At the same time other dogs, to which the same quantity of poison had been administered, but no antidote, met with a death more or less rapid.

These striking results were observed at different times by various persons, notably the Emperor of Brazil and professors of the faculty. Hence, Dr. de Lacerda affirms without hesitation that " permanganate of potassa acts as a true antidote to snake's poison."

Correspondence.

Mr. H. F. Massey, of Williamstown, writes:—" Will you kindly allow me space in your journal to inform Mr. Alexander Hall that the paragraph he refers to in his letter in no way emanated from me? The circulars issued by me state that " I have commenced business in the premises lately occupied by Mr. A. Hall." This by no means infers my having " succeeded" to his business.

CRICKET MATCH.

To the Editor of the Australasian Supplement to the Chemist and Druggist.

Dear Sir—It is the intention of a number of chemists on the south side of the Yarra to arrange a cricket match against a team from the north side. If any of your readers desire to take part in the match, and would kindly send their names and addresses to me, they will be placed before a committee for selection. The match will be played either this or next month, upon a ground to be agreed upon. By kindly inserting this in your journal, you will oblige, yours respectfully,

G. E. Treen.

102 Clarendon-street, Emerald Hill, 9th February, 1882.

Notes and Abstracts.

Ready Method of Preparing Fomentations.—Take your flannel, folded to the required thickness and size, dampened quite perceptibly with water, but not enough to drip, and place it between the folds of a large newspaper, having the edges of the paper lap well over the cloth, so as to give no vent to the steam. Thus prepared, lay it on the heated surface of the stove or register, and in a moment steam is generated from the under surface, and has permeated the whole cloth sufficiently to heat it to the required temperature. This method is often very convenient and efficient where there is no opportunity to heat much water at a time.—*Michigan Medical News.*

Colouring White Flowers.—A correspondent of *Vick's Floral Monthly* says :—A very pretty experiment is performed by putting the stem of a freshly cut tuberose, or other white flower, into diluted scarlet ink for a short time. The liquid will be drawn up into the veins, colouring them in a very pleasant manner. It is also instructive, showing whether a plant is net-veined or parallel-veined. A tuberose coloured not too highly makes a very pretty novelty. I gave one to a young lady, who wore it in a mixed assembly, where it attracted considerable attention. Among those interested was an amateur botanist, who entered into a lengthy explanation of how he supposed the matter to have been accomplished by hybridising, and considerable merriment was caused when the truth was revealed. I discovered this process accidentally, and the ink mentioned is the only colour I have found fine enough to pass into the pores of the flowers."

To Colour Iron Black.—A brilliant black is produced on iron and steel by applying, with a fine hair brush, a mixture of turpentine and sulphur boiled together. When the turpentine evaporates, there remains on the metal a thin layer of sulphur, which unites closely with the iron when heated for a time over a spirit or gas flame. This varnish protects the metal perfectly, and is quite durable.

Stain for Mahogany Cherry.—The most simple and best stain for mahoganising cherry is ground burnt sienna mixed in benzine or turpentine. Apply with a brush or sponge, let it stand for a short time, and clean off with a cloth. It will be better to let it remain in this condition until the following day before commencing to finish.

METALLIC OLEATES AND OLEO-PALMITATES.

Dr. L. Wolff, in a paper read at a pharmaceutical meeting of the Philadelphia College of Pharmacy, recommends the following process for obtaining pure oleates :—

One part of castile soap (sodium oleo-palmitate) is dissolved in eight parts of water ; the solution so obtained is allowed to stand for twenty-four hours, when there will be a considerable deposit of sodium palmitate, while the supernatant liquor, containing mostly sodium oleate, is drawn off and then decomposed with a concentrated solution of a metallic salt, which, if obtainable, should contain no free acid to prevent the formation of free oleo-palmitic acid. The heavy deposit of oleo-palmitate so derived is strained off, pressed out in the strainer, and the adherent water evaporated in a water-bath ; after this it is dissolved in about six to eight times its quantity of petroleum-benzine, and the insoluble palmitate is left to subside while the solution of oleate decanted therefrom is filtered off. The benzine evaporated will yield an oleate that is entitled to that name, as it is a chemical combination, and will remain stable and efficacious.

The oleates, so prepared, he says, present an amorphous appearance, while the palmitates are of a crystalline character. I have noticed a marked affinity of some of the metallic salts for palmitic acid, the absence of it in others is remarkable. Thus, mercury, zinc, bismuth, and lead combine with palmitic acid abundantly ; but iron and copper seem to form an exception therefrom, and while the oleates of mercury, iron, and copper seem to be desirable as therapeutic agents, the oleo-palmitates of zinc, bismuth, and lead appear preferable.

New and Standard Medical Works

ON SALE BY

GEO. ROBERTSON

WHOLESALE AND RETAIL

BOOKSELLER & STATIONER,

33 & 35 Little Collins Street West,

MELBOURNE.

The Cyclopædia of Practical Receipts, Processes, and Collateral Information in the Arts, Manufactures, Professions and Trades, including Pharmacy and Hygiene, by ARNOLD J. COOLEY, 2 volumes ... ... 47s. 6d.

Beasley—The Book of Prescriptions ... ... 7s. 6d.

Beasley—The Druggist's General Receipt Book ... ... 7s.

Beasley—The Pocket Formulary and Synopsis of the British and Foreign Pharmacopœias ... ... 7s. 6d.

Fownes—A Manual of Chemistry, Theoretical and Practical, 2 vols. ... ... 21s.

Mayne—A Medical Vocabulary: being an Explanation of all Terms and Phrases used in the various departments of Medical Science and Practice, giving their Derivation, Meaning, Application, and Pronunciation ... ... 11s. 6d.

Taylor—On Poisons in Relation to Medicine ... ... 18s.

Bloxam—Laboratory Teaching: Progressive Exercises in Practical Chemistry, illustrated ... ... 6s. 6d.

Royle—A Manual of Materia Medica and Therapeutics, illustrated ... ... 17s.

Carpenter—The Microscope and its Revelations, illustrated ... ... 17s.

Dick—Encyclopædia of Practical Receipts and Processes, 6,400 Receipts ... 25s.

Squire—A Companion to the British Pharmacopœia, comparing the strength of its various Preparations with those of the United States and other Foreign Pharmacopœias, &c. ... ... 12s.

Fenwick—The Student's Guide to Medical Diagnosis, illustrated ... ... 7s. 6d.

Savory—A Compendium of Domestic Medicine, and Companion to the Medicine Chest ... ... 6s.

A COMPLETE CATALOGUE OF MEDICAL BOOKS TO BE HAD ON APPLICATION.

GEORGE ROBERTSON,

33 and 35 Little Collins Street West, Melbourne,

AND AT

SYDNEY, BRISBANE, AND ADELAIDE.

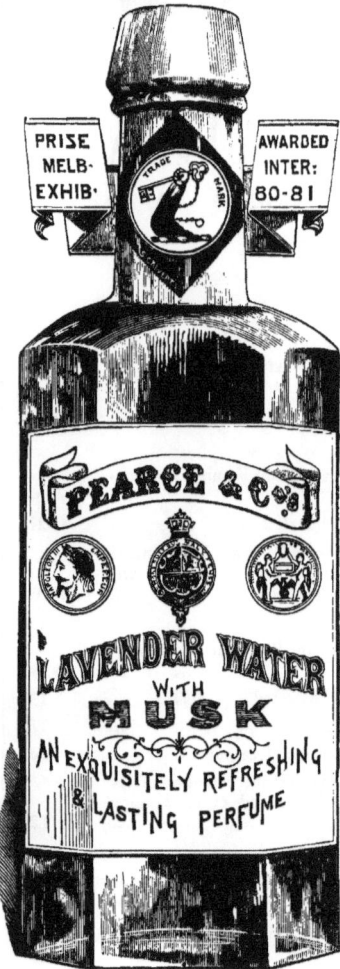

The Chemist and Druggist.

WITH AUSTRALASIAN SUPPLEMENT.

OFFICE: MUTUAL PROVIDENT BUILDINGS, COLLINS STREET WEST.
Published on the 15th of each Month.

THIS Journal is issued gratis to all paid-up Members of the PHARMACEUTICAL SOCIETY OF VICTORIA, and to non-members at Fifteen Shillings per annum, payable in advance. A copy of *The Chemists and Druggists' Diary*, published annually, is forwarded post free to every subscriber.

Advertisements, remittances, and all business communications to be addressed to THE HONORARY SECRETARY OF THE PHARMACEUTICAL SOCIETY, MELBOURNE.

SCALE OF CHARGES FOR ADVERTISEMENTS:

	Per annum.			Per annum.
One Page	.. £8 0 0	Quarter Page	..	£3 0 0
Half do.	.. 5 0 0	Business Cards	..	2 0 0

Special rates for wrapper and pages preceding and following literary matter. Advertisements of Assistants Wanting Situations, 2s. 6d. each.

Advertisements for insertion in the current month should be sent to the office before the 10th.

COMMUNICATIONS for the EDITORIAL department of this journal should be addressed to THE EDITOR, MUTUAL PROVIDENT BUILDINGS, COLLINS STREET WEST, MELBOURNE.

No notice can be taken of anonymous communications. Whatever is intended for insertion must be authenticated by the name and address of the writer—not necessarily for publication, but as a guarantee of good faith.

ANNUAL SUBSCRIPTIONS.

ALL annual subscriptions are now due.

Member's subscription	...	...	£1	1	0
Associate's	...	...	...	0 10	6
Apprentice's	...	...	...	0 5	0

Cheques and Post-office orders should be forwarded to the Honorary Secretary, No. 4 Mutual Provident Buildings, Collins-street, Melbourne.

THE LIBRARY.

THE Library is open daily (Saturdays excepted), from 9.30 a.m. to 4.30 p.m. Catalogue of the books can be obtained on application.

MEETINGS.

THE next meeting of the Council will be held on Friday evening, the 14th April, at 8 o'clock, p.m. The next quarterly meeting will be held on Friday, the 14th April, at 9 p.m. The quarterly meetings are open to all members of the Society.

SPECIAL NOTICE—TENDERS FOR ADVERTISING SPACE.

IN consequence of there being several applications for the front and back pages of the cover of *The Australasian Supplement to the Chemist and Druggist*, it has been decided to put them up for tender. Tenders are invited for the space for a period of twelve months, from 1st April, 1882. For further particulars, conditions, &c., apply to the Secretary at the office of the Pharmaceutical Society, Collins-street.

BIRTHS.

M'BURNEY.—On the 7th March, at 2 Warwick-terrace, Drummond-street, Carlton, the wife of H. G. M'Burney of a son.

PULLING.—On the 27th February, at Waterton, Albert-street, Windsor, the wife of Albert Edward Pulling of a daughter.

WADE.—On the 18th February, at Eglinton-villa, St. Vincent-place, Albert Park, the wife of A. J. Wade of a son. Both doing well.

MARRIAGE.

BAGE—LANGE.—On the 21st February, at All Saints' Church, St. Kilda, by the Rev. J. H. Gregory, Edward, eldest son of Edward Bage, Fulton-street, to Mary Charlotte, eldest daughter of Frederick C. Lange, Alma-road.

PHARMACEUTICAL EDUCATION AND PHARMACEUTICAL EXAMINATION.

RECENTLY Professor Attfield read an excellent paper on " The Relation to each other of Education and Examination, Especially with Regard to Pharmacy," before the Manchester Chemists' and Druggists' Association. It is unnecessary to say that this paper is characterised by its author's eminently clear and practical sense. In England it would seem that the leaders of pharmacy are fully alive to the urgent necessity of an amendment of the Pharmacy Act, but in the present state of affairs in the Imperial Parliament it is probable that some time will be required to get the attention of the Government. There are several of the proposed amendments of the English Pharmacy Act which, fortunately for us, we have anticipated. In England, for instance, there is a generally expressed opinion that the preliminary examination ought to be passed before apprenticeship—a most important and desirable arrangement, and one which we may congratulate ourselves upon having settled. In the mother-country the set of opinion is also in the direction of so altering the law that pharmaceutical students should be compelled to attend a definite course of lectures in recognised schools of pharmacy before presenting themselves for examination. The Pharmacy Act of 1868 prescribed no limitations as to where the candidates should acquire the knowledge necessary to pass. Under our own Act the candidate for the higher examination must produce certificates of having attended lectures in *materia medica*, medical botany, and chemistry; and passed examinations either at the Melbourne University or some school or college of pharmacy recognised by the Board of Pharmacy. So in this respect—*i.e.*, requiring from candidates a certificate of having completed a curriculum at some recognised school of pharmacy—we are in advance of our brethren at home. However, we must seriously consider whether our educational arrangements are up to the proper standard. The provisions of the law are sufficient; but the responsibility of seeing that any school or college of pharmacy now or to be recognised by the Board of Pharmacy is under able and efficient teaching, rests upon the Pharmaceutical Society, as representing the interests of pharmacy and the training in sound knowledge of the youths who are destined to follow us in the practice of our responsible calling. If our readers have read the interesting series of papers on modern pharmaceutical study by Mr. Möller, which we have reprinted recently in our columns, or have followed the debate on pharmaceutical education at the congress which lately met in London, they will have noticed that in all the European states evidence is required that the candidate has gone through a defined educational course; and this curriculum is so complete that the continental pharmacist is now a much more accomplished scientific man than his English *confrère*. As M. Petit said at the Intenational Pharmaceutical Congress, "Whatever may be the literary and scientific studies required from doctors of medicine, the French pharmacists are disposed to accept and even to claim them, in order that they may find themselves in an equivalent position from a social point of view." Some of our antipodean pharmacists are doubtless like the celebrated pococurantist of old—"they care for none of these things." But, as Mr. Johnson told his hearers the other night at the annual meeting—"Why, very soon the children in the State-schools will put to shame some of our apprentices; they will know more of chemistry than the 'chemist!'" Again, the same gentleman said—"When we began our examinations, after the passing of the Pharmacy Act, we found them (the apprentices who came up under the 'modified') very ignorant—deplorably ignorant." But *nous avons changé tout cela.* At the last examination some of the candidates who had been attending lectures, at the School of Pharmacy are reported by the examiners to have displayed a very great advance upon the condition of things formerly manifested.

It is to be hoped that there will be no retrogression under somewhat changed conditions, as far as the teaching staff is concerned, at the School of Pharmacy. We look upon this question as supremely important. We consider that the highest ideal of education ought to be kept before the mind's eye both of teacher and pupil, for depend upon it mere effort to pass examinations will not suffice in the future. The students must "know," to use Huxley's words. And in the present day we think, with Professor Attfield, the model pharmacist—that is, the pharmacist who acts but for the public weel and his own welfare, the man who fears neither the permanent influence of "stores," nor any other form of mere trade competition, is the man who can say—"I guarantee every preparation on my shelves to be trustworthy, either because my professional skill in analysis has enabled me to thoroughly test it, or because it has been made under my own personal supervision from materials which my professional knowledge of botany and chemistry has enabled me to prove to be thoroughly reliable." This is the right tone to speak in, and "unhasting and unresting" must we strive to keep up the standard of pharmaceutical education and examination in this colony. We have taken the lead in this hemisphere, and others will look to us and follow us. At least such is our ineradicable faith, notwithstanding many discouragements, we believe that pharmacy will have a brilliant future, and the pharmacist will, if he is what he ought to be, furnish the class from which, as in France has been the case, are drawn the leading men of science. Did not Scheele, Liebig, and Dumas, and many other eminent chemists, begin life as pharmacists? But, above all, we must strive to bring about "such an improvement of the condition and position of the pharmacist that pharmacy will be the better fitted to be the handmaid of medicine and the trustworthy servant of the public."

The Month.

An attempt has been made to obtain for the chemists and their assistants in Sandhurst some of the privileges of the early-closing system, but the attempt has failed.

The foundation-stone of the new free dispensary to be erected in Church-street, Richmond, was laid on the 21st ult. by Mr. Geo. Coppin, one of the founders of the original institution. There was a large public attendance.

Letters patent were granted by the Solicitor-General on the 13th March to Mr. J. W. Raymond, of Melbourne, sheep-farmer, for his process of and apparatus for phosphorising oats and other grain.

The *Camperdown Chronicle* writes:—"Carrot streated with arsenic, it would appear, are the most effectual and certain specific yet found for the destruction of rabbits. The preparation is being used with greater success than any other means yet resorted to. Every method suggested or recommended for the extermination of rabbits has been used, and none has been found to surpass this in efficacy. The proportion is 1 lb. of arsenic to 30 lbs. of carrots."

The South Australian Government being desirous of establishing an animal vaccine depôt, Mr. Graham Mitchell, F.R.C.V.S., recently proceeded to Adelaide to assist Mr. Chalwin, M.R.C.V.S., the Government veterinary surgeon, in carrying out the details of the scheme. Dr. Gosse, the president of the Adelaide Board of Health, and Dr. Paterson, the colonial surgeon, having acknowledged the value of the assistance rendered by Mr. Mitchell, the Chief Secretary of South Australia, on behalf of the Government, forwarded to that gentleman a substantial acknowledgment in recognition of his services.

NEW INSOLVENT.—Stephen Cox, manufacturing chemist, West Geelong. Causes of insolvency: Withdrawal of co-partner's capital at chemical works, Footscray, and refusal of a certain firm to carry out agreement entered into relating to chemical works at Footscray. Liabilities, £665 12s. 6d.; assets, £96 10s.; deficiency, £569 2s. 6d.

Books, &c., Received—Australian Veterinary Journal, March; *Australian Medical Gazette,* March; *Australian Medical Journal,* February; *European Mail,* January; *Pharmaceutical Journal; Annual Report School of Mines, Ballarat; Prospectus of the Belgian Export Company;* Messrs. H. B. Sleeman and Co.'s *Prices Current; American Journal of Pharmacy,* January and February; *New York Druggists' Circular,* February; *New Remedies,* February; *Therapeutic Gazette,* January.

Mr. a'Beckett has been re-elected honorary attending medical officer of the Melbourne Hospital for Sick Children, and Dr. Snowball has been elected to fill the vacancy caused by the resignation of Dr. Wigg.

We are glad to report that Mr. A. Felton has now quite recovered from his late railway accident.

We are informed that Mr. H. P. Beach, of Chapel-street, Prahran, has relinquished business, which has been purchased by Mr. C. Harrison, a new arrival in the colony.

The new session at the School of Pharmacy commenced on the 6th inst.

A deputation from the Pharmaceutical Society is to wait on the Minister of Lands on the 22nd inst., to make another effort to obtain a site for a school and laboratory.

At the examination for the certificate of the School of Pharmacy, held on the 6th March, the board of examiners complimented one of the candidates—Mr. Wm. Lowe—on the very satisfactory examination passed by him, and expressed themselves as satisfied that Mr. Lowe would one day occupy a position in the foremost rank of pharmacy in this colony. Mr. Lowe obtains the gold medal given by the Pharmaceutical Society of Victoria.

The name of James Egan Wall is to be erased from the Pharmaceutical Register of Victoria. A resolution embodying this recommendation has been forwarded by the Pharmacy Board to his Excellency the Governor-in-Council for approval. It will be remembered that Wall was convicted of a breach of the 15th section of the Pharmacy Act at the Police Court, Sandhurst, on the 23rd January last, and sentenced to be imprisoned for three months.

Meetings.

THE ANNUAL MEETING OF THE PHARMACEUTICAL SOCIETY OF VICTORIA.

THE twenty-fifth annual meeting of the Pharmaceutical Society of Victoria was held at the rooms of the Society, No. 4 Mutual Provident Buildings, Collins-street, on Wednesday evening, the 8th March, 1882.

The president (Mr. Wm. Bowen) in the chair. The following members were present:—Messrs. Thomas, Blackett, Huntsman, Bowen, Hooper, Gamble, Johnson, Cornialdi, Barnard, Treen, Brind, Swift, A. T. Best, Brownscombe, J. C. Jones, Nicholls, F. A. Dunn, Norris, David Jones, Ross, G. Kingsland, B. Baker.

The president read the advertisement calling the meeting.

The minutes of the last annual meeting were read and unanimously confirmed.

The honorary secretary (Mr. H. Shillinglaw) then read the twenty-fifth annual report and balance-sheet, and its adoption was moved by Mr. J. C. Jones.

Mr. A. T. Best made some remarks in reference to the statement in the report in reference to the friendly relationship that existed with the societies in the other colonies, and trusted that there would be some uniformity in the educational standard required in all the colonies, which was much needed.

Mr. J. W. Brownscombe said that in the report it was stated that satisfactory progress had been made at the School of Pharmacy. If that were the case, he should be glad to know why the council had removed it from the Technological Museum.

A general discussion then took place as to the reason that had induced the council to take that step, which was joined in by Messrs. Gamble, Ross, Thomas, Blackett, Hooper, and Barnard.

Mr. Bowen also replied at some length to the remarks of Mr. Brownscombe.

Mr. Norris said he had attended specially to object to the hours at which the lectures were held.

Mr. Blackett remarked that the time was the same as at Bloomsbury-square, and he could not see any hardship in asking students to attend at half-past eight a.m.

The report was then unanimously adopted.

THE PRESIDENT'S ANNUAL ADDRESS.

The president said : In accordance with the usual custom at the annual meeting of the Pharmaceutical Society of Victoria, on retiring from the chair as president, a position which I have occupied for the past twelve months, I will endeavour to refer briefly to some of the more important events which have occurred during that period. In the first place, I beg to thank you sincerely for the courtesy and kindness I have experienced, not only from the council and the members of the society at large, but from the honorary secretary (Mr. H. Shillinglaw), whose invaluable services have rendered the duties of my office of a pleasing character. From the unanimity existing in the council, and the increasing interest felt, as expressed by many members of the society in the proceedings thereof, I conclude the position and future progress of the society may be regarded as established. It is highly gratifying to find the various presentations which have been received, as mentioned in the annual report; they will form a valuable addition to our museum, and I trust the time is not far distant when we shall occupy a building suitable for their reception, and one in which ample provision will be made for the students of our School of Pharmacy in a completely fitted laboratory and lecture-hall, &c. While upon this subject I may mention that during the past month Mr. Blackett, Mr. Shillinglaw, and myself have paid a visit to the Crown Lands Office, for the purpose of ascertaining what sites were available. The result of our labour was that we found five or six, and of this

number one is peculiarly suitable for our requirements; and I have every confidence that if the council, aided by the members of the society generally, will bring to bear in the proper quarter all the influence they can personally command, there will be something more than a mere possibility of securing the object of our ambition. I am much pleased to observe the continued unanimity of feeling and action existing among a portion of our body in Ballarat, and trust the example which this association holds forth will be followed by other districts, for not only do the members of this association meet together for the purpose of discussing subjects mutually interesting, but the unanimity of feeling among them tends to promote their individual prosperity, and to disperse those feelings of reserve and aversion which frequently exist in the absence of social intercourse. Too much praise, therefore, cannot be awarded to the Ballarat Chemists' Association. They have set a noble example to their brethren at large, and one which, I trust, may be followed by other districts in the colony ; and I trust the day is not far distant when the sister societies of the Australasian colonies and New Zealand may assemble together in conference to discuss and pursue our common objects, and have every confidence that such conference may prove no mean element in the constitution and development of society at large. Among the various discoveries and inventions of the past year there is one of such vast importance and brilliancy which will have the effect of casting all others into the shade for the present. I allude to the grand discovery of M. Faure of the power of storing electricity. This discovery has already excited mental action in various directions for the purpose of locomotion ; besides, the day-dream of Mr. Edison has been realised, for electricity has been utilised in Great Britain and the continents of Europe and America, not only for lighting large halls and manufactories, but for dwelling-houses and other buildings of a less pretentious character ; and by the addition of coloured gauze around the lamps, the light is described as one of great beauty. I observe in the report reference is made to the committee which has been appointed to revise the "Sale and Use of Poisons Act," and sincerely hope that some practical legislation will emanate therefrom. I must congratulate the members of the society on the satisfactory report presented by the hon. treasurer (Mr. Gamble), and hope the suggestion which he has made will be received in the same kindly spirit in which it has been made ; for it will be obvious that if the members will pay their subscriptions in advance, and promptly, in accordance with our bye-laws, much good will result. The thanks of the society are due, and I now publicly thank Mr. Blackett for the valuable services which he has gratuitously rendered as editor of our journal—the *Supplement to the Chemist and Druggist*—but I fear the time is coming when other arrangements will have to be made, for it will be too much to expect that he can afford the necessary time, considering his enlarged sphere of usefulness as one of our parliamentary representatives. There is another subject I wish to mention—the desirability of uniting as one body the Pharmacy Board and the Pharmaceutical Council. Such union will be productive of much good, and thus prevent any unpleasantness which may possibly arise. In conclusion, I will ask that the same courtesy and kindness which you have so generously awarded me may be extended to my successor.

THE ELECTION OF MEMBERS OF COUNCIL.

The election of five members of the council, caused by the retirement of Messrs. Best, Gamble, Ogg, Nicholls, and Jones, was then proceeded with. The only candidates nominated were Messrs. Best, Gamble, J. C. Jones, R. Nicholls, and John Ross, who were, on the motion of Mr. Henry Brind, seconded by Mr. Blackett, duly elected.

APPLICATION TO THE GOVERNMENT FOR SITE FOR LABORATORY AND MUSEUM.

Mr. R. Nicholls brought this matter under notice, and urged the members to use all the influence they could with the local members of Parliament.

It was resolved that another deputation wait on the Minister of Lands, and ask him to fulfil the promise made some time ago.

Votes of thanks to Messrs. Kingsland and Rawle, the auditors ; Mr. C. R. Blackett, for his services in connection with the journal ; and to Mr. H. Shillinglaw, the honorary secretary, brought the business to a close.

SYDNEY.

THE monthly meeting of the Pharmaceutical Council of New South Wales was held at the Medical Board Office, Philip-street, on 14th March. Present—the president (in the chair), and Messrs. Abrahams, Guise, Pratt, Larmer, and Row.

The minutes of last meeting were read and confirmed.

Three applications for examinations were received and granted, 23rd March being fixed as the date.

The following applications for membership were granted :— O. Davis, M.P.S., late Great Britain, in business at Woolhara ; J. Mills, Kurragong ; T. H. Mallam, Armidale ; C. S. Gaud, Parramatta ; T. M. Sheridan, Mount Browne, in business prior to the passing of the Sale of Poisons Act, 1876. W. Jesperson, application with a French diploma ; and R. J. Waring, M.P.S., Victoria, of Balranald.

Directions were given in answer to correspondence.

Sundry accounts were passed.

The meeting terminated.

(FROM OUR OWN CORRESPONDENT.)

Two cases of suicide by taking strychnine have occurred in Sydney during the month of February. The first was the wife of a music-dealer named Pognowski, and appears to have been caused by hard drinking. There was no evidence to show how the poison was obtained. The second was the case of Mr. J. G. Thurlow, clerk of petty sessions at the Central Police Court, a gentleman well-known and greatly respected. Deceased appears to have enjoyed good health, and no reason can be assigned for the act, though it was rumoured that pecuniary losses were the cause. On the evening of 10th February Mr. Thurlow was found suffering from the effects of poison. Two men who found him got a van, and drove him to Dr. Power, of College-street, who refused to see him, so they drove to the infirmary, at which place he expired shortly after admission. The jury returned a verdict, "That Joseph Giovanni Thurlow died at the Sydney Hospital from the effects of a self-administered dose of strychnine, which he obtained from the establishment of Mr. Woodhouse, chemist and druggist, William-street, on 8th February." They further added as a rider, "We are of opinion that Dr. Power deserves great censure for his inhumanity in not going out to see deceased when requested to do so." Mr. Thurlow leaves a wife and family of seven.

Robert Malcolm Trauent was charged at the Water Police Court on 23rd February with selling poison to Mr. J. G. Thurlow without having made a faithful entry of the same. The defendant is assistant to Mr. Woodhouse. The sheriff (Mr. Cowper) appeared for the defence, and said that he could certify that it was from no wilful neglect, but rather from the idea that police authorities were exempt from the regulations regarding the sale of poisons. Out of regard to the official position of Mr. Thurlow the usual form was omitted. A fine of 5s., and 4s. 10d. costs, was imposed.

An amusing incident occurred lately before the Licensing Board. A publican was charged with opening his house for the sale of liquor during prohibited hours. The plea was that the customer (a woman) merely came for a dose of castor oil. The Bench, however, ruled that the publican should not sell that or any other beverage in a jug on Sundays.

In the Supreme Court steps are being taken to obtain an injunction to restrain the Technical College from giving instruction in law, political economy, and constitutional history. The parties moving in the matter are the Inspector of Public Charities and the Minister for Public Instruction. These officers consider that the above subjects are not a part of technical education.

Mr. John Rogers has resigned his position as secretary to the School of Arts, an office which he has held for the past fifteen years, during which period the institution has enjoyed great prosperity under his management. It was, however, at the request of the committee that the resignation was tendered.

A series of lectures on "Inorganic Materia Medica" will be commenced on Wednesday, 5th April, at the Technical College by Mr. Fred. Wright. Mr. W. A. Dixon, F.C.S., will also deliver a course of lectures on "Chemistry as Applied to the Arts" during the winter session, and efforts will be made to start a botany class. Mr. Wright has declined an invitation from the committee to deliver a series of popular lectures on

the "Lives of the Chemical Philosophers," assigning as a reason great pressure of work.

Mr. Chas. Lewin, of Cowra, has purchased the business of Mr. Sanders, Lower George-street.

14th March.

NEW ZEALAND.

PHARMACY IN NEW ZEALAND.

"As idle as a painted ship upon a painted ocean" would express the state of pharmacy, or rather the work of pharmaceutical advancement, in New Zealand at the present time.

Our Dunedin friends are said to be the drag upon the wheels. A clause in our constitution says :—"The annual meeting of the general council may be held alternately at Wellington, Dunedin, Christchurch, and Auckland." The last annual meeting of the general council (or delegates) was held at Wellington on the 27th September, 1880, and the next was to have been held at Dunedin in September last. It is now February, 1882, and no arrangement has been made to bring the delegates from the four centres together. It is urged by Dunedin that it is a waste of funds, the travelling and other expenses being too great. Now, in this matter our southern chemists are undoubtedly "too canny," and acting contrary to the best interests of the cause. In order to secure united efforts, and a common understanding, nothing is better calculated to obtain that object than a conference, where the different representatives may meet and cordially discuss matters relating to trade interests and the promoting of pharmaceutical concerns.

The personal acquaintance of members, and the mutual interchange of ideas upon kindred subjects, is certainly worth the proposed expenditure out of the society's funds. Let us hope that New Zealand pharmacists will *unite resolutely* to keep up an interest amongst themselves in matters pharmaceutical. Much remains to be done ; we have only turned the first sod. Our Pharmacy Act requires amendments, and provision must be made for pharmaceutical education. Those who take a pride in their profession should put renewed life into the different local councils, provide local libraries, and adopt a system of reading monthly papers on pharmaceutical subjects.

It is a pleasure to learn that Mr. Barraud, the president of the society, is taking steps to establish a monthly journal of pharmacy, after the style of your valuable publication. Let us wish him success in such a good work.

The New Zealand Pharmacy Board have published their first annual register, and will at once proceed against those in business as chemists and druggists who have not registered. There are not five in the colony against whom this will be necessary ; these individuals may be put down as either wilful or negligent.

Our visitors to these shores from Victoria have been Mr. T. Lakeman, Mr. Rivers Langton, and the Hon. Peter Lalor, the Speaker of the House, who is now amongst us and expatiating strongly upon the beauty of our scenery, and the excellence of our climate.

The present writer will always retain most pleasing recollections of the sociable good feeling existing amongst the chemists in Melbourne, of which he was the honoured recipient some time since.

Auckland, 20th February, 1882.

NOTES ON A HITHERTO UNDEFINED SPECIES OF CYCAS.

By BARON FERD. VON MUELLER, K.C.M.G., M. AND PH. D., F.R.S.

LAST year an opportunity was afforded me by the enlightened editor of this journal, to give the first record of a cycadeous plant, Macrozamia Moorei, from sub-tropical Eastern Australia ; and now I am able, through his concession, to render known another member of the grand order of pine-palms in these pages. Plants of this order are not only of great horticultural and palæontological importance, but they interest likewise chemical and technological investigators, on account of the, as yet, not isolated, highly acrid and perhaps therapeutic principle, and in reference to the large quantity of peculiar starch pervading cycads. Leaving the chemical and industrial inquiries for another time, I confine myself on this occasion to the phytographic record of the new plant. The discovery is due to Mr. Eugene Fitzalan, of Port Denison, whose name has become quite famed through the manifold additions made by him to the knowledge of the north-east Australian flora, and whose attention I had particularly directed to a closer inquiry into the various specific forms of palms and cycads of his district. The new researches were again carried out by that gentleman with much discrimination and zeal.

Cycas Kennedyana.

Stem tall ; leaves very numerous ; leaf-stalks elongated, nearly glabrous, only on their upper part armed with a few spines ; rachis by a single slight curvature gently flexuous, ascendant ; leaf-segments about one hundred on each side, broad-linear, nearly flat, acute and somewhat pungent, rather glaucous on the under page, shining on the surface, glabrous on both sides; all segments, but particularly those towards the summit, decurrent ; the lowest nearly half as long as the middle segments, and not gradually abbreviated into mere spines ; male amentum rather large, oval-ellipsoid, the antheriferous portion of its scales narrowly wedge-shaped, about three times as long as the deltoid, *truncated*, completely velvet-downy, entirely straight and never pointed terminal dilatation ; bare upper side of the antheriferous portion of the scales quite glabrous ; anther-cells extending to the base of the scales, not grouped by any empty space into two areas ; fruit-amentum very large ; stipes of the scales moderately elongated, as well as their rachis velvet-downy ; ovules or fruits on each rachis always only four ; nuts nearly globular, perfectly glabrous.

In the Normanby-Ranges, near Port Denison ; Eugene Fitzalan, Esq.

This new pine-palm is dedicated to His Excellency Sir Arthur Kennedy, G.C.M.G., who for thirty years held the highly distinguished position of Her Majesty's representative in several British colonies, and who now presides over the wide and rich dominions of Queensland. Two other species of cycas, indigenous only to tropical Eastern Australia, were discovered successively during the governorships there of the Marquis of Normanby, G.C.M.G., and of Sir William Cairns, K.C.M.G., and were dedicated at the time to these high dignitaries, with a view of connecting their honoured names also in botanical science with the colony, over which they then ruled.

Cycas Cairnsiana is easily distinguished from C. Kennedyana by the more spiny leaf-stalks, by the narrower leaf-segments with somewhat recurved margins and pale surface, by considerably smaller antheriferous scales with proportionately larger terminal plate, and by nearly glabrous fruit-stalks with only two nuts.

Cycas Normanbyana differs already from C. Kennedyana in simply arcuate raches of the leaves, and in fruit-stalks never bearing more than two nuts.

Cycas media is easily separated from C. Kennedyana by the straight raches of the leaves, and by the fruit-stalks producing always more than four and often eight ovules and nuts. But, irrespective of these distinctive notes, all three are still more marked in difference by the ascendant, sharp-pointed apex of the antheriferous scales, which in C. Kennedyana is entirely absent. Indeed, by the last-mentioned characteristic the new species is also at once separated from the very limited number of South Asiatic and Polynesian congeners, hitherto rendered descriptively known.

NOTES OF THE YEAR 1881.

We extract the following more interesting passages from the "Review of the year 1881," which appeared in the *Pharmaceutical Journal* :—

There has been evidence of a growing opinion that the time has come when the question of branch pharmacies should also be dealt with. As to the desirability of such a course as soon as the time is ripe there can hardly be two opinions, for on several occasions when the society has had to go into a law court to prevent an unregistered person from carrying on a chemist's business with the aid of a qualified assistant, the fact that a registered person can carry on any number of branch shops without employing qualified assistants has evidently appeared as an anomaly to the judges and unfavourably affected their judgments.

A bill was also introduced into the House of Lords, and eventually passed, to amend the law relating to veterinary surgeons. It provided for the establishment of a register and of examinations as a test of qualification for registration,

under the control of the Royal College of Veterinary Surgeons, and it made it penal for any unregistered person, after 31st December, to use any title or description implying that he is qualified to practise veterinary surgery, but it provided for the registration without examination of such persons as had for five years continuously next before the passing of the Act practised veterinary surgery in the United Kingdom.

There have been reported during the year several cases of prosecution under both the fifteenth and seventeenth sections of the Pharmacy Act, the former at the instance of the Council of the Pharmaceutical Society as represented by the Registrar under the Act, and most of the latter at the instance of the Trade Association. The cases that are carried into court do not of course represent the full number of offenders against the Act that are dealt with, the object sought, the cessation of the offence, being frequently attained without the necessity of having recourse to legal proceedings. In one of the cases reported a point of some importance was decided, as to whether a trader could sell to the public poisons supplied to him by a duly qualified chemist and druggist, bearing on the label the name and address of the chemist and druggist, but not that of the owner of the shop in which the poisons were sold. The defendant, an unregistered person, who kept a general shop in Oxford, admitted a sale of red precipitate, but contended that the chemist and druggist whose name and address were on the label was his tenant in respect of one of the windows of his shop and that he, in the sale of drugs and poisons, only acted as an agent. The Oxford magistrates, before whom the case first came for hearing, admitted this plea and dismissed the summons. It was evident, however, that if this decision were allowed to remain unchallenged, another serious rent would have been made in the Pharmacy Act, especially as it was candidly admitted that the multiplication of such agencies was contemplated. The Executive of the Trade Association, who had commenced the prosecution, therefore took the necessary steps for an appeal, which was heard in the Queen's Bench Division before Mr. Justice Grove and Mr. Justice Lopes. At first the judges were inclined to consider the point as one of fact which lay with the magistrates to determine, but after further argument were of opinion that the magistrates had not drawn a proper inference from the facts before them. They held that it was contemplated throughout the seventeenth section that the seller should be the person actually conducting business at the shop where the sale takes place, and that a person living at a distance from the place of sale could not comply, for instance, with the provisions as to the entry of the sale of poisons in the poison-book. They were also of opinion that the Act could be evaded if the word "seller" were construed to mean other than the person who actually conducted the business of a shop. The bearing of this upon the question of branch businesses conducted by unqualified assistants is obvious.

A considerable number of cases of death by poisoning have been recorded during the past year, and the circumstances attendant upon several of them are of particular interest at a time when amendment of the Pharmacy Act is contemplated. The number of deaths resulting from the taking of patent medicines containing poisons, especially the narcotic preparations so widely advertised and used, has attracted attention to the incautious manner in which they are supplied to the public. This has frequently provoked remonstrance from coroners and juries, and the Privy Council has, on more than one occasion, been moved to commend the consideration of the subject to the Council of the Pharmaceutical Society. Although the Privy Council declined to adopt the result of such consideration as presented in the form of the draft bill, there can be no doubt that the present state of public opinion with respect to the supply of poisons furnishes a favourable opportunity of dealing with the subject. The careless manner in which carbolic acid and other disinfectants are left unlabelled or otherwise distinguished has also been the cause of several fatalities.

Some valuable investigations of vegetable substances have been published. Dr. Hesse has examined quebracho bark, and found that it does not contain a trace of his paytine, the alkaloid with which Dr. Wulfsberg had suggested Fraude's aspidospermime was identical. He mentions, however, having separated four other alkaloids, besides aspidospermime, one, which he has named "quebrachine," being present in the bark in larger quantity than that alkaloid. As it is admitted that Fraude's alkaloid is frequently not presented by commercial aspidospermime, the details of Dr. Hesse's results, which will shortly appear in *Liebig's Annalen*, will be welcome. The same indefatigable chemist has supplemented his investigation of *Alstonia spectabilis* bark by one of *A. constricta* bark, in which he has found three alkaloids, with evidence of a fourth. Messrs. Harnack and H. Meyer state that they are able to confirm the suspected existence of two jaborandi alkaloids differing in physiological action. The new alkaloid "jaborine" appears to be readily formed from pilocarpine, and may be altogether a product of alteration ; it is said to be frequently present in commercial pilocarpine, when its physiological action dominates that of pilocarpine ; it is said that perfectly pure pilocarpine has a physiological action similar to that of nicotine, which alkaloid it resembles in yielding pyridine bases upon decomposition ; if distilled with excess of potash a small proportion of a base passes over apparently identical with coniine. Pituri has been investigated by Professor Liversedge, who has arrived at the conclusion that its alkaloid is not identical with nicotine, as alleged by M. Petit. The presence of nicotine in Indian hemp has been also disproved by Messrs. Siebold and Bradbury. Cape tea has been examined by Mr. H. G. Greenish, who has found it to be devoid of theine, but to contain a glucoside and a body giving a green fluorescence in alkaline liquids. *Omphalocarpum procera*, also, has been examined for theine, by Mr. Naylor, with a negative result ; this and the discovery of the presence of bodies analogous to gutta and saponin appear to clear up a doubt as to whether the genus belongs to the Sapotaceæ or the Ternstrœmiaceæ. *Nerium odorum* has yielded to Mr. H. G. Greenish two bitter principles, probably glucosides, and both powerful cardiac poisons, and Professor Warden has signalised the presence of pseudoindican in *Thevetia nereifolia*. Messrs. Wright and Rennie have described, under the name of "glycyphyllin" the sweet principle of the leaves of *Smilax glycophylla*, used in Australia against scurvy. From *Erythrina corallodroenda*, a leguminous tree of which the bark is used in Brazil as a hypnotic, M. Bochefontaine has isolated an alkaloid and named it "erythrine." From another South American plant belonging to the Rutaceæ, the *Xanthoxylum Naranjillo*, said to resemble jaborandi in its physiological action, Dr. Parodi has separated a hydrocarbon analogous to pilocarpine. *Aspidium rigidum*, a Californian fern that has been recommended in the treatment of tænia, has been found by Mr. Bowman to contain a resin and an acid similar to male fern. Further, Mr. T. B. Groves has reiterated a previous statement as to the presence of codeia and narceia in poppy capsules that appeared to have been overlooked.

Enormous strides have been made in our knowledge of the organisms which are now generally admitted to be the determining causes of infective diseases, and sufficient has been published in this journal to show that pharmacists are much interested in the subject. It may be a long time before *Punch's* sketch of a pharmacist being called upon to supply various kinds of these organisms is realised, but what has been done with pepsine and its allies shows that the ferments are not outside pharmacy, and even now the treatment of disease is sufficiently affected to make its mark upon the *materia medica*. Among the chemical substances that have been put forward more prominently during the past year in the antiseptic treatment of disease are resorcin, hydroquinone, cinnamic acid, styrone, and oil of eucalyptus. Amongst other new remedies, chinoline has been recommended as a cheap substitute for quinine ; β-naphthol as a substitute for tar in the treatment of skin diseases ; salicylated camphor in lupus, hydrofluoric acid in goitre, and benzoate of calcium in albuminuria.

The obituary of the year includes several names which were as household words among the pharmacists of Great Britain. Scotland has lost in John Mackay a most indefatigable and genial leader, who for forty years was the directing spirit of the North British Branch as its honorary secretary ; and in Henry Baildon, one who helped in the foundation of the branch and afterwards served in the office of president and as a member of the board of examiners. In England John Abraham and Isaiah Bourdns have passed away, both formerly members of the council, and the latter for a short time vice-president. In John Stenhouse, too, we have lost an eminent chemist who lent lustre to the roll of honorary members of the Pharmaceutical Society. Lastly, William Gowen Cross was the first local secretary to the society for Shrewsbury, and served in that capacity until the time of his death.

PECULIAR PROPERTY OF BROMINE.—A fine tube is half-filled with bromine and hermetically sealed ; on heating, the bromine becomes opaque, so that the tube appears to be filled with a dark red resin.

ANALYSIS OF A SAMPLE OF WATER
Obtained at a depth of 57 feet on the plains of the parish of Marnoo, for the Shire Council of Stawell.

(BY JOHN KRUSE.)

THE appearance clear, with minute black sediment when first uncorked, emitting an odour of hydrogen sulphide ; taste, bitter saline. Sp. gr., 1018. Reaction to test-paper neutral. Amount of saline matter, nearly 1523 grains to the gal., or about 2 per cent.

The saline matter was found to be composed in 100 parts of :—

Sodium chloride ...	...		...	... 80·34
Magnesium do. ...	...		...	... 8·71
Magnesium sulphate	...		...	... 7·23
Calcium do.	...		...	... 3·72
				100·00

PHARMACY BOARD EXAMINATIONS.

THE preliminary examination was held at Melbourne, Ballarat, Sandhurst, and Warrnambool on the 2nd March.

The following are the candidates who passed :—J. J. M. Hemmons, Warrnambool ; Wm. Watson, Sandhurst. At the modified examination, held on the 6th March, 1882, Alric O. Hughes, Greville-street, Prahran, passed.

EXAMINATION FOR THE CERTIFICATE OF THE SCHOOL OF PHARMACY.

THE examination was held at the rooms of the Pharmaceutical Society on the 6th March, before the examiners appointed by the Pharmacy Board (Messrs. Bosisto, Blackett, and Johnson).

William Lowe, Sandridge, and Sidney Victor Say, Carlton, passed in all subjects ; and Thomas S. Woodfull, Prahran, in chemistry (the only subject taken).

THE PHARMACY BOARD OF VICTORIA.

PAPER USED AT THE SIXTEENTH PRELIMINARY EXAMINATION, 2ND MARCH, 1882.

Time allowed—Three hours.

Latin.

Cæsar. De Bello Gallico. (*a*) Lib. I., cap. 19.—Quibus rebus cognitis, quum ad has suspiciones certissimæ res accederent, quod per fines Sequanorum Helvetios transduxissent, quod obsides inter se dandos esse curasset, quod ea omnia sine modo injussu suo et civitatis, sed etiam inscientibus ipsis fecisset, quod a magistratu Æduorum accusaretur, satis esse causæ arbitrabatur, quare in eum aut ipse animadverteret, aut civitatum animadvertere juberet.

(*a*) Translate the above literally. To whom does it refer ?

(*b*) Parse every verb in it fully, omitting participles.

(*c*) What case is each of the following words in, and what is the rule in each case?—Rebus, Helvetios, ea, civitatis, inscientibus, causæ.

(*d*) Write out all the indicative mood, active and passive, of "do," and all the subjunctive active of "facio,"

(*e*) Write out in full the declension of "obses" and "ipse."

(*b*) Lib. I., cap. 31.—Locutus est pro his Divitiacus Æduus : Galliæ totius factiones esse duas : harum alterius principatum tenere Æduos, alterius Arvernos. Hi quum tanto opere de potentatu inter se multos annos contenderent, factum esse uti ab Arvenis Sequaniaque Germani mercede arcesserentur. Horum primo circiter millia XV Rhenum transisse ; posteaquam agros et cultum et copias Gallorum homines feri ac barbari adamassent, traductos plures : nunc esse in Gallia ad C et XX millium numerum.

(*a*) Translate the above literally.

(*b*) Why are the infinitives used throughout ?

(*c*) Write out in full the Latin numerals for which XV, C, and XX are symbols.

Translate into Latin—

(*a*) All these people differ from each other in language, customs, and laws.

(*b*) He says, that all these people differ from each other in language, customs, and laws.

Arithmetic.

1. Multiply £453 11s. 9¼d. by 365.

2. Divide £4 3s. 9d. by 2⅔.

91 grain Troy: how many
water which weighs 1¼ lbs.

½ + 1⅔ — ₂'₅): and if the
money value of the fraction?
n its ⎰ 5·015 — 3·05
... ⎱ ――――――
3 + 1·895
on of £5.
article cost £6 14s. 2d., how
3d.?
ↄ.
case, singular, of "man."
case, plural, of "lady."
:ase, singular, of "who."
ɪdic., active, of "break."
ndic., passive, of "send."
operative, active, of "drive."
Therefore, the poet
7 trees, stones, and floods ;
and *full* of rage,
change his nature.
: in *himself,*
ɪrd of sweet sounds,
s, and *spoils.*
ɪve.
sition on either of the sub-
? Order," attending carefully

N OPEN SURGERIES.
ɪ find that the fatal cases of
ɪwn the attention of medical
ɪe of keeping shops in all
l druggists, where, in virtue
titioners from the provisions
ɪns are sold without proper
:hese shops are often persons
ɔharmaceutical qualification,
cannot be wondered at that
ɪ ensue.
not be out of place to point
1815 contains a specific pro-
l for any person to act as an
compounding or dispensing
ɪlification prescribed by that
7ision of the 17th section
ans of repressing the evil of
:ept by medical men, and it
f the Medical Defence Asso-
ɪ Act could not be turned to
maceutical Journal.

ɪꝺence.

ɪ *Supplement to the Chemist
·gist.*
:tus issued by the Melbourne
ɪ loss to understand how ap-
ɔf the advantages of a course
laboratory at the hours men-
f-past ten a.m. for four days

ely excluded by the regula-
gladly send a student ; but
six months' sojourn in the
a temptations offering in the
·loyed, am at once deterred

d will see how extremely un-
be well filled under existing
ɪe of two lectures a day (on
r a period of, say, six weeks
in which case a youth at the
ɪg the course of it, might be
ɪney to attend the school.
ɪce must obtain his master's
expenses, at the least, will
£12 ; board and lodging, six
ɪotal, £60.
:ion of the matter in your
CHEMIST.

REMINISCENCES OF A PHARMACIST.

(BY J. B. MUMMERY.)

IT has often struck me whilst perusing the pages of this
journal that a little light matter interspersed amongst the
heavier and more valuable, would make its pages more interesting to general readers, without in any way diminishing its
usefulness.

Such matter has occasionally appeared in its columns since
I have been a reader ; and I presume the reason we have not
had more is that there are few articles of such a kind sent in.
Under these circumstances, I have penned a few lines for insertion in the journal if you deem them suitable, and will continue the same as opportunity may offer ; but as my time is
pretty well taken up in attending to the requirements of my
business, my moments of leisure are few and far between. I
have been somewhat puzzled for a title, and have at last hit
upon the one which heads this paper, which, if you think
proper, you can retain, or alter to any one you may deem more
suitable.

I shall commence my recollections with the case of

TAWELL, THE MURDERER.

The career of this individual is known, I dare say, to many
of your readers; but there are some amongst the younger
members of our calling, I doubt not, who have never heard of
the wretch whose infamous deed created a great stir in
England at the time of its occurrence, not only from the
heinousness of the crime and the social position of the
murderer, but from the fact of its being the first instance in
which the electric telegraph was brought into play for the
purpose of arresting a criminal in his attempted flight.

Somewhere about the year 1844 a man named John Tawell,
who was, or pretended to be, a member of the universally
respected Society of Friends, left Sydney with the intention
of spending the remainder of his days in the mother-country.
He had amassed a considerable fortune as a pharmaceutical
chemist in Pitt-street, in the first chemist shop opened in
Sydney. I am not quite sure whether he was the first pharmacist who practised his profession there ; but, considering
the date of his departure, and the same of the establishment
of the colony, it is quite within the bounds of possibility that
he was.

Amongst the passengers by the ship in which Tawell took
his passage to England was a young and pretty widow, with
two or three children ; and as the ex-chemist was either a
bachelor or a widower, it is by no means wonderful that an
intimacy should spring up between them, as it did—an intimacy which ended in a union by no means creditable to either
party.

On reaching England, Tawell took a pretty little cottage at
Slough, near Windsor, in which he placed his paramour and
her children, and where he paid her frequent periodical
visits.

This state of things continued for some time, when Tawell
fell in love with a young lady of good position, when, as a
matter of course, his visits to Slough became less and less frequent,
partly from the effect of counter attractions, and partly from
a dread that they should become known to his intended,
and be the means of breaking off the engagement, until at
last this dread haunted him to such a degree that he formed
the horrible resolve of putting his first love out of the way. In
furtherance of this design, he prepared himself for a last
visit, taking with him a bottle of prussic acid.

Tawell was received with more than usual kindness by the
poor woman, who fancied that his love had been growing of
late somewhat cold, and the heartless wretch, better to disarm
any suspicion on the part of his inamorata, treated her
with feigned increase of affection, and (as seemed to have
been his wont) sent one of the children for some porter.
This having been procured, the murderer managed, during
the woman's temporary absence, to introduce the fatal dose
into her glass. Quite unsuspectingly, the poor victim
swallowed the poison, and in a few minutes was stretched
lifeless on the floor.

The cottage in which this dreadful deed was accomplished
was situated at about a quarter of a mile distance from the
"Slough" railway station, from which place to the metropolis
an electric telegraph had just been erected.

As soon as the wretched man saw that his foul deed was
fully accomplished, he made at once for the railway station.
In the meantime, the cries and screams of the children brought
some of the neighbours on to the scene, and amongst these
was a man who had a little knowledge of chemicals, who

recognised at once the smell of prussic acid, and pronounced the case as one of atrocious murder.

The male portion of the neighbours started off at once in pursuit of Tawell, but arrived only just in time to see the train in which he had taken his seat dash out of the station. On telling the station-master what had happened, that individual, with commendable promptitude, set the telegraph to work, and gave an account of the crime and a description of the murderer, and the result was, that on the arrival of the train in London, a detective was waiting for Tawell, whom he followed to a celebrated restaurant and arrested, just after he had finished a sumptuous tea, and whilst he was, no doubt, congratulating himself on his lucky escape.

The assassin was, of course, locked up for the night, and fully committed, the next morning, to take his trial for wilful murder.

The trial took place at "Aylesbury," and as I was at the time serving a junior-assistantship not very far from that town, I have a lively recollection of the excitement it produced.

The prisoner, of course, employed the very best counsel his ample means could procure, and so confident was he of their ability to get him off (though on what grounds I cannot imagine), that he had engaged to meet and entertain a party of friends at dinner, and had his carriage and pair waiting at the court-house to convey him to his home; but instead of this he was taken back to prison and to the condemned cell.

Tawell was executed in front of the Aylesbury gaol, in the presence of perhaps the largest concourse of people, out of London, who ever witnessed the carrying out of the law's last dread penalty—a penalty, in this instance, I think all who read this account will deem fully deserved.

(To be continued.)

Notes and Abstracts.

SIMPLE MODE OF TEMPERING GLASS.—A Leipsic journal gives a method which it asserts will prevent lamp chimneys from cracking. The treatment will not only render lamp chimneys, tumblers, and like articles more durable, but may be applied with advantage to crockery, stoneware, porcelain, &c. The chimneys, tumblers, &c., are put into a pot filled with cold water, to which some common table salt has been added. The water is well boiled over a fire, and then allowed to cool slowly. When the articles are taken out and washed they will be found to resist afterward any sudden changes of temperature.

PAPER FOR SILVERWARE.—The *Archiv der Pharmacie* gives the following formula for making paper for wrapping up silver. Six parts of caustic soda are dissolved in water until the hydrometer marks 20 deg. Baumé. To the solution add four parts of oxide of zinc, and boil until it is dissolved. Add sufficient water to bring the solution down to 10 deg. Baumé. Paper or calico soaked in the solution and dried will effectually preserve the most highly polished silver articles from the tarnishing action of the sulphuretted hydrogen which is contained in such notable quantities in the atmosphere of all large towns.

TWIN HALF-BROTHERS.—Dr. J. G. Earnest, of Newman, Ga., reports the following unique case in the *College and Clinical Record*, 15th July, 1881:—Amelia, a coal-black negress, aged about forty years, was confined 20th November, 1880, giving birth to twins—one a very bright mulatto, the other perfectly black. The black child was born first, according to the midwife's statement. The mother states that the children were begotten the same night, a negro man having intercourse with her first, and the white man about an hour afterward.

SOME REMARKS UPON MODERN PHARMACEUTICAL STUDY.

(BY H. J. MOLLER.)

(From Pharmaceutical Journal.)

GREECE.

THE pharmaceutical course in Greece resembles that of Italy in many respects. The following communications I have obtained through a correspondence with Professor Xavier Landerer, of Athens, who formerly was pharmacist to the king and from 1835 to 1868 was a teacher of the Greek pharmaceutical students,

In the year 1837 the university in Athens and the pharmaceutical school therewith connected were established, and from 1837 to 1868 it was required that the student should have reached the third class* of the classical school. Then he was two years in a pharmacy as an apprentice (Μαθητὴς τοῦ φαρμακείου), and afterwards he studied at the university for two years more, following the lectures at the pharmaceutical school in chemistry, pharmacy, *materia medica*, toxicology, botany and physics. After this he served as an assistant (Βοηθός) for at least a year, and then passed a final and practical examination.

These rules were changed in the year 1868. The above-mentioned "absolutorial" examination is now required before entrance upon the study of pharmacy, and the student commences immediately to follow the lectures at the university, without any foregoing practical education. Having studied for three years at the university, he spends a year in a pharmacy and then passes the "Major." This is quite the same as that demanded of the Italian "farmacista," and I will, therefore, not tire the reader with a repetition of the whole plan of study, but will refer him to the plan A, given in my remarks on Italy.

Professor X. Landerer, who is himself a German, says in one of his letters to me, that he considers the present standard of Greek pharmaceutical examinations to be quite as high as that of the corresponding ones in Germany.

BELGIUM.

The pharmacy of this country has, as so many other things in Belgium, a French form. On a journey in the spring of 1880 I had opportunity to notice this myself, and to collect a part of the following notes, which I have made more complete through a correspondence with Professor A. Herlant, teacher in *materia medica* at the pharmaceutical institution in Brussels.

In Belgium pharmaceutical study is made at four special pharmaceutical institutes, which are connected with the four Belgian universities in Brussels, Ghent, Louvain, and Liège.

According to the "réglement organique pour la collation des grades académiques de l'université libre de Bruxelles," which I obtained at the questorship of the University of Brussels, the requirements at the pharmaceutical examinations are fixed by Articles 16 and 17 of the law of 20th May, 1876, as follows:—

"(a) The 'candidature† en pharmacie' requires only one examination, which embraces the elements of physics, general chemistry, general and medical botany, mineralogy, and geology, and also a practical test in chemistry.

"(b) The degree of 'pharmacien' (*i.e.*, the 'Major') requires also one examination, but this may be divided in two successive parts if the candidate prefers. The first part embraces the elements of analytical and toxicological chemistry, drugs, posology, and theoretical and practical pharmacy. The second part includes:—(1) Two chemical preparations; (2) Two 'galenical' preparations; (3) A qualitative analysis; (4) A toxicological research (under this also quantitative analysis); (5) An analysis of a remedy and the determination of possible adulteration (by means of chemical and microscopical research); (6) An especial microscopical analysis (of a mixture of different sorts of flour, powder, &c., or of the micrographic characters of a drug)."

After the apprenticeship in a pharmacy, the young man studies two years at the pharmaceutical institutes before he passes the examination for the "candidature en pharmacie," and then two years more before the examination for the title of "pharmacien." In the first two years the students are matriculated at the "faculté des sciences," in the last two years at the "faculté de médecine." The pharmaceutical study at the university thus lasts in all four years; in the last two years the students are instructed in applied micrography. When the diploma as "pharmacien" is obtained, the successful candidate may establish himself when and where he will. By this short communication one can see that pharmaceutical study in Belgium is very well arranged.

(To be continued.)

---

* The third class is the highest, but the final examination of this class (the so-called "absolutorial" examination) was not formerly demanded. This "absolutorial" examination corresponds thus to the German "Maturitäts prüfung," and the French "baccalauréat."

†This degree gives the possessor the right to be an assistant only, and thus corresponds to the German "Gehülfe."

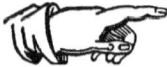

☞ TRADE NOTICE.

Chemist & Druggist.

WITH AUSTRALASIAN SUPPLEMENT.

(Published under direction of the Pharmaceutical Society of Victoria.)

No. 48. { PUBLISHED ON THE 15TH OF EVERY MONTH. }
Registered for Transmission as a Newspaper.

APRIL, 1882.

{ SUBSCRIPTION, 15s. PER ANNUM, INCLUDING DIARY, POST FREE.

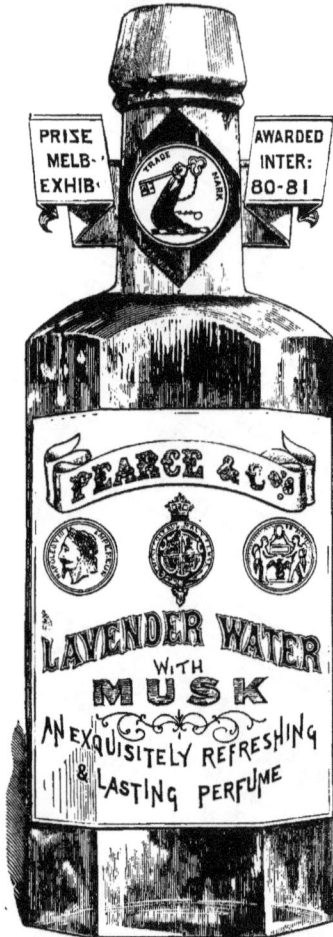

V. 4, no. 48 : 89-96, (April, 1882).

INDEX TO LITERARY CONTENTS.

The Chemist and Druggist.

WITH AUSTRALASIAN SUPPLEMENT.

OFFICE: MUTUAL PROVIDENT BUILDINGS, COLLINS STREET WEST.

Published on the 15th of each Month.

THIS Journal is issued gratis to all paid-up Members of the PHARMACEUTICAL SOCIETY OF VICTORIA, and to non-members at Fifteen Shillings per annum, payable in advance. A copy of *The Chemists and Druggists' Diary*, published annually, is forwarded post free to every subscriber.

Advertisements, remittances, and all business communications to be addressed to THE HONORARY SECRETARY OF THE PHARMACEUTICAL SOCIETY, MELBOURNE.

SCALE OF CHARGES FOR ADVERTISEMENTS:

	Per annum.			Per annum.
One Page	.. £8 0 0	Quarter Page	..	£3 0 0
Half do.	.. 5 0 0	Business Cards	..	2 0 0

Special rates for wrapper and pages preceding and following literary matter. Advertisements of Assistants Wanting Situations, 2s. 6d. each.

Advertisements for insertion in the current month should be sent to the office before the 10th.

COMMUNICATIONS for the EDITORIAL department of this journal should be addressed to THE EDITOR, MUTUAL PROVIDENT BUILDINGS, COLLINS STREET WEST, MELBOURNE.

No notice can be taken of anonymous communications. Whatever is intended for insertion must be authenticated by the name and address of the writer—not necessarily for publication, but as a guarantee of good faith.

ANNUAL SUBSCRIPTIONS TO THE SOCIETY.

ALL annual subscriptions are now due.

Member's subscription	...	...	£1	1 0
Associate's	...	...	...	0 10 6
Apprentice's	...	...	...	0 5 0

Cheques and Post-office orders should be forwarded to the Honorary Secretary, No. 4 Mutual Provident Buildings, Collins-street, Melbourne.

THE LIBRARY.

THE Library is open daily (Saturdays excepted), from 9.30 a.m. to 4.30 p.m. Catalogue of the books can be obtained on application.

BIRTH.

LONGMORE.—On the 29th March, at Kensington, the wife of Francis Longmore, chemist, of a son.

MARRIAGE.

CATTACH—HEWS.—On the 5th April, at the residence of the bride's parents, by the Rev. Thos. Porter, Alexander M. Cattach, son of the late James Cattach, to Eliza, fifth daughter of James Hews, Ryrie-street, Collingwood.

DEATHS.

MURRAY.—On the 3rd April, at the Alfred Hospital, Robt. D. Murray, dispenser, son of the late Andrew Murray, Prince's-street, Edinburgh. Beloved and regretted.

COWL.—On the 31st March, at Walhalla, of phthisis, Gertrude, the beloved wife of R. H. Cowl; aged 23 years.

KERNOT.—On the 26th March, at Milton-house, Newtown, Geelong, Charles Kernot, M.L.A., aged 62 years.

M. YVON ON THE PURITY OF CHLOROFORM.

M. YVON has suggested a new and delicate method of testing the purity of chloroform for anæsthetic purposes. At a meeting of the Paris Société de Pharmacie he read a paper upon this subject, which has been published in the *Journal de Pharmacie et de Chimie*, a résumé of which is given in the *Pharmaceutical Journal* (pp 711, 12), and may be consulted with advantage. We transcribe the following as containing the proposed mode of testing, which would appear worthy of attention :—

Referring to the characteristics requisite for chloroform that is to be used for anæsthetic purposes, as described by Professor Regnault—viz., that it should have a mild odour, be neutral to test paper, give no precipitate when shaken with solution of argentic nitrate, not acquire a brown colour when heated to the boiling point with caustic potash, not blacken when mixed with concentrated sulphuric acid, nor dissolve or consequently become coloured by certain aniline derivatives such as rosaniline or aniline blue—M. Yvon is of opinion that these characters do not constitute a sufficient guarantee of purity unless the boiling point of the liquid has previously been found correct. That he considers to be an absolute necessity, having examined many samples which were not quite pure, although they bore the tests above mentioned. In seeking for further tests of purity, M. Yvon first tried the determination of the boiling point, and by that means was able to classify the samples examined upon under two heads. The first commenced to distil about 59·4° C., the temperature rising gradually to 60·4°, 61·2°, and 63·4° by the time three-fourths had passed over and then rising to 64·4° and even 65·5°. The samples of the second class began to distil at 61°, and nearly eight-tenths passed over at that temperature, after which the temperature rose up to 66°.

Making due allowance for the difficulty of obtaining absolutely precise results by this means, M. Yvon nevertheless felt justified in concluding that the samples examined by him contained substances rather more volatile, and others rather less volatile than chloroform, without, however, affecting the reactions which are accepted as characteristic of the purity of chloroform.

After some further trials of a mixture of bichromate of potash and sulphuric acid M. Yvon finally decided to employ permanganate of potash, as he found that salt was not reduced by pure chloroform. He first used an aqueous solution containing ·025 per cent. of the salt, shaking half a cubic centimetre with 5 cub. cent. of the chloroform to be tested and found that the greater the impurity of the sample the more rapid was the reduction of the permanganate. Subsequently a greater sensibility was given to the permanganate by applying it in the presence of a free alkali. A solution containing 1 part permanganate with 10 parts caustic potash in 250 parts of water has a fine violet colour, which is instantly changed to green by contact with impure chloroform. In testing a great number of samples of chloroform from various sources, M. Yvon did not find any that were free from impurity. With ordinary commercial chloroform the passage from violet to green was almost instantaneous ; with chloroform described as pure it took place within ten or fifteen seconds, and with anæsthetic chloroform within from thirty to fifty seconds.

The Month.

WE may remind our readers that the Royal Society of New South Wales offer a series of prizes, of the value of £25 each, for the best communication, the result of original research, upon eight subjects of colonial interest, one of which, "The Chemistry of the Australian Gums and Resins," must be sent in not later than 31st August, 1883.

The Pharmacy Board have resolved to enforce the fourteenth clause of the Pharmacy Act, and to prosecute persons who neglect to comply with its provisions. The first case brought forward was that of W. F. G. Nettleton, at Warrnambool, who was fined £2 and £1 1s. costs.

At the City Police Court, Adelaide, on the 29th March, a woman was fined for selling milk after the Board of Health had ordered her to desist, in consequence of her having lost two of her sons by typhoid fever. She continued selling milk, and infected some of her customers.

Mr. P. M'Lean, of Brunswick-street, Fitzroy, has added another to the many handsome shops that already exist in the suburbs of Melbourne. The premises, which adjoin the new building of the Bank of Victoria, are situated in Brunswick-street, Fitzroy, nearly opposite Mr. M'Lean's old shop, and are built with the most approved modern conveniences. The shop, which is an exceedingly large one, is fitted in a very elegant manner, the window being specially attractive.

The *Government Gazette* of 30th March announces that the erasure of the name of James Egan Wall from the Pharmaceutical Register of Victoria has received the assent of His Excellency the Governor in Council.

Letters patent have been granted to Mr. F. S. Grimwade, of Melbourne, for a new process for preparing phosphorus.

The half-yearly meeting of the Health Society was held at the Town Hall on the 29th March; his Honour Mr. Justice Higinbotham presided. Several interesting papers were read, the ventilation of the Melbourne Hospital, the use of stimulants, the art of cookery, and the suppression of the smoke nuisance being among the subjects discussed. In order that the general public may have the benefit of the valuable information which from time to time is laid before the society at its meetings, it is intended to publish a volume of the papers in a cheap form.

Some interesting experiments with blasting gelatine have been recently carried out in the open air at the rear of the Technological Museum by Mr. J. Cosmo Newbery. Some of the material is exposed to the direct action of sunlight, to show how it decomposes. Another lot is placed in true shade with ventilation, and a third quantity is placed in cases without ventilation, but with a free circulation of air around the cases. The object of the experiments is to prove in what way these explosives are most likely to deteriorate and become dangerous.

The ordinary meeting of the Microscopical Society was held on 30th March, at the rooms in Collins-street; the Rev. J. J. Halley, vice-president, in the chair. The Rev. J. J. Halley gave a very interesting account of a visit to the zoological station at Naples, presided over by Mr. Anton Dohon, and he also described the magnificent work in course of publication there on the marine fauna of the Mediterranean. Mr. Bage read some notes on recent improvements in microscopy, giving a general *résumé* of the principal changes in the construction of the microscope which have been generally adopted by opticians within the last few years. A number of interesting specimens were exhibited, among which some polycistina, from the "Challenger" dredgings, shown by Mr. Halley, attracted special attention.

The death of Mr. Thos. Cox is announced. Mr. Cox was an old resident of Majorca.

An examination was held on the 31st March at the School of Mines, Ballarat, for the certificate of the school in the subject of *materia medica*.

Mr. Herbert Rocke left for England by the mail steamer "Clyde." Mr. Rocke proposes returning to the colony, *vid* America, about October next.

Mr. Bowen's new premises in Collins-street are being rapidly completed, and he expects to occupy them in a few weeks.

Meetings.

THE PHARMACY BOARD OF VICTORIA.

The monthly meeting of the board was held at No. 100 Collins-street, on the 8th March, 1882. Present—Messrs. Bosisto, Bowen, Blackett, Lewis, Holdsworth, Brind, and Owen; the president (Mr. Bosisto) in the chair.

The minutes of the previous meeting were read and confirmed.

Applications for Registration as Pharmaceutical Chemists.—The following were passed:—Christopher Harrison, Chapel-street, Prahran, certificate from Great Britain; Edward H. Embley, Lonsdale-street, passed modified examination on 4th December, 1879; an interim certificate for six months was granted to Abel James, Geelong, to enable him to obtain his certificate from England.

Removal of Name from Register.—It was resolved that the Governor in Council be asked to sanction the removal of the name of James Egan Wall from the Pharmaceutical Register.

School of Pharmacy.—It was resolved that for this session (March to November, 1882), the board approve and recognise the School of Pharmacy, to be held at No. 6 Hanover-street, Fitzroy, the syllabus of which is submitted this day by the president of the Pharmaceutical Society, subject to the removal at any time to more suitable and convenient premises.

Quarterly Examinations.—The Board of Examiners forwarded their report of the examinations held on the 2nd and 6th March, which was approved.

Several prosecutions were ordered, and it was resolved to enforce the 14th section of the Act.

The ordinary routine financial business brought the meeting to a close.

PHARMACEUTICAL SOCIETY OF VICTORIA.

The monthly meeting was held at the rooms, 100 Collins-street, on Friday evening, 3rd March, 1882. Present—Messrs. Bowen, Gamble, Nicholls, Thomas, Best, Baker, Huntsman, Jones, and Shillinglaw; the president (Mr. Bowen) in the chair.

The minutes of the previous meeting were read and confirmed.

Election of New Members.—The following new members, nominated at the last meeting, were duly elected:—Henry C. Macaulay, Euroa; Edward Thorby Noakes, Rochester; John Henry Reed, 67 Swanston-street; Frederick Cherry, Russell-street, Melbourne.

New Members Nominated.—John Opie, Melrose, S.A.; A. E. Bilton, dispenser Police Depôt; Christopher Harrison, Chapel-street, Prahran.

A large amount of general correspondence, of no special public interest, was dealt with, which, with financial and general business, brought the meeting to a close.

Books, &c., Received.—*Treatise on Chemistry—Non-Metallic Elements*, Vol. 1, Professor Roscoe; *Treatise on Chemistry—Metals*, Part 1, Vol. 2, Professor Roscoe; *Treatise on Chemistry—Metals*, Part 2, Vol. 2, Professor Roscoe; *Treatise on Chemistry—Organic Chemistry*, Part 1, Vol. 3, Professor Roscoe; *First Principles of Chemical Philosophy*, Cooke; Weinhold's *Experimental Physics*, Loewy; *Popular Lectures on Scientific Subjects*, Herschel; *The New Chemistry*, Cooke; Beeton's *Complete Orator*, Ward, Lock and Co.; *Official Record of the Melbourne International Exhibition*, 1880 and 1881; *Druggists' Formulary*, by Kilner, 1881; Kilner's *Modern Pharmacy*, August and November, 1881; Kilner's *Compendium of Modern Pharmacy*, from W. H. H. Lane; *Australian Veterinary Journal*, April; *Australian Medical Gazette*, March; *Australian Medical Journal*, April; *European Mail*, February; *Pharmaceutical Journal*; *American Journal of Pharmacy*, March; *New York Druggists' Circular*, March; *New Remedies*, March; *Therapeutic Gazette*, February.

In the *British Medical Journal* (7th January, p. 8), some cases of poisoning by chromate of lead are recorded, in which the patients were poisoned by inhaling the dust arising in the process of weaving an orange-yellow cloth. Although precautions have been taken to prevent injury to the weavers, the use of the chromate is still continued, and the public therefore are just as likely to suffer in consequence.

DEPUTATION TO THE MINISTER OF LANDS.

A DEPUTATION from the Pharmaceutical Society of Victoria, consisting of Messrs. Bowen, Keogh, Huntsman, Atkin, Jones, Baker, Thomas, Swift, Gamble, George, Hooper, Ross, Best, Nicholls, Shillinglaw, and Messrs. Zox, Blackett, Cook, Macgregor, and Laurens, M.L.A.'s, waited on the Minister of Lands on the 22nd March. The deputation was introduced by Mr. Zox, M.L.A., who shortly placed before the Minister the desire of the society, and said that he felt sure that Mr. Madden would accede to the request of the deputation after he had heard what they had to say. Mr. C. R. Blackett endorsed what Mr. Zox had said. He also desired to point out that in other countries not only was land granted, but every facility given to foster scientific education. Some time since an application was made to the Government on a similar subject, and the deputation were informed that if a suitable site could be obtained the Minister would grant the application. A suitable place had been found, and they were there to-day to ask that the promise might be fulfilled.

Mr. Wm. Bowen, the president of the society, said that they had previously received a promise of a portion of the site on the Eastern Hill adjoining the hospital for sick children, but they had not obtained that. An unnecessary valuable site was not desirable, provided it was central, and as the County Court was about to be sold, the society would suggest that that site be granted, and that they be allowed to take the building at a valuation. Mr. Bowen dwelt at some length on the necessity that existed for a properly organised school of pharmacy. The law obliged all persons to undergo a certain course of study, and there were at the present moment about two hundred apprentices who must attend the school, and this number would be annually augmented by from forty to fifty new apprentices. There was no instruction in pharmacy at the Melbourne University.

Mr. Macgregor, Mr. Cook, and Mr. Laurens, M.L.A.'s, all supported the application.

Mr. Edmd. Keogh reminded the Minister that this was the only application of the sort likely to be made to the Government. It was necessary that persons desirous of becoming chemists should pass certain examinations, and they had to come from all parts of the colony to Melbourne to do so. Parliament having passed such a law, might fairly be asked in the interest of the public to supply a place for them to study in.

The Minister said that when he granted a site to the Medical Society of Victoria he thought he was dealing with all branches of the profession.

Mr. Bowen thought that such a combination would not be likely to work well.

Mr. Madden suggested that a portion of the Exhibition buildings might, with the consent of the trustees, be utilised.

Mr. Blackett said that the objection to this was that they could only have permissive occupancy.

After some further discussion the Minister agreed to grant the society a piece of land—sixty-six feet frontage—near the proposed Women's Lodginghouse, which, he considered, would have the additional advantage of having a frontage to Bowen-street.

The deputation thanked the Minister, and withdrew.

WARRNAMBOOL POLICE COURT.

TUESDAY, 28TH MARCH.

Before Messrs. L. Ogilby (chairman), J. A. Bromfield, and E. Elliget,

Sergeant Hamilton proceeded against W. F. G. Nettleton, for carrying on business as a chemist at Liebig-street, Warrnambool, without being registered under the Pharmacy Act, 1876. Mr. D. Wilkie appeared on behalf of the board, Mr. Higgins appearing for the prisoner.

Mr. Wilkie said the defendant was charged under section 25, sub-section 2 of the Pharmacy Act, with exhibiting the name or title of a chemist whilst not being a registered pharmaceutical chemist, as required by the Act. Section 16 of the same Act provided that the board, in the month of January of each year shall cause to be printed, published, and sold a correct register of the names of all the registered pharmaceutical chemists, and section 17 provided that such register should be accepted as primâ facie evidence in all courts of justice. It would be proved that the defendant did exhibit the title of chemist over the premises in which he was carrying on the business of a chemist, and a copy of the register (produced) would show that his name was not upon it.

Mr. Higgins required to know if this was a private or a public prosecution.

Mr. Wilkie said the summons was served by the police.

Mr. Higgins thought that, under the circumstances, the police would take action in the usual way.

Mr. Wilkie said it was the customary practice for the police to lay the information in such cases.

Mr. Higgins—Yes, and conduct the proceedings also.

Mr. Wilkie did not think that was usual where a solicitor was employed for the prosecuting parties.

Sergeant Hamilton stated that he knew the shop of the defendant in Liebig-street. It had been carried on for some time as a chemist's shop, and the name "Nettleton, chemist," was exhibited over the door. In reply to Mr. Higgins, witness stated that he was prosecuting under instructions from the Pharmacy Board. He had seen defendant's name on the board's register of some years ago. Witness had never made a complaint to the defendant that he was acting illegally.

Harry Shillinglaw, registrar to the Pharmacy Board of Victoria, produced the register of the board on which defendant's name did not appear. The defendant's name had not appeared in the register since the year 1878.

Mr. Wilkie pointed out that section 25 showed the defendant to be liable to a penalty not exceeding £10, and imprisonment for six months.

Mr. Higgins asked if the case was closed, and being informed that it was, he submitted that it must be dismissed. The very section last quoted by the solicitor for the prosecution was fatal to it. The 25th section held that from and after six months after the date of the first appointment of the board any person committing any of the offences enumerated shall be liable to the punishment laid down. In this case there was not a particle of evidence to show that a board had been appointed. At the outset the existence of the board should have been established. That was the very groundwork of the action.

The chairman did not see the objection.

Mr. Higgins submitted that it was as plain as a pikestaff.

The chairman was perfectly aware of the existence of the board.

Mr. Higgins said that was not evidence. There was the proper procedure of the court to be observed. It should have been shown in evidence by the production of the Government Gazette that the board was duly appointed.

Mr. Wilkie would put in the Gazette notice now if the bench would allow it. (Gazette handed up.)

Mr. Higgins submitted that the case for the prosecution was closed, and could not be reopened in this manner.

The chairman said he and his colleagues were just as well satisfied that there was a Pharmacy Board as they were of there being a House of Parliament.

Mr. Higgins persisted that the case had been closed for the prosecution, and, while it was highly necessary to prove that a Pharmacy Board existed, it had not been so proved.

The chairman did not think it was necessary to prove a fact so well known.

Mr. Higgins said there was another point. His client's name was on the register for 1878, and he had received no intimation of its being taken off, nor was he aware that it had been taken off.

The chairman said they were not there to inquire into that. How could section 17 be got over?

Mr. Higgins wanted to know how section 25 could be got over by the bench.

The chairman said the bench had settled that matter.

Mr. Higgins remarked that his client acted in entire ignorance of the law. His name was certainly not on the register, but he was not cognisant of its being off. Why had he not been interfered with before this? The most that he could be guilty of would be the sin of omission, not commission. He had simply neglected to see if his name was on the register or not, and he had received no intimation of its removal from the register. It was not necessary to register every year. It was only in certain cases, such as changing his address, that a member was required to communicate with the board on the subject of registry. Had he known that he was not on the register, he would have taken steps to have his name restored to it before. Perhaps the bench would inflict a nominal fine only, and allow defendant the opportunity of getting reinstated on the register as early as possible.

Mr. Wilkie said the board only asked for a nominal penalty. It would be understood that the defendant must shut his shop at once, and not re-open it until his name appears on the register of the Pharmacy Board, according to the Act.

The chairman said there appeared to be some doubt in the matter as to whether the defendant was cognisant of his offence. The fine would therefore be mitigated to £2, with £1 1s. costs.

The defendant said he considered it a very unjust decision. He would have to go to gaol, for he could not pay.

The chairman said two or three times lately disparaging remarks had been made in that court concerning the decisions of the Bench. He had tolerated them hitherto, but he would do so no longer. If the defendant, or any one else, did not conduct themselves properly in this court, they would be committed for contempt.

Defendant—And Bromfield on the bench too. What right has he there?

The chairman said another remark of that kind would get him quartered in gaol.

The defendant having become silent, the chairman completed the order, recording that distress would follow in default of payment of the fine, and in default of distress, one month's imprisonment.

DEATH OF MR. CHAS. KERNOT, M.L.A.

WE regret to announce the death of Mr. Chas. Kernot, one of the Parliamentary representatives for Geelong, who died at his residence, in Aphrasia-street, Newtown, on the 26th March. His death was not unexpected—he had been ailing for more than twelve months. The deceased gentleman, who was sixty-two years of age, was born at Rochefort, Essex, England, where he carried on business as a chemist prior to leaving for Australia. Mr. Kernot came direct to Victoria about February, 1851, in the ship "Duke of Wellington," one of the vessels chartered by Dr. Lang to bring to these shores a desirable class of colonists. After stopping in Melbourne for a few weeks, he came to Geelong, which has been his home ever since. He first lived in Gheringhap-street, and then started in business as a chemist in one of the shops just above that occupied by Mr. Pardey, the chemist, in Moorabool-street. Being also a practical printer, he combined with his business that of a printer and stationer, in which occupations he succeeded in three years in accumulating considerable wealth, which enabled him to remove to premises at the top of Moorabool-street, and where he confined himself to chemistry. In 1859 his prosperity induced him to erect a comfortable residence in Aphrasia-street, Newtown, at which place he resided up to the time of his death. He was, in 1859 and up to February, 1865, in partnership with his brother, Mr. W. H. Kernot, as chemists and druggists; but at the latter date he retired altogether from active business. From the time of his arrival in Geelong he took a deep interest in everything affecting the general public. He was one of the directors of the old Geelong and Melbourne Railway Company, in which capacity he proved himself a very energetic member. To show that he was not narrow-minded in his views, it may be stated that he was the first to join in the agitation for Sunday trains when the line was under the company's management. Even in January, 1860, when it was proposed to resume the Sunday communication between Geelong and Melbourne, he spoke in support of the movement ; but, at his suggestion, the consideration of the subject was allowed to lapse, as the railway line was about to pass into the hands of the Government. He was the convener of the first meeting of the Geelong Gas Company, in which he retained a very large interest up to the time of his death. The deceased was also for many years a very active member of the directory of the Victorian Woollen and Cloth Manufacturing Company. He proved himself a valuable member of the Hospital Committee of Management. In municipal matters he was equally energetic, and on the 15th November, 1859, he was elected one of the representatives for the Barwon Ward in the Geelong Town Council. He was raised, on the 9th August, 1861, to the office of alderman for Thomson Ward, and on the 9th October, 1864, he became mayor-elect, and took his seat in the mayoral chair on the 9th November of the same year. At the time of his death Mr. Kernot was a Parliamentary representative for Geelong. He entered Parliament about the 13th March, 1868, as a member for East Geelong, when the Darling grant question agitated the

country. After remaining in Parliament as an unpaid member for three years he sought re-election ; but was defeated by the late Mr. J. M. Garratt. He was afterwards elected to fill the vacancy caused by the death of Mr. Richardson. In May, 1877, he was re-elected ; but in February, 1880, he was defeated for Geelong by Mr. Chas. Andrews, whom he beat in the election which took place in July of the same year, and remained a member of Parliament up to the time of his death.

REMARKS ON A NEW CASUARINA.

By BARON FERD. VON MUELLER, M. & PH.D., K.C.M.G., F.R.S., F.G.S., &c.

THE order of Casuarineæ is only a small one, restricted to one genus and comparatively few species. Bordering, as it does, alike on the Coniferæ and on the subordinal groups, which constitute the complex of Amentaceæ, it has great morphologic interest. Paleontologically forms of Casuarina are known from the tertiaries of Britain, pointing to the existence of this kind of tree in Europe prior to the glacier epoch. Utilitarian considerations lead us to value our Australian species for superior fuel, especially as their growth can be effected even in arid waterless wastes. Potash is yielded by them in fair percentage ; cattle like to browse on the foliage, and are occasionally sustained on it in times of severe drought, the acidulous taste of the branchlets being evidently pleasant to pastoral animals ; the organic acid, thus obvious, could by turned to special applications ; the remarkable structure of the wood and even the trachenchyma of the seedshell of the fruitlets, interests the anatomist ; while I have shown already at the International Exhibition of 1867, that the foliage of Casuarinæ can easily be converted into pulp for paper-mills. As any addition therefore to our knowledge of the specific forms of this genus is of more than ordinary interest, the account of a new species will be acceptable. It was obtained by Mr. F. M. Bailey, of Brisbane, and has been named by us

Casuarina inophloia, F. v. M. and Bailey.

Arborescent ; aged bark disintegrating into long narrow somewhat fibrous particles ; branchlets very thin, slightly streaked, not prominently angular, almost imperceptibly downy ; whorls of rudimentary leaves bearing 7-9 semilanceolar acute teeth ; fruit-amenta cylindrical-ovate, or sometimes shortened to an almost globular form, constantly depressed at the summit ; axis densely beset with straight pale-brown hair ; bracts obliterated ; bracteolar valves of the fruitlets rather small, semi-ovate, nearly blunt, short-exserted, enlarged by a very thick dorsal rather angular appendage of vertical slight cleavage, and of nearly as much protrusion as that of the valves themselves ; appendages and valves very slightly downy ; nutlets (when young) pale, the terminating membrane (then) about as long as the nucleus.

In the southern portions of Queensland, near Roma, F. M. Bailey ; near Toowoomba, C. Hartmann.

This species is nearest allied to the common southern C. distyla, especially to that variety which, on account of its slender branchlets and small bracteolar valves, was formerly distinguished as C. paludosa. Our new species is however of taller growth, the bark is less solid, the branchlets are neither prominently streaked nor conspicuously furrowed, the fruit axis is very hairy, the bract under each fruitlet is not distinctly developed, the dorsal protuberance of the bracteolar valves is comparatively much thicker and by partial incision somewhat doubled. Furthermore, the fruitlets below their membranous appendage are in age probably not almost black. The flowers of either sex (not yet seen) may also be different. From C. corniculata the species now described is already separated by wanting distinct bracts and by the dorsal appendage of the bracteoles not being long and sharply pointed. But there can be no doubt, that our new plant is identical with the one, which Dr. Leichardt passingly mentions under the name of C. villosa, in the diary of his famous journey overland to Port Essington, p. 49 (1847), as occurring on Robinson's Creek, at Expedition Range. Still, Mr. Bailey justly observes, that this appellation is misleading, the bark, though very fibrous, not being villous in the accepted scientific sense of that term. It is remarkable that this tree should have escaped notice since Leichardt's time—a fact demonstrating how much yet needs to be done for the further investigation of the Australian flora, even in long-settled districts, for which researches pharmaceutical gentlemen more especially should render every local aid.

Review.

A compendium of Modern Pharmacy and Druggists' Formulary, containing the recent methods of manufacturing and preparing elixirs, tinctures, fluid extracts, &c., &c., and miscellaneous information indispensable to the pharmacist. Second edition. By Walter B. Kilner, pharmaceutist, Springfield, Illinois. H. W. Bokker, printer, 1881.

THIS work, which we have upon our table, has evidently been compiled with great care and much earnest labour; although written more particularly for the American pharmacist, it contains a mass of information, and a very large number of formulæ, which will be found useful to British and Australian pharmacists. The author says in his preface, "Many of the working formulæ have been kindly donated by eminently successful pharmaceutical chemists of great learning and wide experience." Many works have been published making great pretensions to accuracy, but have been found, although costly, unreliable. We do not think that the same criticism can be applied to this work.

In Chapter II., devoted to the comparison of the metric and United States measures, very simple rules are given for converting one denomination into the other, and we are glad to see that our American cousins are gradually preparing the way for the adoption of the metric system. Elixirs would seem to be great favourites in the United States. These compounds are very numerous, but the basis is the simple elixir, a sort of flavoured sugared spirit, and are doubtless of German origin. The formulæ for these preparations are, as "the sands upon the sea-shore, innumerable;" but our author has carefully selected the best. We notice one elixir of *eucalyptus globulus* containing 2 oz, of the leaves to the pint, associated with cherry bark and liquorice. The therapeutical value of eucalyptus leaves is now well understood, and is lower than a few years ago, but in a compound containing cherry bark, it would be somewhat difficult to test its medicinal action and value. There are 302 formulæ for elixirs, many of which have appeared from time to time in the various pharmaceutical journals. It ought to be borne in mind by readers that nearly all the quantities given are in Troy weight. In concluding our notice of this work we cannot do better than quote the compiler's remarks in the preface to the second edition. "It is not the aim or intention of the author to supply the place of the United States Pharmacopœia, or text book of like character, but to furnish a work of ready reference, and compilation of unofficial formulæ, as well as those of an official character, from the cream of the drug and medical publications of the world, that will be of use to the profession." We have observed one or two typographical errors, such as "startling" for "starting" (page 5), and "correct" for "correctly" (page 14). The book is well printed on good paper, and strongly bound.

INTERLOPERS.

ONE would have supposed the Pharmacy Act of Victoria encompassed the calling of a chemist and druggist sufficiently to guard it against all interlopers, but it appears such is not the case, and their representatives, be they the Board of Pharmacy or the Pharmaceutic Society, will have to be on the alert if they wish to keep the coast clear against the invasion of their rights and privileges.

Representations have been made to the Board of Pharmacy on one or two occasions that shopkeepers of various denominations have set portions of their premises apart for the sale of drugs, under the superintendence of some impecunious chemist (who, very likely, for some reason or other, cannot trade in the usual way), and thus not only doing an injury to the regular authorised pharmacist, but opens the door for a perversion of trade.

If once such a deviation is allowed, then away must go all that we have been contending for during the last quarter of a century, and the Act becomes null and void. It was bad enough for the Pharmacy Board to be compelled, by the provisions of the Act, to register as pharmacists all those who before its passing had any pretentions to the sale of medicines, the which has in many instances legalised charlatans to keep an open shop. The Pharmacy Act, to a certain extent, actually broke down under such circumstances; and it is to be regretted the board were compelled to admit, as it were, to holy orders, such as were never intended.

The framers of the Pharmacy Act also, no doubt, thought that every title under which a chemist could trade legally had been invoked to prevent false pretences; but the cunning which is inherited specially by persons without knowledge, serves them also in this particular, and an evasion of the Act is practised by persons calling themselves "professors." This term has, unfortunately for the public, been omitted both in the Medical and Pharmacy Acts, and the consequence is that men such as Mr. Fisher (the bonchcidist) practice medicine under this title.

SURGEON-DRUGGISTS.

WE were perfectly surprised and equally disgusted to find that on one of the metropolitan goldfields the medical men are in the habit of making up their own medicines. Out of about a dozen surgeons only two are found who give their patients prescriptions to be made up by chemists. Each of the others have dispensaries and dispensers, and up to a very short period some of them also sold drugs and even patent medicines. Is it, then, to be wondered at if pharmacists resort to various means of obtaining a living outside their legitimate calling? The profession of medicine should be above this double-dealing, and ignore it, as they are apt to do when they hear of a druggist prescribing over his counter. We know of one instance where the surgeon receives his fee for consultation, hands his patients the prescription with a significant indication they can have it made up in the adjoining dispensary. They then find that another charge is made for the medicine, and the prescription is detained unless demanded by the patient. Actions like these on the part of medical men tend to generate a bitter feeling between the faculty and the chemist, which might be easily avoided if a course were adopted calculated to cement rather than estrange them; and for the good of both it is hoped that a better understanding will be arrived at. We believe that a much better system prevails in Ireland, where the apothecary is to the physician what the solicitor is to the barrister, and the system is found to work well.

ECONOMY OF FUEL, AND SMOKE ABATEMENT.

(Read by C. R. Blackett, M.L.A., before the Australasian Health Society, 29th March, 1882.)

AT the present time this question is exciting a considerable and increasing interest among intelligent persons; and I do not know any subject of more importance to us in Victoria than the economical use of fuel, more particularly coal. In England, Professor Jerons has long ago drawn public attention to the gradual exhaustion which is going on of the available coal supply as a reason for using the utmost care in consumption; and in the present day, when the light of scientific knowledge is spreading more and more, it is to be hoped that the principles involved in the proper and complete combustion of fuel will be adopted as much as possible; and when it is universally recognised that an economical use of fuel not only adds to the national wealth, but assists to abate the unhealthy and disagreeable "smoke nuisance," its importance cannot be over-estimated. Moreover, as the colony of Victoria, according to all the geological knowledge at present possessed, not having any very rich or extensive coal seams, and is dependent upon New South Wales for her supplies, ought to exercise a powerful influence over all who take an interest in our industrial progress.

This question has its sanitary aspects, and our society, which has already done so much to spread the knowledge of the applications of exact science to the improvement of the health of the community, may do good service by again impressing upon the public mind this important matter.

It may be considered by some that the smoke nuisance has not yet assumed a sufficiently aggravated form in our city, with its light and bright atmosphere, to cause the necessity for any active measures to be taken for its suppression. But, although at present the large towns of Victoria are, compared with London and other great cities, not greatly suffering, we have to remember that in a very few years the evil will greatly and rapidly increase, and so the health of the people will be affected; and our public buildings, upon which we are spending so much, will also be seriously disfigured and injuriously acted upon. Inside buildings the injury to pictures and works of art ought also to be taken into consideration, so great is the deleterious action of the corrosive gases given off during the combustion of coal, such as sulphurous acid. There are other products of combustion which have a prejudicial influence upon health—namely, carbonic acid and oxide, carburetted hydrogen, sulphuretted hydrogen, sulphide of ammonium, bisulphide of carbon, phosphoretted hydrogen, &c.

So great has the smoke nuisance become in England that the National Health Society have appointed a committee to examine the question. That committee, presided over by Mr. Ernest Hart, has brought up its report. Professor Chandler Roberts, F.R.S., chemist to the Royal Mint, undertook to make an examination of existing methods of combustion of coal in household grates and in furnaces. The committee also made complete arrangements for a smoke abatement exhibition at South Kensington, for the purpose of trials of apparatus and fuels, the objects sought being—

1. A better utilisation of coal and coal products.
2. To determine, practically and scientifically, the means which are actually available for heating houses as at present (and as may be constructed), without producing smoke.
3. To enable the committee to examine the subject generally, and report for public information upon the relative adaptability of the various coals and appliances to the different requirements of every class of the community.
4. To afford reliable information upon which to base sufficient and equitable amendments of the existing laws regarding smoke.
5. To enable the committee to ascertain and make known the comparative value of existing appliances for the utilisation of gas for heating purposes, and generally bringing together the available material for determining how far smoke may be prevented, and to test numerous inventions, many of which are little known.

The smoke abatement exhibition has taken place, and judging by the reports—extracts from which I shall give—it has been eminently interesting and successful.

A few words upon the nature of fuel may, perhaps, be fittingly introduced here, as well as some remarks upon the subject of combustion and its products—smoke, &c. First—Fuel.—All substances chemically termed combustible may be considered as fuel; but the term is usually applied to organic bodies, such as wood, coal, and peat. Now, all these substances are chiefly composed of carbon and hydrogen. Both these elements combine with great rapidity with oxygen, and the intensity of the chemical action is so great that heat and light are produced—the carbon producing carbonic dioxide and the hydrogen water, the oxygen of the atmosphere being the agent or supporter of combustion. Wood is the fuel most used in France. In Paris the use of coal is very restricted and generally objected to; indeed, the bright, clean beauty of the buildings in that city could not co-exist with coal smoke. The French have, also, a great dislike to coal, on sanitary grounds. For cooking, charcoal is very generally used; the fire is rapidly lighted, and when done with put out—so careful is the French housewife not to waste anything. Of peat we need not say anything, as it is not known here. Coal is by far the most valuable source of heat, and is compounded of chemically altered vegetal matter and mineral substances, such as arsenic, sulphur, iron, lime, &c., &c.

Combustion, or burning, takes place when certain conditions are favourable; and when coal, or wood, or gas is burnt, the oxygen of the air combines with the carbon and hydrogen, as above mentioned. If the oxygen of the air is supplied in the exact proportion to the carbon and hydrogen, we get perfect combustion, and no escape of combustible gases could then ensue, nor of carbonaceous matters which we generally call smoke, and the greatest amount of heat would be obtained; but these conditions are in ordinary grates and furnaces never or rarely approached. Coals are thrown on to the fire in thick layers, reducing the temperature of the fire, and causing at once the production of heavy volumes of smoke. This thick bed of superincumbent fuel also impedes the draught of air. The heated air is deoxidised by the ignited fuel on the bars, and no oxygen is available for a considerable time to act upon the dense mass of fuel, although the temperature may be sufficient to distil off the hydrocarbons, which pass away into the chimney, and so much valuable heating power is lost. Smoke is a compound of various gases and solid particles in a very fine state of division—nitrogen, steam, carbonic oxide, carbon, and is the result of imperfect combustion.

In early times the citizens of London had a great dislike to smoke, as they considered it injurious to health. In 1306 Parliament petitioned King Edward I. to prohibit the use of coals, or,

as it was then called, "secole." It was afterwards made a capital offence to burn "secole" within the city. A man was actually executed for the crime of burning "secole" contrary to the law.

Evelyn dedicated a book to Charles II., entitled *Fumifugium*, in which he affirms his belief that Old Parr might have lived more than 150 years if he had not come to London, and had his digestion spoiled by "*smoake*" (*Westminster Review*, January, 1882). Theodore Hook once spoke of London as "that sink of sin and sea-coal."

Although Melbourne, as we have said above, is never likely to suffer to the extent complained of in London and other great cities of Europe, as dense fogs are rare in our warmer and lighter climate, yet many people find the prevalence of smoke particles very disagreeable indeed, and injurious to health; and if it can be shown that by better methods of combustion and the more scientific utilisation of fuel, we can not only add greatly to our wealth, but render our cities and towns more healthy and pleasant to live in, we shall have the great satisfaction of knowing that a great public service has been rendered; and although many difficulties may meet us, yet undoubtedly intelligent perseverance will ultimately triumph over all.

(To be continued.)

Correspondence.

KILNER'S *DRUGGISTS' FORMULARY.*

To the Editor of the Australasian Supplement to the Chemist and Druggist.

DEAR SIR—On behalf of the publishers I beg to hand you a copy of Kilner's *Druggists' Formulary* and supplements Nos. 1 and 2 for your review, and be kind enough to add same to your library. I bespeak for this work a careful perusal and a full review. I shall do myself the honour of handing you the other supplements as they are issued from time to time. Price, with supplements, as fast as issued, £2 2s. per copy.—Very respectfully yours, W. H. H. LANE.
28th March, 1882.

REMINISCENCES OF A PHARMACIST *(Continued).*
(By J. B. MUMMERY.)
DR. CRONIN'S CASE.

IT is not my intention to rack my memory for every case of poisoning, by accident or design, which came under my notice in the old land, and dish them up as news for my readers in the new; but there was one which occurred shortly before my leaving England, which caused a great commotion at the time, and, as it bears materially on a point which affects the interests of pharmacists all the world over, I shall be pardoned, I think, for narrating it.

Dr. Cronin was a medical man in good practice in London, not far from Leicester-square, where I was then living. He was one of those practitioners (of whom, happily, we have few, if any, in the colony) who, though doing a rattling thing by the practice of their professions, covet the profits of the retail chemist, and yet affect to consider it *infra dig.* to openly keep a shop for the sale of drugs.

This Dr. Cronin, did virtually keep such a shop, but borrowed a fictitious name, under which to carry it on; and naturally desiring to have the dispensing of his own prescriptions, resorted to the questionable practice of writing them, in a character known only to himself and his assistant, and kindly intimating to his patients the fact that the shop round the corner was the only one where his prescriptions could be made up. This, they found, after presenting them at various establishments, to be the case, and were, per force, obliged to patronise the doctor's dispensary.

On one occasion, Cronin was called in to see and prescribe for a young lady of title, about eighteen or nineteen years of age, beautiful, accomplished, and on the point of being married.

The prescription was written in the usual way, and the parents of the patient, disregarding the doctor's advice, or order, to take it to his own shop, sent it, as a matter of course, to their family chemist. The young man into whose hands it came for compounding managed to make out, or guess, at all the components, except the menstruum, which was indicated as peach-water. This article taxed the wits of the dispenser, a young and somewhat inexperienced hand; so calling the shop-boy, he gave him a paper with the name of the required article written on it, and desired him to go to a well-known establishment in Oxford-street for the same. As the sender did not mention what the peach-water was for, and the messenger could give no information, the assistant, thinking it was for flavouring, sent the essence of bitter almonds. When the boy got back with the bottle, the sender, who was waiting for it, completed his task by filling up, without in any way testing, or even tasting, the liquid, which had been supplied. The result may be guessed. The young lady died shortly after the first dose, a victim to cupidity on one part and stupidity on the other.

I am not aware whether any punishment was meted out to either doctor or chemist; but the former, as almost a matter of course, lost his practice and the name of Cronin, once famous was heard no more. He disappeared from London, and probably from England, to die in obscurity.

"FAREWELL, FAREWELL TO THE DEAR OLD LAND, HURRAH, HURRAH FOR THE NEW!"

If any one had told me at the time of Tawell's execution that it was probable that I should ever stand behind the counter in the very shop in which that notorious criminal had made his (to use a colonialism) pile, I should have given them very little credit for skill in fortune-telling. Yet this event did actually come to pass in the year 1853; but of this anon. Chemists in this colony, and those at the present day at home, know nothing, except by hearsay, of the direful drudgery which was the lot of those whose business it was to minister as assistants in chemists' shops to the wants of those who suffered from any of the numerous ills to which humanity is heir. From earliest dawn to the latest hour of the night it was one continued round of toil. They were not allowed to sit down until the principal lights were turned out, at ten o'clock, and not even then until every drawer was filled to replotion with pennyworths of sticking-plaster, salts, magnesia, or rhubarb, as the case might be ; they were not allowed at any time during the long, long day to go to the door for a breath of fresh air, lest it should be thought by passers-by that there was a moment in the sixteen hours when the shop was without a customer. Not one holiday, or even half a one, from one year's end to another ; two or three hours every alternate Sunday being about the amount of relaxation considered necessary for a chemist's assistant in enlightened, anti-slavery England in the middle portion of the nineteenth century.

I am afraid that my brother chemists in this land of freedom will think that I am drawing an exaggerated picture of the miseries of an assistant pharmacist in olden days. If they do so, all I can say is that their lot was a happier one than mine. I am writing my *own* reminiscences.

This kind of life (irksome enough, no doubt, to all subordinates in the drug business) was particularly unsuited to my taste, which inclined in a remarkable degree to out-door exercise, and I yearned for adventure by sea and land ; for, as a boy, I had devoured *Crusoe*, admired *Mungo Park*, and perused Campbell's *Travels in Africa*, until I fear they were more familiar to me than my "catechism."

With such tastes and aspirations, it will not be wondered that the land of my birth became distasteful to me, or that I came to the determination to turn my back on it, and set my face towards other lands, where I could earn my bread literally by the sweat of my brow in wild and untried regions under a sunny sky.

(To be continued.)

PHARMACEUTICAL NOTES.
(BY ROBERT F. FAIRTHORNE, PH.G.)

UNGUENTUM AQUÆ ROSÆ.—The ointment of rose-water of the United States Pharmacopœia, prepared according to the directions given in that work, is, in most respects, justly regarded as a satisfactory preparation. It is not, however, entirely unobjectionable, and the directions can be so modified that those engaged in the manufacture of it will be assisted thereby. The length of time required to produce an ointment such as the apothecary desires is often quite a serious tax upon his patience, and in order to lessen this I would recommend it to be made in the following manner :—All the ingredients employed are put into a wide-mouthed bottle, placed in a hot-water bath, and allowed to remain until the solid portion is melted, then the bottle is taken out, and, having tightly corked or stoppered it, the mixture is thoroughly shaken ; a uniform emulsion will result, which is to be agitated until solid.

The resulting ointment will be found smoother and more uniform than that produced by stirring, and the operator will find less exertion required, and will have also the advantage of knowing exactly the right moment when it is proper to stop agitation by solidification taking place. If in making it, three times the quantity of the ingredients ordered by the Pharmacopœia are used, an ordinary preserving jar, with a cover that screws on, will be found a very convenient vessel to use.

COLD CREAM, AND A CHEAP SUBSTITUTE FOR OIL OF ALMOND.—One of the objections to the rose-water ointment of the Pharmacopœia is its unstable character. It seldom remains in good condition more than two weeks, by which time in many cases it will be found rancid and the rose-water often separated in globules, giving it an unsightly appearance. For those reasons it has been customary amongst the druggists to make a substitute for it which is called cold cream, either with much less rose-water or without any, or by substituting a small amount of glycerine for it.

The use, however, of oil of sweet almonds has been almost universally retained. This oil is certainly unobjectionable, but can be replaced in making the unofficial ointment by a much cheaper one, which is sold by the wholesale druggists under the name of nut-oil. This is obtainable at about one-fourth the price of the former, to which it bears a very close resemblance in colour, odour, and other characteristics. I have used it, and found it quite satisfactory, and offer the following formula to those who would like to try it :—

Take of Nut-oil	...	...	¼ lb. avoirdupois
Spermaceti	...	...	3 oz. „
White wax	...	...	1¾ oz. „
Rose-water	...	...	½ oz. „
Oil of rose	...	...	18 drops

Make an ointment in the same manner as suggested above. If a very white cold cream is desired, the addition of 25 grains of borax will produce it.

In this place I would remark that all, or nearly all, the ointments and cerates of the Pharmacopœia can be advantageously made by agitation, and more expeditiously than by the ordinary method.

A SOLID GLYCERINE PREPARATION.—The very extensive application of glycerine renders it desirable to present it in many different forms, and two very convenient ones will be produced by the following formulæ :—

Take of French gelatine	...	...	120 grains
Glycerine	...	...	1½ fl. oz.
Water	...	...	½ fl. oz.

Cut up the gelatine in small pieces, and, having added it to the water in a wide-mouthed vial, melt it by means of a water bath, then add the glycerine, which must be warmed ; shake the mixture, pour into moulds, and keep in a cool place until solid. It can then be taken out and wrapped in either tin-foil or waxed paper. This makes a clear, elegant, ice-like preparation, and can be applied to the skin, which should be previously moistened with water. If used for toilet purposes, a drop of oil of rose can be added whilst the ingredients are fluid.

An article having more resemblance to a cerate, or to stick pomade, in which glycerine predominates, can be made by taking—

French gelatine	...	...	100 grains
Starch	...	...	60 „
Glycerine	...	...	12 fluid drachms
Water	...	...	4 „

Add the gelatine to the water, and proceed as in the other receipt. Rub up the starch with the glycerine, and having heated the mixture on a sand-bath in a capsule, with constant stirring until it becomes translucent through the starch dissolving, add the solution of gelatine to it, and pour into moulds. If for toilet purposes, it can be perfumed and moulded of a cylindrical form by pouring it into wide glass tubes closed at the bottom with corks. In order to remove it from them, take out the cork, and, having warmed the tube by pouring a little hot water over it, blow through the tube, when the solidified gelatine will fall out. This is placed on a sheet of glass, and kept cool until the outside has become solid. This can be applied to the skin without previous wetting, and has a singular cerate-like consistence.—*American Journal of Pharmacy.*

SYRUPS FOR SODA WATER—ORANGE AND LEMON.—Very superior syrups can be made in the following manner :—Take the peels of six oranges or lemons ; cut them very thin ; make a tincture of them by macerating in 6 fluid ounces of alcohol for three days. Having filtered it, pour it on 1 lb. (avoirdupois weight) of sugar contained in an evaporating dish or other suitable vessel, and allow the alcohol to evaporate spontaneously. When dry dissolve in half-pint of water in which, if orange syrup is to be made, 1½ ounces of citric acid—if lemon, 2 ounces of the acid and 2 drachms—are to be dissolved. This mixture, added to 11 pints of simple syrup, will produce fine flavoured syrups, which keep well.

SECRET REMEDIES.

In considering the subject a distinction should be made between "secret remedies" and "specialties." A "specialty" may be defined as any substance or product which, prepared according to an official formula, realises an improvement in the art of pharmacy, and presents special therapeutic advantages. A "secret remedy" is any simple or compound substance or medicine employed in the treatment of disease, which has not received official sanction or publication, and which has not been prepared for a particular case upon a medical prescription. One is the product of the professional skill and practical sense of the pharmacist, and is generally met with in competitions and industrial exhibitions. The other is a product of charlatanism and an inordinate desire to acquire a fortune rapidly; it makes itself known especially by advertisements in the public prints. Even if the remedies of which neither the basis nor the proportions are known ought to be rejected from therapeutics, genuine specialties, which mark a progress in the pharmaceutic art, or are intended to facilitate the administration of certain medicines, might, up to a certain point, be admitted. The distinction between a specialty and a secret remedy is not, however, always easy to establish.

The public has acquired a taste for secret remedies, and will continue to take them; secret remedies enjoy a prestige that imposes upon the public, and it will be difficult to fight against this infatuation. The word public is here used in the widest sense, as including the learned as well as the ignorant. And it is certain the public will have secret remedies as long as it has incurable invalids haunted by the hope of being healed or having their pains assuaged. The medicine that would appear without any value if it were given simply under the cover of the pharmacist, with his label, becomes a panacea, and imposes upon the public as soon as it is noisily advertised and covered with a stamp and a specious prospectus; if, in addition, it be prescribed by a medical man, the confidence becomes unlimited.—*Pharmaceutical Journal.*

INQUEST.

Mr. MAUNSELL held an inquest on 6th March, at the Travellers' Rest Hotel, Gerogery, on the body of William Francis Wilkes, chemist. The following evidence was taken:—James E. Britton deposed: I first met the deceased in Albury on the 20th February, when he informed me he was hard up; that he was a chemist by profession, and had been managing a shop in Chiltern. He told me his father was a medical man in England, and that he was expecting money from home. I saw the deceased the last time alive about a quarter of a mile from Brown's Springs Station. He used to eat large quantities of salt and drink a great deal of water. He had a good appetite. Jesse Young, boundary rider, deposed: I found deceased lying dead on a rock about a mile from the station on Tuesday last. He was lying on his face, and there was no appearance of any struggle. There was no blood on him. Henry Lucas, manager of Brown's Springs Station, corroborated the evidence of last witness. His hat and clothes were found half a mile from the place where he was found. Deceased had only his trousers on; no shirt. Dr. J. Leonard, duly qualified medical practitioner, deposed: I find nothing to account for death, but from the evidence given I believe him to have died from exhaustion consequent on exposure. I think he must have had delirium, and, probably, had been drinking heavily recently. The jury found the cause of death was exhaustion and exposure.

VICTORIA PHARMACEUTICAL SOCIETY'S MEDAL IN GOLD.

SCHOOL of pharmacy prizes presented by the Council—Chemistry ("elementary and practical"), botany, *materia medica*, and pharmacy.

At the end of each term a gold medal will be offered for competition. Students who have attended more than one term will be ineligible to compete. The medals can only be taken by students who have worked in the laboratory for not less than 75 per cent. of their period of study, and who are connected with the Society as registered apprentices of the same. On receiving the report of the examiners, the Council will award the prizes.

Notes and Abstracts.

FOWLER'S SOLUTION.—Dannenberg does not regard the algaceous growth, occasionally observed in this liquid, as being of any importance concerning the arsenic present; but he directs attention to the gradual oxidation, in partly filled bottles, of the arsenious to arsenic acid, as was shown by Fresenius many years ago. According to Frerichs and Woehler arsenic acid is far less poisonous than arsenious acid, and it is obvious that it cannot be immaterial which of the two compounds is present. Fowler's solution should be prepared only in small quantities and preserved in well-stopped vials.—*Phar. Centralhalle,* 1881, p. 319.

PREPARATION OF SODIUM ETHYLATE.—Hager gives the following directions:—100 grams absolute alcohol are placed into a glass flask of 350 ccm. (about 12 ozs.) capacity; small pieces of the metallic sodium of the size of a pea or bean are then gradually added, and the flask is closed with a cork, through which a long open glass tube passes for the purpose of condensing the alcoholic vapours evolved during the reaction. The addition of sodium is continued, until 12 grams of the metal have been used, repeated agitation being required towards the end of the process. The hot thickish liquid is now poured into a porcelain dish, the flask is rinsed out with a little hot alcohol, any undissolved sodium is carefully removed, and the liquid is heated until, after cooling, it will completely solidify, when the mass is rubbed into a fine powder and carefully preserved. Thus prepared, it contains some alcohol in combination, which may be expelled by heating it to 200° C. In contact with water it is decomposed into alcohol and sodium hydrate. Its action is milder than that of caustic soda, and it is more conveniently applied than the latter. Richardson's sodium ethylate is a clear solution of 1 part of the above compound in three parts of absolute alcohol. Freshly prepared it is colourless; but brown yellow if made from old ethylate.—*Ibid.,* p. 359.

ELASTIC ADHESIVE PLASTER.—Dr. W. P. Morgan, in a communication to the Boston *Medical and Surgical Journal,* states that he has been trying to obtain an elastic adhesive plaster that, when attached to the skin, should yield to the movement of the muscles and parts beneath without the sensation of stiffness or an uncomfortable wrinkling. Not being able to obtain an article of this description, he procured some india-rubber, and, giving it a coat of plaster such as is recommended in Griffith's *Formulary* under the name of "Boynton's Adhesive Plaster" (lead plaster 1 lb., resin 6 drachms), he found the material he wished. After using it as a simple covering for cases of psoriasis, intertrigo, &c., he extended its use to incised wounds, abscesses, &c., and found it invaluable. Placing one end of the strip of plaster upon one lip of the wound, and then stretching the rubber and fastening the other end to the opposite lip of the wound there is perfect apposition of the several parts, the elastic rubber acting continually to draw and keep the parts together. When unable to get the sheets of rubber, one may use broad letter-bands (sold by stationers), by giving them a coat of plaster.—*Ohio Medical Journal,* September, 1881, p. 136,

A valuable paper, by M. Paul Bert, on the administration of anæsthetics, has recently been read before the Academy of Sciences (*Comptes Rendus,* Vol. xciii., p. 768). M. Bert finds by experiment that if an anæsthetic be mixed with variable quantities of atmospheric air there comes a point at which an animal made to breathe such an atmosphere exhibits anæsthesia, and that this point bears a definite relation to the point at which the anæsthetic proves fatal. In experiments made upon dogs, mice, and sparrows, using chloroform, ether, amylene, and bromide and chloride of ethyl, it was found that the fatal dose was double that required to produce insensibility. In the case of protoxide of nitrogen the ratio is one to three. The result shows that chloroform acts not by the quantity inhaled, but by the amount of air mixed with it. This important result, although the experiments had not then been made upon mankind, shows that in all probability careful observation made by those who have the administration of chloroform in their hands may reduce its use to a minimum of risk and that in the future it may be employed with scientific precision. An instrument by which the amount of admixture of air and chloroform could be easily regulated before inhalation seems therefore to be a desideratum.

INDEX

Australasian Supplement to Chemist and Druggist.

VOL. IV.

FROM MAY, 1881, TO APRIL, 1882.

All letters to the Editor will be found arranged under the head of Correspondence.

INDEX—(Continued).

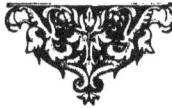

Chemist & Druggist.

WITH AUSTRALASIAN SUPPLEMENT.

(Published under direction of the Pharmaceutical Society of Victoria.)

No. 49. { PUBLISHED ON THE 15TH OF EVERY MONTH. }
Registered for Transmission as a Newspaper.

MAY, 1882.

{ SUBSCRIPTION, 15s. PER ANNUM, INCLUDING DIARY, POST FREE.

PEARCE'S LAVENDER
With Musk.

PRISE
MELB.
EXHIB.

AWARDED
INTER:
80-81

TRADE MARK

PEARCE & Cᵒˢ

LAVENDER WATER
WITH
MUSK
AN EXQUISITELY REFRESHING
& LASTING PERFUME

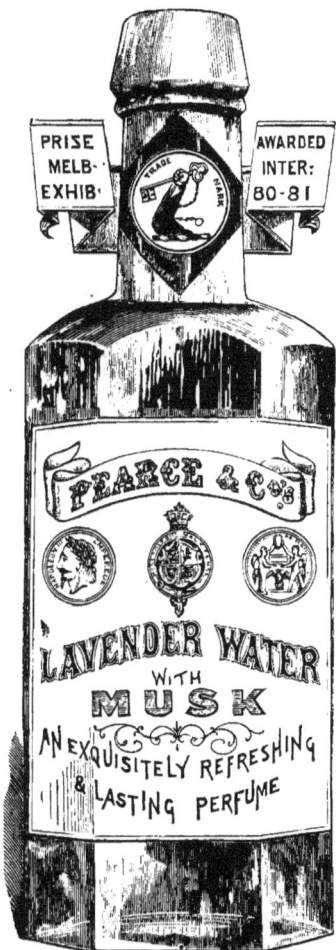

THIS is a well-known fragrant Perfume, and from its cheapness may be used lavishly.

Sprinkled about the Room, or used in a Bath, it will be found most refreshing and invigorating.

As a perfume for the handkerchief, its peculiar fragrance and exquisitely penetrating odour, so delightfully refreshing in hot climates and grateful to the invalid, render it one of the Standard Perfumes of the day.

PROPRIETORS:

HEMMONS, LAWS & Cᵒ.
WHOLESALE DRUGGISTS,
RUSSELL ST., MELBOURNE.

The Chemist and Druggist.

WITH AUSTRALASIAN SUPPLEMENT.

OFFICE: MUTUAL PROVIDENT BUILDINGS, COLLINS STREET WEST.

Published on the 15th of each Month.

THIS Journal is issued gratis to all paid-up Members of the PHARMA-CEUTICAL SOCIETY OF VICTORIA, and to non-members at Fifteen Shillings per annum, payable in advance. A copy of *The Chemists and Druggists' Diary*, published annually, is forwarded post free to every subscriber.

Advertisements, remittances, and all business communications to be addressed to THE HONORARY SECRETARY OF THE PHARMACEUTICAL SOCIETY, MELBOURNE.

SCALE OF CHARGES FOR ADVERTISEMENTS:

Per annum.		Per annum.
One Page £3 0 0	Quarter Page ..£3 0 0	
Half do. 5 0 0	Business Cards .. 2 0 0	

Special rates for wrapper and pages preceding and following literary matter. Advertisements of Assistants Wanting Situations, 2s. 6d. each.

Advertisements for insertion in the current month should be sent to the office before the 10th.

COMMUNICATIONS for the EDITORIAL department of this journal should be addressed to THE EDITOR, MUTUAL PROVIDENT BUILDINGS, COLLINS STREET WEST, MELBOURNE.

No notice can be taken of anonymous communications. Whatever is intended for insertion must be authenticated by the name and address of the writer—not necessarily for publication, but as a guarantee of good faith.

THE LIBRARY.

THE Library is open daily (Saturdays excepted), from 9.30 a.m. to 4.30 p.m. Catalogue of the books can be obtained on application.

PHARMACEUTICAL SOCIETY OF VICTORIA.

ANNUAL SUBSCRIPTIONS.

ALL annual subscriptions are now due.

Member's subscription	...	...	£1 1 0
Associate's	...	...	...	0 10 6
Apprentice's	...	...	...	0 5 0

Cheques and Post-office orders should be made payable to the Honorary Secretary, No. 4 Mutual Provident Buildings, Collins-street, Melbourne.

HARRY SHILLINGLAW, Hon. Sec.

WANTED,

FOR THE MELBOURNE PUBLIC LIBRARY, a complete File of the *Chemist and Druggist*, with Australasian Supplement, from May, 1878. Will any Member supply?

BIRTH.

BOULLY.—On the 6th instant, at Howard Place, Sandhurst, the wife of James Boully of a daughter.

DEATHS.

BRIDGE.—On the 25th March, at Maldon, Essex, England, the Rev. Robert Lee Bridge, B.A., aged 86 (father of Richard Barnes Bridge, Chemist, &c., formerly of Bright and Wangaratta, Ovens District, Victoria), for nearly 50 years Incumbent Rector of St. Mary's Parish, Maldon, Essex.

ADAMS.—On the 7th instant, at Heathcote, Edward Adams.

EXCHANGE OF CERTIFICATES.

LAST July the council of the Pharmaceutical Society of Victoria decided by a resolution to communicate with the Pharmaceutical Society of Great Britain with reference to the question of the exchange of certificates of registration and qualification as "pharmaceutical chemists." The reply of the secretary (Mr. Bremridge) has been received, to the effect that the council has considered the matter, and find "that there are no statutory provisions under the Pharmacy Acts of Great Britain empowering the registrar to place any name on the register except on the production of certificates of skill and competency, signed by the respective boards of examiners appointed by the council of the society, and approved by the Privy Council." Undoubtedly this was correct enough, and was perfectly well known by the council of the Pharmaceutical Society of Victoria; but the object and intention on our part was to see if the pharmaceutical authorities of the mother-country were disposed to take steps to enable, under proper conditions, our Pharmacy Board to exchange certificates. It is well known also to us whose term of apprenticeship in England dated at a time anterior to any Pharmacy Act in England, and whose period of pupilage even expired before that legislative measure was placed upon the English statute-book, that the highly accomplished and most scientifically educated French or German pharmacist, whose education is infinitely superior and more extensive than the English pharmaceutical chemists can pretend to be, cannot exchange or reciprocate certificates, but must, forsooth, submit to be examined by those, able as they are, who would not presume to consider themselves their superiors. When the Pharmacy Act in England was passed, thousands of persons in business at the time were registered, and we in Victoria were in justice compelled to follow the same precedent. The desire of the Pharmacy Board of Victoria is, and has always been, to make the standard of education as high as in the mother-country, and we think that at the present time we have fairly realised that object. In the last numbers of the *Pharmaceutical Journal*, in an article upon "Pharmaceutical Registers," attention is drawn to our recent proposal for the consideration of the question of the exchange of certificates, from which we make the following extract:—

The opportunity may also be taken to refer to still another Pharmacy register, that of the colony of Victoria, issued by the Pharmacy Board constituted under the Act passed in December, 1876. This register, which, like the Irish register, recognises only one qualification, that of "pharmaceutical chemist," contains 623 names, and as a proposal has recently been put forward for reciprocity in the recognition of the qualifications granted in the colony and this country it may be of interest to devote a few lines to the analysis of this list. It would appear that of the 623 persons now registered as "pharmaceutical chemists" under the Victoria Act only three have become qualified by having passed the "major" examination of the Victoria Board; 540 have been registered without examination, in virtue of having, before the passing of the Act, either for not less than two months carried on the business of a chemist and druggist or homœopathic chemist in keeping open shop for the dispensing of prescriptions, or having been employed for not less than three months as dispensing assistants in such shops, or for not less than three years as dispensing chemists in hospitals or other public institutions. Another 44 became qualified through having passed a "modified" examination provided for persons who have served an apprenticeship of not less than three years that commenced prior to the passing of the Act. Of the remainder, 34 are registered in virtue of qualifications under the British Act and two in virtue of German qualifications. It is only right to state, however, that in Victoria a candidate before becoming entitled to present himself for the "major" must have served a four years' apprenticeship and attended one course of lectures and passed examinations in *materia medica*, medical botany, and practical chemistry at the Melbourne University or some other recognised school; so that sufficient time has hardly elapsed to allow this provision to come into play. Twelve certificates have been issued under the Sale of Poisons Act to unqualified persons—five of whom appear to be Chinese—resident four miles from a registered chemist, and permission has been granted to four widows and executrices of pharmaceutical chemists to carry on business for twelve months ending with the present year.

We cannot, however, expect the realisation of our wishes at once. It is only right that the leaders and authorised guardians of pharmaceutical education in England should carefully guard their diplomas against deterioration, and we only hope that the discussion of our proposition may lead to some salutary results in the future; certainly it ought to make us determined on our part that our standard of education shall not be allowed to fall below that which is now considered essential to the proper discharge of the important and responsible functions involved in the practice of pharmacy.

The Month.

WE are authorised by Messrs. George Lewis and Sons, of No. 5 Collins-street West, the well-known chemists, to state that there is not a particle of truth in the report that their business was about to be disposed of. It is not, and never was, in the market.

The manager of the Warrenheip Distillery Company gave some interesting particulars with respect to that industry before the Tariff Commission. He stated that the company now turned out 72,000 gallons of whisky, gin, and spirits of wine annually, which they sold at 4s. 6d. per gallon in bond, but as a duty of 4s. per gallon was allowed by the Government, they were, as a matter of fact, protected at the rate of something like 100 per cent. The amount represented by this differential duty was within £1600 of the total value of the company's yearly operations; but this, Mr. Walker asserted, was made up by the consumer getting his spirits so much cheaper.

The ordinary meeting of the Microscopical Society was held on Thursday evening, the 27th April. The Rev. J. J. Halley, vice-president, occupied the chair, and there was a fair attendance of members. Mr. Geo. Matthews was nominated as a country member. Mr. W. M. Bale described a convenient form of stage micrometer, which is not in use among English microscopists, but a modification of which is much used on the Continent. Mr. W. W. Allen exhibited and described a lichen from the Cape Otway ranges, a member of the genus Cladonia, known as the coral lichen. The Rev. J. J. Halley gave a very interesting account of his visits to the principal microscopical societies in England, particularly the Royal Microscopical Society, the Quekett Club, and others. Some interesting exhibits were laid before the meeting, particularly specimens of meridion mounted in situ, shown by the Rev. J. J. Halley; some sections of Australian plants double-stained, by the Rev. T. Porter; and one of Zeiss' variable low-power objectives, exhibited by the same gentleman. Among the other specimens exhibited, Trichina spiralis, in human muscle, shown by Mr. Halley, attracted special attention.

The annual report of Dr. O. H. Schomburgk, the curator of the Botanical Gardens, Adelaide, notes the fact that during the past season the frosts were the most severe on record, yet the temperature in the sun was the highest yet known. It also states that rust-proof wheat has proved a success, and recommends also that drought-resisting fodder plants and the Californian phylloxera-resisting vines should be cultivated. The small farmers are recommended to give up growing wheat only. A Government grant is asked for to slope the Torrens bank. A lengthy appendix is printed with the report, proving the influence of trees upon climate.

The second annual *conversazione* of the Field Naturalists' Club of Victoria was held at the Royal Society's Hall on Wednesday night. About 200 ladies and gentlemen attended. The Rev. J. J. Halley, one of the vice-presidents, was in the chair. In the unavoidable absence of Professor M'Coy, president of the club, his address was read by the Rev. J. J. Halley. The society was stated to have made satisfactory progress during the year, and it now numbered 140 members, including many of the first scientific men in the colony. The chairman gave a short and interesting lecture on "The Beauties and Curiosities of Protophytes, a First Form of Plant Life." Mr. H. Watts spoke of "Microscopic Life around Melbourne." Bad drainage developed certain unhealthy forms of this life, which were productive of disease. He mentioned the localities where malaria of this kind was most rampant. Among them was Sandridge Bend, which he regretted to see had been named as a site for the proposed contagious diseases hospital. That swampy land was highly unsuitable for the purpose. During the evening the company were invited to inspect the museum in the lower hall. The collection was a large and varied one, in an excellent state of preservation. It was formed of the contributions lent for the occasion by members and friends, upon whom the exhibition reflected much credit. Among the most admired specimens were some birds of paradise of gorgeous plumage, handsome cases of Australian birds, both waders and the parrot tribe, reptiles, beetles, eggs, shells, ferns, and butterflies.

Mr. F. S. Grimwade (Messrs. Felton, Grimwade and Co.) has been elected president of the Chamber of Commerce, and on taking the chair delivered an unusually interesting address.

Four fires occurred during the month in chemists' establishments—a very unusual occurrence.

Mr. John Lamb, 47 Elizabeth-street, North Melbourne, has closed his shop.

Mr. Tom Luke, a new arrival in the colony, is about commencing business at Shepparton.

Mr. Thos. Ingham, of Rockhampton, Queensland, whose name is well known in connection with euphorbia, pilulifera, has been on a visit to Melbourne.

Messrs. Rocke, Tompsitt, and Co. are the successful tenderers for the supply of medicine and photo-lithographic chemicals to the Government for 1882-3.

Mr. W. W. Caught has taken over the business of the late Mr. Griffiths, St. Kilda.

Messrs. Blogg and Grist have established a new chemical manufacturing firm in Melbourne.

The death of Mr. F. B. Spicer, late of Morwell, Gippsland, is announced. Mr. Spicer died in Hobart, where he was well known.

The next quarterly examination of the Pharmacy Board will be held in June, the dates are—preliminary examination, 8th; modified, 12th; and practical pharmacy, 13th June.

Mr. Fred. Cherry, formerly traveller for Messrs. Hemmons, Laws and Co., has purchased Mr. H. C. Armstrong's business at Hay, N.S.W.

The Pharmacy Act and regulations, and the Poisons Act and regulations for the sale and custody of poisons, have just been published in a neat and handy form—price, one shilling ; by post in Victoria, 1s. 6d.; neighbouring colonies, 1s. 8d. They can be obtained at the office of the Pharmaceutical Society, 100 Collins-street.

Meeting.

PHARMACEUTICAL SOCIETY OF VICTORIA.

THE monthly meeting of the council of the Pharmaceutical Society of Victoria was held at the rooms, 100 Collins-street, on Friday, the 14th April.

Present—Messrs. Bowen, Hooper, Blackett, Nicholls, Thomas, Jones, Best, Baker, Huntsman, Ross, and Shillinglaw.

The president (Mr. Wm. Bowen) in the chair.

The minutes of the previous meeting were read and confirmed.

The first business, after the confirmation of the minutes, was the election of office-bearers for the year 1882-3.

PRESIDENT.

Mr. C. R. Blackett said that he thought they could not pay a higher compliment to the retiring president than to re-elect him to the position he had so ably filled during the past year. The interest and attention Mr. Bowen had given to affairs of the society was well known to all the members, and he had, therefore, great pleasure in proposing the election of Mr. Bowen as president for the ensuing year.

Mr. Bowen, while thanking the members of the council for their kind expression of feeling, said that he thought that some other member might aspire to the office of president. He was, however, quite willing to leave the matter in their hands; and if it was their unanimous wish that he should retain the position, he would be happy to accept it. The motion was then seconded by Mr. J. C. Jones, and carried unanimously.

VICE-PRESIDENT.

Mr. B. Baker said he had much pleasure in proposing the re-election of Mr. J. Turner Thomas as vice-president. The motion was seconded by Mr. Hooper, and carried unanimously. Mr. Thomas briefly returned thanks.

TREASURER.

On the motion of Mr. Huntsman, seconded by Mr. Best, Mr. Henry Gamble was unanimously re-elected treasurer.

Mr. Bowen remarked that the office of treasurer was one that should be changed as seldom as possible. They must all feel grateful to Mr. Gamble for the admirable manner in which he managed the finances of the society, which were now in an exceedingly satisfactory condition.

HONORARY SECRETARY.

Mr. Bowen said he had great pleasure in moving the re-election of Mr. Harry Shillinglaw. His duties as president had been very much lightened by the valuable assistance he had received from Mr. Shillinglaw. The motion was seconded by Mr. Blackett, and carried unanimously.

The ordinary business was then proceeded with.

Election of New Members.—The following were duly elected :—John Opie, Melrose, South Australia ; A. E. Bilton, Police Depôt, St. Kilda-road ; C. Harrison, Chapel-street, Prahran ; H. B. Given, Milparnika, N.S.W.

Nominations.—R. S. D. Morgan, Wood's Point ; Thos. Luke, Shepparton ; John Warrington, Echuca.

Apprentices Elected.—A. C. Lock, Fitzroy ; C. L. Henshall, Seymour.

On the motion of Mr. A. T. Best, a special vote of thanks was recorded to the members of Legislative Assembly, Messrs. Zox, Cook, Macgregor, Laurens, and Blackett, for their valuable assistance in connection with the application to the Government for a site for a museum, school, and laboratory.

Correspondence, &c.—A letter was read from Mr. H. A. Glyde, of Deniliquin, New South Wales, resigning his membership. The resignation was accepted, subject to Mr. Glyde returning his diploma, which, on ceasing to be a member, reverts to the society.

The following letters were also read :—

"5 Collins-street East, 4th May, 1882.

"Gentlemen—Allow me to congratulate you, and the members generally, on having obtained so favourable a site for the proposed new ' school of pharmacy,' and trust no time will be lost in erecting a suitable building. My object in writing is to suggest that a direct appeal be made to the trade for donations to a building fund. If we can only raise a few hundred pounds, it would be a grand thing to open our new school free from debt.—I am, yours, &c.,   "GEO. LEWIS.

"To the Council of Pharmaceutical Society of Victoria."

"Melbourne, 30 Collins-street East, 19th April, 1882. "H. Shillinglaw, Esq., hon. sec. Pharmaceutical Society of Victoria.

"My Dear Sir—Will you kindly convey to the council of the Pharmaceutical Society my appreciation of their vote of thanks, and to assure them that my services will always be placed at their disposal when required ?—I remain, my dear sir, yours faithfully,   "E. L. ZOX."

Appointment of Lecturer on Pharmacy at the Melbourne University.—Moved by Mr. Blackett, and seconded by Mr. Best —" That as it is understood that the council of the University have it in contemplation to reconsider the advisability of appointing a lecturer on pharmacy, the council of the Pharmaceutical Society beg to respectfully intimate to the council of the University, that in the event of the appointment of a lecturer being decided upon, they have the honour to recommend Mr. E. L. Marks as a fit and proper person to undertake the duties appertaining to the aforesaid lectureship."

Financial and general business brought the meeting to a close.

Books &c., Received.—*Australian Veterinary Journal,* May ; *American Journal of Pharmacy,* March ; *Pharmaceutical Journal,* March ; *Year-Book of Pharmacy,* 1881 ; the *Druggists' Circular,* New York, April ; Messrs. Burgoyne, Burbidges and Co.'s *Monthly Circular,* March ; *European Mail,* March ; *Analyst,* March ; Messrs. Sleeman and Co.'s *Drug and Export Chemical Circular,* February.

SCHOOL OF MINES, BALLARAT.

A VERY successful term has just been brought to a close by a *conversazione,* in which councillors, lecturers, old and new students, governors, and subscribers joined. Several lecturettes were given, with experiments, and a number of the philosophical apparatus belonging to the school exhibited and explained, including the school's microscopes, with a number of slides, illustrative of each branch of natural history. The classes have in each case been well attended ; in the chemical laboratory every place was taken. One of Dr. Usher's students presented for examination in *materia medica,* and passed well. This is the first examination under the Pharmacy Board ; but as the school is exceedingly well provided with the means of instruction in this branch, there will doubtless be many more candidates before long.

In the telegraphy class thirteen presented for examination, of whom *nine* passed, two with credit. The museum, with its very varied contents, is resolving itself into splendid order under the able hands of Professor Krause, and will be a means of educating the student and the general public such as is not often found outside a metropolis. It is already of great importance to the class in mineralogy and geology. The classes in mathematics are growing in importance, as are also those in mechanical drawing. These subjects are not valuable to the miner only, but are specially applicable to the wants of the artisan and the workman in every department of labour.

In the chemical and metallurgical departments the laboratories are open day and evening, except Wednesday evening, for practical work, when pharmacy, mining, agricultural, and general students may attend. In addition to the evening-class lectures a lecture is given on Tuesday afternoons to pharmacy students (who are also exercised in the whole of "Attfield"); on Wednesday afternoons to 150 State-scholars of upper forms in chemistry, to be followed by other subjects (the Council have resolved to award some free scholarships in connection with this class); on Saturdays for State-school teachers from eleven to twelve o'clock in chemistry, from ten to eleven o'clock being devoted to practical work. During the term a dozen lectures on chemistry and electricity have been delivered by the laboratory assistants to the various mutual improvement societies of the district. These lectures have always been well attended.

The Chemical and Electrical Industries Society, started some time ago by the vice-president, continues to meet fortnightly. During the term a course on applied chemistry was delivered, together with a variety of lecturettes.

Arrangements are being made to deliver a series of lectures on chemistry and metallurgy to the miners in the neighbourhood of Redan.

A further series of popular lectures is also being organised to be held in the school, Mr. Ellery having been invited to deliver the first on the electric light.

A very large number of donations have been made to the school, including books, pamphlets, and museum specimens; £50 from the Hon. Francis Ormond, and £50 from Messrs. Ham, Goodall, Morey, and Stoddart, for the purchase of the Preshaw collection. The new term commences on Monday, 24th April.

COUNTRY DRUGGISTS.

WE are informed that in many of the country towns where surgeons make up their own medicines prescriptions are few and far between, unless they are dispensed for visitors, or are in the possession of those residents who have sought advice from Melbourne physicians. It consequently transpires that pharmacists are shorn of one of the most lucrative portions of their business, and great dependence has to be placed upon the sale of drugs and patent medicines.

Now, since the Americans have poured such a continuous stream of the latter article into this market, combined with a more copious supply from England, this trade has assumed unusual proportions; and in some measure the sale of them would make up for other deficiencies, if confined to those who naturally consider it one of their rights. Unfortunately, however, the mutual stores, the friendly societies' dispensaries, and the grocers are gradually absorbing into their business much of this trade also, and, for the sake of diverting custom, are underselling the druggists. Thus, unless some remedy can be suggested for this evil, a druggist will shortly be left as the sole admirer of his gold-labelled bottles and show jars. Previous to the passing of the Pharmacy Act, and when its provisions were being considered by the society, it was suggested that a clause should be inserted whereby the sellers of patent medicines should pay an annual license fee, but it was strongly opposed by the metropolitan druggists, as likely to imperil the passing of the bill, but, as a remedy against the incursions of other traders, it is a pity that some such enactment was not adopted, and sooner or later it must come to pass, if the trade in them is valued.

A custom that helps to place this class of business in the hands of storekeepers arises from the fact that a druggist's shop is never frequented with the same regularity that other shops are, and as such medicines as Cockle's and Holloway's pills enter largely into household arrangements, orders are given for them along with groceries.

The home druggists make the same complaint, and a regular correspondence has for some time been carried on in the columns of the *Chemist and Druggist*, with a view to remedy this state of things; various methods have been proposed, and the most likely one is to combine other trades with the business.

It is very certain that country druggists might do this with every degree of satisfaction so far as regards having time at their disposal, but most of them are wanting in inclination; and if it were entertained at all, a very different class of shops would be required. However, in these days of protection in this colony, something is requisite, and with the high class of education that is now needed to fit persons for the position of a chemist, the sooner a change comes the better.

THE RUSSIAN JEWISH RELIEF FUND.

MESSRS. BOWEN, Thomas, and Shillinglaw (the president, vice-president, and hon. secretary of the Pharmaceutical Society), waited on Mr. E. Z x, M.L.A., the treasurer of the fund for the relief of persecuted Jews in Russia, on the 27th April, and presented that gentleman with a cheque for £30, being the amount collected among the members of the society. In making the presentation Mr. Bowen said that the society had selected this mode of expressing their appreciation of Mr. Zox's services as the one they thought would be most agreeable to his feelings.

Mr. Zox said he felt great pleasure in having given the application to the Government for a grant of land for a museum, school, and laboratory; the establishment of such an institution was a matter of national importance. He could only assure them that his services would always be at their disposal when required.

OCCURRENCE OF BASSORA-GUM IN CYCADEÆ.
(BY C. R. BLACKETT, M.P., HON. MEMB. PH. S., AUSTRIA.)

BARON VON MUELLER, the Government botanist, in the course of his scientific researches upon some hitherto undefined species of cycadaceous plants, being anxious to examine the gum exuded by Macro-zamia Fraseri, collected by Mr. John Forrest, the Australian explorer, and Macro-zamia Miguelii, procured by the Rev. Dr. Wools, requested me to make an examination as to the character of this gum.

It would seem that hitherto it has not been recorded that a kind of gum is exuded by cycadaceous plants, although the abundance of a peculiar starch in the stems of the Australian Macro-zamias has been noticed in various publications, and also in the pages of this journal by Baron von Müeller. This gum is similar to bassora and cherry gum, is secreted both from the stem and fruit-cones of the Macro-zamias; in general appearance it is not unlike gum acaciæ, it is very tough and of a brownish colour. In the experiments upon these gums from M. Fraseri and M. Miguelii, it was found that they were with difficulty fractured, and swell up and soften on being macerated in cold water, becoming transparent gelatinous masses, and not rapidly dissolving; by long-continued digestion in boiling water, the less soluble matter is gradually brought into solution; the clear solution dried at 100° C. forms a clear and hard gum, adhesive to the touch of the slightly moistened finger. The addition of potassic hydrate renders the gum readily soluble, but darkens the colour considerably. In water, acidulated with H_2SO_4 it is soon dissolved, and a flocculent precipitate is formed, and after boiling for a short time the presence of sugar was detected on the addition of Febling's copper test, absolute alcohol produced only a slight turbidity in the watery solution. The latter will keep undecomposed for several days, and dries up very slowly; therefore, this gum, even if more adhesive, could not be used as a substitute for gum arabic. Ferric chloride produces no action upon the solution whatever. The ash yielded was found to be equal to 1·75 per cent., and composed of lime, iron, sodium, potassium, carbonic acid, sulphuric acid, and chlorine.

This gum is therefore analogous to Bassora-gum, or tragacanth, and similar gummous exudations of plants, whether it can be used instead of gum tragacanth has yet to be tried. This gum was not found to possess any of the deleterious acridity which pervades the sap of the cycads generally, and which renders their fruit, in a raw state, poisonous. Since writing the above, I find that Dr. Pareira, in his *Materia Medica*, p. 288, Vol. 3, under Cycas, says—"A clear mucilage, which converts into a gum like tragacanth, exudes from fresh wounded plants of several species of cycas."

Gum of Bassora, which appears to be the produce of a cactus, is white and honey-coloured, mealy, and silvery on its surface, and in the form of somewhat flattened and elongated masses. It is insipid, and crackles between the teeth. In water it swells up to a transparent jelly, but only a small portion dissolves. The soluble portion contains arabin, amounting to about one per cent. of the gum; the insoluble portion contains Bassorin. It dissolves with the aid of heat in potash and weak acid.—*Watts' Dic.*, p. 955.

Baron von Müeller informs me that he "has just obtained a specimen of gum from Brachychiton ramiflorum, which behaves like the Bassorin gum of the Cycadeæ." He also says :—"In my travels I have noticed gummous exudations from all the Brachychitons and Sterculias in Australia, including the famous "bottle-trees," and I have no doubt that the gum of the various Sterculia trees of the tropics of Asia, Africa, and America consists of Bassorin, one species from Western Africa being described by Professor Lindley as Sterculia tragacantha, on account of the tragacanth-like gum exuding from its stem and branches. Whether by chemical action this Bassorin gum can be turned to important practical uses has yet to be seen."

CHINESE METHOD OF MANUFACTURING VERMILION.
(BY HUGH MACCALLUM).

THERE are three vermilion works in Hong Kong, the method of manufacture being exactly the same in each. The largest works consume about six thousand bottles of mercury annually, and it was in this one that the following operations were witnessed:—

First Step.—A large, very thin iron pan, containing a weighed quantity (about fourteen pounds) of sulphur, is placed over a slow fire, and two-thirds of a bottle of mercury added ; as soon as the sulphur begins to melt the mixture is vigorously stirred with an iron stirrer until it assumes a black pulverulent appearance with some melted sulphur floating on the surface ; it is then removed from the fire and the remainder of the bottle of mercury added, the whole well stirred. A little water is now poured over the mass, which rapidly cools it ; the pan is immediately emptied, when it is again ready for the next batch. The whole operation does not last more than ten minutes. The resulting black powder is not a definite sulphide, as uncombined mercury can be seen throughout the whole mass ; besides, the quantity of sulphur used is much in excess of the amount required to form mercuric sulphide.

Second Step.—The black powder obtained in the first step is placed in a semi-hemispherical iron pan, built in with brick, and having a fireplace beneath, covered over with broken pieces of porcelain. These are built up in a loose porous manner, so as to fill another semi-hemispherical iron pan, which is then placed over the fixed one and securely luted with clay, a large stone being placed on the top of it to assist in keeping it in its place. The fire is then lighted and kept up for sixteen hours. The whole is then allowed to cool. When the top pan is removed the vermilion, together with the greater part of the broken porcelain, is attached to it in a coherent mass, which is easily separated into its component parts. The surfaces of the vermilion which were attached to the porcelain have a brownish-red and polished appearance, the broken surfaces being somewhat brighter and crystalline.

Third Step.—The sublimed mass obtained in the second step is pounded in a mortar to a coarse powder, and then ground with water between two stones, somewhat after the manner of grinding corn. The resulting semi-fluid mass is transferred to large vats of water, and allowed to settle, the supernatant water removed, and the sediment dried at a gentle heat ; when dry, it is again powdered, passed through a sieve, and is then fit for the market.—*Government Civil Hospital, Victoria, Hong Kong, China.*

Correspondence.

To the Editor of The Australasian Supplement to the Chemist and Druggist.

SIR—What is the best composition for marking linen, such as sheets, towels, counterpanes, such composition to stand plenty of washing ? I have tried some three or four kinds, but none seem to stand. The letters required to be some three-quarters of an inch or an inch long ; consequently it will take some quantity of fluid. It must be inexpensive— that is to say, a reasonable price.   M. P. S. V.

11th May, 1882.

To the Editor of The Australasian Supplement to the Chemist and Druggist.

SIR—I should feel very much obliged to you, and I am sure the trade generally would feel much obliged to you also, if you would inform me through the medium of the journal whether our ordinary fire insurance for stock-in-trade and fixtures includes stock, bottles, show-jars, &c., as I have been recently advised that unless specially named in the policy as "utensils, show-jars, &c.," the offices will repudiate any claim for these articles in the event of their being destroyed by fire.—Yours respectfully,   CHARLES RUBIN.

To the Editor of The Australasian Supplement to the Chemist and Druggist.

DEAR SIR—Will you kindly inform me under what disability does an unregistered assistant lie in regard to the Poisons and Pharmacy Acts, and also what extra liability does the employé of an unregistered person incur ? There are still some assistants who are entitled to register on passing the modified examination, yet they do not avail themselves of it. There certainly ought to be some limit to this, and perhaps if employer and employed are made acquainted with their respon-

sibilities the evil will be remedied. The employment of unqualified assistants is unfair, both to the public, whom the Pharmacy Act is designed to protect, and to those who have to pass a severe examination before being permitted to dispense medicines.—I am, yours truly,   SANITAS.

To the Editor of The Australasian Supplement to the Chemist and Druggist.

SIR—I have often thought that, considering how much the success of the prescriber depends upon the exact execution of his instructions by the dispenser, there should be frequent communication between the two ; yet, as a matter of fact, hardly any communication at all exists—except across the counter. I believe if by some means the physician's wishes could be made known to the pharmacist, that the latter would take every pains to give them effect. This would lead to the improvement of old remedies and to the adoption of new, and also to greater uniformity. The subject is a wide one, having many aspects, but at present I must limit myself to mentioning a few simple matters upon which misunderstanding exists, and which, if medicine and pharmacy are to be considered sciences, should speedily be removed. Ether chloroform or spirits of ether chloroform is variously dispensed as 1 in 8, 1 in 10, or 1 in 20, and some prescribers intend one and some the other strengths. When "sodæ carb." is written the bicarbonate is often meant, and it is sometimes difficult to determine which. When "oz. of potass bromid" is ordered, as 437½ grains are contained in the official ounce, that quantity ought to be dispensed, but many prescribers mean the old troy ounce of 480 grains. These discrepancies might be largely added to, but I must now only refer to one more difficulty which occurs in this direction ; but it is perhaps the most important of all, because it matters not how exactly a prescription may be dispensed if the patient takes half or twice as much as the doctor intends. About five years ago I sent a circular to every medical man in Victoria, asking him if he attached any other values to the terms tea, dessert, and tablespoon than one, two, and four drams respectively, to kindly let me know. I further suggested that the terms fluid ounces and drams should be substituted for spoonfuls, &c. I received replies thanking me for the suggestion, and approving of the plan I then adopted me of giving a measure with each prescription, but no one disputed the generally accepted values. Still I find that no material alteration has occurred in practice ; and while the now-replies to my circular proved that Victorian medical men at any rate mean a tablespoonful of four drams, their patients still continue in most cases to use four, five, six, or even seven drams, according to the make of the family spoons. Nor is this all, for even where 2 ozs. is written some dispensers interpret it as a tablespoon, and the patient uses his own discretion as to the size—some believing in large, others in small doses. This I think unwarrantable ; but it is nevertheless the fact, and to remedy such anomalies more frequent interchange of opinions is needed between the two branches of the healing art.—Apologising for trespassing so far, I am, yours truly,   ALFRED J. OWEN.

POISONING CASES.

A GATEKEEPER employed on the railway at Footscray, named Thomas O'Connor, aged forty-five years, was admitted at the Melbourne Hospital on the 9th April, suffering from strychnine poisoning. It appears that O'Connor, who had been suffering from despondency for some days, consequent upon hearing that he was to be removed from his position, purchased four grains of strychnine from Mr. Stephens, chemist, Footscray, in the morning, on the plea that he desired to poison a dog. The poison was obtained in the regular way in the presence of a witness, and no suspicions were entertained that the purchaser contemplated suicide. On returning to his home O'Connor proceeded to eat the strychnine, but was prevented from taking the whole four grains by his young son, who obtained assistance and conveyed him to the hospital.

An attempt was made to commit suicide on the 9th April by a man named Robert Miller, aged twenty-seven years, residing at Cardigan-street, Carlton, by taking a large dose of poisonous liniment. It was stated by Miller's friends that he had been drinking heavily for some days, and while recovering from the effects of the bout he drank a quantity of liniment, consisting of belladonna and camphor, from the effects of which he almost immediately became unconscious. He was removed to the Melbourne Hospital, where he was successfully treated.

An attempt was made to commit suicide by a woman named Bridget Heffernan, aged twenty-one years, living at Little Lonsdale-street, on the 10th April, by taking a quantity of rat poison. She had been drinking heavily for some time, and while under the influence of liquor she purchased a quantity of rat poison and drank it in some beer. She was immediately removed to the Melbourne Hospital and successfully treated by the medical staff.

A case of supposed suicide was reported to the police on the 24th April, at Ballarat. A man whose name is supposed to be Joseph Preston, but whose identity is not established, who said he had come from the neighbourhood of Horsham, where he had been at work, went into M. Thetaz's wine shop, and complained of being unwell. After he had been there some time, he was seen to swallow something from a phial, and then throw the latter into the fireplace. The bottle had contained chlorodyne, which he had obtained during the day from a chemist in the Main-road. He was then removed to the hospital, where he died.

FIRES.

ABOUT half-past two o'clock on the 22nd April, the watchman on duty at the establishment of Messrs. James M'Ewan and Co., ironmongers, observed smoke issuing from the premises of Messrs. Evans and Wormall, surgical instrument and cutlery dealers, and at once gave the alarm at the Insurance Brigade station. On arrival it was found that a quantity of benzine was on fire, and it was with the greatest difficulty that it was extinguished. One of the men, named Langridge, was burned about the legs by the bursting of one of the bottles containing the fluid. The stock in the shop was damaged, but it was covered by insurance in the Victoria Company to the extent of £400. The stock of Mr. Leighton, portmanteau maker, in a lower portion of the premises, was slightly damaged by water.

A fire broke out on the premises of Messrs. E. Rowe and Co., wholesale druggists, George-street, on the 22nd April, and damage was done to the amount of £1000. Through the exertions of the firemen, the fire was confined to one story. The stock was insured for £1450 in the New Zealand Insurance Company, and £500 in the Mercantile Mutual.

A fire occurred at the premises of Messrs. Marshall Brothers, chemists, Market-street, Sydney, on the 25th April, in consequence of some spirits of wine used in the manufacture of syrups catching fire. The damage amounts to £60. A youth named Oswald Dawson was seriously injured, but it is thought he will recover.

A rather alarming discovery was made about half-past two o'clock on the 17th April, by Mr. Thomas Webb, stationer, of Hare-street, Echuca. He was lying down reading and found that the room was filled with smoke. A thorough search of his own premises failed to reveal the source of the smoke, but it was eventually found to be issuing from Mr. Warrington's premises (the Millewa dispensary) which is situated next door. Mr. Webb at once communicated with Constable Harris, who rang the firebell. The firemen turned out with praiseworthy promptitude and soon had two lengths of hose playing into the shop. It was impossible to discover the seat of the flames for some time, owing to the dense smoke which filled the compartment; so the whole place was deluged with water. Mr. Warrington had a very large stock of chemists' and druggists' goods, fancyware, &c., and a great proportion of this was ruined by the flooding the house was subjected to. It is possible that fire was caused by spontaneous combustion through the agency of acids. The Millewa dispensary is situated in the centre of the best block of buildings in Hare-street, and had the fire once firmly established itself a dreadful conflagration would have followed. When the fire was discovered, Mr. Warrington was out driving and the house was empty. We understand that the house and stock was insured.

REMINISCENCES OF A PHARMACIST (Continued).

(By J. B. MUMMERY.)

IT was not my good fortune to be blessed with wealthy relations, nor had I (to use an old saw) been born with a silver spoon in my mouth; but I managed, nevertheless, to scrape a sufficient sum together with which to pay my passage to Sydney in a very humble way.

The vessel in which I sailed was, although A1 at Lloyd's, far from being a clipper; for these fast-sailing crafts were then unknown. Ships were built with sea-going qualities, and carrying capacity was then considered of more account than speed, and four months from England to Australia was considered a quick passage.

I am not going to bore my readers with an account of the voyage, which presented no features of unusual interest, but content myself with saying that after a run of 117 days from port to port (112 of which were passed out of sight of land), the good ship by which I was a passenger entered Sydney Heads on the 1st day of February, 1849; and never to my dying day shall I forget the magnificent prospect which regaled the sight of myself and fellow-passengers as we sailed up the magnificent harbour of "Port Jackson."

Four months at sea, with no change in the prospect of sky and water, gives every one a longing to tread the solid earth again; and had it been but a bleak and barren land we were approaching, we should have felt our hearts yearn towards it; but being one of earth's fairest paradises—as the approach to Sydney really is—I cannot find words to express the delight which we all felt at the magnificent prospect which met our gaze, as promontory after promontory was passed, and the city at last burst upon our view, with the early morning mist drawing up from it like a vast curtain.

It will readily be believed that we passengers lost no time in decking ourselves in our best attire, and making for the shore; and here I found myself in a little difficulty as regards the state of my exchequer, which was certainly at low-water mark, for all my worldly resources in the shape of money were represented by nearly the smallest silver coin extant—namely, a fourpenny piece; for just before leaving England I had the misfortune to fall in with a couple of sharpers, who, in the most insinuating manner possible, had eased me of the few shillings I had remaining after procuring the necessary outfit for the voyage. However, I was by no means disheartened, for I had unlimited faith in the resources of the land I had come to, and confidence in my ability to avail myself of them. So, borrowing a sovereign from one of my fellow-passengers, I laid a few shillings out in a good square meal, and then proceeded to write an advertisement, which I took to the office for insertion in the next day's Herald, with, however, but very slender expectation of an immediate answer, for chemists' shops in the colony in those days were certainly few and far between. I was more fortunate, however, than I expected, for the evening's post the next day brought me two letters from gentlemen who were anxious to accept my proffered services, one in the city, the other in Maitland, a town on the Hunter River, about 150 miles from Sydney. I accepted the former, and the next day saw me installed as assistant to a medical man in tolerable practice, who, residing in the outskirts, had a retail shop in the city; and it was to reside at and manage the latter that I was engaged. The salary was not large; but as it was more liberal than what I had been accustomed to in England, I was satisfied on that score; but there was another on which I certainly was not—that was, regarding the duties required of me. I found the daily routine of business too much like that at home, and the hours of relaxation very little, if any, better than they were in the land I had just left, and I came to the determination to stay just long enough to get a few pounds together, and then follow the bent of my inclination by making a start for the interior.

I stayed with the doctor about three months, when I bade him adieu rather unceremoniously, and turned my back on civilised life for a spell. It was on a Saturday, I remember well, when my week's notice expired, and the same evening I hired a barrowman* to carry my worldly effects (which were all then packed in a moderate-sized trunk), to the Hunter River steamers' wharf, where I booked myself as a passenger for Newcastle. These steamers left at the unseemly hour of eleven p.m., and usually arrived at Newcastle by daybreak the following morning.

It is not my intention to give a narrative of personal adventure, apart from such as may have a bearing on the interests of our profession, for two reasons; first, because such has already been published, and may be read in the Australian Journal, of the years 1872-3. Secondly, because I apprehend

* Barrowmen, in the days of which I am writing, had their regular stands in the streets, as cabs have here, and where they waited with their one-wheeled vehicles for any odd job which might turn up. This was before the days of parcels-delivery carts. There was such a stand in King-street, nearly opposite our door.

that a record of the kind would not be suitable for these columns. Suffice it to say that, for a period of something over three years, my desire for the ups and downs of a roving life were realised to their fullest extent, in the then almost untrodden regions of the far interior.

Although I had bidden, as I thought, a final adieu to the pestal and mortar, my three years in the bush was not altogether passed out of the odour of drugs, for as I was two hundred and fifty miles further out than any person pretending to medical knowledge, I had a medicine chest of course, and was often called upon to administer to such ailments as hardy bushmen are liable to, and as an evidence of what persons of education in the wild bush may be called upon to do at times, I may mention the following incident.

A poor young fellow, well connected in Sydney, who had joined an exploring party, on the look out for new grazing country, had taken a violent cold during the journey, and was brought into a station, about forty miles from ours, in a dying state, and I was sent for to see him as a matter of course.

I saw at once, on my arrival, that nothing could be done for him beyond relieving his pain, which I was able to do by the aid of remedies which I had brought with me, and he lingered a day or two, and then died. As he was possessed of some property, I acted as his lawyer, as well as his doctor, by helping him to draw up his will, and when all was over, I assisted in making his coffin, took a hand at digging his grave, and finally read the burial service over his remains. Thus having practised in this one case, the professions of law, physic, and divinity, as well as the callings of undertaker and sexton.

One wearies, however, of bush life, and I was thinking of a return to civilisation, when the gold-diggings broke out. I caught the fever, like almost every male persons in New South Wales, and in the year 1852 I was one of the many who rushed headlong to the then famous Forest Creek.

I must pull up here, or my "Reminiscences" will be getting into the adventurous track, and I shall find myself doing what at the commencement of the present paper I have promised not to, but will merely state that, after about six months' delving, I returned to Sydney with a sum which I thought might, with economy, suffice to start me in a shop of my own.

As, however, my available capital was something under £100, I was rather dubious of the advisability of trying to make a start on so little; and whilst I was revolving the question of doing so in my mind, my eye caught an advertisement in the Sydney Morning Herald for an assistant, and I decided to apply for the billet, which I did at once, and was accepted.

My success in this matter being due, I expect, more to the circumstance of the dearth of chemists' assistants than to anything else, for I had no testimonials or recommendations to produce.

(To be continued.)

ECONOMY OF FUEL, AND SMOKE ABATEMENT
(Continued).

(Read by C. R. Blackett, M.L.A., before the Australasian Health Society, 29th March, 1882.)

IN an ordinary domestic fire about seven-eighths of the heat of combustion goes up the chimney, about one-half going up with the smoke, a quarter by the open space about the grate, and the remaining eighth in the unconsumed carbon of the smoke itself. The report of the committee of the Board of Health in England laid down the requisites of a theoretically perfect fireplace. It recommended with respect to the domestic fireplace, that the smokeless fire-grate designed by Dr. Arnott should be adopted; that polished surfaces to the fireplaces should be used for reflecting heat; that ash-pans and sand ash-pits should be used for cleanliness and ornament; that the smoke apertures should be at the back of the grate; that fire-brick should generally be used for the interior of grates, and the fireplace so arranged that the fire should be seen from the largest possible number of points in the room, and that a good frontage of fire-surface should be exposed. They also recommend that a supply of fresh air should be given in proximity to the fire; and further, that the domestic fire-grate should be studied for warming purposes only, and not for ventilation. In the last number of the *Westminster Review*, and in the *Sanitary Record* for 15th December and 15th January, very complete details are given of the numerous inventions which have been introduced for economising fuel

and abating the smoke nuisance. A condensed abstract of some of these may be acceptable and useful.

Dr. Arnott's grate, arranged upon thoroughly scientific principles, is spoken of as the best grate, as a non-producer of smoke and for economy of fuel. It may be described as a lidless coal-box under an ordinary grate, the fire being upon the top of the box, as in an ordinary grate. The fire is replenished from below by raising a false bottom in the box by means of a rack with holes in it, to which a rachet is attached, and the poker as lever. The box being air-tight, there is no through draught, but combustion takes place upon the top of the coal only, while the fuel is gradually prepared for combustion and for incandescence from below. The hydrocarbons given off as combustion progresses have to pass through the incandescent carbon of the fire when the temperature is sufficiently high (about 2·400 F.) to ensure their perfect combustion upon meeting, as they do, the oxygen about the open top of the box; the coal-box should be, for a small room, 8 or 10 inches deep, to hold 20 or 30 pounds of coal. There should be a throttle-valve placed in the chimney-flue about on a level with the mantelpiece to regulate the draught. Dr. Arnott also recommended a ventilator in the chimney-flue, near the ceiling, to purify the air of rooms in which gas is burnt; there is also a blower attached to stimulate the draught. This grate will burn for many hours without replenishing, and is especially valuable in the sick-chamber, as no noise is caused by putting coals on the fire. For the prevention of draughts, air supplied under the hearth will be found effectual. Mr. Engert's grate, described in the *Times* of 15th January, 1881, is effective. Its general features are similar to Dr. Arnott's. Mr. Engert places his coal-box at the back of the fire, instead of the bottom. Another grate is described in which the coal is forced into the bottom of the fire by a screw, with steeped pitched blades. Another, upon the right principle, has a spherical grate revolving easily upon legs, acting as axes; by reversing the grate, the green coals remain at the bottom, resulting in complete combustion of smoke. There is the "Little Wonder" grate of Mr. Cornforth, arranged with fire-bars and tubes, perforated with holes, so that hot air is brought into complete contact with the fuel, and mingles with the hydrocarbon at a high temperature, ensuring perfect combustion.

Dr. Siemens has lately designed a gas and coke grate "which appears admirably suited to assist in the solution of the domestic smoke problem." Drawings of this grate were given in *Nature*, November, 1880, page 25, a few months since. But the use of gas and carbon, in the form of half-coked coal, is worthy of attention. A new *califère Parisien* has been brought out by Mr. Mangin, of Paris, which, it is said, embodies most of the excellencies of previous stoves, with safeguards against down draughts.

The Calebrooke Company have devoted much attention to the stove and grate department of their business. Their new patent "Kyrle" fire is said to be a complete success, minimising, if not entirely abolishing, smoke.

The principle to gasify the fuel before combustion is at the basis of all good smoke-consuming grates. Time will not allow me to quote the description given of other grates; they are so numerous and can be referred to at leisure in the journals, the dates of which I have given.

Gas apparatus for heating and cooking has been vastly improved of late, and many very interesting inventions and improvements are reported, and can be found in the above-mentioned magazine in its reports upon the smoke-abatement exhibition at Kensington. Judging by the accounts given in the very able report of the sanitary record there has been a wonderful amount of energy and scientific intelligence devoted to this problem. There are some simple appliances for attaching to any ordinary open fire-grate which deserve the attention of those who are not willing to revolutionise their system of domestic heating, such as Gray's patent false back, which secures a chamber of air behind the coals. This simple appliance would be suitable for small tenements.

The improvements in furnaces, boilers, and apparatus used for manufacturing purposes demand especial attention from all the large consumers of coal in our factories. Messrs. J. and J. M'Millan (Glasgow) have invented a fuel-feeding apparatus, automatic in action, "raising the fuel to the bottom of the fire; it is bound to enter it at one point only, and, therefore, cannot be misplaced."

For full information upon the numerous and important inventions and improvements in furnaces, attention is directed to the report of the *Sanitary Record.*

Notes and Abstracts.

ADULTERATION OF DRUGS IN ENGLAND.—The Society of Public Analysts report that the percentage of adulteration of drugs examined in 1880 was 16 per cent., against 28 per cent. in 1879. In most cases the pharmacists were not the delinquents. Many of the instances were of paregoric destitute of opium, sold by small shopkeepers who were not pharmacists, and therefore prohibited by the British Pharmacy Act from dealing in an article containing poison. A curious distinction—the shopkeeper may sell paregoric without opium, while the pharmacist must sell paregoric with opium.

THE TESTING OF OIL OF BITTER ALMONDS.—This substance is frequently adulterated with artificial oil of bitter almonds (essence of mirbane or nitro-benzol). This adulteration is best detected by the reaction by which it yields aniline under the influence of nascent hydrogen, which the genuine oil does not. The test is applied in the following manner :—To an alcoholic solution of the oil some fragments of granulated zinc are added, and then about half its volume of strong hydro-chloric acid, after which the solution is gently warmed. An energetic reaction ensues, which should be allowed to proceed for about five minutes. The liquid which now contains, if nitro-benzol was present, chloride of aniline is poured off from any undissolved zinc and treated with an excess of strong solution of caustic potash until the precipitate at first formed is redissolved. The aniline thus set free is extracted from the liquid by agitation with ether, the ethereal layer is removed, placed in a test-tube with an equal bulk of water, and a few drops of a cold solution of bleaching powder added, when a splendid mauve colouration will be produced, the intensity of which depends upon the amount of nitro-benzol originally present in the sample under examination. Boyveau gives the following as the characters of the genuine oil. The specific gravity varies from 1·043 to 1·060, while some specimens of spurious oils had a specific gravity of 1·019 to 1·080. The genuine oil, if mixed with an equal volume of sulphuric acid, turns red, but remains limpid and clear. The spurious oil, on the other hand, turns dark red in colour, and then becomes brown, at the same time becoming dull and thick, and finally congealing to a brownish mass.—*Sanitary Engineer of New York.*

IMPURE WATER.

THE following valuable suggestions made by Dr. Lowe, of Lynn, Norfolk, deserves the attention of travellers and pharmacists. We quote from the *Pharmaceutical Journal,* p, 488:—"He points out the great danger of contracting typhoid fever by total abstainers and travellers, from drinking impure water. His experience led him, when travelling, always to carry a small case containing a kettle and spirit lamp, and invariably to boil water before drinking it; also to apply Nessler's test to it. He suggests that if 10 or 15 drops of that reagent were enclosed in a thin glass capsule and hermetically sealed, the fluid would keep for a length of time, and a dozen or so packed in a box would form a valuable addition to a travellers' outfit. One of the capsules, broken in a wineglass, and a spoonful or s) of the suspected water added, would show at once if it were of a dangerous nature, and might thus be the means of saving life."

RULES FOR THE CARE OF THE EYES.

1. ALWAYS have an abundance of steady light for any work which you may have on hand. Do not work in a poor light.

2. Avoid a glaring light. It is as bad as too little light.

3. Let the light come from the side, behind, or above, *but not from the front.*

4. *Never read or use the eyes closely during twilight.* Put up your book when the sun goes down. Do not sew black goods at night. Do not work with the microscope at nights.

5. Never use a flickering light when reading or writing.

6. Avoid suddenly passing from the shade into a bright and glaring light.

7. When using artificial light, it is always beneficial to wear a shade *over* the eyes, which will cut off all direct light from them ; the desk or table should be covered with a light blue paper or cloth.

8. Use a lamp with a good, large burner, *the best oil,* and try to obtain as white light as possible. *A student's lamp is worth all it costs to the poorest student.*

9. Hold the head erect ; and at such a distance from the lamp that it will not be heated by it. When the head and eyes are hot, bathe with pure cold water. Do not bend over your work.

10. *Whenever the eyes pain on using, or are fatigued, or the images are blurred, stop using them.* Look up and away from the work frequently, and in bad cases study only by daylight, or not at all for a week or more.

11. Do not confine the eyes too closely to the work. Hold the book at least twelve inches from the eyes ; this will prevent growing nearsightedness.

12. Avoid books poorly printed, with small type, and on poor paper.

13. Do not use the eyes for reading when riding on the cars, in a carriage, or when walking, &c.

14. Never read when lying down.

15. Do not read during convalescence from any debilitating diseases.

16. Keep all patented eye-washes out of the eyes, and avoid all quack eye-doctors. The eye is too precious an organ to be trifled with.

17. Keep all soap out of the eyes ; be especially careful of children in this respect.

18. When the eyes are inflamed sleep much and thus restore them.

19. In all cases of weak-sight, near-sight, and far-sighted, squinting, or cross-eye, have the eyes carefully examined by a competent oculist, and follow his advice implicitly. When glasses are prescribed, procure and wear them.

20. *Avoid coloured glasses and goggles,* unless prescribed by a physician competent to judge of your condition.

21. Have all diseases of the eye treated early and skillfully, and remember that the well eye sympathises with the diseased one, and you may lose both unless early attention is given to the matter. Diseases of the eyes in which a large amount of matter forms are dangerous, and patients so affected should be careful to get no matter from the diseased eye into the well one, and they should have a separate basin and towels for washing purposes.—*Accident and Emergencies.*

JUST PUBLISHED.

Price—One Shilling ; by post, sixpence extra.

The Pharmacy & Poisons Acts ;

WITH THE

REGULATIONS OF THE PHARMACY BOARD,

AND THE

SALE AND CUSTODY OF POISONS.

Copies can be obtained at the Office of the Pharmaceutical Society, No. 4 MUTUAL PROVIDENT BUILDINGS, COLLINS STREET WEST.

MAJOR EXAMINATION.

IN accordance with the provisions of clause 40 of the Regulations to the Pharmacy Act, an EXAMINA-TION IN PRACTICAL PHARMACY before the Board will be held at this office on MONDAY, the 12th JUNE, 1882, at Eleven o'clock a.m. Candidates must give to the Registrar notice of their intention to present themselves for examination, together with their indentures of apprenticeship, the certificates required by Section 18, Sub-section 4, of the "Pharmacy Act 1876," and the fee of three guineas, ten days prior to the day.

HARRY SHILLINGLAW,

Melbourne,   Secretary and Registrar.

12th April, 1882.

[handwritten: Launched Stereopticon microscopes] 12-13.

[SUPPLEMENT ONLY.]

Chem. & Drugg. Aust. Suppl.
Vol. 5, no. 50: 9-20.
(June, 1882)

Chemist & Druggist.

WITH AUSTRALASIAN SUPPLEMENT.

Vol. 5. (Published under direction of the Pharmaceutical Society of Victoria.)

No. 50. { PUBLISHED ON THE 15TH OF EVERY MONTH. }
Registered for Transmission as a Newspaper.
JUNE, 1882.
{ SUBSCRIPTION, 15s. PER ANNUM, INCLUDING DIARY, POST FREE

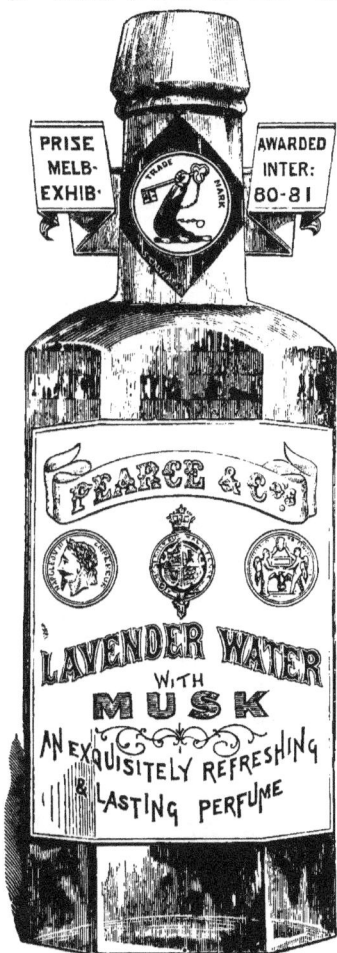

The Chemist and Druggist.

WITH AUSTRALASIAN SUPPLEMENT.

OFFICE: MUTUAL PROVIDENT BUILDINGS, COLLINS STREET WEST.
Published on the 15th of each Month.

THIS Journal is issued gratis to all paid-up Members of the PHARMA-CEUTICAL SOCIETY OF VICTORIA, and to non-members at Fifteen Shillings per annum, payable in advance. A copy of *The Chemists and Druggists' Diary*, published annually, is forwarded post free to every subscriber.

Advertisements, remittances, and all business communications to be addressed to THE HONORARY SECRETARY OF THE PHARMACEUTICAL SOCIETY, MELBOURNE.

SCALE OF CHARGES FOR ADVERTISEMENTS:
	Per annum.			Per annum.
One Page	.. £8 0 0		Quarter Page	..£3 0 0
Half do.	.. 5 0 0		Business Cards	..2 0 0

Special rates for wrapper and pages preceding and following literary matter. Advertisements of Assistants Wanting Situations, 2s. 6d. each. Advertisements for insertion in the current month should be sent to the office before the 10th.

COMMUNICATIONS for the EDITORIAL department of this journal should be addressed to THE EDITOR, MUTUAL PROVIDENT BUILDINGS, COLLINS STREET WEST, MELBOURNE.

No notice can be taken of anonymous communications. Whatever is intended for insertion must be authenticated by the name and address of the writer—not necessarily for publication, but as a guarantee of good faith.

THE LIBRARY.

THE Library is open daily (Saturdays excepted), from 9.30 a.m. to 4.30 p.m. Catalogue of the books can be obtained on application.

PHARMACEUTICAL SOCIETY OF VICTORIA.

ANNUAL SUBSCRIPTIONS.

ALL annual subscriptions are now due.
Member's subscription	...	...£1	1	0
Associate's	...	...	0 10	6
Apprentice's	...	...	0 5	0

Cheques and Post-office orders should be made payable to the Honorary Secretary, No. 4 Mutual Provident Buildings, Collins-street, Melbourne.

HARRY SHILLINGLAW, Hon. Sec.

WANTED,

FOR THE MELBOURNE PUBLIC LIBRARY, a complete File of the *Chemist and Druggist*, with Australasian Supplement, from May, 1878. Will any Member supply?

THE SALE OF POISONS AS PATENT MEDICINES.

"THE subject of patent medicines containing poison has been so frequently commented on of late, and the practice of allowing them to be sold without a poison label being attached has been so strongly condemned by medical men and by the press, that there is reason to believe that this subject will before long receive the attention of the legislature.

"It is chiefly from this point of view that we think it will be useful to place before our readers an account of what took place at an inquest held at Devonport, to inquire into the cause of death of a child aged two years and seven months, who died suddenly on Good Friday. According to the evidence given, the child had been in good health for some three months previous to its death, with the exception of a cold, to relieve which the mother gave him, on the recommendation of a neighbour, several doses of the preparation sold under the name of 'linseed compound.' On the Friday, after the child was put to bed, some red marks were observed on its face; and, as it was thought the child was in a fit, a spoonful of brandy was given, together with a warm bath, after having which the child died in a few minutes. It was further stated that, though the child did not usually sleep during the afternoon, it had frequently gone to sleep since it had been taking the medicine, and had slept more than usual during the past week.

"The evidence of the medical man who was called in to see the child had reference only to the *post-mortem* examination, as he was, when first sent for, engaged with a patient that he could not leave. His observations led him to conclude that death was due to narcotic poisoning, the symptoms being such as are invariably produced in such cases. At the same time, it appears from the report that the doctor also said there was some difficulty in reconciling the evidence with the presumption of narcotic poisoning, but it is not quite clear what was here referred to. As regards the medicine given to the child, the doctor stated that a bottle of what the mother had administered was given to him, and he described it as bearing a notice on the label in the words, 'Registered under the Sale of Poisons Act,' apparently inferring that these words applied to the preparation in the bottle. This view was also adopted by the coroner, who spoke of the medicine as containing something that made it a registered poison. This, however, was evidently a mistake, for the words referred to merely indicate that the makers of the article are registered under the Pharmacy Act. It is strange that such a mistake should have been made by the medical man who gave evidence in this case; but as regards the coroner there is perhaps less room for surprise on this account, as he was not a medical man.

"In another part of the medical evidence we find it stated that the medicine in question is 'a dangerous narcotic,' the effects produced by it are similar to laudanum, and that he 'believed a number of children had been killed by its use unknown to the parents.' These are strong statements, and would seem to point to the necessity for the use of a poison label as a precautionary measure. We give them as they appear in the newspaper report, and are unable to say on what grounds they were based. It may, however, be inferred from the doctor's remarks on the danger of administering opium to young children, that he has reason for thinking the preparation he spoke of contains opium, and that on that account it was open to the objection of bearing a label which, in his opinion, was misleading, since linseed contains no poison, and is one of the most harmless medicines known.

"The remarks of the coroner were chiefly directed to this point, exonerating those who had used the medicine while unaware of its character, and blaming those who prepared it, as well as the Government for allowing it to be sold in such a manner as to mislead people. The jury returned a verdict in accordance with this direction, and requested the coroner to communicate with the Home Secretary, for the purpose of pointing out the danger of allowing patent medicines containing poison to be sold freely with labels not clearly defining the danger of taking them and with a name indicating harmlessness. Though the account given of this case in the newspaper reports we have seen is not altogether free from obscurity in some respects, it is probable that the general expression of opinion to the Home Secretary in regard to the sale of poisons as patent medicines will not be without good effect."—*Pharmaceutical Journal.*

The Month.

AT the request of the honorary general secretaries to the British Pharmaceutical Conference the following circular has been sent to every chemist on the *Pharmaceutical Register* of Victoria:—

"Sir—The annual meeting of the Conference will this year be held at Southampton, commencing on Tuesday, the 22nd of August, at 10.30 a.m. precisely. The following subjects are suggested for investigation. The Executive Committee hope that you will undertake to work on one or more of the questions, or upon others that may occur to you. The committee, anxious to add new subjects to this list as others are worked out, will be glad to receive from you any questions that may have presented themselves as desirable for investigation. Authors are specially requested to send the titles of the papers they intend to read, to the secretary British Pharmaceutical Conference, Bloomsbury-square, London, W.C., as soon as possible, or not later than two or three weeks before the annual meeting. The subjects will then be publicly announced, and thus full interest secured. All manuscripts of papers should be in the hands of the Executive Committee at least ten days before the meeting."

"Yours faithfully,
"F. BADEN BENGER,
"MICHAEL CARTEIGHE, } *Hon. Secs.*"

THE CHEMISTS OF ECHUCA:—A meeting of the resident chemists in Echuca having been convened by Mr. Calder, of Hare-street, for the purpose of considering the advisability of forming an association to decide upon hours of closing, and other matters affecting the interests of the chemists in this district, the meeting took place on the 22nd May; present— Mr. Warrington, in the chair, Mr. Calder, and Mr. Grace, the latter representing the new firm of Messrs. Grace and Co. A letter was read from Mr. Strong, of High-street, stating his inability through illness to attend; another letter was read from Mr. Fairthorne declining to attend, and giving a reason which it was considered could only have arisen from an erroneous impression as to the objects of the meeting. After some discussion it was decided, as only three of the chemists of Echuca were represented, to abandon the formation of an association for the present.

The recent great advance in the position of the advocates of the germ theory is amusingly illustrated by an episode in the pathological section of the Medical Congress, recorded in the *Medical Times and Gazette.* Dr. Bastian, in a speech, had alleged that wherever tissues are deprived of vitality, or have their vital power lowered, organisms can originate spontaneously. M. Pasteur said he had not understood Dr. Bastian's remarks, but it had been explained to him that that gentleman advocated the spontaneous generation of organisms, and, turning to Dr. Bastian, he asked if this were true. Not receiving an immediate negative, M. Pasteur raised his hands and exclaimed, "Mon Dieu! mon Dieu! est-ce que nous sommes encore là? Mais, mon Dieu, ce n'est pas possible!" and then in a vigorous speech proceeded to demolish Dr. Bastian's arguments.

THE ACCIDENT TO MR. FRED. FAIRTHORNE.—The many friends of Mr. Frederick Fairthorne will be glad to hear that somewhat reassuring news was received yesterday concerning the recent injury to his eye. Dr. Bowen, the well-known Melbourne oculist, holds out some hopes of the ultimate restoration to sight of the injured optic. At present it is useless, although the opacity is not so intense as it was. An operation will be performed when all inflammatory and other disturbing symptoms have disappeared. One eye only was hurt, the other being perfectly sound. The accident was caused by the bursting of a tube of nitrate of amyle, which is a very volatile chemical, the warmth of Mr. Fairthorne's hands, it is supposed, provoking an expansion of gases to a greater extent than the tube could bear. Whether a minute splinter of glass or the nitrate of amyle caused the injury to the eye, is undetermined as yet.—*Launceston Examiner,* 5th May.

An amusing scene occurred a few days ago in a chemist's shop not many miles from Brunswick-street. A young lady entered and had a prescription made up, and during the time required examined various articles in the show cases around. When paying for the drugs she inquired the price of some soap which had taken her fancy, and the assistant being unable to answer called the proprietor. This gentleman came forward all smiles and smirks. "Ah!" he said, "that is a beautiful soap; quite a new article; most excellent for babies, miss; most excellent for babies!" "Oh! I presume it is what you use, then," the young lady retorted, and left the chemist staring after her with astonishment and vexation. "Confound her impudence," he muttered, as he turned and found the assistants almost exploding in their efforts to control their laughter.

Mr. G. M. Reid, formerly of Castlemaine, has passed his second medical examination at the Edinburgh University.

In another column Mr. J. Holdsworth, of Sandhurst, advertises a number of patent and proprietary medicines for sale or exchange.

The business for some years carried on by Mr. J. Warrington at Echuca has been sold to Dr. Grace, of West Melbourne.

Mr. A. A. Rigney, who for a number of years acted as dispenser at the Sale Hospital, has resigned his appointment and purchased the business of Mr. D. M. T. Lerew at Shepparton.

Another business has changed hands, Mr. Peddington, who for the last nine years has been assistant with Mr. J. Walton, of Gertrude-street, Fitzroy, having recently purchased Mr. W. Witt's business in Carlton.

Mr. J. C. Jones, Campbell-parade, Richmond, announces having taken his son, Mr. J. C. C. Jones, into partnership. The firm will in future be J. C. Jones and Son.

Dr. Thomas Hopper, of Carngham, has been good enough to forward a complete copy of the *Chemist and Druggist* from May, 1880, for the Melbourne Public Library.

Messrs. Rennick, Kemsley and Co., 55 Little Collins-street West, desire to bring under notice that they have just received a number of binocular and minocular microscopes from the well-known manufacturer, Henry Crouch, of London.

Meetings.

THE PHARMACY BOARD OF VICTORIA.

THE monthly meeting of the Board was held at No. 100 Collins-street, on the 10th May. Present—Messrs. Brind, Lewis, Blackett, Bowen, and Owen; Mr. Brind in the chair.

The minutes of the previous meeting were read and confirmed. Apologies were received from Messrs. Bosisto and Holdsworth.

Application for registration approved—William Ball, 96 Swanston-street.

Apprentices indentures registered—F. Waller, Sandhurst; C. S. E. D. Carlisle, Hawthorn; Richard Derry Bowen, Melbourne.

The following cases were considered:—W. F. G. Nettleton, Warrnambool, application to be restored to the pharmaceutical register. Mr. Nettleton attended personally before the board to support his case. After due consideration, the board declined to restore Mr. Nettleton's name. The second and third cases considered were those of Edward Fisher, Sandhurst, and J. T. Weaver, who appeared to have their indentures registered although more then twelve months had elapsed since their execution.

The board decided that the indentures were illegal, and could not therefore be recognised. The applicants would require to pass the preliminary examination and enter into new indentures.

Names erased from the register :—The names of the following deceased persons were erased from the register—F. B. Spicer, Thomas Cox, H. E. E. Bewley, R. D. Murray, and F. Wilkes.

The gold medal of the Pharmaceutical Society.—The examiners recommended that the gold medal given by the Pharmaceutical Society should be awarded to Mr. William Lowe.

Financial and general business brought the meeting to a close.

THE PHARMACEUTICAL SOCIETY OF VICTORIA.

THE monthly meeting of the council was held at the rooms, 100 Collins-street, on the 2nd June. Present—Messrs. Bowen, Baker, Gamble, Nicholls, Thomas, Hooper, Best, Huntsman, Swift, Jones, and Shillinglaw.

The president, Mr. Wm. Bowen, in the chair.

The minutes of the previous meeting were read, and—[?] from the calyx petals red; pod hairy. Habit, calyx, and fruit-valves almost of Bossiæa ; calyx also much like that of the section Euchilus of Pultenaea; affinity to Sphaerolobium more distant, the habit and foliage being quite different, the calyx dissimilar in form and not spotted, the bracteoles far removed for the calyx, the style thinner less twisted and without any appendage, the ovary hairy and the pod not spherical. From all these genera Euchilopsis is moreover separated by its dimorphous anthers, by which characteristic it approaches Templetonia and Hovea, thus connecting the tribe of Podalyrieæ with a portion of that of Genisteæ by an intermediate genus. Among Indian plants, recently added as indigenous to the Australian flora, are also some Leguminosæ, for instance, Desmodium reniforme, obtained at Carpentaria.

QUARTERLY EXAMINATIONS OF THE PHARMACY BOARD.

THE examinations were held as follows :—

The MAJOR EXAMINATION, on 6th June.

Sidney Victor Say, St. Kilda, pharmaceutical meant[?]—Gazette, May ; Geological Survey of Victoria, by F. M'Coy, Decade 2, 4, 5, and 6 ; Analyst, April ; Pharmaceutical Journal, March ; Elements of Agricultural Chemistry and Geology, Johnson and Cameron ; European Mail, April ; Messrs. Burgoyne, Burbridge and Co.'s Circular, April ; Australian Veterinary Journal, June ; Australian Medical Journal, May ; Catalogue of Microscopes, Objectives and Accessory Apparatus ; the Melbourne University Calendar, 1881-1882 ; New Remedies, April and May ; Scientific American, April ; Therapeutic Gazette, March and April.

SYDNEY.

PHARMACEUTICAL SOCIETY OF NEW SOUTH WALES.

THE monthly meeting of the Pharmaceutical Council was held at the board-room, Philip-street, on Tuesday, 16th May, 1882, at 11 a.m.

Present—Mr. A. J. Watt, in the chair, and Messrs. Turner, Row, Guise, and Abraham, the president arriving towards the close of the meeting.

The minutes of last meeting were read and confirmed. Letters were read from Mr. Fred. Wright regarding the society's lectures, and the proposals therein contained were entertained ; and from Mr. Josiah Parker, of Orange, applying for the registration of his son's indentures of apprenticeship to himself, which was granted.

The applications for membership from Mr. H. A. Rose and F. C. Rose were granted on condition of their complying with clause 5 of the constitution. Mr. Alex. Daglish was admitted a member, he having been for many years in business prior to the passing of the Act.

The application of Mr. C. G. Steedman from New Zealand was postponed for the examination of the candidate, and the date of the next examination was fixed for 1st June.

It was decided to hold the annual meeting at the board-room on the evening of the 14th of June.

A letter was read from Mr. Edward Row, resigning his seat on the board. The resignation was accepted with great regret, and a unanimous vote of thanks was passed to Mr. Row for his past services.

The meeting then was brought to a close.

TWO druggists have suffered loss from fire during the past month, one on Tuesday, 25th April, at Messrs. Marshall Bros., of Market-street. A bottle of alcohol took fire and burst in consequence of being stood near a gas-stove. By the prompt and courageous action of one of the proprietors the fire was soon quenched and a heavy loss averted. The second case was a Chinese apothecary in Goulburn-street, supposed to be caused by fireworks kept in stock. The damage would have been comparatively small had it not been for the quarrelling of the firemen and the reckless use of water. The loss is estimated at £1000.

The committee of the School of Arts have appointed Mr. John Henderson, late British Vice-Consul at Hamburg, to the office of secretary.

Mr. W. A. Dixon, F.C.S.. F.I.C., is delivering a series of chemistry lectures at the Technical College. These lectures are free, and attended by audiences varying from one to three hundred. What this lecturer lacks in eloquence he makes up in the sound scientific teaching which distinguishes his utterances from the childish prattle that is so often palmed off upon the Sydney public under the name of "Popular Science."

The Technical College Committee have all the machinery ready for a School of Pharmacy, but it is feared that want of patronage will cause the scheme to be a failure. Not a single pupil has been registered for the botany class.

The resignation of Mr. Edward Row from the Pharmaceutical Council is received by the trade with very great regret, Mr. Row having been widely known and highly esteemed by the profession.

NEW ZEALAND.

PHARMACY BOARD OF NEW ZEALAND.

A MEETING of this board was held in Christchurch on the 10th May, with daily sittings throughout the week. Present : Messrs. C. D. Barraud (Wellington), president ; G. Aickin (Auckland), J. V. Ross (Christchurch), T. M. Wilkinson (Dunedin), and J. A. Allan (Wellington), secretary.

The president, in his opening remarks, stated that up to the present time there had been 234 chemists and druggists registered under the Pharmacy Act of New Zealand ; and that as soon as examinations were established in the four centres proceedings would be instituted against all unregistered chemists carrying on business. It was determined to hold examinations simultaneously at Auckland, Wellington, Christchurch, and Dunedin, the first to be held the first week of July, due notice of which would be given to intending applicants for registration. It was resolved "that the modified examination of the British Pharmaceutical Society be adopted for the present standard, and that a higher standard, the syllabus of which was arranged, should come into operation, in whole or part, with the new elective board in January, 1884." It was agreed to communicate with the pharmacy boards of Victoria, New South Wales, Queensland, and Tasmania, ascertaining the standard of efficiency necessary to insure mutual recognition. A series of text-books for the use of students in pharmacy was approved, and it was ordered that the conspectus of education required by the board should be printed and circulated through the local registrars, and that every facility should be given to place pharmaceutical education on an efficient and permanent footing. The official register of registered chemists for 1883 will be bound up in pamphlet form with the Pharmacy Act of 1880, the Sale of Poisons Act, 1871, and the syllabus of education, text-books, &c.

The resolutions adopted will no doubt convince the chemists throughout the colony, as well as the public, that the provisions of the Pharmacy Act, 1880, are being energetically carried out, so far as circumstances permit ; and also afford some guarantee that the future pharmacist in New Zealand shall, at all events, possess a good education, and be thoroughly efficient in his profession.—New Zealand Times, 22nd May.

PHARMACEUTICAL SOCIETY OF NEW ZEALAND.

THE second annual meeting of this society was held this year in Christchurch, at Coker's Hotel, on the 11th and 12th May. Present—Messrs. C. D. Barraud and Allan (Wellington), T. M. Wilkinson (Dunedin), Graves Aickin (Auckland), and Messrs. J. V. Ross, Bonnington, Irving, Douglass, and Parsons (Canterbury).

The president (Mr. C. D. Barraud) gave an interesting address containing a retrospect of the society's work, and indicating a line of policy for the future calculated to increase the interest taken in the society's proceedings and promote the welfare of pharmacy in this colony. As the constitution of the society provides that the annual meetings shall be held alternately at Christchurch, Auckland, Dunedin, and Wellington, he thought it only right that he should resign his position, and that a Christchurch president be elected, with the head office also in that city.

On the motion of Mr. Aickin, Mr. J. V. Ross was unanimously elected president for the year. The newly elected president then proposed, in the most cordial terms a flattering vote of thanks to Mr. C. D. Barraud (the retiring president), for his unremitting labours at Wellington in promoting the new Pharmacy Act. Carried unanimously. The secretary, Mr. J. A. Allan, of Wellington, also tendered his resignation, which was reluctantly accepted.

A high tribute of commendation, accompanying a vote of thanks, was paid to Mr. Allan by the members present for the efficient energy devoted to the interests of pharmacy and pharmaceutical education.

Mr. C. M. Brooke was elected secretary, and Mr. M. M. Irving treasurer.

It was resolved that the annual subscription be reduced to one guinea, and to assistants half-a-guinea.

The offer of Mr. J. O. Morgan, the proprietor of the English *Chemist and Druggist*, to supply copies of that publication to registered members, through the society, at reduced rates, and afford space in its columns for New Zealand correspondence was accepted, and Mr. Aickin, of Auckland, was appointed to edit and receive communications for transmission through the colony.

The president of the Victorian Pharmaceutical Society was elected an honorary member of the Pharmaceutical Society of New Zealand.

It was proposed by Mr. Barraud, and carried unanimously —"That a cordial vote of thanks be recorded and forwarded to Messrs. C. R. Blackett, M.P., Joseph Bosisto, M.P., and Harry Shillinglaw, secretary Victorian Pharmacy Board, for their willing and generous assistance in promoting the working of the Pharmacy Act by valuable information freely supplied at all times."

The sum of £100 was voted for the purchase of books as the nucleus of a reference library, to be equally divided between the local centres of Christchurch, Dunedin, Wellington, and Auckland.

The introduction of medicinal plants for educational and industrial purposes was considered highly desirable, and the secretary requested that each of the several domain boards throughout the colony asking them to co-operate.

After a vote of thanks to the president, the proceedings terminated.—*New Zealand Times*, 22nd May.

NOTES ON SOME LEGUMINOUS PLANTS.

(BY BARON FERDINAND VON MUELLER, K.C.M.G., M. PH. D., F.R.S.)

IN striving through a long series of years to perfect a system of Australian plants, it was always cheering to the writer to contemplate, that in the course of time medicine and pharmacy could take advantage of these phytographic researches, whenever occasion arose to test any particular plants in reference to its therapeutic value, or its physiological effect, or its chemical constituents. In giving solidity to any such experiments it is necessary, that the investigator should be able to trace with facility the vegetable material under his examination to the exact plant, which afforded the drug, in order that only the genuine species might be utilised elsewhere. Let it not be supposed, that comparatively few of the plants of Australia are possessing medicinal value—contrarily, it may be anticipated, that multitudinous kinds are destined, in a vegetation so rich as ours, to serve for the purpose of *materia medica*. To give a new impetus to original inquiries of this kind, the *pharmaceutic profession* is more particularly

called on to afford some help; and it ought to be an object of every pharmacist, to *form a complete collection of the plants indigenous in his district*, as a step towards the medicinal test of any roots, bark, foliage, flowers or seeds, obtainable from the surrounding native vegetation. The systematic acquaintance with the names of all the plants indigenous anywhere will lead to some rational comparisons with allied plants of other countries, where the therapeutic value of kindred sorts has become established. But in methodic proceedings of this kind also the general knowledge of the flora of the country would be advanced, the regional distribution of known species would be further traced, and with due acknowledgment of the source of information be placed on record. In newer countries for settlement, such botanic inquiries would have for a series of years yet the additional charm of bringing many absolutely new plants under notice, while the characteristics of others from augmented material, to which every pharmaceutic gentleman might contribute easily enough, would be better understood for future editions of our flora. As an instance in this respect, a few notes on such conspicuous plants as the leguminosæ are now offered, showing that even among the stately plants still new forms might be gathered, not merely in distant and unsettled localities, but even near our towns and harbours. Thus the environs of Cooktown furnish as new a highly ornamental Labichea, of which the description is subjoined.

"Most excellent for hahies!" "Oh! I presume it is what you use, then," the young lady retorted, and left the chemist staring after her with astonishment and vexation. "Confound her impudence," he muttered, as he turned and found the assistants almost exploding in their efforts to control their laughter.

Mr. G. M. Reid, formerly of Castlemaine, has passed his second medical examination at the Edinburgh University.

In another column Mr. J. Holdsworth, of Sandhurst, advertises a number of patent and proprietary medicines for sale or exchange.

The business for some years carried on by Mr. J. Warrington at Echuca has been sold to Dr. Grace, of West Melbourne.

Mr. A. A. Rigney, who for a number of years acted as dispenser at the Sale Hospital, has resigned his appointment and purchased the business of Mr. D. M. T. Lerew at Shepparton.

Another business has changed hands, Mr. Peddington, who ... ... nine years has been assistant with Mr. J. Walton, ...

Podopetalum.

Calyx ... ... deltoid teeth of nearly equal length, the two upper approximated, all slightly overlapping in bud. Petals all free, the upper renate, hulching towards the middle, tapering into a stalklike base of moderate length; the four other petals reaching somewhat beyond the upper one, spatular or orbicular, obovate, almost equilateral, attenuated into a long stalklike base. Stamens ten, free; anthers oblong, centrifixed. Disk adnate, reaching to half the height of the calyx-tube, ten-furrowed. Style filiform at first involute. Stigma very minute, terminal. Ovary long-stalked, narrow, without partitions inside. Ovules 6 to 7. Fruit unknown. Leaves pinnate; leaflets large, lanceolar, the uppermost single. Stipules deciduous or obliterated; stipelles none. Racemes paniculated; bracts minute, deltoid persistent; bracteoles rudimentary; petals pink.

Podopetalum differs from the South American genus Bowdichia, to which it closely approximates, in less distinctly developed bracteoles, in not strictly valvular teeth of the calyces, and in not almost round anthers. From Castanospermum it is readily separated by the terminal position of the flower-bunches, by the not almost toothless calyces, and by the petals not being extremely short-stalked. From Sophora and Ormosia it differs already in the longer-stalked petals, none of which dimidiated or auriculated; from Ormosia besides in no portion of the stigma being lateral or dentigerous. Moreover, from all these genera very possibly it may recede widely in characteristics of pericarp and seeds.

While it is thus shown, that yet entirely new forms of plants might be gathered in many parts of Australia, I should like to demonstrate also on this occasion, by some striking example, how much yet remains to be done to follow up the characteristics of even long-known plants in detail. Thus, already in 1837 the illustrious Bentham defined from Baron von

Huegel's West Australian collections an exceedingly pretty leguminous plant as Euchilus linearis ; but noticing subsequently also some affinity of this plant to Sphærolobium, he referred it in 1864 (*Flora Australiensis* II., 67) to that genus. On still closer examination I recognised the necessity of assigning to this Euchilus or Sphærolobium, full generic rank, and have thus defined the new genus as follows :—

Euchilopsis.

Upper lip of the calyx very large, deeply divided into two cuneate-orbicular upwards not angular lobes ; lower lip minute, cleft into three equal semilanceolar segments ; tube very short, upper petal renate, orbicular, not callous ; lateral petals slightly shorter than the upper, little exceeding in length the lower petals ; the latter anteriozely connate at their upper portion, somewhat pointed ; stalklike base of the lateral petals and of the upper one very short ; stamens ten, perfectly free ; filaments slightly dilated from the middle to the base ; anthers alternately longer and shorter, the five longer hasifixed. Style setaceous, glabrous, without any appendage Stigma minute, terminal. Ovary short-stalked, biovulate. Pod obliquely orbicular-ovate, moderately compressed, outside foveolar-rough, 1-2 seeded. Funicle very short. Strophiole none. A dwarf half-shrub ; leaves scattered, coriaceous, linear, with revolute margin ; pedicels axillary, solitary or sometimes in pairs, as long as or longer than the flowers ; bracts basilar, stipulelike, minute, deltoid ; bracteoles, smaller still, distant from the calyx petals red ; pod hairy. Habit, calyx, and fruitvalves almost of Bossiaea ; calyx also much like that of the section Euchilus of Pultenaea ; affinity to Sphaerolobium more distant, the habit and foliage being quite different, the calyx dissimilar in form and not spotted, the bracteoles far removed for the calyx, the style thinner less twisted and without any appendage, the ovary hairy and the pod not spherical. From all these genera Euchilopsis is moreover separated by its dimorphous anthers, by which characteristic it approaches Templetonia and Hovea, thus connecting the tribe of Podalyrieæ with a portion of that of Genisteæ by an intermediate genus. Among Indian plants, recently added as indigenous to the Australian flora, are also some Leguminosæ, for instance, Desmodium reniforme, obtained at Carpentaria.

QUARTERLY EXAMINATIONS OF THE PHARMACY BOARD.

The examinations were held as follows :—

The MAJOR EXAMINATION, on 6th June.
Sidney Victor Say, St. Kilda, passed.

PRELIMINARY EXAMINATION was held at Melbourne, Ballarat, and Sandhurst, on 8th June. Seventeen candidates presented themselves, and the following passed :—

J. Canstoun	Sandridge
H. G. Mau	Sandhurst
E. Fisher	Sandhurst
F. Waller	Sandhurst
James T. Weaver	Emerald Hill
A. F. Davy	Melbourne
Edgar Wing	Echuca

For the MODIFIED EXAMINATION five candidates presented themselves on the 12th June. The following passed :—

Lewellyn Best	Fitzroy
George Phillips	Hamilton

SCHOOL OF MINES SCIENCE SOCIETY, SANDHURST.

AT the annual meeting of members of the School of Mines Science Society in Sandhurst, Mr. E. L. Marks, lecturer on chemistry, read the following very interesting paper, which was illustrated by copious sketches on the black-board, and by some well devised experiments :—

"The study of any subject is greatly facilitated by method, and whether we take up history, literature, the fine arts, or natural science, by dividing and subdividing we obtain a clearer insight as to how one portion depends upon or influences another, or how they reciprocally act, placing ourselves by such a system in a position to survey the completed subject, by uniting the hitherto separate parts, which, like the disjointed pieces of a dissected map, were until then but so many valuable yet isolated fragments. In studying any branch of natural science, we constantly find that collateral information is required to thoroughly explain it. Constant reference is at the same time made to some other branch. For instance, in botany we are referred to chemistry, medi-

cine, physiology, physics, geology, meteorology, &c,, hence we must conclude that there is no sharp line of demarcation anywhere ; indeed, the various branches of science touch at so many points, so constantly interlace, that an acquaintance with all is requisite for the thorough comprehension of any one, just as there is a correlation of the physical forces for chemical action. Heat, light, magnetism, and electricity are thought to be but modifications of some one force, differing only in the manner in which the effects are produced, or according to circumstances in operation ; for chemical action may produce heat and light. Heat will effect chemical decomposition with the evolution of light. Electricity may arise from and will also occasion chemical action ; will again elicit those phenomena, the effects of the calorific. Luminous and actinic rays of the sunbeam are apparent to us in our daily intercourse with Nature, and in every case motion results. Now, motion may be due to the vibration of particles, and will itself occasion sound and colour. Hence it is easier, as well as more philosophical, to regard nature as a whole, for as Pope tersely says :—

> From Nature's chain, whatever link you strike,
> Tenth or ten-thousandth, breaks the chain alike.

If, now, we desire to know *how* a plant grows—by what metamorphoses its constituents are assimilated, by what means the material of its structure are disseminated throughout its system—we require to do more than watch its growth, since at that stage of its existence it is the outcome of many combined agencies. It is a congeries of something and not a single body, hence we must look to the source of the fabric to unravel its history :

The origin of a plant is the cell ; the complete fabric is an organism ; the various parts are organs ; the constituents of organs, cells. What these are I propose to indicate, with the assistance of a few sketches and collated facts from the best available sources.

A cell is a small self-supporting body, that takes up its food through a membrane from without ; inwardly, by a process of diffusion called endosmose—*endon*, inwards ; *osmos*, impulsion. For such an operation to take place there must be a difference in the density on each side of the septum, or a difference in their character ; the thinner liquid then passes with force to mingle with the thicker, this passing outwardly more slowly by an exosmotic movement. To illustrate this statement I have here a tube, one end closed with moistened bladder ; the other with a cork, carrying a long capillary tube. Some tinted alcohol is poured in, and the system is now immersed in water. Under these conditions the water will quickly diffuse inwardly by endosmose, as shown by the rising column of liquid, the alcohol very slowly, by exosmone into the water. That substances capable of permeating such a membrane must be in a liquid or gaseous condition will be evident, since no solid particles, however fine, could possibly pass through. Now, vegetable cells contain liquids of different densities and composition—acid, alkaline, starchy, sugary ; hence, such exosmotic movement must be always going on.

By endosmose, therefore, water holding mineral substances obtained from the soil in a state of solution, penetrates the wall of the cell, ascends by capillary attraction, and under the influence of the vital principle, from one cell to another, through the entire plant, from the root to the leaves. Cells placed near the extremity of the roots contain a highly charged solution of these mineral salts, and, absorbing more water from the soil, dilution takes place ; the second cell then absorbs some of the contents of the first, transmitting them to the third, and so on from cell to cell, the solution depositing in its passage solid matters in the cells it traverses. Arrived at the leaves, much water is given off by evaporation and by transpiration through the stomata that thickly stud those organs, chiefly on the under surface. The crude juice is now exposed to the influence of the carbonic acid gas in the air ; its quality is altered ; part returns downwards through the back to the root to reascend and complete a circulation.

The typical cell is spherical ; through pressure from its neighbours it assumes various shapes, as shown by these sketches ; but in any case it may be regarded as a cavity enclosed by a thin membrane or wall. An inflated bladder will recall the idea. The cell-wall is the part that forms the skeleton of the plant ; that gives toughness to it. It is a continuous membrane, and frequently marked with dots, rings, lines, spheroidal threads, or a kind of network, thought to be due to the unequal absorption of water.

The general term for this membrane is cellulose. Its chemical composition is $C_6H_{10}O_5$. It is the most abundant of the solid parts of plants, and the origin of many substances transformed out of it. In its purest state it is known to us as cotton, this being the "hairs surrounding the seeds of the cotton plant (*Gossypium herbaceum*). Husks of seeds, flax, and fibres generally are varieties of cellulose.

If by pressure cells lengthen in one direction, they frequently have pointed ends; if much lengthened tubes are formed, such form the greater portion of the wood of the plant. When the length and diameter are much increased, vessels result; when by pressure or other cause a mass results, formed by many cells adhering, we get cellular tissue, or parenchyura. If the vessels are very long, with pointed ends, the tissue is prosenchyura; and when the walls are much thickened, elongated, and flexible, the result is pleurenchyura (*pleura*, the side), on account of the support such ribs give to various parts. Pleurenchyura forms the woody fibre of plants, the material of which ropes, cordage, and mats are formed, and from which the more delicate parts have been removed by maceration in water—as in the cases of hemp, flax, bass. If maceration in water be carried much further pulp results, and hence cellulose is readily converted into paper. Pleurenchyura is characteristic of vascular plants ; in those entirely cellular— as fungi, algæ, &c.—decay under the action of water speedily sets in and disrupts them, hence probably the reason that their fossil remains are so rare, whilst plant remains of vascular vegetation are often met with. As cellular tissue is thus composed of an aggregate of cells of various shapes, it is evident they cannot touch on all sides, hence unfilled parts must exist ; such are called intercellular spaces ; they contain air.

Coming now to the interesting question as to what cell-contents are at the outset, the growth of a plant will assume a clearer aspect. Firstly there is a transparent liquid or sap. Within this is a roundish body called the nucleus or cytoblast (*blastos*, a germ), and enclosing the nucleolus. There is also a thick viscid granular slimy body called protoplasm, an essential of living cells, always in motion absent from dead cells. Protoplasm contains water and organic matters, and especially organic matters containing nitrogen. It is the most important of cell-contents, as out of it new ones are formed.

Here is also contained the substance called chlorophyll, or leaf-green, either as a layer or in granules. This is the source of all the green colour in plants. It is only developed under the influence of light, or more strictly under the influence of the red and yellow rays—the rays exciting heat and luminosity —whilst when plants are subjected to the influence of the actinic rays only, by being grown under blue or violet glass screens, they become quite blanched. For the development of chlorophyll, iron is found by experiment to be essential ; deprived of iron it ceases to form. If, then, ferruginous matters are administered, it is quickly produced, and the plant becomes green. Hence it would appear that plants, like animals, are subject to anomia, the same remedy also effecting a cure. From chlorophyll, under various circumstances, the colours of plants are produced. The variegation in leaves is due to alteration or absence of this principle ; so are the gorgeous tints of plants, as seen in the "fall of the leaf." Advantage is taken by gardeners of the fact that light is essential to formation of chlorophyll in the cases of asparagus and celery, for by earthing-up these plants and thus excluding light, the secluded parts become quite blanched. Many efforts have been made by chemists to utilise chlorophyll as a colouring agent in confectionery, the charming tones of green not being readily imitated safely ; but chlorophyll, although apparently pure green, is composed of two distinct principles— phyllo-cyanic and phyllo-xanthic—into which the green quickly resolves itself, nor should we be surprised at it speedily undergoing organic changes since it is from it that Nature forms her varied colours. The two series of colours just mentioned were ingeniously tabulated by De Candolle into the cyanic, or blue, and the xanthic, or yellow green, composed of blue and yellow, occupying the middle, whence the two series diverge thus :—

Red	⎫	Blue-green	⎫
Orange-red		Blue	
Orange		Blue-violet	
Yellow-orange	⎬ Xanthic series	Violet	⎬ Cyanic series
Yellow		Violet-red	
Yellow-green		Red	
Green	⎭		⎭

Beyond indicating the above, I need not deviate further except to mention that chlorophyll is strongly fluorescent— that is, it displays, when properly illuminated and viewed at an angle, a spectral colour not ordinarily visible. Sir John Herschel referred the phenomenon to epipolic dispersion, or dispersion of the rays of light from the first surface of the fluid, irrespective of the gross bulk. Fluorescence derives its name from having been first studied in Fluor spar. but it is a property enjoyed by a great many organic and inorganic bodies. In the present case we have a red fluorescence, in quinine a fine blue, as also in kerosene oil ; in tannine there is a green. And just as there are sounds too deep to be audible, too shrill to be perceived by us, so there are colours ordinarily invisible until the vibrations producing them are so controlled by these fluorescent bodies as to bring them in a condition to stimulate the optic nerve. Advantage may be taken of this property in analysis to detect admixtures. Thus, tannine fluoresces, whilst pure mustard does not. Should the sample be fluorescent, it must be sophisticated with a foreign body, probably tannine. When cells become matured, in addition to cell-sap, protoplasm, and chlorophyll, they contain a great variety of other substances. The pulp of an orange contains citric acid. In the potato the cells are filled with starch, a body readily recognised by the blue colour formed on adding iodine to it, as may be observed here. Starch varies physically, according to its source ; and by the microscope the starch from maize, wheat, potato, arrowroot, sago, tapioca, &c., may each be distinguished, but chemically it has the same composition as cellulose $C_6H_{10}O_5$, and from starch many proximate principles are formed, such as sugar, dextrin gum ; hence it may be regarded as a reserve food for the formation of these and other active matters. Then we have wax, oils, fats, resins, balsams, as the contents of cells. In the grass family silica is found ; in rhubarb, onion, squill, banana, crystals of oxalate of calcium are met with ; but far the most important of cell-contents, physiologically considered, is albumen, corresponding to white-of-egg, a body rich in nitrogen, and serving for the support of the young plant, as in the egg it does for the young chick during incubation. It is to albumen in vegetables that a ropy appearance is due when an infusion of herbs is heated, and coagulating at a temperature of 160 degs. F., it rises as a scum, or sinks as dregs, enclosing within its meshes all suspended matters ; thus liquids are clarified. Albumen also contains sulphur, the cause of mustard spoons and egg spoons, when of silver, becoming discoloured.

Frequently in medicinal infusions it is desirable to exclude starch and albumen, as that is not dissolved in cold water. Whilst this coagulates by heat, a cold infusion subsequently heated will remain clearer and brighter than if otherwise made.

The growth of a plant is the aggregate result of the enlargement and multiplication of cells. In a fungus the growth is especially rapid, but in any case the continuous growth depends upon the constant growth of new cells. Each cell is thought to grow by intersusception or the intercolation of fresh particles between those already formed, and not as is the case with shells by the deposition of layers on the inside. Ordinarily cells are microscopic objects. In the cotton, however, they may be one or two inches in length ; in the lemon they are about half-an-inch long, still longer in the shaddock. Their multiplication takes place in several ways, either the entire protoplasm is consumed in forming a new one out of those already formed as in a swarm-spore, or two cells in close proximity transfer protoplasium matter from one to another through a tube, or again by a kind of budding as in the grass plant, small, independent cells being thrown off.

Under varying conditions modifications in the form and structure of cells must take place to produce the great variety we see in nature. Then there are fibres and vessels through which nourishment is conveyed, these often having spiral vessels inside, or tubes fashioned into rings. In some vessels is found the true juice of the plant or latex, a fluid becoming white on exposure to the air. Assafœtida is such a juice exuding from an umbelliferous plant growing in Persia, Afghanistan, and the Punjaub ; the milky exudation from a freshly cut dandelion stalk is another example of latex.

The epidermis is composed of a layer of tubular cells, the cuticle of another layer above this. Stomata or breathing pores are cells thickly studding the under surface of the leaf. These are also present on the stem, the epidermis, and the flower, but absent from the root. Hence by this means the true root may be distinguished from the under-ground stem.

Various appendages formed of altered cells, and called trichomes, are distinguished as hair bristles, prickles, and scales, each characterised by qualities indicative of these organs, according to length, position, hardness, &c.

The brown, chafflike substance on ferns, called rameuta, from resembling chips or shavings, is formed of greatly elongated cells. When cells secrete peculiar substances they are called glands; in the orange they secrete a fragrant oil; in the nettle an irritating fluid; in the sun-dew a viscid solution; in an acacia a kind of honey, and so on."

The foregoing remarks are to serve as a stimulus to such members as have leisure to pursue this fascinating branch of natural science.

Legal and Magisterial.

MAGISTERIAL INQUIRY.

A MAGISTERIAL inquiry, touching the death of Edwin Adams, chemist and druggist, Heathcote, was held by James Christie, Esq., J.P., at the Heathcote Hotel, on the 10th May, when the following depositions were taken:—

Henry Scobell, sworn, deposed—I am a legally qualified medical practitioner, residing at Heathcote. Knew the deceased, Mr. Adams, and was in his company from one till a quarter to three o'clock yesterday afternoon, when I was called away. He made a hearty dinner, and when I left him was sitting by the fire reading a paper; he appeared to be in his usual state of health. When I returned home at six o'clock I heard that I had been sent for to see him, and that he was dead.

Daniel Pammenter, sworn, stated—I am an hotelkeeper, residing at Heathcote. Knew the deceased Mr. Edwin Adams, who resided opposite the hotel, and carried on the business of a chemist and druggist. He was a frequent visitor at the hotel, and occasionally had his meals here. About seven minutes past five o'clock yesterday evening, I saw him come from the garden, shut the gate, and walk along the verandah, apparently in his usual health. A few minutes after Mary Young called me to see the deceased, whom I found lying across the chair with his feet on the floor, and his head nearly touching the floor with a paper on the table before him, he appeared to have been reading. Lifted him up and immediately sent for medical assistance. Did not at first think he was dead, but as I could not find any signs of his breathing, and as he did not come to, I thought he was dead. Have known deceased for over twenty years. Reported the matter to the police at once.

James Charles M'Kee, sworn—I am a legally qualified medical practitioner, residing at Heathcote. I was called to see the deceased about a quarter past five o'clock yesterday evening. When I arrived, and examined him, I found life extinct. Have since made a *post-mortem* examination of the body, and found the immediate cause of death was serous apoplexy. His heart was healthy, but his liver was very much enlarged, and the kidneys contracted. There was food in the stomach, and the stomach had a healthy appearance. The amount of serous effusion into the brain was sufficient to cause instantaneous death.

A decision was given to the effect that death resulted from serous apoplexy.

PROSECUTION UNDER THE PHARMACY ACT.

AT the City Police Court, Ballarat, on the 20th May, before Mr. J. C. Thomson, P.M., and a full bench of honorary magistrates, Alfred Perkins was proceeded against by Detective Hyland, under the Pharmacy Act, 40 Vict., No. 558, clause 25, subsection 1. The clause referred to applies to any person, not being a registered pharmaceutical chemist, who carries on or attempts to carry on business as a chemist or druggist, or homœopathic chemist, or either. The maximum penalty for an infringement of such regulation is a fine of £10 and imprisonment in adition for six months.

Mr. Gaunt appeared for the defendant; Detective Hyland conducted the case.

The first witness called was Mr. Harry Shillinglaw, registrar of the Pharmacy Board of Victoria. He produced the *Gazette* containing the formal appointment of the board, also his own appointment as registrar. Witness produced the register of pharmaceutical chemists duly qualified under the Act, and deposed that he did not know defendant. No such name as that of Alfred Perkins appeared on the register.

To Mr. Gaunt—The name of Robert Dixon Bannister, of Ballarat, appears on the register as a pharmaceutical chemist of Victoria.

Constable Corrigan, of Ballarat West, gave evidence to the effect that on the 16th inst. he purchased from the defendant, at a shop in Sturt-street, a bottle of medicine. Witness gave defendant the piece of paper produced. Perkins then asked him if he would like a homœopathic preparation, to which he replied in the affirmative. Defendant then gave witness the bottle of belladonna produced, for which he paid one shilling.

To Mr. Gaunt—Had never been in the shop before to my knowledge. I received the prescription from Detective Hyland. Do not know who wrote it. The label on the bottle produced is "Belladonna—Posion. This bottle is labelled poison in conformity with the Act for the Sale of Poisons. R. D. Bannister, dispensing chemist, 5 Sturt-street." The shop has all the appearance, both outside and inside, of being a dispensing chemist's shop. I was supplied with the medicine by defendant, from which fact I would presume he was a dispensing chemist.

Mr. Gaunt—So you would term Messrs. Eyres Bros. dispensing chemists for selling bluestone or arsenic to their customers?

Witness continued.—I do not know whether I can buy the same at any shop. Do not know whether I could get it at Hammond's. Have never seen belladonna retailed in public-houses or groceries.

Mr. Shillinglaw, re-examined, stated that if the contents of the bottle were belladonna they were poison. Belladonna was not a patent medicine. No storekeeper had power to sell poisons without authority.

To Mr. Gaunt—I am not a chemist.

Mr. H. Brind, who was next examined, stated that he had been a chemist for a number of years. Storekeepers had no authority to sell belladonna. He supposed what was in the bottle produced was a preparation. Was not acquainted with defendant. Belladonna was used both externally and internally. If what was in the bottle was strong, it would be a poison. Knew the whereabouts of Mr. Bannister's shop. Mr. Bannister had not been carrying on business there personally for the last two or three years. Witness knew that he was in Sydney receiving a salary.

To Mr. Gaunt—Mr. Bannister had not been occupying the shop at least for twelve or eighteen months to my knowledge. I do not know that he was paying rent for it, or deriving profits therefrom. Captain Bloomfield informed me that Mr. Bannister was occupying a position of profit in Sydney.

Detective Hyland stated that he knew defendant personally to have been connected with the shop during the last three or four years. Witness served the summons in the present instance on the 17th inst., at the shop. Witness told defendant he was instructed to take proceedings, as he was not registered under the Pharmacy Act. Defendant, in reply, then said he knew that he was in a false position, but that he had been studying for the last five years at the School of Mines, in order to pass the necessary examination. He stated that he was about to write to the board to ask if he would be allowed to pass a modified examination. Defendant also informed witness that Mr. Bannister was in Sydney, and had not been in Ballarat since the Melbourne Exhibition, and that the business was for sale. Perkins also stated he had asked Mr. Bannister to give him increased facilities, and that he had had sufficient experience in the shop to pass an examination. Witness noticed, on the left hand wall when entering the shop, printing to the following effect :—" R. D. Bannister, late C. Pleasance, homœopathic chemist." The shop, to all appearances, was a chemist's shop, and had within it coloured bottles, &c,

To Mr. Gaunt—I have not known Mr. Perkins to make up the prescriptions of a legally qualified medical practitioner. The writing on the paper produced by Constable Corrigan is not a prescription. I did not write on the paper—" 1s.—Belladonna." I do not think it necessary to tell you who did. The paper should not have been put in as evidence. It was merely asking for a shilling's worth of belladonna. I will not tell you who wrote the prescription unless directed to do so by the bench. I asked a chemist to write it for me, and he did so.

This closed the proceedings for the prosecution, and Mr. Gaunt submitted that no case had been made out. There was nothing in the Act under which the complaint was brought to prevent any person selling drugs, and if he (Mr. Gaunt) so chose he could keep in his chambers Turkey rhubarb or jalup, and physic his clients, if it would do them any good. There was no evidence to show what was sold by defendant to Corrigan. Belladonna had its uses besides for physic, and was sold to ladies, who used it for their eyes, in order to enhance their beauty. Mr. Gaunt further pointed out that not long ago Mr. Hammond sold homœopathic preparations, and he was bound to say there was not a shop up country where there would not be seen Gould and Martin's homœopathic cases. So far as the evidence went, he maintained the case must be dismissed, as the intention of the Act was to prevent unqualified persons from compounding medicines. He submitted that no case had been made for the prosecution, but that the evidence, in fact, had made clean the defendant's own case.

Mr. Thomson stated the magistrates were of opinion that no breach of the Act had been proved, and the case was therefore dismissed without costs.

Mr. Gaunt then informed the bench that Mr. Bannister had been communicated with by telegram, and that steps would at once be taken to obtain the services of a qualified person until Mr. Perkins had qualified himself by passing the necessary examinations.

THE FAILURES OF POLICE PROSECUTIONS AT BALLARAT.

THE prosecution of Mr. A. Perkins, at Ballarat, for non-compliance with the provisions of the Pharmacy Act by keeping an open shop, not being registered, broke down through sheer carelessness, or want of knowledge, on the part of the police, who appeared to prosecute unassisted by an advocate, whilst the defendant was aided by learned counsel in the person of Mr. Gaunt, barrister, and late police magistrate, who appeared to be well acquainted with the Act. Everything went wrong from the beginning. The sergeant of police, who usually conducts cases in the police court, was objected to by the defendant's counsel, and the detective officer who had charge of the case was unprepared, or unused to such proceedings, and was consequently hamboozled by Mr. Gaunt. Mr. Shilling-law could not give any evidence as an expert, and, with the exception of Mr. Brind, who gave evidence as to the defendant's identity, no other witnesses were called; consequently Mr. Gaunt, having overawed the detective, had the rest of it all his own way, and took advantage of the court by saying "the Pharmacy Act did not prevent any one selling drugs; even he himself could keep a stock in his office for the benefit of his clients if he thought fit to do so." And so he could if he liked to give them away; but he must not use the title, or sell those scheduled as poisons, and that was the point the prosecution had in view. Belladonna is a poison, and is in the second schedule *as not to be sold except under certain conditions.* It was selected by the police for purchase on that account; and although labelled "Poison," this point was neglected by the prosecution, and so the case fell through. Now, if a solicitor had been employed, things should have been different. In the first place, two summonses should have been served upon the defendant—one for keeping an open shop, and the other for selling poisons. And if this had been done I doubt if even the most astute lawyers would have saved their client from the penalties; but as the case stands now, aided by what the police magistrate concurred in from the bench, persons not being druggists will feel inclined to set the Pharmacy Act at defiance, and nothing else but a good stiff case of poisoning will set the public against that proceeding. Even as it was, after the case was decided defendant's counsel admitted what would have proved the case for the prosecution—"That Mr. Bannister had been communicated with, and had obtained *a duly qualified person to conduct the business until Mr. Perkins had passed his examination.*"

REMINISCENCES OF A PHARMACIST.

(*Continued.*)

"A SYDNEY CHEMIST OF THE OLDEN TIME" AND A SHORT ASSISTANTSHIP.

I PRESENTED myself punctually at eight o'clock the next morning, according to orders, and as the principal had not yet put in an appearance, took a seat in front of the counter and a good look about me. I was aware that this was the identical shop in which the notorious "Tawell" (whose career I sketched in my first paper) had made his fortune, and it will not be wondered at that I regarded with curiosity the bottles and jars on the shelves, many, and indeed most, of which had been often touched by his murderous hands.

The shop, which was double fronted and low pitched, and which bore every mark of antiquity, was devoted to the united businesses of chemist and grocer, distinct counters and fittings embracing each side of the shop as you entered from the street, the windows, of course, being decorated in a suitable manner.

After sitting for some time taking mental stock of the place Mr. F——, the proprietor, made his appearance fresh from the breakfast-table, from which he had evidently risen in a bad humour, for he said to me rather snappishly, "Oh, *you've* come, have you? well, don't sit there staring about you, but get to work;" an order which, of course, I immediately obeyed, although I could not help thinking that a more gentlemanly tone could have been used without in any way detracting from his portly dignity, for portly he was, but by no means ungainly-looking, although his clothes and general appearance were antique and in keeping with the establishment. I saw but little of him, however, for he was out nearly all the morning, but on the one or two occasions on which he did come behind the counter his manner was decidedly pompous and overbearing. His son, a lad of eighteen or nineteen years of age, was with me, and seemed to be equally at home behind the counter. This young gentleman was a decided chip of the old block, not having a very extensive knowledge of drugs and chemicals, but any amount of assurance, as people of this class usually have, and put on airs which seemed to say—"I must keep you at a distance; you are only an assistant, but I am the son of the boss."

As I had always been treated in England as one of the family in every situation which I had held, I was not prepared for the kind of reception which awaited me at the dinner table. Young F—— had relieved the grocer's assistant and myself that we might partake of the mid-day meal, and we went in together for that purpose. At the head of a very long table Mr. F—— and the family were discussing their dinner. To these I was not introduced, but, under the directions of my guide, I sat down before one of the two plates of half-cold meat at the extreme end of the table. That this was to be our *allowance* was attested by the fact that all the dishes appertaining to the meal had been removed. A glass of water, placed beside each plate, on a board where ale and porter bottles were still standing, spoke to the fact that in this establishment at least Jack was by no means reckoned as good as his master.

At tea the same routine was observed. A few slices of bread and butter of the boarding-school stamp, and a cup of (*tea*, I was going to say; well, if it was, it must have been of the third or fourth generation) being our portion.

I do not recollect at this distance of time the exact hour at which the shutters were put up, but know that as there were no lights in the shop and occasional customers were served up to half-past eleven, that was the actual time at which the business of the day was supposed to come to an end.

I had been all alone for more than an hour (for the grocery assistant left at ten), when the errand boy brought in a stretcher, mattress, &c., and proceeded to make his bed behind the counter, when he leisurely undressed himself, and, bidding me a sleepy "Good night," turned in.

Just as I was wondering whether I was expected to follow the boy's example behind my own counter, Young F. came in and graciously inquired if I took suppers. Having replied in the affirmative, I was treated to a slice of thick bread and a morsel of bad cheese, with a glass of water from the best tap; and having disposed of this sumptuous fare, the worthy head of the establishment conducted me in person to my dormitory. This, I found, was at the very bottom of the yard, over a sort of scullery, and adjoining the stable. Here, having ascended by means of a ladder, my conductor left me to repose. The furniture of the chamber was not luxurious. It consisted of a rickety bed, a chair the worse for wear, and wash-basin and ewer, mounted on an old packing case. There was no carpet on the floor; but an old sack cut in two was laid down by the side of the bed. There was a very scant supply of bed-clothes, and I knew that I was wretchedly cold all the night; but towards morning I fell asleep, and hardly seemed to have done so when a voice, which I recognised as belonging to F., senior, asked me if I was going to sleep all day; and as it was then pitch dark, he left the candle which he carried, and told me to look sharp and present myself in the shop. When I got downstairs I found the gas alight, and the boy sweeping and dusting, in which duties I was, of course, expected to join.

I did not go to breakfast that morning, as I had had enough of Mr. F. and his amiable son. And as soon as the latter gentleman made his appearance, and suggested that I should send for my traps, I respectfully begged to be excused, and left the service, after a short assistantship of twenty-four hours.

STARTING A SHOP UNDER DIFFICULTIES.

I was so thoroughly disgusted with the twenty-four hours' service of the eminent "Mr. F——, chemist, druggist, grocer, &c.," that I determined to make a start for myself at all hazards, and, as I was not known to many persons in the city of Sydney, and could not reasonably expect much assistance in the credit line, I had to make my ninety odd pounds go as far as possible ; and to this end set myself to work to fit up with my own hands a small shop which I had secured in the rising suburb of Newtown.

This I was able to do with tolerable neatness, for a three years' residence in the bush, where almost my first act had been to build my own house, had made me a tolerable adept at the carpenter's art. I found it, however, a much easier task to procure the wood for shelving than I did to get the necessary bottles, &c., to put on them after they were up ; and those of my younger brethren who have started in business within the past ten or fifteen years, and found our splendid wholesale establishments capable of supplying their every want, from a pillbox to the most elaborate specie jar, will smile when I tell them that day after day I searched Sydney, from one end to another, to procure a few narrow and wide-mouthed bottles, suited to the requirements of an ordinary shop, with the result of obtaining one here and one there, kindly raked out from some outhouse or other, the whole forming such a rascally collection when arranged that I was ashamed to let daylight on them by taking down the shutters ; and I was nearly giving way to despair, when good luck caused me to turn into a china shop in desperation. This was about the last place I should have thought where I should be likely to find my requirements. Yet, strange to say, find them here I did, to the mutual joy of the storekeeper and myself—he, because he had found a purchaser for what he told me he had long considered a dead stock, and I, because they were the very identical things I most coveted. There was about a gross of them altogether, and when labelled in gold (which I was fortunately able to do myself, or they would have remained unlettered), they put on a tolerably respectable appearance. Such a thing as an ointment, or even an extract jar, was not to be thought of ; and I was fain to make shift with some yellow culinary affairs, purchased at the crockeryware shop where I had picked up the bottles ; and then, having laid in a stock of drugs and patent medicines, as extensive and varied as my limited means would permit, I took down my shutters, and became at once a full-fledged chemist and druggist, announcing this fact by letters over the door and window, which cost me the last penny of capital. But my difficulties did not end here ; all my pills had to be rolled singly by hand, for such a thing as a pill machine was not to be purchased for love or money. Leeches were unobtainable ; and on inquiring for seidlitz boxes I was told that I should have to make my own, as most—or, I should say, all—of the chemists at that period were doing. (The reader will please to remember that I am writing of the latter end of 1852, when the industries of box-making, leech-gathering, &c., were unknown.) This, however, I did not find an arduous task, for I had, of course, ample leisure for the work, and the stationers' shops supplied the materials. As the diggings, both in New South Wales and Victoria, were then in their zenith, people had plenty of money to spend, and, what is more, were not afraid to spend it ; and as there was no fear of offending a customer by asking too much, prices ran high, and I was soon enabled to renew my stock on a much larger scale.

(*To be continued.*)

Correspondence.

PARCELS POST—NEW REGULATIONS WANTED.

To the Editor of the Australasian Supplement to the Chemist and Druggist.

SIR—As doubtless there will be some alteration in postal matters ere long, will you kindly allow me to draw attention to a want felt very generally by druggists—that is, the convenience of sending small quantities of liquids through the post.

At present the public generally are debarred from doing so ; but I venture to think that it affects our calling to an extent far beyond any other. In districts where there are no railways, and sometimes no conveyance but that of a packhorse, this regulation is a complete handicap to business ; for to send small parcels otherwise than through post entails upon the customer a cost of more than the article itself. I could give numberless illustrations of this anomaly, but will content myself with mentioning the fact, and hope that it may be the means of bringing about some concession, and would ask your aid, sir, likewise that of the Pharmaceutical Society, which, being ably supplemented at the proper time by that of our worthy M.L.A.'s, Messrs. Bosisto and Blackett, may possibly be the means of conferring a boon that would be widely appreciated.—I am, sir, yours, &c.   J. TIPPING.
Bairnsdale, 9th June, 1882.

STEAMY WINDOWS.

To the Editor of The Australasian Supplement to the Chemist and Druggist.

SIR—In the *Chemist and Druggist* of December, 1881, appears an article on the above subject, and no doubt in this colony, especially in the cold districts, chemists' windows are affected in the same manner during the winter months. The plan I have adopted is to open the slides of the windows about four inches, and let them remain so while the lights are burning, which, of course, is only at night, when dust and flies cannot cause extra labour in cleaning, as they are rarely to be seen in winter. I find this plan answer very well ; my windows always appear bright, and entirely free from the nuisance.—I am, yours respectfully,   COUNTRY CHEMIST.

"SUMMUM JUS, SUMMA INJURIA."

To the Editor of The Australasian Supplement to the Chemist and Druggist.

SIR—We have just got over what is termed the first representative meeting of pharmacy in New Zealand, and, as Victorian chemists are interested to some extent, I crave space in your valuable journal for a few remarks thereon.

The Pharmacy Board of New Zealand are great on "reciprocity," which, if I understand the word, means equal mutual rights or benefits, to be yielded or enjoyed ; but I have not yet been able to find the dictionary that will bear out the construction put upon the word by the Pharmacy Board of New Zealand, which is that we must be admitted to all the rights and benefits enjoyed by our Australian brethren, and having nothing to offer in exchange, nothing can be expected from us beyond our bare assurance that we are splendid chemists and highly respectable people.

A registered chemist of Victoria, whose certificate is dated 1881, applied for admission, and was refused. When the subject was being considered, a member of the board remarked that the Victorians admitted all kinds and conditions of men, or words of similar import ; and a resolution was passed to the effect that only Victorians who have passed the examination be admitted in New Zealand.

This, I think, for cool assurance would be difficult to surpass. It is virtually saying to the Pharmacy Board of Victoria— "You are not competent to determine who are eligible for registration. Gentlemen who have been twenty years in business in Victoria cannot be admitted here, and, to insure our standard of superiority, none but chemists by examination need apply."

I must not omit to mention that our first puny attempt at examination is to take place some time in July next.

If the gentleman who indulged in this high falutin will step down from his self-erected pinnacle of pharmaceutical pre-eminence, I will show him another phase of the subject, which from his elevated position he has evidently overlooked.

There are about two hundred and thirty chemists in New Zealand, amongst whom are a fair sprinkling of "all kinds and conditions" of men, comprising carpenters, watchmakers, bakers, &c., who are full-fledged registered pharmaceutical chemists of New Zealand, and are with this gentleman co-equally entitled to all the rank, dignity, and titles of the profession.

It would not be difficult to run down the names and place your finger upon some to whom the *British Pharmacopœia* is a sealed book. There are yet more such to come, and the

Pharmacy Board of New Zealand cannot, dare not, refuse registration.

Nearly one-third of the registered chemists of New Zealand are in this district, and I can say that they are unanimous in condemning the action of the board in this matter.

It would be very interesting to know how many pharmacies there are in New Zealand where a youth could be sufficiently instructed in the art and mystery of the profession to enable him to pass the *modified examination* of the Victorian Pharmacy Board. I venture to say that before you counted your fingers once over their number would be exhausted, and I should not be surprised if the first finger proved to be one too many.—Yours very truly,   NATRIUM.

Dunedin, 31st May, 1882.

To the Editor of The Australasian Supplement to the Chemist and Druggist.

DEAR SIR—In my letter last month a number of printer's errors crept in, which must have made my meaning anything but clear. Perhaps the best way to correct them will be to re-write the misinterpreted portions. In referring to the necessity for more frequent communication between prescriber and dispenser, I mentioned as examples the following cases wherein misunderstanding often occurs:—Chloric ether is dispensed variously, as 1 in 8, 1 in 10, or 1 in 20, according to the dispenser's fancy. The sign ℥i. is taken by some to be 480 grains, and by others 437½ grains. The last, being its official value, is strictly correct, but many prescribers are known to mean the former. Many similar discrepancies exist; but the dose is the part of the prescription where the greatest error occurs. A doctor who orders a tablespoonful must mean some definite quantity; but the amount taken varies greatly, according to the fancy of the patient or the size of his spoons. Some years ago I suggested that fluid drams or ounces should be ordered in all cases, supposing that the dispenser would then feel bound to supply the means for accurate measurement; but I find many dispensers interpret these terms teaspoonful or tablespoonful without any qualification, so that the prescriber's attempt to secure accuracy fails. I will not trouble you further at present, but hoping that the matter will be taken up, I am, yours truly,   ALFRED I. OWEN.

To the Editor of The Australasian Supplement to the Chemist and Druggist.

SIR—In your issue of March a paragraph appears stating that carrots treated with arsenic are a certain specific for the destruction of rabbits. You will oblige by publishing the mode of preparing the poison.—Yours, &c.,

Invercargill, 4th May, 1882.   E. B. JONES.

[1 oz. of arsenic dissolved in q: suff: sub-carbonate of soda to 30 lbs. of carrots.—*Ed.*]

REPLIES TO CORRESPONDENTS.

CHARLES RABIN.—According to law "fixtures, utensils of trade, &c." are not included in insurance upon "stock-in-trade."

"SANITAS."—As to the question, "What extra liability does the employé of an unregistered person incur?" an "unregistered person" has no legal right to practise pharmacy, and therefore cannot employ any one. Unregistered assistants have no right to dispense medicines or sell poisons. If a pharmaceutical chemist employs an unqualified person, he is liable and responsible for all the assistant does. If an assistant is registered, he is responsible, and the principal also.

A PHARMACEUTICAL CURRICULUM FOR GREAT BRITAIN.

THE proposed curriculum for pharmaceutical education in England, decided upon by the committee appointed by the council, is as follows. It will be observed that it closely resembles our own:—

"First, that candidates for examination be required to produce evidence of apprenticeship or pupilage of not less than three years under some duly registered chemist and druggist.

"Second, that the preliminary examination, or its equivalent, be passed prior to apprenticeship or pupilage. In regard

to this recommendation, it was suggested that the object in view might in most cases be ensured by not permitting a candidate to present himself for the minor examination until three years after he had been certified to have passed the preliminary.

"Third, that candidates upon presenting themselves for the minor examination shall, in addition to the requirements above mentioned, produce evidence to show that they have, within the time then present and the date of their preliminary examination, attended a course of lectures on chemistry, a course of lectures on botany, a course of lectures on *materia medica*, and a course of instruction on practical chemistry, of the scope and character defined in certain syllabuses presented with the report. With respect to the authoritative recognition of the lectures and teaching referred to in this recommendation, the committee recommended that the council should, at its discretion, recognise and accept certificates from those public schools of sciences throughout the country of which the principal, or dean, or other corresponding officer or authority, shall have satisfied the council that their scope of teaching on the required subjects includes the points enumerated in the above-mentioned syllabuses, as well as from other schools in which it shall have been proved to the satisfaction of the council that the teaching is of sufficient excellence in kind, and of the scope indicated in the syllabuses. It was suggested that, from time to time, a list of such recognised schools should be published.

"The fourth recommendation of the committee was that the minor examination should be divided into two parts, with an interval of not less than six months between the first and second portions of it. It was proposed that the first portion should be a written examination, to be conducted under suitable regulations in London, Edinburgh, and certain provincial centres to be agreed upon by the council, and that it should consist of the translation of prescriptions from Latin into English and from English into Latin, also of pharmacy and theoretical chemistry and botany. Candidates would not receive any certificate on passing this part of the examination, but would be entitled to present themselves after an interval of not less than six months for the second part of the examination, which it was proposed should be essentially *viva voce* and experimental, comprising chemistry and practical chemistry, botany and *materia medica*, and practical dispensing.

"The fifth recommendation was that these proposed regulations should come into operation on the 1st of January, 1886."

Notes and Abstracts.

HOW TO DISTINGUISH SALIVA SPOTS IN CLOTHES FROM OTHERS OF SIMILAR APPEARANCE.—Dr. Cervera gives a simple mode of distinguishing salivary stains from spermatic and others of similar appearance with which they may be confounded. This distinction is often of importance in medico-legal cases. The piece of cloth containing the spot is by capillarity moistened with a saturated solution of ferric chloride. Chemical reaction will give rise to a blood-red colour in the case of saliva, but not in stains due to other fluids. Carotid saliva, especially after meals, contains the sulpho-cyanide of potassium, a substance which strikes an intense red colour in contact with ferric salts, although these may be present only in minute quantity. Such reaction does not take place in the case of pus, nasal or vaginal mucus, spermatic or gonorrhœal fluid.—*Cron. Med.-Quir de la Hab.*

WORSE THAN PRESCRIPTION LATIN.—According to *Harper's Weekly*, the members of the New York Medical Club were invited to an entertainment a few years ago by Dr. H. D. Paine, of that city, in the following terms:—"'SCIENS, SOCIALITE, SOBRIETE.'—DOCTORES—Ducum nex mundi nitu Pancs; triticum at ait. Expecto meta fumen tu te & eta beta pi. Super attento, uno. Dux, hamor clam pati, sum paratos, homine, ices, jam, &c, Sideror hoc. Anser. 'FESTO REASONAN FLOAS SOLE.'"

ANTI-ASTHMATIC POWDER.—

Potassæ nitratis	} aa ℥ ss.
Pulv. anisi fructus	
Pulv. stramonii folior	℥ j.

Misce. A thimbleful of the powder placed on a plate is pinched into a conical shape and lighted at the top. It burns like a pastile, and is held near the patient, who inhales the fumes.—Jas. Sawyer, M.D., in *British Med. Journal.*

The remedy for snake-bites recommended by Dr. Lacerda, which has recently attracted considerable attention, is already experiencing the fate, in part, of all its predecessors, in having to submit to adverse criticism. M. Vulpian states (*Comptes Rendus*, xciv., 613) that when 1 per cent. of permanganate of potash is injected hypodermically into a dog it is almost immediately decomposed, a brown deposit of the binoxide taking place in a limited circle round the puncture. He therefore thinks that such a solution could be of little service except in very recent bites. Further, he found that the intravenous injection of 0·5 gram of permanganate was itself sufficient to cause the death of a small dog in from ten to twenty hours.

A new antidote to strychnine has been discovered by Messrs. Greville, Williams and Waters (*Proc. Royal Society*, xxxi., p. 162) in β lutidine, which is produced in the distillation of cinchonine with caustic potash. A frog first treated with β lutidine and then dosed with strychnine was not tetanised ; in another, in which tetanus had been induced by the administration of strychnine, the spasms were found to pass off when β lutidine was given ; and when both bases were simultaneously given no effect was produced.

The results of some experiments as to the evaporation of glycerine have been put on record by M. Couttolenc (*Répertoire*, x., 73). He states that if heated in a water-bath to 90 degs. C., glycerine will lose in five hours any water it may contain, and that then the evaporation of the glycerine proceeds regularly at the rate of about 0·00317 gram per square centimetre of surface exposed. This proportion is increased by the admixture of sand, and rapidly diminished by the lowering of the temperature. The more water there is present in the glycerine the greater is the quantity of glycerine carried off in the evaporation, but the quantities are not in regular proportion.

Mr. A. R. Bennett has described before the Glasgow Philosophical Society a cheap form of voltaic battery, which well deserves notice. The battery consists of a zinc and iron combination in caustic soda solution. In the specimen shown the containing vessels were an Australian meat can containing iron borings and a porous cell holding caustic soda solution, together with a piece of sheet zinc. The electro-motive force of this new battery is 1·23 volts., or practically the same as the Leclanche form (1·30 volts.). A practical comparison of the "Bennett" and the Leclanche cells was made by setting each cell to ring an electric bell of five ohms resistance. The Leclanche cell vibrated the bell hammer continuously for twenty days, while the "Bennett" cell vibrated a similar bell hammer continuously for thirty-one days, or a difference in favour of the "Bennett" cell of eleven days. A detailed description of this new battery will be found in the *Electrician* of 25th February and 4th March, and in the *English Mechanic* of 10th March.

Mrs. Mulhall, in *Between the Amazons and Andes*, gives a curious account of the origin of the name of the celebrated botanist, Bonpland. Visiting the house of one of his friends at Corriente, she came across a manuscript in Bonpland's writing, which begins :—"I was born at Rochelle on 29th August, 1773. My real name was Amadé Goryand. My father —a physician—intended me for the same profession. It was on account of my great love for plants that he gave me the *sobriquet* of 'Bon-plant,' which I afterwards adopted instead of my family name."

In Italy the disease known as pellagra, and which is said to be as fatal in that country as consumption is in Great Britain, has been attributed to the exclusive use of maize or Indian corn for food, especially when damaged grain has been ground. According to the recent researches of Lambroso (*Revue Scientifique*, 20th January, 1882), the substance which causes the symptoms characteristic of the disease is not the spore of the fungus which is formed on the grain, but an active principle which can be obtained from it by a process analogous to that by which ergotine is obtained from ergot of rye. This substance is called by its discoverer "pellagrozeine." A tincture made from damaged maize, taken in doses of six grams daily, was found to produce in twelve workmen all the symptoms characteristic of incipient pellagra. It has been noted by Stambio that the majority of those who, suffering from this disease, commit suicide, do so by drowning. This would seem

to arise from the pleasure experienced in seeing and touching water, which is one of the symptoms characteristic of the disease.—*Pharmaceutical Journal and Transactions.*

The danger that may arise from grocers selling even such simple medicines as Epsom salts is shown by a recent case of poisoning recorded in *British Medical Journal* (p. 304). A man intending to take Epsom salts took what he supposed to be that article, but was nitrate of potash, obtained at the village grocer's, noticing at the time, however, that it had not the usual "sour" taste. In large doses nitrate of potash acts as an irritant poison, and the man, consequently, barely escaped with his life. The remedies used were thin milk gruel, copious warm water enemas, one-quarter grain of morphia every three hours, followed by a dose of castor oil.

At Auckland some experiments in tea culture, made under the auspices of the Acclimatisation Society, have been very successful, an excellent infusion having been obtained. The plant grows luxuriantly in the ordinary soil of Auckland.

Acacia p. 25-20.

[SUPPLEMENT ONLY.]

Chem. & Drugg. Aust. Suppl.
v. 5, no. 51: 21-28, (July, 1882)

THE
Chemist & Druggist.

Vol. 5 · No. 51, WITH AUSTRALASIAN SUPPLEMENT.

(Published under direction of the Pharmaceutical Society of Victoria.)

No. 51. { PUBLISHED ON THE 15TH OF EVERY MONTH.
Registered for Transmission as a Newspaper.
JULY, 1882.
{ SUBSCRIPTION, 15s. PER ANNUM, INCLUDING DIARY, POST FREE.

FELTON, GRIMWADE & Co.

☞ *Since our Circular of JUNE 7th—*

We have landed Supplies of **INDIA-RUBBER GOODS,** invoiced at from 15 to 20 % advance, and from this date we shall have to increase our List Price to that extent.

We call attention to following Quotations :—

Bals. Copaib., 4s. per lb.; gallon tins, 3s. 9d.
Bismuth Sub. Nit., Howard's, 10s.; 7 lbs., 9s.
Camphor, Eng. refined, per lb., 1s. 10d.; for bell, 1s. 9d.
Ferri Cit. c. Quinæ, No. 3, 2s. per oz.; 25 ozs., 1s. 9d.
     ,,   ,,   Howard's, 3s. 6d. per oz.; in lb. bottles, 51s. per lb.
Hyd. Bichlor., 3s. per lb.; 28 lbs., 2s. 6d.
Iodine, re-sublimed, 1s. per oz.; 14s. per lb.
Ess. Lemon Super., in 60-lb coppers, 11s. per lb.
    ,,   ,,   in W. quarts, 12s. 6d. per lb.
    ,,   Medium, in   ,,   11s. per lb.
Ol. Sant. Flav. Opt., in 1-lb. bottles, 28s. per lb.
Opium, Colonial (containing 11% Morphia), 34s. per lb.; 7 lbs., 33s.
Pot. Bromid., Howard's, 1-lb. bottles, 2s. 9d.; 4-lb. bottles, 2s. 6d.; 28 lbs., 2s. 4d.;
    under drawback for export, 3d. less.
Pot. Iodid., Howard's, per lb., 11s.; 7 lbs., 10s. 6d.; 28 lbs., 10s.; under drawback
    for export, 10d. less.
Quinine, Howard's, 12s. 6d. oz.; 10 oz., 12s.; 25 oz., 11s. 6d.
    ,,   Whiffen's, 12s. oz.; 10 oz., 11s. 6d.; 25 oz., 11s.

BISULP. CARBON, in 5-gallon drums, 1s. per lb.
BORO-GLYCERIDE, C.3, H.5, B.0.3, 5s. per lb.

JULY 19th, 1882.   FELTON, GRIMWADE & CO.

Printed by Mason, Firth & M'Cutcheon, 51 & 53 Flinders Lane West, Melbourne.

INDEX TO LITERARY CONTENTS.

The Chemist and Druggist.

WITH AUSTRALASIAN SUPPLEMENT.

OFFICE: MUTUAL PROVIDENT BUILDINGS, COLLINS STREET WEST.
Published on the 15th of each Month.

THIS Journal is issued gratis to all paid-up Members of the PHARMA-CEUTICAL SOCIETY OF VICTORIA, and to non-members at Fifteen Shillings per annum, payable in advance. A copy of *The Chemists and Druggists' Diary*, published annually, is forwarded post free to every subscriber.

Advertisements, remittances, and all business communications to be addressed to THE HONORARY SECRETARY OF THE PHARMACEUTICAL SOCIETY, MELBOURNE.

SCALE OF CHARGES FOR ADVERTISEMENTS:

	Per annum.			Per annum.
One Page	..£8 0 0	Quarter Page	..£3	0 0
Half do.	.. 5 0 0	Business Cards	.. 2	0 0

Special rates for wrapper and pages preceding and following literary matter. Advertisements of Assistants Wanting Situations, 2s. 6d. each.
Advertisements for insertion in the current month should be at the office before the 10th.

COMMUNICATIONS for the EDITORIAL department of this journal should be addressed to THE EDITOR, MUTUAL PROVIDENT BUILDINGS, COLLINS STREET WEST, MELBOURNE.

No notice can be taken of anonymous communications. Whatever is intended for insertion must be authenticated by the name and address of the writer—not necessarily for publication, but as a guarantee of good faith.

THE LIBRARY.

THE Library is open daily (Saturdays excepted), from 9.30 a.m. to 4.30 p.m. Catalogue of the books can be obtained on application.

PHARMACEUTICAL SOCIETY OF VICTORIA.

ANNUAL SUBSCRIPTIONS.

ALL annual subscriptions are now due.

Member's subscription	...	...	...£1	1	0
Associate's	...	...	... 0	10	6
Apprentice's	...	...	... 0	5	0

Cheques and Post-office orders should be made payable to the Honorary Secretary, No. 4 Mutual Provident Buildings, Collins-street, Melbourne.

HARRY SHILLINGLAW, Hon. Sec.

BIRTH.

HUGHES.—On the 16th June, at 61 Elizabeth-street North, the wife of Albert E. Hughes, pharmacist—a daughter.

JONES.—On the 13th July, at Bay-street, Sandrige, the wife of Walter Jones, Chemist, of a daughter.

DEATHS.

ANGIOR.—On the 19th June, at High-street, Northcote, William Frederick, youngest son of Samuel and Sarah Jane Angior, aged 2 years and 2 months.

AUMONT.—On the 27th June, at 92 Wellington-street, Collingwood, Louis Philippe Aumont, pharmaceutical chemist, aged 37.

The Month.

IN Mr. E. L. Marks's paper on "Vegetable Cells," that appeared in our issue of June, some typographical and clerical errors crept in; but as they are almost self-corrective, our readers have doubtless been at once able to remedy the oversight.

A private letter received by the executive secretary to the Bordeaux Wine Commission in this colony states that all the wines shipped here arrived in first-class condition. Owing to the casks being plastered at the ends the bulk wines landed undeteriorated, while some of the wines from other colonies not so treated reached Bordeaux in an inferior state.

A fire broke out at Ipswich, Queensland, early on Saturday morning, 1st July, destroying the premises of Smith Bros., drapers; Melvin, confectioner; Finch, greengrocer; and Von Lossberg, chemist. The fire originated in Lossberg's shop, it is supposed by a dog, accidentally shut in, breaking a bottle and causing the exposure to the air of an inflammable chemical. Von Lossberg's stock was insured in the National and New Zealand offices for £500.

The dean of the Faculty of Medicine (Dr. Halford), with Mr. L. L. Smith and Dr. Le Fevre and the medical students of the University, visited the Model Farm, and carefully inspected the whole process of animal vaccination. Mr. Graham Mitchell showed the students a calf which had been vaccinated during the previous week, pointing out how the lymph was taken and preserved on points, tubes, and glasses. A fresh calf was then vaccinated, and the lymph transferred to the arms of thirty-three persons, including seventeen students.

The analytical chemist appointed by the Government to examine any doubtful teas which might be imported has reported to the Commissioner of Trade and Customs that he has examined nine hundred cases submitted to him from the cargoes of the steamers "Killarney" and "Douglas." These cases were intercepted by the experts, on the ground that they were of a very low and doubtful character; but the analytical chemist, after an examination, has come to the decision that they are genuine teas, and may be passed into the colony for consumption. He reports, also, that he is now engaged in examining and testing some low-class teas which arrived in other vessels than the two mentioned.

Two young men, named Joseph Langley and George Ryder, were committed at the sittings of the Central Criminal Court in May last, before his Honour Mr. Justice Williams, on a charge of conspiracy to defraud. The two defendants had victimised a number of persons in the suburbs by representing that Langley was a medical man, and by selling to their patients some medicines which it was said would cure all manner of diseases. At the trial Mr. Justice Williams, who presided, reserved a case for the opinion of the full court as to whether there was any evidence of conspiracy. This special case was heard in the Supreme Court, but no counsel appearing on behalf of the defendants, and the court, without calling on the Crown prosecutor, decided that there was evidence of a conspiracy, and therefore affirmed the conviction. Langley had been sentenced to seven weeks' imprisonment, and Ryder to three weeks' imprisonment, which punishment they will now have to undergo.

On the 29th June Mr. Bosisto asked the Commissioner of Railways whether the chief medical officer has yet reported to him on the subject of colour-blindness in railway signalmen; and, also, whether he will adopt (as other countries are doing) the complete "tests of sights," as resolved upon and recommended by the late International Medical Congress, for stokers, drivers, and others connected with railway signalling. Mr. Bent, in reply, said that reports had been obtained from the chief medical officer and Mr. Rudall, who attended the recent International Medical Congress. When the men on the Hobson's Bay lines were medically inspected by Mr. Bent's directions, it was found that the usual percentage suffered from colour-blindness, and they had been removed to positions where an ability to distinguish colours correctly was not required. The recommendations of the chief medical officer are to be acted upon in the application of tests.

The death of Mr. L. P. Aumont, of Collingwood, is announced.

Messrs. Felton, Grimwade and Co. have forwarded a donation of £100 in aid of the Working Men's College.

The Microscopical Society now meet in the rooms of the Pharmaceutical Society.

Mr. William Vale, who for the last two years has been dispensing to Dr. M'Gillivray, Sandhurst, has been appointed to the vacancy at the Friendly Society Dispensary, Sandhurst.

Mr. J. T. Poock has purchased the business of Mr. R. Anderson, at Colac. Mr. Anderson retires from the business in consequence of failing health.

At the last meeting of the council of the Pharmaceutical Society of New South Wales, Mr. Frank Senior, J.P., was, by a unanimous vote, elected president for the ensuing year.

At the annual meeting of the New Zealand Pharmaceutical Society the president of the Pharmaceutical Society of Victoria was elected an hon. member.

Mr. Churchus, who for some time has been carrying on business at Coleraine, has disposed of his business to Mr. J. P. Nicholas. Mr. Churchus goes to Casterton, having taken over the business of Mr. T. F. Blackburn. A new establishment will be opened at Nhill by Mr. Blackburn.

An action has been commenced in the County Court against Messrs. Rocke, Tompsitt and Co., by C. F. E. Brown, stock and station agent, of West Melbourne, for the recovery of £49, damages for injuries caused to his horse in Bridge-road, Richmond, by the carelessness of their servant.

The Tariff Commission will sit on the 19th inst., when acids, drugs, chemicals, patent medicines, &c., will be dealt with. Messrs. Bowen, Thomas, Atkin, Wallworth, and Jones have been nominated to attend on behalf of the trade. We shall give a full report of the examination in our next issue.

The window in Mr. Bowen's new premises in Collins-street, one of the largest sheets of plate glass in Melbourne, was accidentally broken while pulling down the iron shutters the second day after it had been in. Luckily for the owner, it was insured, and was at once made good by the company.

A daring burglary was committed at an early hour on the 24th June on the premises of W. J. Bentley, chemist, West Maitland. The shop was completely ransacked, but little was taken out of it. The burglars, who had evidently been searching for money supposed to be on the premises, have been arrested.

Mr. Ellery, the Government astronomer, delivered the third of the winter course of lectures at the School of Mines, Ballarat, on the 6th instant, the subject being "The Sun's Distance, and the Transits of Venus." Mr. J. Oddie, the vice-president of the school, presided, and there was a large attendance. Mr. Ellery, who treated his interesting subject in a clear and popular manner, and illustrated it by numerous diagrams and a suspended orrery, received a cordial vote of thanks.

Mr. J. T. Poock, on his departure from Yass, was presented by a number of friends with a handsome watch and ring. The *Yass Evening Tribune* of the 22nd June says :—"Not only as a chemist has Mr. Poock won for himself a good name in Yass, but as a vocalist he has proved himself to be almost without an equal in town, having materially assisted at various concerts and entertainments that were got up in aid of different local charities. We feel sure that he will make a name for himself wherever he is located, both as a dispenser and a private citizen ; and the sentiments of the whole community are only being echoed when we express a hope that health, wealth, and prosperity may attend him in whatever place he may decide to settle."

Meetings.

THE PHARMACY BOARD OF VICTORIA.

The monthly meetings were held at 100 Collins-street on the 14th June and 12th July.

Present—Messrs. Bosisto, Blackett, Brind, Bowen, Holdsworth, Lewis, and Owen.

The president, Mr. Bosisto, M.P., in the chair.

The minutes of the previous meetings were read and confirmed.

Applications for Registration as Pharmaceutical Chemists. —The following were passed :—William Simpson, 117 Collins-street ; Spencer Smithson Dunn, Gover-street, North Adelaide ; Tom Luke, Shepparton ; Robert Shanklin, Maffra,

Gippsland. Registered by virtue of certificates from Pharmaceutical Society, Great Britain—Carl W. H. Helms, Geelong ; L. W. Tschoepe, Middle Brighton ; Paul Kleesattel, Fitzroy. Registered under certificates from Germany Universities— A. O. Hughes, Yass, N.S.W. Geo. Phillips Hamilton Llewellyn Best, Fitzroy, passed the modified examination. Sydney Victor Say passed major examination. Wm. Geo. Weaver, Hobart, and Sarah Fairthorne, Echuca, in business before the passing of the Act.

Apprentices' Indentures Registered. —James Tonkin Weaver, Emerald Hill ; John Cranstoun, Sandridge ; and John A. Hawkes, Warrnambool.

In reference to the cancelling of indentures, it was resolved that in all cases where indentures are cancelled by mutual consent they must be subscribed to by all the contracting parties, in the presence of a witness, before they are forwarded to the board.

Prosecution under the Sale and Use of Poisons Act. —The registrar was instructed to prosecute in the case of John Digby, Emerald Hill, for the illegal sale of poison. It was also resolved that in all cases where the Pharmacy or Poisons Acts are known by any registered pharmaceutical chemist to be evaded the board will pay all ordinary expenses incurred in obtaining evidence for the prosecution.

Correspondence. —From the secretary of the Pharmacy Board of New Zealand, asking whether the present or the future standards recommended to come into operation in January, 1884, are such as would meet with reciprocal recognition of diplomas from the Pharmacy Board of Victoria. A sub-committee was appointed to deal with the letter, and report at the next meeting. A letter was received from the secretary of the Medical Society of Victoria, bringing under notice the conduct of two suburban chemists who are practising medicine and surgery. The cases were referred for legal opinion, with a view of prosecuting the offenders. Communications were also read from the chief medical officer, Fiji ; Mr. C. H. Keogh ; the police, Melbourne, Warragul, Emerald Hill, and Drysdale.

A certificate under the Poisons Act was granted to T. Montgomery, Mortlake.

The honorary treasurer submitted the balance-sheet to the end of the financial year, 30th June, which was ordered to be audited.

Routine and general business brought the meeting to a close.

THE PHARMACEUTICAL SOCIETY OF VICTORIA.

The monthly meeting of the council was held at the rooms, 100 Collins-street, on the 7th July. Present—Messrs. Bowen, Baker, Nicholls, Huntsman, Ross, Swift, Jones, and Shillinglaw.

The president, Mr. Wm. Bowen, in the chair.

The minutes of the previous meeting were read and confirmed.

Nomination of New Members. —The following were nominated :—A. M. Cattach, Collingwood ; S. S. Dunn, North Adelaide ; R. Williams, Punt-road ; apprentice, W. J. Bowen.

It was resolved that counsel's opinion be taken in reference to the prosecution of persons who have ceased to be members, and who still exhibit the diploma of the society.

A communication was read from the secretary of the Pharmaceutical Society of New Zealand, stating that the president of the Victorian Pharmaceutical Society had been elected an honorary member of the Pharmaceutical Society of New Zealand, and that a vote of thanks was also carried unanimously to Messrs. C. R. Blackett, M.P., Joseph Bosisto, M.P., and Harry Shillinglaw, secretary Victorian Pharmacy Board, "for their willing and generous assistance in promoting the working of the Pharmacy Act by valuable information freely supplied at all times."

It was resolved that the thanks of the society be forwarded for the honour conferred.

The Tariff Commission. —A letter was received from the Tariff Commission stating that the next items under consideration would be drugs, chemicals, &c.

At the conclusion of the business the president presented to Mr. Wm. Lowe the gold medal of the society for the best examination passed during the year 1882. Mr. Lowe served his apprenticeship with Messrs. Wm. Ford and Co.

Books, &c., Received. —*Calendar of the Pharmaceutical Society of Ireland* for year 1882 ; Messrs. Burgoyne, Burbridges and Co.'s *Export Price Report*, May ; *European Mail*

for May and June ; *Fragmenta Phytographiæ Australiæ*, Vols. 7, 8, 9, and 10 ; *Magnetic Survey of Victoria*, from 1858 to 1864 ; *Natural History of Colony of Victoria*, decades 1 to 6 ; *Deutch-Amerikanische Apotheker-Zeitung*, May ; *New York Druggists' Circular*, June ; *American Journal of Pharmacy*, May ; *Therapeutic Gazette*, May ; "Proceedings of the American Pharmaceutical Association," 1881 ; *Scientific American*, 6th, 13th, 20th, and 27th May ; Messrs. Sleeman and Co.'s *Export Drug Circular*, May ; *Chemical News*, May ; the *Quarterly Journal of the Microscopical Society of Victoria*, August, 1879, May, 1880, April, 1882.

SYDNEY.

PHARMACEUTICAL SOCIETY OF NEW SOUTH WALES.

THE annual meeting of the Pharmaceutical Society of New South Wales was held on Wednesday evening, 14th June, in the boardroom of the society, Phillip-street. The meeting was very largely attended, being the most successful annual gathering held since the society came into existence. The president, Mr. F. Senior, J.P., occupied the chair. The secretary, Mr. W. T. Pinhey, having read the advertisement calling the meeting, the following report was submitted :—" Your council, in submitting their sixth annual report, desire to record the gratifying result of their efforts during the past year. They have pleasure in stating that during the past year the names of thirty-four new members have been enrolled, an indication that the society is gaining increased confidence amongst those interested. They have to report also the engagement by them of Mr. Frederick Wright to deliver at the School of Arts a course of twelve lectures, which met with unqualified success, the attendance having exceeded the most sanguine expectations, and those who attended them having expressed themselves satisfied, and benefited by the same. Arrangements have been made with Mr. Wright to deliver a second course of lectures, which will commence next month. The council have, during the past year, added many valuable works to the library on *materia medica*, pharmacy, and chemistry, by purchase and gifts, and they would seriously urge upon associates and apprentices the propriety of making greater use of all the means afforded for their mental improvement. The members have been supplied, gratuitously, during the past year with the *London Chemist and Druggist*, which they, the council, are led to believe is fully appreciated, as containing much valuable and reliable information of importance to the chemist. The council anticipated that during the last session of Parliament a bill would have been introduced to have the effect (as stated in the last annual report) ' of raising the status of the chemist, and giving assurance to the public that in future none but those qualified to deal in or dispense medicines will be permitted to do so.' In this they have been disappointed, but they will use all the means at their command to get it accomplished during the coming session. The council have thankfully to acknowledge the report for the past year of the *American Journal of Pharmacy*; also, from the Pharmaceutical Society of Victoria, the last annual report and *Supplement to the London Chemist and Druggist*, &c. It is earnestly hoped that the pharmaceutical chemists will heartily co-operate with the council in providing means to extend the usefulness of your society, which, although yet in its infancy, promises to be one of the permanent institutions of the land, in which the public as well as the chemist have unquestionably a direct interest."

Mr. Wm. Larmer, in moving the adoption of the report, said that it certainly commended itself for their approbation. It was as exhaustive as it was possible for it to be, and the statement made in it as to the financial affairs of the society very satisfactory ; and he felt sure that in the future the efforts put forth by the council would be equally as worthy of praise, and would be equally as appreciated. He had heard it said that the calling of the medical man was almost divine ; surely, if that were so, the calling of the chemist was equally so, for he compounded the medicines that were administered, and life and death lay in his hands. However, be that as it might, he could not say the calling of the chemist was a fortune-making one. Chemists were too greatly handicapped, various causes militating against their success. One of these causes was medical men dispensing their own prescriptions. He thought this *infra dig*. The motto of the two bodies should be "live and let live." Another matter was that of wholesale chemists doing a retail business. The chemist's

business, he remarked, was also limited. He could not offer his wares, as did those in other trades, by advertising "an alarming sacrifice ;" hence his privileges needed to be the more closely conserved. The council of the society, however, were doing their best to promote the welfare of the trade. Some of the members were getting grey in the service, and when the time came that they should be succeeded by others he hoped their successors would also receive the help the present members had received from their excellent secretary, whose judgment and experience were so great that the speaker hardly knew what they would do without him.

Mr. J. Henry, in seconding the adoption of the report, referred to the subject of medical men in the city and suburbs dispensing their own medicines. If they were in their own right as medical men to dispense medicines, he would be content ; but he objected to their doing so on the grounds they stated—first, that they could not trust most of the chemists and druggists to keep pure medicines ; secondly, that they charged enormously for their medicines. As to the first charge, it was untrue, and he was sure many of the chemists were more competent to make up medicines and understood their physiological action better than many medical men. As to the second charge, it was also untrue. Then there was also the charge made against them by the doctors that they practised. Well, for his part, not having a license to kill, he preferred sending all the patients to the medical men. He contended, not that it was unfair for medical men to dispense their own prescriptions, but that it was unfair for them to do so on the grounds that chemists were dishonest men, who would not give good medicines, and that they were extortioners. He referred to the necessity of the young chemists in their midst endeavouring to attain a high status of education. He would indeed wish to see them reach that of a medical degree, and then no such charge as that it was dangerous to allow a chemist to dispense medicines could be made against them by the medical men. In conclusion, he paid a tribute to the secretary, to whom the society, he thought, owed a great deal of its present prosperity.

Mr. F. Wright entered a protest against what had been said by the mover of the motion as to the wholesale houses doing a very large retail trade. Even if it were so, the remedy lay with the chemists and druggists in taking unanimous action, and in ascertaining from the wholesale houses if their manner of carrying on trade was injurious to the retailers or not. He felt sure the proprietors of wholesale houses would in every way meet the wishes of the trade in this respect. As to dispensing, he believed the method to be adopted in bringing about an alteration in this respect was by raising the standard of education ; in fact, giving the chemist such an education as would enable him to deal with elementary analyses, and enable him to detect adulteration, &c.

Mr. A. J. Watt thought the less they said about the wholesale houses retailing the better. The matter had been represented to the proprietors of those places of business on several occasions. The number of wholesale houses that retailed was very large.

Mr. W. Pratt thought they should do all in their power to bring about a better feeling between the medical men and the druggists. He also advised a higher status of education for their young men.

Mr. William Parker, of Balmain, thought there was little use in blustering or speaking unkindly of the medical men. If they alluded to them at all it should be done as quietly as possible. If they wished to keep pace with the times it was not to be done by raising a quarrel between the two bodies.

The president said that he must say he agreed to a great extent with what had been said by Messrs. Larmer and Henry.

The motion for the adoption of the report was then put and carried.

The treasurer (Mr. A. J. Watt) read the financial statement, showing that the sum of £67 12s. 3d. was lodged to the society's account in the Bank of Australasia, which, with £200 to its credit invested in the Building Society, gave a total of £267 12s. 3d. to the credit of the society.

The statement was adopted.

Mr. J. S. Abraham, the retiring member of the council, was re-elected ; and Mr. M'Carthy was elected to the council board in the room of Mr. Edward Row, who had resigned.

Mr. M'Carthy returned thanks for the honour done him.

Messrs. J. A. Row and H. Sadlier were appointed auditors, and in recognition of the honour returned their thanks.

The chairman then, in accordance with the annual practice, delivered an address. He said :—I think we must all agree our report and balance-sheet are both favourable; in fact, much more so than were any previous ones. You will see we have still over £200 invested. This would have been very much increased but for our expenditure on three important items—namely, £48 on additions to our library, £40 for supplying the *Chemist and Druggist* to the members, and £25 for providing lectures. You will allow that the council have acted very wisely in these matters. If you will just peep at our little library you will see what a good beginning we have made ; indeed, I consider that we may be justly proud of it. The council have determined to go on purchasing all the new works pertaining to chemistry and pharmacy ; and here I must thank our old friend Mr. Pinhey for his very valuable contribution of about fifty volumes of admirable works, many of which are now out of print. I have also to thank our Victorian friends for their regularity in forwarding their *Supplement*, which I am sure all will find adds to their stock of knowledge. The addition of thirty-four new members to our list shows that confidence is increasing amongst our professional brethren in our endeavours to raise the status of dispensing chemists. On two matters I cannot help expressing my regret. The first is at finding so few young men applying for books. However, the fault is not ours. I have uttered warnings before, and if young men who will be obliged to pass our examinations will not indulge in a moderate amount of reading, the fault will be their own ; for although our examinations are simple, but practical, it is simply lamentable to see the miserable exhibitions of pharmaceutical knowledge made at such times. The other matter of regret is that we are yet without our amended bill. I believe pressure of business in Parliament is still the cause. However, your council will not lose the slightest opportunity of getting it before the House. It is only six years since our society was formed, and very soon after we obtained our present Poisons Act. I think this was very smart work compared with what has been done in the old country, where the parent society was many years without being a legally recognised body, and where 264 years have elapsed before our pharmacopœia has become what I may call matured, though certainly not yet perfected. While on the subject of pharmacopœia, I will give you a few jottings I have taken on this subject from the meeting at York last year, and also from Bell and Redwood's *Progress of Pharmacy*. The first pharmacopœia was published by the College of Physicians of London in the year 1618. This was the very first step taken towards reducing the process of pharmacy to a regular standard for the guidance of dispensers of medicine. It was, however, a very imperfect production. Subsequent editions were published by the college in 1621, 1632, 1639, 1650, 1677 ; in 1721, 1746, 1788 ; in 1809, 1815, 1824, and 1836. The first *Edinburgh Pharmacopœia* was published in 1699. New editions appeared in 1722, 1736, and 1744, and a few years afterwards Dr. Lewis published an English translation under the title of the *Edinboro' New Dispensatory*, and other editions followed in 1755, 1774, 1788, and in 1803, 1804, 1806, 1813, 1817, 1839, and 1841. The first *Dublin Pharmacopœia* was published in 1794, and another in 1805. These were circulated among the members of the college only. The next was published in 1807, and was for general circulation. This work which had been several years in preparation, was chiefly completed by Dr. Percival, at that time professor of chemistry in Dublin University. Another edition appeared in 1826, chiefly completed by Professor Donovan, whom I hope, is known to all of you as the introducer of the well-known Liquor Donovani, and the last edition in 1850. Then last, but not least, came in 1864 the amalgamated edition, known as the *British Pharmacopœia*, which, I believe, is considered universally as a great improvement in various ways on its predecessors, but still far from perfect. The next step has been to endeavour to establish a universal pharmacopœia. In the history of pharmacy one of the most important events which has happened for some time has been the great meeting last year, at York, of pharmacists from almost all parts of the pharmaceutical world. The attention of this meeting was engaged on several matters of the highest importance to pharmacists in Australia, as well as in the older countries of the world. The only one I shall dwell on is the production of a universal pharmacopœia. The importance and utility of this have been generally acknowledged by pharmaceutical associations in Europe, America, and Australia ; by International Medical Congresses at Petersburg in 1874, Brussels in 1875, Geneva in 1877, and Amsterdam in 1879. The Pharmaceutical Congress at Petersburg made a great advance in this direction by entertaining a draft of a universal pharma-

copœia prepared by the Pharmaceutical Society of Paris ; but none of these congresses led to any real improvement. The Geneva Congress of 1877 ended in establishing an international committee, and the pharmacological section of the Amsterdam Congress of 1879 contented itself with inviting the Pharmaceutical Society of Paris to communicate the draft of its new pharmacopœia, so as to have it printed in the transactions of their congress ; in short, these congresses have failed in two important particulars—the introduction of a universal pharmacopœia and an international uniformity in medicine as desired by the American Medical Association. It seemed, therefore, desirable that the Geneva committee should be augmented by pharmaceutical and medical experts capable of securing the co-operation of countries not yet represented, and of confining its attention exclusively to the creation of a universal pharmacopœia. The following points were suggested for the particular consideration of the committee, the settlement of these points forming the necessary basis for a universal pharmacopœia. These points were—The languages, weights, measures, temperatures, nomenclature, arrangement, contents, uniform regulations as to the degree of purity required, methods of testing important drugs and chemicals, and, lastly, a table of maximum doses. It was suggested the language should be Latin ; the weights and measures should be the French decimal system ; the temperatures on the Centigrade scale ; strict uniformity in the botanical and other names of drugs, in the nomenclature of chemical compounds (adding the molecular formula where possible) and in the Latin terms for all galenical preparations ; the arrangement to be alphabetic or systematic, or a combination of both, like the last *French Pharmacopœia* ; the contents to be limited to remedies of high importance and in general use, supplements to be appended for particular countries; uniform regulations for degrees of purity, methods for testing, and, finally, a table of maximum doses. These would form the nucleus of a universal pharmacopœia. A general agreement having been arrived at on the above points, it was considered desirable for the whole congress to employ their influence in their respective countries in revising their own pharmacopœias in harmony with these suggestions. In this way the introduction of a universal pharmacopœia would be greatly assisted, and immediate advantages would be conferred on medical practitioners in all countries. A comparison of all European pharmacopœias would form the basis of the preliminary compilation. It seems now settled that the final results of all these deliberations are that, for the present, they relinquish the too difficult proposal of a universal pharmacopœia, and adopt the more limited scheme of equalising the strength of the preparations of the most potent drugs generally employed in medical practice. I think all this seems very like the mountain in labour bringing forth a mouse. Still it ought to teach us a salutary lesson in patience. If all these eminent societies for so many years have been striving in vain for an improved pharmacopœia, we may well go on hoping and trusting that each year will bring us an improved Pharmacy Bill ; and you may rest assured that your council will lose no opportunity of helping on that very desirable object.

The thanks of the meeting were moved to the committee of the Technical College for the manner in which the society had been permitted to use its room for the delivering of lectures. It was decided to forward a letter to the committee in accordance with this resolution.

The thanks of the meeting were also given to Mr. Pinhey for his valuable gift of fifty volumes of books to the library, the collection containing many very rare works now out of print ; also to Mr. Parker, of Balmain, for his gift of two volumes of *Coolcy's Cyclopædia* ; and also to Mr. W. H. H. Lane, for his gift of books to the same object.

Each of these gentlemen acknowledged the courtesy. Mr. Lane, in doing so, remarked that he had travelled through the colonies, and visited all the pharmaceutical societies therein, and believed the New South Wales Society to have the largest library of any of them. It had about one-third more books than the Victorian Society, and he believed the latter was the older society of the two. He had some more works which he would be glad to present to the society.

Mr. F. Wright stated that there was great dissatisfaction in the minds of the associates and apprentices on account of their partial and meagre representation in the society ; and having discussed the matter they thought that, with the permission of the society, it would be wise to form a sub-society, to be called the "Students' Pharmaceutical Society," the president of which would be the president of the principal society, and its vice-presidents the board of pharmacy. A committee would also be elected. The object of this subsociety would he to discuss matters of interest in pharmacy and chemistry, and to form such classes for instruction as might be useful in promoting the knowledge of members. This scheme, he thought, would be of great advantage, not only to the main society, but it would also have a good effect in the education of the students. He mentioned that the Technical College had formed a class for botany, hut not a pupil had applied to be enrolled. He offered as a prize to the student of the new society who should pass the best examination on chemistry a three-guinea set of chemical instruments.

The president was sorry to say that the young men did not take their studies to heart as they should. The examinations were comparatively a farce, and yet none of those who presented themselves seemed to have thought of reading up. He thought to compel them to do so the examination should be made much more difficult.

Mr. Lane offered a prize to the student who would pass the best general examination in the detection of adulteration in drugs, &c., a first-class student's microscope, with objectives and other fittings.

The meeting was terminated by a vote of thanks being passed to the chairman.—*Sydney Morning Herald*, 16th June, 1882.

THE monthly meeting of the Parmaceutical Council was held on Tuesday, 20th June, at the boardroom, Philip-street. Present :—Mr. W. T. Pinhey (in the chair), and Messrs. Senior, Watt, Abraham, Guise, and Larmer.

The minutes of last meeting were read and confirmed. Report of proceedings at the annual meeting, together with the annual report and balance-sheet, was laid on the table, and the board ordered the same to be printed and circulated.

The secretary reported that the council was now complete by the election of Messrs. Abraham and Macarthy at the annual meeting.

The council then proceeded to the election of a president for the ensuing year. It was moved by Mr. Guise, and seconded by Mr. Abraham—"That Mr. F. Senior be president for the ensuing year." Carried unanimously.

It was proposed by Mr. A. J. Watt, and seconded by Mr. Larmer—"That Mr. Abraham be treasurer for the ensuing year." Carried unanimously.

A vote of thanks was passed to Mr. A. J. Watt for his services as treasurer during the past twelve months.

Applications for membership were received from Mr. Parkinson (of Paddington), Mr. Osmond (of George-street), Mr. F. Ryan (William-street), and Mr. J. Butterfield. Mr. Parkinson and Mr. Osborne were admitted members. The application of Mr. Ryan was referred to the Medical Board. The application of Mr. Butterfield was postponed for the examination of the candidate.

The indentures of C. C. T. Magee, apprenticing him to Mr. Hudson, of Corowa, were received for registration.

The meeting then adjourned.

THE annual meeting of the Pharmaceutical Society, held on the 10th of June, was by far the most successful gathering that the trade has ever held in the colony. The increased interest shown in the proceedings speaks well for the future of the society.

In some of the speeches made at the meeting reference was made to the large trade done by the wholesale houses with persons whose custom, the speakers thought, should go to increase the profits of the retail chemist. For instance, the doctors are supplied with drugs on the same terms as the druggists, and thus are encouraged by the wholesale houses in the pernicious practice of dispensing their own medicines. The furniture polisher, the blacking manufacturer, and the cordial maker, or even the tobacconist, can purchase the articles required in their business at the wholesale drug warehouses, and thus the retailer is robbed of what he considers his legitimate business.

In the daily papers great outcry has been raised to the practice of medical men dispensing their own medicines. The fact is, the medical men get their sons or daughters, their stableman or their kitchen girl, their coachman or their governess to do the work, and if the public only knew by whom the medicines were at times compounded, they would hesitate a little before they entrusted their lives into such hands.

Messrs. Elliott Bros. have taken additional precautions to prevent private persons buying articles under the pretence that they are in the trade, or are buying the goods for use in their business. No employé is allowed to make any purchase without special permission from a member of the firm.

12th July, 1882.

THE MICROSCOPICAL SOCIETY.

THE monthly meeting of the Microscopical Society was held on 29th June, at eight p.m. There was a good attendance, and the chair was occupied by the Rev. J. J. Halley, vice-president. The secretary acknowledged the receipt of a number of journals and other publications. The Rev. T. Porter read a paper describing his method of preparing and mounting double-stained plant sections, and illustrated it by a number of specimens, very beautifully executed, principally stained with carmine and aniline green. Mr. Barnard also sent a series of sections of native and other woods, showing double staining with carmine and picric acid. The Rev. J. J. Halley described and exhibited a new form of turntable designed by him, in order to provide a simple and ready means of clamping a slide in any position, either central or eccentric. Mr. Halley also made some remarks on the use of starches as adulterants, &c., and presented a series of seventeen slides of various starches for the society's cabinet. Mr. W. W. Allen exhibited a recent microscope by Hartnack, furnished with an adjusting binocular eye piece, and a very complete set of objectives and accessories. Mr. J. F. Bailey distributed among the members present some valuable microscopic material, principally obtained during the voyage of H.M.S. "Challenger," comprising several samples of globigerina, radiolarian, and diatomaceous ooze, dredged from depths varying from one and a half to nearly three and three-quarter miles ; also, coral sand from Raimie, North Australia, and from the coast of Bermuda, containing many forms of foraminifera.

REMARKS ON AUSTRALIAN ACACIAS.

(BY BARON FERD. VON MUELLER, K.C.M.G., M. & PH.D., F.R.S.)

THE great genus Acacia claims in the whole range of Australian vegetation the particular attention of pharmacists. Irrespective of the durable and hard yet pliable timber for carriages, furniture, casks and implements supplied by some of the large arboreous species, several Acacias furnish like the sandal tree scented wood likely available for the distillation of oil ; others in not a few cases yield bark extraordinary rich in mimosa-tannin, while many kinds exude gum, rivalling in some instances with the best gum Arabic. Furthermore a multitude of Acacias in all parts of Australia exhale a fragrance, widely wafted through the air by their flowers, when such successively burst forth from various species in spring and early summer. It is more particularly to the latter quality of the Acacias, that it is wished to direct the practical interest of pharmaceutic gentlemen all over Australia on this occasion, as still further experiments have to be carried on for ascertaining whether the subtle fragrant principle could be concentrated and isolated by any process, not impairing so much the delicate odour as the heat of ordinary distillation, or simpler and more expeditious as the "eufleurage" method. Possibly the vapours of the cheaper kinds of pleasantly odourous essential oils, such as that from the peels of the sweet orange, might at very moderate heat in a vapour-still be passed through Acacia blossoms, thus to produce new cosmetics of mixed essential oils ; or even perhaps the aid of good-sized air-pumps might be invoked, to withdraw the delicate fragrance from the selectest kinds of flowers of this kind also, to be condensed by some apt absorbent. Not all Acacias however possess an odour of pleasantness and strength ; therefore it would be well, if the various species were studied in their fresh state locally all over Australia. The importance of this also for other industrial as well as systematic purposes will be apparent, when it is stated, that of about 450 species known from all the warmer regions of the globe, fully 300 are endemic in Australia. Of these however a considerable number remain imperfectly described, either the well developed flowers or the ripe fruits being as yet unknown. As a further contribution to the systematic of this, the largest of all genera of Australian plants, the descriptions of a few new species are offered, by which means the search for additional novelties may also become stimulated for the perfection of works on the Australian flora.

Acacia adnata.—Branchlets slightly angular, short-downy; phyllods small, glabrous, oblique-rhomboid, mucronate-pointed, 3-4-nerved, with broad adnate base sessile, the anterior side produced into a blunt angle with a minute gland; stipules bristly; peduncles axillary, solitary, bearing a single globular flower-head, finally twice or thrice as long as the phyllode; pods broad-linear, compressed, glabrous, straight along the sutures; seeds very small, rhomboid or ovate-roundish, black, not shining; their areoles very minute; strophiole cymbiform, not much shorter than the seed, parallel to the valves, longer than the straight capillary funicle.—Near the Irwin River; F. v. M.—Already the broad adnate base of the phyllods distinguishes this from every species of the small group, to which the allied A. deltoidea belongs. Flowers unknown.

Acacia Gilesiana.—Glabrous; branchlets slightly angular; phyllods straight, pale, thickly filiform, not compressed, rigid, acute, not mucronate, traversed by several exceedingly fine longitudinal nerves; stipules obliterated; racemes short, axillary and terminal, bearing 2-4 flower-heads; pods rather broad, compressed, wavy along the sutures; seeds ovate, placed longitudinally.—Near Mount Eba; E. Giles.—Foliage more like that of many Hakeas than that of any Acacia; as a species nearest to A. rigens. Flowers and ripe fruits unknown.

Acacia sessiliceps.—Branchlets not angular, at first silky; phyllods thinly filiform not or slightly compressed, longitudinally streaked and faintly furrowed, pointed but not mucronate; stipules obliterated; flower-heads axillary, generally solitary; lower bracts ovate-lanceolate, forming a minute involucre; sepals spatulate-linear, at first high-connate; corolla not streaked, about half as long as the calyx; pods rather broad, moderately compressed, almost circularly twisted, very thinly silky, slightly wavy along the outer suture; seeds placed longitudinally, rather large, clasped at the base by the short strophiole; funicle yellowish.—Near the Finke River; Rev. H. Kempe.—Allied to A. rigens. Ripe fruit unknown.

Acacia Kempeana.—Arborescent; branchlets faintly angular; phyllods rather short, falcate-oblong, blunt, between the few slightly prominent longitudinal nerves closely subtle-streaked; stipules and gland obliterated; spikes axillary, generally solitary, short-stalked, much shorter than the phyllods; flowers glabrous, nearly three times as long as the very thin but rhomboid-laminulated bracts; calyx short-toothed, nearly three times shorter than the unstreaked corolla; pods rather short, flat, oblique-oblong, smooth, rounded-blunt at the summit and base, suddenly short-stalked; valves almost membranous; seeds placed transversely, shining-black, three times shorter than the width of the valves; strophiole extending not beyond the basal portion of the seed, cymbouscupular; funicle twisted beneath the strophiole.—Between Youldeh and Ouldabinna, Jess. Young; near the Finke River, Rev. H. Kempe; between the Warrego and Maranoa, Barton.—Nearest to A. aneura.

Acacia cibaria.—Branchlets not angular, slightly silky; phyllods rather long, thick, rigid, broadly linear, very finely many-nerved, of greyish hue, curved-apiculated; stipules and gland obliterated; spikes axillary, solitary, short-stalked, not elongated; flowers slightly short-hairy; bracts rhomboid towards the summit, very thin towards the base, surpassed in length by the flowers; sepals narrow, free, hardly half as long as the unstreaked corolla; pods straight, cylindrical, longitudinally streaked; seeds placed lengthwise, oblong, their two areoles minute; strophiole very short, cupular, occupying only the basal portion of the seed; funicle closely twisted beneath the strophiole.—Between the Darling River and Barcoo, Dr. Beckler; near the Murchison River, Ch. Gray; near the Gascoyne River, Oliver Jones.—A tall shrub or small tree, allied to A. aneura in foliage, but very different as regards fruit. The aborigines use the seeds very largely for food, wherever this species occurs. The fruits from near Shark Bay are much larger and the seeds brownish, not black. It is the "Wonuy" of the natives.

Legal and Magisterial.

THE RECENT PROSECUTIONS UNDER THE POISONS ACT.

THE prosecution of Mr. A. J. Wade, chemist, of Emerald Hill, and his assistant, for illegally selling poisons, "points a moral," and should be inwardly digested by all druggists who are either in business for themselves or assisting others. In fact, the development of the Pharmacy Act chiefly depends upon druggists themselves as to whether it should be a means of elevating the trade, or allowing it to remain as of yore. Most pharmacists will, I venture to say, incline towards doing what the Act was intended to produce. It is astonishing, however, to find persons openly setting it at defiance, and engaging those to assist who are not legally competent, thus not only rendering themselves liable to penalties, but producing other unpleasant consequences not easily forgotten.

It is also astonishing to find what an amount of penalties an unregistered chemist acting as an assistant renders himself also liable, and subjects his employer; although the latter (if not imposed upon), knowing the consequences, is more to blame than the former—for in the eyes of the law every employer is supposed to know who or who are not registered. Possibly chemists in general are not aware that a complete registry for each preceding year is published annually, and can be purchased from the registrar for one shilling. The case in point was one of the most flagrant, and showed that the derelict did not even know the rudiments of his business; for long before the selling of poisons became penal every druggist, for his conscience' sake, labelled the article "poison." This was even neglected; and whether the strychnine was coloured or not report does not say. Evidently the purchaser was not known, and the sale of it was unregistered. Without knowing whether the strychnine was coloured or not, the seller rendered himself liable to four penalties, besides that of his employer.

The prosecution, it is to be hoped, will have the effect of making druggists more careful as to the class of assistants they employ; for without this care it is impossible for the Board of Pharmacy to carry out the provisions of the Act.

In the prosecution of Mr. Perkins, of Ballarat, referred to in our last, it is consoling to find the proceedings were not instituted by the board, but that they originated with the police, who were entirely answerable for their failure; and it also discloses the absence of an advocate or a solicitor to conduct the case; for, without doubt, it would be far better not to prosecute at all than to lose a case for the want of getting it up properly, as in the latter case it rather stimulates than prevents others to rebel.   J. H.

PROSECUTION UNDER THE SALE AND USE OF POISONS ACT.

AT the Emerald Hill Police Court on the 20th June, before Messrs. Foote, Stead, Mouatt, and Twentyman, J.P.'s, a young man named John Digby, in the employment of Mr. A. J. Wade, a pharmaceutical chemist, carrying on business in Clarendon-street, Emerald Hill, was charged, under the third section of the Sale and Use of Poisons Act, 1876, in that he, not being a duly qualified chemist, did sell a poison to one James Lee, on the 12th inst. Mr. D. Wilkie appeared to represent the Pharmacy Board and the police, and Mr. Daley for the defendant. In opening his case, Mr. Wilkie referred to the number of accidents which had recently occurred through the careless sale of poisons. The first witness was Alexander Thomas Waugh, who deposed that he had been with the deceased Lee on the evening before his death, and had seen him enter the shop of Mr. Wade. About two o'clock in the morning he was awakened by the cries of deceased, who was in convulsions. At the inquest it was found that he had died of poisoning by strychnine. Senior Constable Rogers deposed that on the morning of the 13th inst. he went to a house in Chester-street, and, on making a search, found the wrapper produced, on which the word "poison" was printed, and "strychnine" written underneath. Witness made inquiries, and learned from Digby that on the previous day a man had come into the shop and asked for sixpence worth of strychnine to poison rats. Digby did not like to serve him, as Mr. Wade was temporarily absent from the shop. In a short time the man called again, and was served with the article. Witness found no entry of the sale in the poison-book. There was also no name on the label. Digby afterwards proceeded with witness to the house in Chester-street, and identified the dead man as the person to whom he had sold the poison. Defendant acknowledged the handwriting on the wrapper to be his. This closed the case for the prosecution. Mr. Daly contended that Digby was not responsible for the sale, having made it on behalf of his employer. It was pointed out, however, that by section 10 the assistant was made as liable as the master, and that if the assistant made the sale he was held to be the seller. Mr. Wade testified that the defendant was his junior assistant.

Digby had received no instructions from him concerning the sale of poisons, but witness had thought him qualified to act in his absence. The Bench considered the case proved, and fined the defendant £5, with £2 2s. costs. A nominal fine of 10s. in each case, with costs, was inflicted on Digby for the infringement of sections 5 and 6, which required that an entry of the sale should be made, and the name of the vendor on the wrapper. Mr. Wade was fined 10s., under the sixth section, the other summons being withdrawn.

At the City Court on 28th June, before Mr. Call, P.M., and a bench of magistrates, a magician and illusionist, named Martin Beaufort Tolmaque, was brought up on remand, charged with obtaining goods and money from Mr. William Ball, chemist, Swanston-street, by means of false pretences. The evidence for the prosecution was that on the 16th inst. the prisoner visited Mr. Ball's shop, and stated that he had just received an engagement to appear in conjunction with Lynch's troupe of bellringers, but was unable to do so in consequence of having a bad cold, and he asked for something to remove it. Mr. Ball made him up a gargle, for which he charged 2s. 6d., and the prisoner tendered a cheque for £2 2s. on the Bank of New South Wales, purporting to be signed by Henry Lynch, which he said had been given to him by the proprietor of the company of bellringers. Witness cashed the cheque, and gave the prisoner £1 19s. 6d. in change, but when he presented it at the bank it proved valueless, and a warrant was subsequently issued for Tolmaque's apprehension. It transpired that the prisoner had not been engaged to appear with the bellringers, and that he had only waited upon Mr. H. Lynch, at Prahran, on the 19th inst., and asked for something to do, after the cheque had been dishonoured. The cheque was dated "June 14th," and was made payable to "Herr Tolmaque." The prisoner did not deny the facts stated, but alleged that the cheque had been given to him by some unscrupulous persons in the profession who wished to do him an injury, and who had threatened to "put him away." Mr. Call said that if the prisoner was an honest man he would have returned the money to Mr. Ball on discovering that the cheque was valueless, and he consequently sentenced him to seven days' imprisonment.

PHARMACY BOARD EXAMINATIONS.

In order to afford intending candidates some idea of the character of the examination before the Pharmacy Board, we publish the last examination papers :—

PRELIMINARY EXAMINATION.—8th June, 1882.

Time allowed, three hours.

LATIN.

1. Translate into English :—
(a) Eo opere perfecto præsidia disponit, castella communit, quo facilius, si se invito transire conarentur, prohibere possit,
(b) Divico respondit: Ita Helve stitutos esse uti obsid a

ARITHMETIC.

Every step in the work should be clearly and neatly shown, and all results should be reduced to their simplest form.
1. How often is five inches contained in one mile ?
2. Multiply £8 16s. 9½d. by 5, divide £118 9s. 7½d. by 9, and find the difference between the results.

3. Simplify— $\dfrac{\frac{1}{2\frac{3}{4}}}{\frac{1}{7} + \frac{1}{4} + \frac{1}{7} + \frac{1}{7\frac{1}{4}} + \frac{1}{8\frac{1}{7}}}$

4. Multiply 1·075 by ·39 : Divide ·0012123 by ·09, and find value of ·75 of £3·75.
5. Write out Troy weight : If nine silver spoons weigh 2¼ lbs. Troy, find the weight in grains Troy of 36 such spoons.

ENGLISH.

1. What is a relative pronoun ? Name those used in English.
2. What is an inflexion ? What inflections are used in forming the possessive case, singular and plural ?
Write the possessive case singular of bridge, who, pony.
3. Point out the grammatical errors in the following sentences, say what rule of grammar each violates, and write each sentence in the correct form :—
(a) Let you and I go to town.
(b) John can write as good as Charles.
(c) Who did you lend the money to ?
4. Parse, with full syntax, every word in the sentence— "All is not gold that glitters."
5. Write a short piece of composition on—The Value of Time ; or, Kindness to Animals, paying great attention to spelling and punctuation.

THE MODIFIED EXAMINATION.—12th June, 1882.

Questions on Materia Medica.

Time allowed, one hour and a half. Examiner, J. Bosisto.
1. Name six plants yielding essential oils of the B.P.—(1) Write the names in English and in Latin ; (2) give their natural orders ; (3) habitat.
2. Name two plants yielding fixed oils of the B.P.—(1) Give their natural orders ; (2) the part of the plant supplying the oil; (3) the processes employed to procure it.
3. Describe the root of monkshood, and the difference between it and horseradish.
4. Gamboge.—From what tree, and how obtained ?
5. Musk.—(1) What is it ? (2) state the varieties and adulterations.
6. Annatto.—Name the tree and the part supplying it.
1 and 3 answered well will obtain extra marks.

Questions in Practical Pharmacy.

Time allowed, one hour. Examiner, C. R. Blackett.
1. Give the officia' Latin names and chemical formulæ of—(a) Potassium carbonate ; (b) calcium chloride ; (c) dilute phosphoric acid ; (d) Epsom salt.
2. (a) How are volatile oils usually obtained ? (b) how are fixed oils usually obtained ? (c) how would you test a volatile oil for the presence of alcohol ? and how for that of a fixed oil ?
3. What excipient would you use in making pills of—(a) sulphate of quinine ; (b) aloes, rhubarb, and extract of nux vomica ; (c) potassium bromide ; (d) chloral and camphor ?
4. (a) Define a gum resin, giving its characteristic ; (b) name not less than three which are official.
5. Criticise and explain the following:—

R Plumbi acetatis gr. x
Infusi rosæ. ad. fl. ℥ vi,
Rosæ
Syrupi fl. ℥ ii.
R Resinæ podophylli 0·50
Elaterini ... 0·50
Ext. nux vom. ... 2·00
Misci fiant pilulæ viginti,
8. One morning and night.

6. What causes bumping in distillation, and how may it be prevented ?

Correspondence.

SIR—I beg to draw your attention to a subject which, I think, deserves notice—viz., the time allowed for answering questions in the preliminary examination, three hours being insufficient. To work out the arithmetic paper *properly* would take an hour and a half, leaving only the same time for the other two subjects.

If the candidate is at all nervous he is sure to get flurried, knowing he has to do it in so short a time, thereby greatly decreasing his chance of success.

Hoping you will kindly insert the above—I am, yours, &c., Victoria, 18th June, 1882.　　ONE WHO HAS TRIED.

[The time allowed is the same as in England for no more difficult paper.—EDITOR.]

SIR—Seeing an account of the accident to Mr. F. Fairthorne, by the bursting of a tube of nitrite of amyl in this month's *Chemist and Druggist*, and having once broken one myself, I should feel obliged if you would inform me as to the best way of opening the tubes.—Apologising for the trouble given, I have the honour to be, your obedient servant,

Murtoa, 23rd June, 1882.　　WM. T. WARBRECK.

[The tube containing the nitrite of amyl should be wrapped in a folded cloth, and then the end gently scratched with a sharp file and broken off.—EDITOR.]

REMINISCENCES OF A PHARMACIST—(*Continued*).

(BY J. B. MUMMERY.)

"TWO EARLY CUSTOMERS."

I WAS fortunate in procuring the good-will of the only medical man in the place, who was glad to have a person on the spot capable of dispensing his prescriptions; and he readily promised his support. And, as I was a total stranger to most of the people, it was arranged at the doctor's own suggestion that he should place upon his prescriptions a certain mark indicating those of his patients to whom credit might safely be given; and the want of this mark was the means of introducing me under somewhat laughable circumstances to a gentleman of exalted position, who afterwards became one of my most influential and appreciated customers.

A few days after opening my shop, a young woman, apparently of the "servant gal persuasion," presented a prescription of Dr. B——'s for a Mr. Holt. It was only a small affair, half-a-dozen pills, I think. At all events, the charge was eighteenpence, which sum as the young lady did not happen to have about her, and the prescription lacked the magical mark, which was to be "open sessame" to the pages of my ledger, I started her off for the cash, which she brought in due conrse, got the pills, and departed, and I thought no more of the matter.

The next day a gentleman called, who, after making some trifling purchase, said—"So you would not trust me eighteenpence last night." I of course made the best excuse I could, saying that as I was a stranger I did not know the good marks from the bad. "Well," he replied, "I don't blame you. I should most likely have done the same had I been in your position; but I may tell you that my name is generally considered good here, for eighteenpence at all events, he added, laughingly. My name is Holt, as you see by the prescription. Thomas Holt, usually dubbed honourable, and my position at present is that of 'Colonial Treasurer.' Now I suppose you will trust me to the value of this prescription, and, if so, you can make it up and send it down to 'Camden Villa.'" Of course I replied that I should be only too happy to open an account with the honourable gentleman, which I did; and Mr. Holt became, not only, as I said

before, one of my firmest supporters, but a kind and valued friend, with whom after-circumstances brought me in frequent contact.

My introduction to another of my customers, a wealthy merchant, was made under circumstances quite as peculiar, although of a different nature.

Exactly opposite my establishment was the mansion of Mr. R——, a member of the largest importing firm in Sydney, This gentleman had never been in my shop to my knowledge, nor had I ever had a prescription for any member of the family, although I knew there was sickness in the house, for I saw the doctor's carriage go in every day. I was foolish enough to be awfully annoyed at this, for I was young and inexperienced then, and imagined (as many young beginners do at the present day) that because I had opened bandy to them, every person in the place was in duty bound to close their connection with shops in the city, where they had been dealing perhaps for years, and transfer their custom then and there to mine.

Well, one day the morning coach brought a parcel for Mr. R——, directed to my care, from a well-known firm of chemists in Sydney, and the address was written on one of their labels; and the fact of its containing medicines was announced on shaking it by the gurgling sound of liquid, and the rattle of pills. This riled me not a little. I thought it bad enough to be overlooked in the dispensing line, but to be made use of as a receiver for goods from a firm in the same line I was not going to stand, so I gave the parcel back to the driver of the coach, on its return journey, and desired him to leave it at the place he obtained it from. 'Buses run now every five minutes, but in those days there was only a coach twice a day, and hardly had I sent the parcel off when a servant girl came and asked if anything had come from town for Mr. R——. I told her yes, of course, and what I had done with it, adding, with perhaps more truth than prudence, that it was like her master's impudence to have his medicines consigned to my care. Whether she told him this I cannot say; but the same night I was called up by Mr. R——, who informed me that one of his children was bleeding profusely from leech-bites, and that he could not stop the blood, and asked me what he should do.

I was on the point of telling him that he had better go to Sydney and call up the chemist that he got the leeches from, but I did not do so. I simply gave him some lint, with instructions how to use it, and desired him to call me again if its application did not prove effectual. He thanked me, and asked what he had to pay. "Nothing," I said; "I do not charge for advice." Nevertheless he replied, "You can't live by *giving* it." Thereupon he advanced to the counter as if for something he had left, and again thanked me and bade me good-night. On preparing to extinguish the gas, I saw Mr. R—— had placed a couple of half-crowns on a glass case. These I took up and thankfully appropriated.

The next day, after the doctor's visit, I received a prescription to dispense, and opened an account with the worthy merchant, and then and there began a connection which lasted for many years; and if I did not get the whole of his business, I had quite enough to make Mr. R——'s quarterly cheque an agreeable and useful arrival.

(*To be continued.*)

of poisoning by strychnine. Senior Constable Rogers deposed that on the morning of the 13th inst. he went to a house in Chester-street, and, on making a search, found the wrapper produced, on which the word "poison" was printed, and "strychnine" written underneath. Witness made inquiries, and learned from Digby that on the previous day a man had come into the shop and asked for sixpence worth of strychnine to poison rats. Digby did not like to serve him, as Mr. Wade was temporarily absent from the shop. In a short time the man called again, and was served with the article. Witness found no entry of the sale in the poison-book. There was also no name on the label. Digby afterwards proceeded with witness to the house in Chester-street, and identified the dead man as the person to whom he had sold the poison. Defendant acknowledged the handwriting on the wrapper to be his. This closed the case for the prosecution. Mr. Daly contended that Digby was not responsible for the sale, having made it on behalf of his employer. It was pointed out, however, that by section 10 the assistant was made as liable as the master, and that if the assistant made the sale he was held to be the seller. Mr. Wade testified that the defendant was his junior assistant.

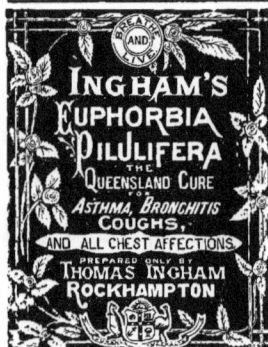

FELTON, GRIMWADE & CO.,
Melbourne.

☞ **LANDED**

Ex R.M.S.S. "SUTLEJ"

Savon Veloutin Violets
Tartrate Chinoline, 1-oz. bottles
Salicylicate Chinoline, 1-oz. bottles
Galante's Annular Pessaries, Esmarch's Bandages and Spray Producers
Atkinson's White Rose and assorted Pomades, Soap, and Sachets
Do.   Stephanotis and Assorted Sachets.

Orient Steamer "AUSTRAL"

Atkinson's Assorted Essences, stoppered, and Sprinklers, 1-oz. 2-oz., 4-oz., 8-oz., 16-oz. sizes
Atkinson's Rondeletia and Eau de Cologne
Grossmith's Assorted Perfumery Cabinets
Tortoiseshell, I.R., Buffalo, and White Horn Rack, Dressing Combs
Arm Slings, Vaccinating Shields
Carlvert's Carbolic Soaps
Do.   do.   Tooth Powder
Do.   do.   Acids, Nos. 1, 2, and 5
Super Essence Lemon, 60-lb. coppers.

S.S. "CATANIA"

Pepper's Sulpholine Lotion
Do.   Taraxacum and Podophyllin
Maltine Manufacturing Co.'s Maltine
Do.   do.   do.   with Beef and Iron
Do.   do.   do.   with Peptones
Do.   do.   do.   Ferrated
Do.   do.   do.   with Hypophosphites
Do.   do.   do.   with Cod Liver Oil
Do.   do.   do.   with Iron, Quinine, and Strychnine.

R.M.S.S. "MIRZAPORE"

Large assortment Kent's Tooth, Badger Shaving, Nail, and Hair Brushes
Tome's nickel-plated Forceps
Perfume Caskets, plush, glass, painted china, &c.
Corbyn, Stacey & Co.'s Menthol
Do.   do.   Gurgun Balsam
Do.   do.   Spts. Nucis Juglandis
Do.   do.   Liq. Rosæ Dulc.
Ferris and Co.'s Glycerole of Nitrate of Bismuth.

[SUPPLEMENT ONLY.]

p. 56.

THE

Chemist & Druggist.

WITH AUSTRALASIAN SUPPLEMENT.

(Published under direction of the Pharmaceutical Society of Victoria.)

No. 55. { PUBLISHED ON THE 15TH OF EVERY MONTH. }
Registered for Transmission as a Newspaper.

NOVEMBER, 1882.

{ SUBSCRIPTION, 15s. PER ANNUM, INCLUDING DIARY, POST FREE. }

HEMMONS, LAWS & CO.

Wholesale & Manufacturing Druggists,

Importers of Drugs, Chemicals, Botanic Herbs, Druggists' Sundries, &c.,

HAVE JUST LANDED

Ex "SIKH" (from London).

A large assortment of Medicated and other Lozenges, from Messrs. Joseph Terry & Sons, York, England.

Pulv. Rhei. E. I. Opt
„ „ E. I. Super.
„ Aloes Bbd.
„ „ Socot
Ferri Ammon. Tart.
„ „ Cit.
„ Limat
Pot. Acetat.
„ Cyanid.
Sodæ Acet. Pur.
Pulv. Myrrh Tky. Opt.
„ Scammony, Aleppo and Virgin
„ Gallæ
White and Orange Shellac
Ol. Rorismar, Juniper, Cassia, Origani
„ Sassafras, Succini, Theobromæ

Ol. Amygd. Ess., Amygd. Dulc.
„ Sinapis, Menthæ Viride
„ Carui. Ang., Lavand. Ang.,
Mitcham, Neroli
Otto, Virgin and commercial
Pulv. Jalapæ, Acid Gallic, P. Cassia, Colocynth
„ Canella, Ipecac., Card. Min., Carui
„ Sang Drac, Acid Tannic, Sabinæ
Pulv. Catechu Pal., Zingib. Jam. Opt., Acacia Tky.
„ Oss Sepiæ, Hellebore Nig., Antim Pot. Tart.
Pil. Hydrarg., Glob Prunella, Gum Mastich
Coccus Cacti, Gum Ammon. Gutt., Guaiaci
Gum Assafætida, Sang Drac, Benzoin

Zinci Chlor., 1 oz.; Sulph. Hypochlor., 1 oz.
Sodæ Carbolas, Liq. Pepticus, Benjer's
Liq. Pancreaticus, Benjer's
Ess. Pine Apple, Pear, Ribston Pippin
Hyd. Oleat, Hyd. Oleat c. Morph., Acid Oleic
Tonquin Beans, Fol. Coca., Pulv. Guarana
Amyl. Nitrite, Zinci Sulphocarb.,
Pulv. Opii Tky.
Succ. Belladon., Conii, Scoparii, Rhamni, Succ. Digitalis, Cetaceum Opt., Magnes Sulph.
Sulph. Sub., Pulv. Lini. Aug., Pulv. Lini. c. Oleo Ang.
Pot. Bichrom., Cupri. Sulph., Ferri Sulph., &c., &c.

Ex "SORRENTO."

Silverlock's Labels	Cotton Wool	White Covd. Pots (all sizes)	Absorbent Cotton
P. O. Boxes (nested)	Waterproof Sheeting	Antiseptic Gauze	Fletcher's Concentrated
Throat Sprays	Blister Pots (1 and 2 oz.)	Stag Lint	Liquors

From Messrs. KEITH & CO., New York (ex "SIAM," S., from London).

Collinsonin	Juglandin	Leptandrin	Stillingin
Cornin	Lupulin	Sanguinarin	Colocynthin
Euonymin	Lycopin	Scutellarin	Taraxacine
Gelsemin	Podophyllin	Senecin	

From Messrs. W. R. WARNER & CO., Philadelphia, (ex "SIAM," S., from London).

A large and complete stock of their Sugar-coated Pills, Fluid Extracts, and other specialties.

NOW LANDING.

Ex "SHANNON" (from London).

Burnett's Fluid, No. 1, 2, and 3
Savory & Moore's Datura Tatula, No. 1 and 2
Savory & Moore's Medicinal Pepsino

Eno's Fruit Salt
Kay's Cue Cement
„ Coaguline
Alpaca Pomade, No. 1 and 2

Liq. Santal Flav. Co., Hewlett's
Mist. Pepsine c. Bismuth „
„ „ „ (sine opii)
Liq. Quinæ Sulph. Amorph.

INDEX TO LITERARY CONTENTS.

The Chemist and Druggist.

WITH AUSTRALASIAN SUPPLEMENT.

OFFICE: MUTUAL PROVIDENT BUILDINGS, COLLINS STREET WEST.

Published on the 15th of each Month.

THIS Journal is issued gratis to all paid-up Members of the PHARMA-
CEUTICAL SOCIETY OF VICTORIA, and to non-members at Fifteen Shillings
per annum, payable in advance. A copy of *The Chemists and Druggists'
Diary*, published annually, is forwarded post free to every subscriber.

Advertisements, remittances, and all business communications to be
addressed to THE HONORARY SECRETARY of THE PHARMACEUTICAL SOCIETY,
MELBOURNE.

SCALE OF CHARGES FOR ADVERTISEMENTS:

	Per annum.		Per annum.
One Page	..£8 0 0	Quarter Page	..£3 0 0
Half do. ..	.. 5 0 0	Business Cards	.. 2 0 0

Special rates for wrapper and pages preceding and following literary
matter. Advertisements of Assistants Wanting Situations, 2s. 6d. each.

Advertisements for insertion in the current month should be sent to the
office before the 10th.

COMMUNICATIONS for the EDITORIAL department of this journal should be
addressed to THE EDITOR, MUTUAL PROVIDENT BUILDINGS, COLLINS STREET
WEST, MELBOURNE.

No notice can be taken of anonymous communications. Whatever is
intended for insertion must be authenticated by the name and address of
the writer—not necessarily for publication, but as a guarantee of good faith.

The Annual Dinner

OF THE

PHARMACEUTICAL SOCIETY OF VICTORIA,
in aid of the BENEVOLENT FUND, will be held
on WEDNESDAY, the 13th DECEMBER, 1882, at
Clement's Café, Swanston-street, at Eight o'clock p.m.

Tickets, £1 1s. each, can be obtained from any member
of the Council, or from

HARRY SHILLINGLAW, Hon. Sec.

PHARMACEUTICAL SOCIETY OF VICTORIA.

ANNUAL SUBSCRIPTIONS.

The attention of members is directed to clause 13 of
the Laws.

Subscriptions for the current year must be paid on or
before the 31st December, 1882, or membership will
cease.

HARRY SHILLINGLAW, Hon. Sec.

BIRTH.

LUKE.—On the 12th October, at Shepparton, the wife of T. Luke, chemist,
of a daughter.

MARRIAGE.

TREACY—WALTON.—On the 27th September, at St. Francis's, by Rev. M.
M'Kenna, Richard N. D., eldest son of Martin Treacy, Esq., brewer,
Wagga Wagga, late of Geelong, to Minnie, eldest daughter of the late
George Walton, chemist, Geelong.

SECRET REMEDIES.

THE *Pharmaceutical Journal* would have a line drawn between secret remedies and specialties. A "specialty"
is defined by that journal to be " any substance or product
which, prepared according to an officinal formula, realises
an improvement in the art of pharmacy, and presents
special therapeutic advantages." "A ' secret ' remedy is
any simple or compound substance or medicine employed

in the treatment of disease, which has not received official
sanction or publication, and which has not been prepared
for a particular case upon a medical prescription." One
is, according to this author, the product of the professional
skill and practical sense of the pharmacist, and is generally met with in competitions and industrial exhibitions.
The other is the product of charlatanism, and an inordinate
desire to acquire a fortune rapidly ; it makes itself known
especially by advertisements in the public prints. The
Pharmaceutical Journal goes on to say that even if the
remedies of which neither the basis nor the proportions
are known ought to be rejected from therapeutics, genuine
specialties, which mark a progress in the pharmaceutic
art, or intended to facilitate the administration of certain
medicines, might, up to a certain point, be admitted.
The distinction between a specialty and a secret remedy is
not, however, always easy to establish.

To these remarks of our contemporary we can only say,
Go on, brother; your aim is in the right direction, but there
seems to be a mist in front of your mental vision that needs
clearing up before you can see the difference between
scientific pharmacy and the unscientific nature of some of
these " specialties " that you seek to shield from the
righteous condemnation of an outraged pharmaceutical profession. Specialties are never officinal preparations. One
objection we have to them is that they are not prepared
after officinal formulæ, nor are they improvements in the
art of pharmacy, and many of them have never yet been
proven of any special therapeutic advantage. If the
author means to designate official preparations as " specialties," we challenge his authority for so doing. There is a
marked difference between the officinal preparations of the
pharmacopœia and the various " specialties " that flood
the market. Surely the writer in the *Pharmaceutical
Journal* is able to see the broad line of demarkation that
separates " specialties " from officinal preparations, the
formulæ for which are published in the *Pharmacopœia*.
By his own definition the writer classifies " specialties "
with secret remedies, for a secret remedy is one " which
has not received officinal sanction or publication." And
is not this classification usually correct ; for what difference is there, except in degree, between a "specialty," the
name of which is claimed as private property, and the formula of which is nowhere published so that any one else
may manufacture it, and a remedy *all* knowledge of which
is concealed from the public eye ?

It would seem to us, however, that a better standard has
been fixed between science and secrecy than that given by
this writer. It is not necessary that a thing should receive
officinal sanction, or be recognised in the pharmacopœia
as officinal, to be scientific ; and a remedy that is not thus
sanctioned is not for that reason necessarily a secret
remedy, as this writer seems to infer. The standard to
which we refer is that required by the patent laws of the
United States in the giving of patents upon mechanical

inventions. For a thing to be regarded as scientific by this standard, exact knowledge of it, whereby any one else can manufacture the same thing, must be published. No "specialty" can mark a progress in the pharmaceutic art unless this demand is complied with ; no "specialty" that does not come up to this requirement can be admitted ; and we do not think that we overstate when we say that any "improvement in the art of pharmacy presenting special therapeutic advantages, the product of professional skill and practical sense of the pharmacist," is acceptable to both the medical and pharmaceutical professions, and if its claims to merit are proved, there can be no reason for not admitting it. But proprietary "specialties," the names of which are claimed as trade-marks, and the art of the manufacture of which can be nowhere found in literature, cannot be admitted from the very nature of the case. To admit them would be to ruin scientific nomenclature, seriously injure medical literature, and encourage a system that weighs down all progress in the science of pharmacy like the old man of the sea. If pharmacy is to be a science, it must conform to the demands of science ; if those who practise the art wish it to be known as a profession, they must be professional. Secrecy is not science, and the hiding of knowledge for trade purposes is not professional. A pharmacist's standing in his profession is in exact proportion to his record as a scientific man. The question is, what has he done to advance knowledge in pharmacy and to benefit his profession? It is required of him to publish full knowledge of all the improvements and discoveries he may make in the art for the benefit of his science, and receive compensation therefor in the demand thus created for medicine manufactured by a member of the profession of so much "professional skill and practical sense." Not until this ideal is realised can pharmacy be regarded either as a science or a profession.—*Therapeutic Gazette.*

The Month.

THE following are the arrangements for the quarterly examinations to be held in December next. Modified, 4th ; school certificate, 5th ; preliminary, 7th ; practical pharmacy, 8th.

The Pharmaceutical Register of Victoria for 1883 is now in course of preparation, and we are requested to notify that, in accordance with the thirteenth section of the Pharmacy Act, a number of names of those persons who have neglected to comply with that section will be omitted.

The triennial election of the members of the Pharmacy Board of Victoria will be held early in the month of February, the board retiring by effluxion of time in January, 1883. The returning officer notifies in another column the date of nomination. All the retiring members are eligible for re-election.

The annual dinner of the Pharmaceutical Society of Victoria will be held at Clement's Café on Wednesday, the 13th December next. Arrangements are being made by the committee to make it a success, and it is expected that the attendance will be far larger than on any previous occasion. A number of gentlemen from other colonies are likely to be present. Cards can be obtained from any member of the council, or at the office, 100 Collins-street.

Mr. J. Bosisto, M.L.A., who proposes spending a fortnight in South Australia, left for Adelaide on the 15th inst. Mr. Bosisto may be reckoned amongst the pioneers of South Australia, as he landed there over thirty-four years ago, and prior to his arrival in Victoria he carried on business as a chemist there. Mr. Bosisto while in the neighbouring colony will visit the principal olive and forest plantations, with the view of making himself acquainted with the systems of cultivation adopted, Olive planting has been attended with great success in South Australia, and Mr. Bosisto has always advocated the establishment of a similar industry in Victoria, certain districts being admirably adapted for that purpose.

Mr. James Greenwood, M.A., died at his residence, Paddington, Sydney, on the 7th November, from an overdose of chlorodyne. The deceased gentleman was forty-nine years of age, and a native of Nottingham. He came to the colony as minister of the Baptist Church, Bathurst-street, and remained in that position until the time when the Public School League was formed in Sydney, and an agitation for "free, secular, and compulsory education" was carried on throughout the country. Mr. Greenwood was the soul of the league, and owing to the prominent position he occupied on the education question he was elected to the Legislative Assembly in 1877 as one of the members for East Sydney. For a considerable time he was a contributor to the *Sydney Morning Herald* and *Echo.* The deceased gentleman leaves a widow and several children.

We are requested to state that the following names will be omitted from the Pharmaceutical Register for 1883 for non-compliance with the thirteenth section of the Pharmacy Act:— W. P. Green, Queenscliff ; Paul Bohrdt, Islington-street, Collingwood ; William Fraser, Rochester ; John Dolphin, East Brunswick ; W. S. Siddall, Footscray ; Richard Zoepfel, 20 Islington-street, Collingwood ; James C. Nicholson, George-street, Fitzroy ; F. H. Newth, Rockhampton, Queensland ; James F. Donaldson, Footscray ; J. B. Barker, Best-street, North Fitzroy ; William Craig, Ballarat ; Andrew Chadwick, Campbell-parade, Richmond ; Charles Finch, 190 Wellington-street, Collingwood ; John T. Osmond, Sydney, New South Wales ; C. V. L. Florance, Willunga, South Australia ; Jane Veal, Johnston-street, Collingwood ; J. H. W. Stevens, South Yarra ; George C. Powell, Footscray.

Messrs. Rocke, Tompsitt and Co. are the successful tenderers for the supply of drugs to the Melbourne Hospital for the year 1883.

Messrs. Simpson and Davenport have purchased the business of Mr. John Ross, 63 Collins-street. Mr. Ross goes to Sale, Gippsland.

Mr. T. M. Wilkinson, of Dunedin, N.Z., is in Melbourne, on his way to England ; he leaves in the ship "Melbourne," early this month.

The will of the late Mr. Henry J. Long, of Bourke-street, Melbourne, was proved on the 2nd November ; the property was sworn at £1803.

From Messrs. Parke, Davis and Co., Detroit, Mich., we have received a number of their publications, which will receive due notice in a future issue.

The resignation of Mr. John Ross as a member of the council of the Pharmaceutical . Society was received and accepted at the last meeting of the council.

Messrs. Felton, Grimwade and Co. have just issued the first number of a new price-list, which is by far the best and most complete list of the sort that has ever been issued in the colonies. The typographical portion has been done by Messrs. Mason, Firth and M'Cutcheon, on whom it reflects great credit.

The firm of Main and Geyer, who for a number of years have carried on business at 9 Hurdlay-street, Adelaide, have dissolved by mutual consent, and Mr. W. James Main has been taken into partnership. The business is now carried on at the new premises, 56 King William-street, and the style of the firm in future will be Main and Son. Mr. W. J. Main having been in the business for the last thirteen years warrants an assurance of the success of the new firm.

Meetings.

PHARMACY BOARD OF VICTORIA.

THE monthly meeting was held at 100 Collins-street on the 8th November; present—Messrs. Bosisto, Blackett, Bowen, Brind, Holdsworth, and Lewis; the president, Mr. J. Bosisto, M.P., in the chair.

The minutes of the previous meeting were read and confirmed.

An apology was received from Mr. A. J. Owen.

Applications for Registration as Pharmaceutical Chemists.— The following were passed by the board :—John Newton Woolcott, Ballarat, and John Frederick Grace, West Melbourne, certificates from the Pharmaceutical Society of Great Britain; John William Queale, Kyneton, certificate from the Pharmaceutical Society of Ireland ; Sarah Ann George, Brunswick, an assistant before the passing of the Act.

Apprentices Indentures Registered.—Pierce Butler, apprentice to Henry Trumble, Sandhurst.

School of Pharmacy, Ballarat.—The examiners reported that they had held an examination for the school certificate, and passed the candidates who attended. They have also placed on record their appreciation of the very satisfactory manner in which the school is conducted.

Names Erased from the Register.—The names of the following deceased persons were erased from the Pharmaceutical Register of Victoria :—John Wm. Yeats, St. Arnaud ; Henry James Long, Melbourne.

Prosecutions under the Sale and Use of Poisons Act.—The registrar reported that cases had been taken in Melbourne, Emerald Hill, Carlton, Fitzroy, Collingwood, and Prahran, and in every case convictions had been obtained. He also reported that a number of other cases in country districts would shortly be proceeded with.

Quarterly Examinations.—The following are the examination fixtures for December :—The modified, 4th December ; for the school certificate, *materia medica*, botany, and chemistry, 5th December ; preliminary, 7th December ; practical pharmacy, before the whole board, 8th December.

Amendments to the Poisons Act.—The amendments were further discussed, and will be finally dealt with at the next meeting.

The Pharmaceutical Register for 1883.—Authority was given to print and issue.

Election of Board.—The registrar was instructed to notify to the returning officer that the board retire by effluxion of time in January, 1883.

Correspondence.—Letters from the following persons were dealt with :—Captain Adams, Seymour ; the police, Whittlesea, Stawell, Epping, Healesville, Nhill, Terang, and Williamstown ; Wm. Boardman ; Redford and Co., Warrnambool ; the executors of the late Mr. George Wilson, Sale ; Newman, Buninyong ; Calder, Echuca ; Ryan, Wells, and Hawkridge.

Financial and general business brought the meeting to a close.

THE PHARMACEUTICAL SOCIETY OF VICTORIA.

THE monthly meeting of the council was held at the rooms, 100 Collins-street, on the 3rd November. Present—Messrs. Bowen, Hunstman, Hooper, Nicholls, Baker, Thomas, and Shillinglaw.

The president, Mr. Bowen, in the chair.

The minutes of the previous meeting were read and confirmed, and an apology was received from Mr. Gamble.

The following new members were duly elected :—William Stephens, Footscray ; Wm. Ball, Swanston-street, Melbourne ; Geo. F. Webb, Chapel-street, Prahran. A. C. Richards, Swan-street, was also elected as an associate.

The following were nominated as new members :—Richard B. Bridge, Essex, England ; J. N. Woolcott, Echuca ; Richard C. Hill, Franklin, Tasmania.

The Tariff Commission.—A communication was addressed to the Tariff Commission by Mr. Bowen, making certain propositions in reference to the duties on preparations of opium.

Correspondence.—A letter was read from Mr. John Ross, forwarding his resignation as a member of the council, which was accepted with regret. A communication was also received from Mr. C. M. Brooke, the secretary of the Pharma-

ceutical Society of New Zealand, intimating that the council of the New Zealand society would at their next meeting consider the desirability of distributing a copy of *The Australasian Supplement to the Chemist and Druggist* to all their members. Mr. F. Baden Benger, honorary general secretary of the British Pharmaceutical Conference, forwarded a letter of thanks for the kind assistance rendered in the distribution of the circulars, &c., of the conference.

Annual Dinner.—The Dinner Committee reported that there was a prospect of an excellent attendance at the dinner to he held on the 13th December next. The Land and Building Committee also submitted a most satisfactory report, and it is expected that the matters will be shortly finally arranged.

Financial and general business brought the meeting to a close.

BOOKS, &C., RECEIVED.—*Australian Medical Journal*, September ; *Chemical News*, September and October ; *European Mail*, September ; Messrs. Sleeman and Co.'s *Export Drug and Chemical Circular*, August ; *American Druggists' Circular*, September ; *New Remedies*, September ; *Therapeutic Gazette*, August ; *American Journal of Pharmacy*, September ; *Scientific American*, September ; *Australasian Medical Gazette*, October ; *Natural History of Victoria*, Decade 7 ; Messrs. Rocke, Tompsitt and Co.'s *Monthly List of Drugs, &c.;* Messrs. Felton, Grimwade and Co.'s *Market Report and Prices Current* ; *Pharmaceutical Journal*, August ; *Nature*, August ; *Analyst*, September ; *Annual Report of the Homœopathic Hospital*, 1882 ; *Australian Sugar Planter*, November.

SYDNEY.

PHARMACEUTICAL SOCIETY OF NEW SOUTH WALES.

THE monthly meeting of the Pharmaceutical Council was held at the board-room, Philip-street, on Thursday, 19th October ; present—the president (in the chair), and Messrs. Larmer and Pratt.

Applications for membership were received from Messrs. H. J. Tracy (M.P.S., Vic.), J. Bradbury (M.P.S., Vic.), F. Rich (of Walgett), and E. Vangetti (of Parramatta). The two former were admitted, and the two latter were informed that they must be examined.

Applications for registration of indentures were received from F. Rich, of Walgett; A. Rogers to H. A. Glyde, of Deniliquin ; J. H. Fort to A. J. Watt, Sydney ; H. Poole to J. H. Reid, of Paddington ; and Mr. W. E. Gavin. The first four applications were granted, the application of Mr. Gavin was postponed until a satisfactory proof of education should he forwarded.

The examiners' report of the late examination was laid on the table.

The secretary reported that the society's library had been insured in the Sydney Mutual Insurance Company for £200. The monthly accounts were passed, and the meeting closed.

PHARMACY IN NEW SOUTH WALES.

THE sixth of a series of lectures on "Practical Pharmacy" was delivered to the students of the Pharmaceutical Society on the 23rd October, at the Technical College, by Mr. F. Wright. Mr. W. Larmer presided. The lecturer briefly reviewed the past course. There are 28 groups of preparations in the British Pharmacopœia ; 18 of these are liquid and 10 solid. The 18 liquid preparations are subdivided into the alcoholic and the aqueous classes ; the 10 solids are subdivided into those for internal administration and those for external application. The last of these subdivisions called for their attention at this last lecture of the course. The members of this group are 5 in number—viz., unguenta, emplastra, suppositoria, cataplasma, and charta. There are 34 ointments in the Pharmacopœia, and of these 19 have inorganic substances as their active ingredients. The vegetable kingdom is represented by 13, and the animal kingdom by 2, although substances from the animal kingdom form the basis of all ointments. The 14 plaisters are, with 3 exceptions, modified forms of lead plaister. Of the 7 suppositoria, 3 should he prepared with soap or starch, and the remainder with lard, wax, and cocoa butter. Linseed meal enters into the composition of 5 out of the 6 official cataplasma. The varying strengths of the preparations were then given in tabular form. The lecturer, in conclusion, referred to the new Act that the Board of Pharmacy are preparing. They were sparing no pains in laying the foundations of the profession, but the veterans of pharmacy in our colony will soon be passing away, and we are in danger of having to fill their places with men lacking their matured experience and professional attainments. Especially we should study scientific methods of working, and put forth a great effort to rescue our profession from the hands of ignorant quacks. Mr. Wright thanked the members of the Pharmaceutical Council for their kindness in presiding at the various lectures, and the Technical College Committee for the use of their hall. Mr. W. Larmer said that the lecture was at once the last and the best of the series. A more practical, instructive, and entertaining lecture he had never had the pleasure of listening to. The lucid manner in which the subject was handled by the lecturer did him great credit, and he was sorry that so admirable an address was delivered to so comparatively small an audience. In the name of the Pharmaceutical Council he thanked Mr. Wright for the manner in which he had discharged his duty as their lecturer during the late session. We are given to understand from the president of the Pharmaceutical Society that the standard of qualification for chemists and druggists is being steadily raised, and no expense will be spared in placing a thorough knowledge of their business within the reach of every registered apprentice. The society's library is the finest of its kind in the southern hemisphere, and as soon as the Act to amend the present Poisons Act is passed a school of pharmacy will probably be formed, when public lectures will be delivered upon all subjects relating to pharmaceutical chemistry.

DEFINITION OF A NEW SPECIES OF EUCALYPTUS;

BY BARON VON MUELLER, K.C.M.G., M. & PH.D., F.R.S., F.G.S., &c.

IN the vegetation of all Australia the eucalypts are of higher interest to the pharmaceutic profession than any other generic group of plants; and this importance is enhanced by the wide and copious distribution of this genus over all parts of our great southern continent. As shrubs, and still oftener as trees, the eucalypts offer on many places material in extraordinary vastness for the collection of kino or tannic sap, as well as for the distillation of oil, irrespective of their affording such factory-products, as tar, pitch, kreosote, potash, acetic acid, alcohol and various dyes, which come not generally within the immediate province of pharmacists, not to speak of the ready and very payable gathering of the tiny seeds of the leading timber-yielding and anti-miasmatic species for demands abroad. It is however of moment, that the particular properties of the very numerous species of this genus should be much further investigated locally, than has hitherto been possible; for although mainly through Mr. Bosisto's enterprising exertions the oil of several kinds of eucalypts became accessible to the whole pharmaceutical world, and also to special branches of technological industry, there remains yet much to be learned even in this respect by additional researches, particularly on species occurring only in regions as yet scantily settled or hitherto not even colonised. Certainly numerous species of eucalyptus have become well defined botanically during the last ninety years, but many others remained imperfectly known, and in all likelihood a few absolutely new kinds will yet be discovered. A wish is therefore expressed on this occasion, that these highly useful kinds of trees should become the subject of special studies by medical or pharmaceutical practitioners, particularly in outlying districts, so that biomorphically and geographically the range of each congener may be traced. To give an instance of the characteristics, on which mainly the distinctions of forms in this genus is depending, the diagnosis of a yet unrecorded species is subjoined. Notes on stature, bark, wood, geologic relation, time of flowering, form of young seedlings, and other details not observable in transmitted specimens, facilitate the recognition of specific forms in this very intricate genus.

Eucalyptus Foelscheana.

A dwarf tree, or only of shrubby growth; branchlets robust, not angular; leaves scattered or exceptionally opposite, on rather short stalks, ovate or verging into a roundish form, sometimes very large, always of firm consistence, blunt or at the summit slightly pointed, greyish-green on both sides, not much paler beneath; their primary veins very divergent or almost horizontally spreading, numerous and thus closely approximated, but subtle and therefore not prominent; the circumferential vein contiguous to the margin of the leaf; oil-dots concealed or obliterated; umbels four to six-flowered or rarely three-flowered, forming a terminal panicle; calyces pear-shaped, on longish or rarely short stalks, faintly angular, not shining; lid not so broad as the tube of the calyx, very depressed or sometimes conspicuously raised towards the centre, tearing off in an irregular transverse line, long retained and soon reflexed from the last point of adherence; stamens all fertile, bent inward before expansion; filaments yellowish-white, some of the outer dilated towards the base; anthers (when fresh) almost cuneate-ovate or the inner more oblong and the outer slightly cordate, all bursting anteriorly by longitudinal slits; connective reddish, with a slight dorsal turgidity towards the summit; style much exceeded in length by the stamens; stigma not dilated; fruit large, urceolar, not angular; valves generally four, nearly deltoid, inserted much below the narrow edge of the fruit, at last deeply enclosed; fertile seeds large, terminated by a conspicuous membrane; sterile seeds very slender.

Near Port Darwin, on sandy soil; Mr. Paul Foelsche. Found also in other northern portions of Arnhem's Land, by Mr. J. M'Kinlay. Specimens without fruit, brought by R. Brown in 1802, during Captain Flinders' expedition from Carpentaria, may also belong to *E. Foelscheana*, although the leaves pass into a lanceolar form.

The species, above defined, is flowering already at the height of 18 inches (as is the case also with *E. cordata* and *E. vernicosa*), therefore when still quite young, producing then a comparatively large cluster of blossoms; the full grown tree seldom exceeds a height of 20 feet, and always remains of cripply stature. Stem-diameter to nine inches, or rarely more; bark, dark grey, rough; leaves of young plants often twice or even thrice the size of those of old trees. *E. Foelscheana* belongs to the series exemplified by *E. terminalis.* In some respects it is allied to *E. latifolia ;* the leaves however are larger and not decurrent at the base; the petioles are comparatively shorter and, as well as the branchlets, less slender; the peduncles and pedicels are thicker and less angular; the calyces larger, not roundish-blunt at the base, and therefore not passing suddenly into a pedicel of upwards unincreased thickness; the fruit is much larger, at least twice as long as broad; and considerably contracted towards the summit, thus not almost semiovate; the flowers of the real *E. latifolia* are as yet unknown, and may prove different from those of the *E. Foelscheana*, though their anthers, seen as remnants, show the same form.

EXAMINATION OF A SO-CALLED "NON-ALCOHOLIC WINE."

(BY EDWARD LLOYD MARKS, LECTURER ON CHEMISTRY AND BOTANY, SCHOOL OF MINES, SANDHURST.)

A BOTTLE of such wine having been submitted for examination, a portion was carefully distilled from a new flask into a new receiver, until about half the quantity was condensed. Some of the distillate warmed in a test tube gave off an inflammable vapour, burning with an almost colourless flame. To another portion some solid iodine was added, together with hydrate of sodium; to a third a solution of iodine and the alkali; in both cases a yellow crystalline precipitate shortly subsided, showing under the microscope most beautiful stellate plates of iodoform (CHI_3). According to the equation in *Attfield's Chemistry*, the text-book for my pupils $(C_2H_6O) +$

$$4 (I_2) + 6 (N'a\, \overset{\_}{HO}) = (CHI_3) + 5 (N'a\, I') + (N'a\, \overset{\_}{CHO_2}) + 5 (H'_2O'').$$

23rd October, 1882.

THE CAUSE OF CONSUMPTION,

MR. ELLERY, F.R.S., president of the Royal Society, made the following observations upon the recent discoveries in relation to the cause of tuberculosis. Allusion is made to Mr. Wm. Thomson's writings and theories published some years ago in a work entitled, *Histo-Chemistry and Pathogeny of Tubercle.* Koch's microscopic researches would seem to give strong support, if not proof, of the assumption that tuberculosis is the result of a *materia morbi* in the form of a bacillus. This question is one of great interest and of supreme importance to Australians, as the prevalence of pulmonary consumption is by Dr. Thomson reported to be more prevalent in Victoria than in some countries. "It has been estimated that about one-seventh of the human race die of tubercular disease, or consumption, as it is called, and, further, that of the deaths in middle life fully one-third are caused by this fatal disease. This dreadful scourge has gone on, and still goes on, unhindered, at least to any marked extent, by any human effort, backed up by all the advanced medical science of the day. By hygienic precautions and a more profound knowledge of the disease, there is little doubt that of late years it has been in some small degree successfully opposed; nevertheless, those who know most of it cannot but acknowledge our comparative helplessness in the face of this enemy. But knowledge is strength. Consumption is now admitted on all hands to be contagious. For the last twenty years the contagiousness or infectiousness of this disease has been suspected, and various experimenters have more or less satisfactorily demonstrated its high probability. Creighton, Burdon-Sanderson, Giboux, Martin, and more recently Klebs, Cohnheim, and others advanced still another step in the same direction, but it has remained for Professor Koch, of Breslau, now chief of the imperial medical department of Berlin, to demonstrate it as a germ disease, transmissible by inoculation, and that its contagiousness is due to a form of bacillus, one of those low orders of germs which appear to be at the bottom of many diseases to which the human as well as other animals are prone. Now, assuming this to be the case, such knowledge gives great strength, for the modes of resisting contagion offer at once a prospect of in some degree stemming the onward course of this destroyer. And, again, if it should be further shown, as we may reasonably hope, that being a contagious germ disease it is not an hereditary one, then we may cheerfully anticipate that science will find effective weapons to check the spread of this fatal disease. Speaking of this brings to my memory a *brochure* published six years ago (1876) by Mr. Wm. Thomson, of South Yarra, entitled, *Histo-Chemistry and Pathogeny of Tubercle*, which I referred to in a former address. In this pamphlet he discusses at length the pathogeny of tubercle, and gives his reasons for concluding it to be a purely germ disease. On page 27 he says—" The idea of micrococci being in any way associated with the process of tuberculosis is a recent one; and the explanation of their mode of operation is, at least as far as I am aware, now for the first time in the history of pathology attempted, with what degree of success remains to be seen." What has now been demonstrated by Koch was undoubtedly indicated as of the highest probability in Thomson's pamphlet of 1876, and reiterated at greater length and with fuller illustrations in another pamphlet in 1879, and afterwards by Cohnheim in his work on the *Contagiousness of Tubercle*, published in 1880, who says—" We must look forward to the day when the '*tubercle corpuscule*' shall have been discovered in the form of a minute organism."

We understand that a great divergence of view has taken place between Koch and Pasteur upon the question of the cause of tuberculosis. Dr. Thompson was first led to adopt the theory which he propounded some years ago (and which has been, it is assumed by some, adopted by European etiologists) by reasoning from analogy. As the scab disease in sheep is caused by the acarus scabæii, and ringworm by the presence and propagation of a microphylion on the skin, &c., so he concluded that typhoid, consumption, &c., were caused by specific germs.

BOTANICAL EXCURSION OF THE STUDENTS OF THE MELBOURNE SCHOOL OF PHARMACY.

At the end of August an excursion was proposed to and accepted with delight by the students generally; but one could notice that some faces became overshaded as from a cloud of difficulty hovering in the distance that would likely prevent them from participating.

A *concilium* was at once held to choose the locality to be visited, and the *animus* exhibited in studying maps and railway lines was such as could not be surpassed by a council of war, having under consideration the strategy of an attack.

It was decided to traverse *per pedes apostolorum* the coastline from Cheltenham to Brighton Beach railway station, a distance of eight or nine miles; and Tuesday, the 29th of August, was fixed for the excursion.

The nine o'clock train took us in about an hour to Cheltenham, situated a couple of miles from the bay, and we at once followed the road leading straight towards it, and within a few minutes, on both sides of the road, groups were busily engaged in collecting, studying, and discussing botanical specimens.

The sandy soil, alternating with clayey patches in close proximity to the beach, produces a flora with the physiognomy in which heaths and their consorts predominate, and some members of the *Epacridcæ* family became soon visible.

The beautiful *Epacris impressa*, with its different roseate tints was very rare, while specimens of the white flowering species of *Epacris* were as common as *Erica Tetraliæ* and *Calluna vulgaris* in the heath districts of the old country. The other *Epacridcæ* we found were *Styphelia virgata* and *Correa speciosa*. This latter, the Australian Fuchsia, we met in many large and handsome specimens; and intermixed with these undershrubs we frequently came across *Bossiæa cinerea*; but only rarely another leguminous plant the *Hovea heterophylla*, by some called the Australian Forget-me-not, and occurring in great abundance about Oakleigh. Of *Kennedya prostrata* we found specimens creeping over six feet of ground, and covered profusely with its splendid scarlet-coloured corollæ.

Only a solitary but magnificent representative of *Acacia Latrobei* was discovered, and of the very many indigenous *Mimoseæ* we collected specimens of *Acacia armata, A. oxycedrus, A. longifolia*, and *A. suaveolens*.

Of the *Droseraceæ* family we found *Drosera Whitackeri*, with its large and *Drosera granduligera*, with its crimson petals; and of *Drosera Menziesii* we noticed a specimen thirty-six inches high climbing around the branches of a *Correa viridis* in a fantastical manner.

The lily tribe was represented by thousands of specimens of *Anguillaria Australis*—this very pretty and to botanists highly interesting Spring messenger. We found all the different varieties—the staminate, the pistellate, the hermaphrodite, and the uniftoral forms—and scarcely less frequently occurred the bright yellow blooming *Hypoxis glabella*.

Of the *Ranunculaceæ* we met besides the *Ranunculus aquatilis*, that beautiful diœcious creeper, *Clematis microphylla*, of which, in one instance, we found specimens of both sexes running high up a *Banksia*, encircling and embracing each other in a most tender fashion.

Although the order *Orchidaceæ* is represented by numerous genera in the locality, we found only the modest little Jack-in-the-box, *Pterostylos conninna*, growing in groups of many specimens under Tea-tree hedges.

Only a few specimens were found of *Tetratheca ciliata, Caulinia prostrata, Cassythe pubercens, Comesperma volubilis, Cræpedia Richei, Pimelia phylicoides, Helichrisum scorpioides, Diuris pedunculata*, and *Isopogon ceratophyllum*.

Pteris aquilina abounds in Australia like in many other parts of the globe; the other *Filices* we found were *Adianthum æthivpica* and *Cheilanthes tenuifolia*.

As dear old friends of my younger days, and involuntary dwellers in Australia, sharing the fate of many other individuals of the species *Homo sapiens*, I introduced to my little party *Fumaria officinalis, Malva rotundifolia, Urtica urens, Vicia hirsuta*, and *Marrubium vulgare*, and they were cordially received, quite in a sense of " *Les amis des vos amis sont nosamis.*"

The day was a glorious one, and the impressions received among the umbrageous groves on the high cliffs overhanging the beach, with a view of the magnificent mirror-like and endless expanse at the bay, found a vent in the exclamation of David :—

> *Opera Jehovæ magna !*
> *Exposita omnibus, qui delectantur illis ;*
> *Gloriosum et decorum opus ejus.*

About four o'clock we arrived at the Brighton Beach station, well pleased with our collections and general success, carrying with us pleasant and, I believe, non-evanescent recollections of the many happy incidents of this first botanical excursion—viz., the luncheon in the boat on the beach, the plunge into the sea, the lonely fishermen's huts, the meeting at the Red Bluff, &c.; and in parting we were repeating the adopted device—*Fratres pharmaceutici conjuncti vivant !*

It is contemplated to visit in November the locality of the giant specimens of *Eucalyptus amygdalina* in the forest near Fernshaw, and we cordially invite all those that feel inclined to join.

I embrace this opportunity to express my opinion that it is hardly fair to both student and teacher not to allow the former sufficient time for his studies, or to detain him from joining the botanical excursions, which are of such vital importance, as it is in the field where we best find opportunities to exercise, apply and improve our botanical knowledge; while at the same time a love for the pure pleasures connected with the collecting, studying, and preserving botanical speci- mens is created.   JOHN KRUSE.

Obituary.

MR. HENRY JAMES LONG.

THE death of Mr. Henry James Long, of 183 Bourke-street East, Melbourne, which took place on the 6th of last month, removed from us one of the earliest and most respected of our colonists, and lessened the number of the best-known mem- bers of our profession. Mr. Long was a native of Bath, Eng- land, and came to this part of the world with his family in 1839, when only seven years of age. His father, Mr. D. R. Long, had been in business in Bath for some years, and he emigrated hither when, as need hardly be said, this colony was in the very early days of its existence. He built the well- known establishment at the corner of Bourke and Stephen streets, when that part of Melbourne was still in the "bush" stage, and he was regarded as having made a somewhat hazardous experiment by starting a business "quite out into the country," where he could not, his friends told him, expect to get much custom. At that time Melbourne hardly existed east of Elizabeth-street ; Richmond, where Mr. Long at first lived, was the only suburb, and the journey thither was through thick forest. Mr. H. J. Long was trained to his father's business, and in 1854 he was taken into partnership, and the firm then became known as D. R. Long and Son. In 1857 the elder Mr. Long retired, and Dr. Neild, who, on coming to the colony in 1853, had given up the regular practice of his pro- fession, joined Mr. H. J. Long, and, until 1861, when Dr. Neild resumed practice, the firm was Long and Neild. It then again became Long and Son, and so continued until the melan- choly occurrence which caused the death of the junior partner.

For many years the firm carried on an extensive wholesale business as well as enjoying a large retail connection, princi- pally among the old colonists, to whom the Messrs. Long were well known, and by whom they were greatly respected. Indeed, there are very few instances in this city of a building continu- ing to be devoted for so long a time to its original purpose as this corner has been. "Long's, the chemist's," in fact, has come to be quite an institution; and while nearly every other house in the street has changed its business—some a great many times—this remains exactly as it was years before the goldfields era began, and, as Mr. H. J. Long's eldest son has been educated to the business, and will carry it on, it is not likely there will be any change for some time to come.

And Mr. H. J. Long himself never diverged into any pursuit other than that of a pharmaceutical chemist. He thoroughly understood his business, and was fastidiously conscientious in the practice of it ; and in the dispensing branch of it, we need hardly say, the importance of care and conscientiousness cannot be overrated. Neither did he ever permit himself to take any part in public affairs, although, as an old colonist, being so com- pletely familiar with the progress of Victoria, he would have been very useful, especially in municipal work. Privately, how- ever, he took a warm interest in whatever concerned the general weal and in the brotherhood to which he belonged. His relations with the medical profession were of the best kind, for he held decided views upon the obligation of the pharmacist to limit himself to his specific duties.

His sudden death by an overdose of morphia caused a pain- ful regret in the minds of his many friends, and to his relations it was necessarily a most distressing shock. He left a widow and five children, the eldest of whom, as has been said, will continue the business to which he has been brought up, so that the familiar corner will, in all probability, retain the appearance to which the public have so long been accustomed.

WE regret that we have to announce the death of Professor Dr. Fredrich Wöhler, the illustrious chemist, at the age of eighty-three years. This eminent man passed away on the 23rd of September, after a short illness, to use the language of one of his friends who lives in our midst, "a sad and irrepar- able loss to science and to his wide circle of friends ; but the lustre which this bright spirit shed on chemical science can never be dimmed."

REMINISCENCES OF A PHARMACIST.

(BY J. B. MUMMERY.)

(Continued.)

A CHARGE OF EMBEZZLEMENT.

THE other case I mentioned, as occurring to myself, was of quite as outrageous, although of a different nature.

Some years after I had served the public in the capacity of postmaster, and more than twelve months after resigning its duties, I happened to be riding in the neighbourhood of Cook's River, and drew up at a water-trough outside a public-house for the purpose of refreshing my steed. During the few minutes in which the animal was quenching his thirst, a man (evidently a shoot and three-quarters in the wind) emerged from the hotel, and commenced forthwith to pour upon me a regular cataract of abuse. His language was by no means fit for ears polite, and it was fortunate that there were no houses near, so that his vituperation was poured out to but few, if any, hearers beyond myself.

As the man was a perfect stranger to me, and I could not recollect ever having seen him before, I came to the conclusion either that he had mistaken me for some one else, or that he was an escapee from "Tarban Creek." The solution of the matter, however, came in due time, and it was this :—The irascible individual informed me that three or four years previously he had duly placed in my hands a letter, directed to his friends in "Old Ireland," and as no answer had been returned to the epistle, the sender had not sense enough to account for the fact, in any other way, than that the postmaster had pocketed the sixpence and destroyed his letter.

The gentleman in whose service the young lady who wanted the postmaster to open his letter had been, was the son-in-law of a famous character in convict history, whose chequered career was brought to a close at Newtown some twenty or twenty-five years ago. This was no less a personage than

MARGARET CATCHPOLE, THE SUFFOLK GIRL.

Many of my readers have, no doubt, read a book under the above title. The work is now, I think, almost extinct ; I know that I have made many attempts of late years to procure a copy, but without success. I read it myself on the voyage out to Sydney, but this was long before I knew the heroine, and con- sequently it did not possess the same interest for me as it would have done afterwards, but for the information of such of my readers as have not seen the book in question, I will relate in brief the circumstances as they occur to my recollection.

A noted smuggler of the name of Laws, I think (or something sounding like it), got into trouble over his nefarious business, and would undoubtedly have fallen into the hands of the officers of the law, and paid the penalty of his misdeeds (which penalty in those days, I believe, was death), but for the heroic devotion of his sweetheart, a girl whose name is mentioned above.

This young female, with a true woman's love, thinking of nothing but the danger to the object of her affections, pressed a horse into the service, and rode the animal a great distance in a marvellously short space of time for the purpose of aiding in some way her lover's escape. This she accomplished under circumstances which not only made her name famous from one end of England to another, but even caused her to be regarded as a heroine in humble life. As, however, the steed did not belong to Margaret, but to a gentleman who had an objection to parting with it, even for such a purpose as aiding in a smuggler's escape, she was taken up, tried, and sentenced to transportation.

What became of her quondam lover I do not recollect, but Margaret, after serving her sentence in New South Wales, married a well-to-do squatter, who had become enamoured of her personal charms, with whom she lived for many years a most exemplary life. When her husband died he left her well-provided for, and with a family of sons and daughters, some of the former occupying at this day posts of honour and influence in the sister colony.

I have at this moment a lively recollection of a venerable lady, with hair as white as driven snow, possessing even at her advanced age traces of former beauty, who used to drive up to my door in a carriage and pair worthy of the Governor. This was "Margaret Catchpole," the Suffolk girl.

A MEMORABLE EVENT.

Of all the varied scenes which arise to my memory after the lapse of many years there are none which present themselves to my mental vision with such distinctness as the memorable wreck of the ship "Dunbar."

As most of the events connected with that lamentable affair have appeared from time to time in various journals, it will not be necessary for me to allude to them further than to chronicle some with which I was personally connected, and which, I do not recollect having before seen in print, and which, I am afraid, speak more for the curiosity of the gentler sex than either their humanity or their decency.

Nearly every one now is cognisant of the fact that about twenty-five years ago (I forget the exact date) a fine new ship called the "Dunbar" went down close to Sydney Heads through a fatal mistake of the captain's, and that every soul on board save one found an immediate and watery grave.

This occurred, if I recollect aright, on a Friday night, and the following Sunday I determined to go down to the Heads and have a look at the wreck. I had expected that there would be many of the masculine gender who would be touched with the same inclination as myself ; but I was not at all prepared for the scene which met my gaze when I got fairly on the road. Vehicles of every conceivable description had been pressed into the service of excited sightseers, and the whole distance from George-street to the Heads (as I subsequently found) was literally alive with carts, cabs, 'busses, private carriages, and pedestrians—men, women, and even children, trudging along with a pertinacity which could only be equalled by passengers on the road to Flemington on Cup Day.

On arriving at the Heads I found an immense concourse of persons, of all ages and of both sexes, gathered at the edge of a cliff overlooking the scene of the catastrophe ; and here a sight met my gaze which I shall not forget to my dying day—a sight which, I am sorry to record, was witnessed, not only by strong, stout-hearted men, able and willing to render assistance should such have been required, but by women and children, whose sole object must have been a morbid desire for sickly sight-seeing, and whose presence could only have been a hindrance to those whose painful occupation I will endeavour to describe.

On a flat ledge of rock, fully two hundred feet below the spectators, a man was standing nearly naked. A line was round his body, one end of which was held by his friends above. The end of another line, also held by his mates, he grasped in his left hand ; and, thus equipped, waited for the influx of the waves, nearly every one of which carried on to the rocky platform on which the man was standing portions of the mangled bodies of the unfortunates who had perished in the wreck. These mangled portions of humanity having been secured by the man on the rock before the retreating waters could carry them back to the deep, were made fast to the line, and, having been drawn up, were placed in a large black box. This box when filled was replaced by another, and thus were gathered together and subsequently interred portions of the bodies of the passengers and crew of the ill-fated ship "Dunbar."

(To be continued.)

Legal and Magisterial.

ECHUCA POLICE COURT.
TUESDAY, 24TH OCTOBER, 1882.
(Before Mr. Graham Webster, P.M.)
CASE OF ALLEGED ARSON.

JOHN FREDERICK FAULKNER GRACE, chemist, was charged with feloniously and maliciously setting fire to the house of Mrs. Shields. Mr. Conant appeared for prisoner. Mr. Penne-father, instructed by Mr. Akehurst, appeared for the prosecution, and explained the circumstances of the case.

Detective Hayes, stationed at Echuca, deposed that on the 14th inst. he went to Mrs. Shields' premises in company with Constable Rogers. In consequence of something he heard he went to the railway station, and told Grace there had been a fire at the house he lived in, and in consequence of statements made he wished him to come back. Grace asked if the place was burnt down. He said—"No, only the back portion." Prisoner then said—"What a d—— shame." They then went back at prisoner's own request. Took prisoner to the police station and read the warrant to him. He made no statement. Searched prisoner, who had three keys (produced) on him. One opened No. 3 door, and another the back door of the

front cottage. The third did not open any of the doors. The fire appeared to have originated in No. 3 room, and went towards No. 2. Found a match in the right-hand corner of No. 3 room, amongst some rubbish. By Mr. Conant—The match was damp when he picked it up. (His Worship was of opinion the match had never been lit.) Had no warrant to arrest Grace at the railway station. Looked at the lock of the door.

A quantity of other evidence was taken, and the prisoner was committed to the first gaol delivery. Bail was allowed in his own recognisance of £200 and two sureties of £100 each.

TESTING OF BENZOIC ACID.

C. SCHNEIDER has modified Schacht's method of testing benzoic acid, sublimed from Siam benzoin, by using 16 (instead of 5) drops of half per cent. solution of potassium permagnate, which is completely decolourised, and after eight hours the liquid remains colourless (*Phar. Zeitung*, No. 20). The artificial benzoic acids, or such sublimed with Siam benzoin, or prepared from benzoin by the wet process, do not effect the complete reduction of the test solution, and in the presence of cinnamic acid the odour of benzaldehyde becomes apparent. The sublimed acid, carefully preserved in dark-coloured bottles, does not lose this deoxidising power on keeping.

Mr. Jahns having noticed the strong reducing power of vanillin upon permanganate, experiments were also made with this compound and with mixtures of vanillin and toluol-benzoic acid. Such mixtures, more particularly those containing one-tenth, one-twentieth, or one-thirtieth of vanillin behave very similar to sublimed benzoic acid ; but, aside from the peculiar odour, the liquid, after eight hours, is of a distinct yellow colour, and contains a deposit of colourless or slightly-coloured crystals.

The author regards the permanganate test as well adapted for distinguishing benzoic acid, sublimed from benzoin, from the acid of other sources, and from that which is contaminated with cinnamic acid ; but he advocates its preparation by the pharmacist.—*Archiv d. Phar.*, June, 1882, pp. 401—403.

Professor Ed. Schaer has likewise made a series of comparative experiments with benzoic acid of different origin and permanganate, following Schacht's directions, and arrived at the following conclusions :—

1. Benzoic acid, sublimed from benzoin, exerts a striking reducing action, both in acid and alkaline solution, upon permanganate solution, not shared by benzoic acid of other modes of preparation, or only in a limited degree. The non-officinal benzoic acids give, in alkaline solution, at first a green colour.

2. Benzoic acid, prepared from benzoin with lime, behaves like the artificial acid, and resembles the sublimed acid in its reducing action only if prepared from the residues of sublimation or from benzoin containing cinnamic acid.

3. The acid prepared from benzoin with lime does not, by sequent sublimation, acquire the reducing action of genuine flowers of benzoin.

4. Non-officinal benzoic acids acquire, by sublimation with benzoin, the reducing action upon permanganate ; but even with an addition of 20 per cent. of benzoin before the sublimation, the action is by far less pronounced that that of the official acid.

5. Cinnamic acid possesses an energetic reducing action in acid and alkaline solution, and in mixtures with non-officinal benzoic acids modifies the behaviour of the latter.

6. Benzoic acid, which does not reduce permanganate in acid solution, and causes with it a green colour in alkaline solution, does not acquire the property of instantaneously reducing the permanganate, even when mixed with 10 per cent. of cinnamic acid ; the reduction takes place only after several minutes.—*Archiv d. Phar.*, June, 1882, pp. 425—430.

LECTURE ON AGRICULTURE.

THE lecture on the " Science of Agriculture," by Mr. Marks, of the School of Mines, delivered on the show ground on the 26th October, was listened to by a very large audience. The speaker was introduced by the Hon. Mr. M'Bain. The Minister of Agriculture presided. The Minister of Mines and the Hon. R. Clark also appeared on the platform, and at the close the latter gentleman spoke in high terms of what had been heard. The lecture itself was attentively listened to, and commenced with the value of science to the farmer, and ran through the various points of interest in agriculture. The effects of disforesting, deficient drainage, manures, rotation, food of plants, functions of their organs, the applications of geology, meteorology, botany, and chemistry were severally discussed. A word was said on behalf of the birds; the value of chemical fertilisers, the utilisation of waste, the formation of new industries, &c., were forcibly spoken of. A vote of thanks, cordially responded to by the audience, showed their appreciation of the lecturer's remarks.

Correspondence.

To the Editor of The Australasian Supplement to the Chemist and Druggist.

SIR—Respecting the assertion of your amusing correspondent "Natrium," in your October number, that "if the chemists and druggists of Otago could have foreseen the position of pharmacy in New Zealand in September, 1882, there would have been neither Pharmacy Act or Pharmacy Board in existence," I would simply repeat the remark of Sir Joseph Banks when he boiled a potful of fleas, and the result was unsatisfactory to that distinguished naturalist—"Fleas are not lobsters." So Otago is not New Zealand, nor its pharmacists omnipotent.

PAKEHA TACOOTA.

Wellington, N.Z., 4th November, 1882.

Notes and Abstracts.

CARBOLIC ACID TURNING RED.—The cause of this change is not exactly known, but is generally attributed to the presence of ammonia and nitrous compounds in the atmosphere. A deep red colour would not be admissible, but a slight pinkish tint is not considered objectionable in carbolic acid intended for internal use.

UTILISING LIQUID CARBONIC ACID.—Krupp, the great gun manufacturer, is said to be employing at his works a very ingenious way of recovering the coils of guns which have become useless. He beats the barrel to redness, and then introduces liquid carbonic acid. The cold thus produced causes shrinkage, and allows the coils to be removed.

THRIFT AND SCIENCE.—The *Univers* professes to explain the mystery of the collection of used postage-stamps. It states that the indigo used in printing them being rather expensive, the French post-office itself buys back the old stamps, and skilled chemists are employed to extract the indigo, so that it may be again employed in making new stamps.

TO PULVERISE ZINC.—Zinc becomes exceedingly brittle when heated to nearly its melting point. To reduce it to powder, therefore, the best plan is to pour melting zinc into a dry and warm cast-iron mortar, and as soon as it shows signs of solidifying pound it with the pestle. In this way it may be reduced to a very fine powder.

TO DETECT ALKALIES IN NITRATE OF SILVER.—Stolba recommends the salt to be dissolved in the smallest quantity of water, and to add to the filtered solution hydrofluosilicic acid, drop by drop. Should a turbidity appear an alkaline salt is present. But should the liquid remain limpid, an equal volume of alcohol is to be added, which will cause a precipitate in case the slightest trace of an alkali be present.

REMOVAL OF PLASTER-OF-PARIS BANDAGES.—Dr. F. H. Murdock, of Bradford, Pa., says:—"A very convenient way to remove a plaster-of-Paris bandage is as follows:—Take a strong solution of nitric acid, and by means of a camel's hair pencil paint a strip across the bandage at the most desirable point for division. The acid will so soften the plaster that it may be readily divided by means of an ordinary jack-knife."

ABSORPTION OF POISONS BY PLANTS.—Late experiments by Prof. Phillips appear to confirm the theory of Freytag, that plants absorb all soluble matters indiscriminately through their rootlets, and that the absorption of poisonous metals causes no disturbance until a certain degree of concentration is reached, when the plant rapidly withers and dies. It is thus of the greatest importance to prevent any crop-growing soil from becoming impregnated with any poisonous elements.

INDELIBLE ANILINE MARKING INK.—Dissolve 1 oz. of cupric chloride in 3½ ozs. of distilled water, and add 1¼ ozs. of common salt, and 1⅛ ozs. aqua ammonia. One volume of this solution is then mixed with four parts of a solution prepared as follows: Aniline hydro-chlorate, 3¾ ozs.; distilled water, 2½ ozs.; gum arabic solution (gum 1 oz., water 2 ozs.), 2½ ozs.; glycerine, 1¼ ozs. The greenish liquid resulting is an excellent indelible ink for linen, although the characters written with it do not develop a full black colour until after exposure to the air for a day or two if not hot pressed.

USE OF PYROGALLIC ACID.—M. Vidal, after using pyrogallic acid with care in the treatment of psoriasis, has tried a salve with good effect to heal phagedenic ulcers and to cicatrise chancres. He applied it to the ulcer daily for three days, and states that the pain caused is only moderate, and lasts but from eight to ten minutes. The formula he recommends is acid pyrogallic 20 grams and lard or vaseline 100 grams.—*Bull. Soc. de Thérap.*

IODOFORM INSANITY.—According to Max Schede (*Centralblatt für Chirurgie*, No. 3, 1882) the use of iodoform externally, particularly in children, has been attended by marked psychical symptoms, even at times amounting to true insanity. General mental confusion has in at least two instances been traced to it, recovering when local applications of iodoform to wounds have been removed, and reappearing on their reapplication. He has had also one case of deep melancholia result from its use, two cases of raptus melancholicus, and the three cases of simple depression. It is probable that iodoform only has these effects in patients of a neuropathic diathesis.—*Chicago Med. Review*, 15th March.

MOSQUITO OIL.—A correspondent from Sheepshead Bay, a place celebrated for the size of its mosquitoes and the number of its amateur fishermen, recommends the following as a very good mixture for anointing the face and hands while fishing:

Oil of tar	1 ounce.
Olive oil	1 ounce.
Oil of pennyroyal	½ ounce.
Spirit of camphor	½ ounce.
Glycerine	¼ ounce.
Carbolic acid	2 drachms.

Mix. Shake well before using.

MM. Weber and Thomas, of the French army (*Lancet*, p. 152), state that they have prepared tow in a chemically pure state, of perfect whiteness, soft, very elastic and readily absorbent, easily impregnated with antiseptics, and cheap. It is obtained by treating ordinary tow with caustic soda, and afterwards washing with solution of hypochlorite of soda to bleach it, the alkali being subsequently removed by hydrochloric acid. The cost of the tow is stated to be 1½ fr. to 1¾ fr. per kilo, or when carbolised 2 fr. to 2½ fr. per kilo. To impregnate it with carbolic acid, a solution of three parts of the acid in two of alcohol is sprinkled on sheets of filter paper laid between sheets of tow and placed in a closed box. In forty-eight hours the acid is said to pass entirely into the tow. The tow is thus made to contain 10 per cent. of carbolic acid. The medical papers are now largely discussing phthisis from various aspects, and it is within the limits of possibility that the pharmaceutical chemist may be called upon to provide test solutions for detecting the *Bacillus tuberculosus*. It may be as well for him to know therefore that Dr. H. Gibbes, curator of the King's College Museum, London, publishes, in the *Lancet* (p. 183), a new method of detecting the *Bacillus tuberculosus* in phthisical sputa, which he says he has found more successful than either Koch's or Ehrlich's process. The solutions he uses are those of magenta crystals, and chrysoidin, and the formula given is:—Magenta crystals, 2 grams; pure aniline, 3 grams; alcohol, specific gravity ·130, and distilled water, 20 cubic centimetres. The aniline is dissolved in the spirit and then rubbed up with the magenta in a glass mortar, adding the spirit gradually until all is dissolved, then adding the water slowly while stirring. The solution should be kept in a stoppered bottle. The solution of chrysoidin is a saturated one in distilled water, a crystal of thymol being added to preserve it. Dilute nitric acid, made of one part of commercial acid and two of distilled water, is used to remove the excess of colour after using the magenta stain. According to Dr. Gibbes the bacilli, when mounted, can be detected with daylight by an ordinary quarter-inch objective, and a one-eighth dry glass will show with the same illumination that they are rows of spherical bodies.

J. BOSISTO

LABORATORY: RICHMOND, MELBOURNE

By whom the Eucalyptus preparations were first introduced, both in Australia and Europe, and to whom has been awarded the Silver Medal of the Society of Arts, London ; the Gold Medal of the Sydney International, the Gold Medal of the Melbourne International Exhibitions, and Prize Medals from the various European, American, and other Australian Exhibitions, dating from the first of his investigations of this vegetation in 1853, and published in the Transactions of the Royal Society of Victoria, Exhibition Reports, &c.

OL. EUCALYPTI ESS.

Obtained from the Amygdalina Odorata species ; the Eucalyptus Oil of Commerce.

FOR EXTERNAL USE. A valuable remedy for Rheumatism, Lumbago, Sciatica, Sprains, Chilblains, Whooping Cough, Croup, Asthma, Bronchitis, Sore Throat, Chronic Hepatitis, and all other painful affections where a stimulating application is required.

MODE OF APPLICATION FOR RAPID EFFECT. Apply the Oil with much friction, until a glow of warmth is established.

FOR A SOOTHING AND STEADY ACTION. Shake well together a tablespoonful of the Oil with half-a-pint of warm water, saturate a cloth with this, and apply over the painful part—repeating, if necessary, in half-an-hour.

FOR INTERNAL USE. For Coughs, Asthmatic and Throat Affections — 5-drop doses on loaf sugar occasionally.

This Oil is a thorough **DEODORANT** and **DISINFECTANT**, and an antiseptic of great power. A few drops sprinkled on a cloth and suspended in a sick room renders the air refreshing ; and for disinfecting and deodorising, a tablespoonful of the Oil added to two or three pounds' weight of sawdust, well mixed and distributed, will speedily produce a purifying effect.

BOSISTO'S EUCALYPTUS OIL is the genuine Essence of the Tree, and all labels bearing the name of Bosisto and the Parrot Brand may be relied on.

As Mr. Bosisto finds that inferior and unreliable Oils, obtained without discrimination from various or uncertain species or Eucalyptus, are being vended in the place of his Ol. Eucalyptus Amygdalinæ, he cautions buyers and the trade, in ordering, to specify

BOSISTO'S EUCALYPTUS OIL.

All original jars and bottles bear the certificate, signed, "J. Bosisto & Co.," together with the Trade Mark, "Parrot Brand," on yellow ground.

WHOLESALE AGENTS:

Felton, Grimwade & Co.,

31 FLINDERS LANE WEST, MELBOURNE.

Chem & Druggy (Aust. Sup.)
v. 5, no. 56 : 61-68, (Dec., 1882)

THE Chemist & Druggist.

WITH AUSTRALASIAN SUPPLEMENT.

(Published under direction of the Pharmaceutical Society of Victoria.)

No. 56. { PUBLISHED ON THE 15TH OF EVERY MONTH. }
Registered for Transmission as a Newspaper.

DECEMBER, 1882.

{ SUBSCRIPTION, 15s. PER ANNUM, INCLUDING DIARY, POST FREE.

HEMMONS, LAWS & CO.

55 & 57 RUSSELL STREET, MELBOURNE,

Wholesale Druggists, & Druggists' Sundriesmen,

MANUFACTURERS OF PURE CHEMICALS, PHARMACEUTICAL, PHOTOGRAPHIC, AND OTHER PREPARATIONS,

IMPORTERS OF

Drugs, Chemicals, Essential Oils, Fruit Essences,

AND DRUGGISTS' SUNDRIES.

"New Remedies stocked as soon as introduced."

PROPRIETORS OF

PEARCE'S LAVENDER WATER WITH MUSK.

,,   TOILET VINEGAR.

,,   ROYAL STANDARD PERFUMES.

,,   INDIAN INSECT POWDER.

,,   SALICYLIC SOAP.

,,   FULLERS' EARTH, &c.

H. L. & CO. *desire to state that they have just opened up Goods ex* "SHANNON," "CARLISLE CASTLE," "CONNAUGHT RANGER," *and* "AFGHAN," *comprising large parcels from the well-known houses of*
MESSRS. HOWARDS & SONS,
       SAVORY & MOORE,
          BATTLEY & WATTS,
             MALTINE MANUFACTURING CO.,
                THOS. WHIFFEN & SON,
and are in receipt of regular shipments, their Stocks in every br
being carefully and well assorted.

55 & 57 RUSSELL STREET, MELBOURNE

The Chemist and Druggist.

WITH AUSTRALASIAN SUPPLEMENT.

OFFICE: MUTUAL PROVIDENT BUILDINGS, COLLINS STREET WEST.

Published on the 15th of each Month.

THIS Journal is issued gratis to all paid-up Members of the PHARMA-
CEUTICAL SOCIETY OF VICTORIA, and to non-members at Fifteen Shillings
per annum, payable in advance. A copy of *The Chemists and Druggists'
Diary*, published annually, is forwarded post free to every subscriber.

Advertisements, remittances, and all business communications to be
addressed to THE HONORARY SECRETARY OF THE PHARMACEUTICAL SOCIETY,
MELBOURNE.

SCALE OF CHARGES FOR ADVERTISEMENTS:

	Per annum.		Per annum.
One Page	..£8 0 0	Quarter Page	..£3 0 0
Half do.	.. 5 0 0	Business Cards	.. 2 0 0

Special rates for wrapper and pages preceding and following literary
matter. Advertisements of Assistants Wanting Situations, 2s. 6d. each.

Advertisements for insertion in the current month should be sent to the
office before the 10th.

COMMUNICATIONS for the EDITORIAL department of this journal should be
addressed to THE EDITOR, MUTUAL PROVIDENT BUILDINGS, COLLINS STREET
WEST, MELBOURNE.

No notice can be taken of anonymous communications. Whatever is
intended for insertion must be authenticated by the name and address of
the writer—not necessarily for publication, but as a guarantee of good faith.

PUBLIC NOTICE.

MESSRS. HEMMONS, LAWS & CO. desire to notify
that business will be carried on as usual at 55 & 57
RUSSELL-STREET, MELBOURNE.

MARRIAGE.

ANDERSON—OGLE.—On the 2nd December, at the residence of the bride,
by the Rev. E. H. Du Bois, William Ross Anderson, receiver, paymaster,
and clerk of courts, Maryborough, to C. Florance Ogle, daughter of Mr.
Frcdk. Ogle, chemist, Maryborough.

DEATHS.

OGG.—On the 10th December, at his residence, Walsh-street, South Yarra,
Charles Ogg, chemist, of this city and South Yarra, in his fifty-sixth
year.

PULLING.—On the 24th November, at Coburg, Alexander Frederick, aged
forty-three years, chemist, eldest son of the late Charles Pulling, wholesale druggist, Melbourne.

STEPHENS.—On the 30th November, at Footscray, William Bell, only son of
William Stephens, chemist, aged fourteen months.

The Month.

THE council of the Pharmaceutical Society of Victoria have
concluded the purchase from the Government of the building
at present in the occupation of the County Court in Swanston-
street. The purchase is deemed in every respect a very satisfactory one for the society.

We regret to announce that a meeting of the creditors of
Messrs. W. Hood and Co., wholesale chemists, Elizabeth-street,
Melbourne, was held on Tuesday, 19th December, at Scott's
Hotel, and an approximate balance-sheet was presented,
showing liabilities amounting to £6413. The assets are set
down at £7561, leaving a surplus of £1148. The estate was
assigned to two of the principal creditors, Messrs. M'Lean and
Gotch, and Messrs. Davey, Cole and Flack were appointed
accountants.

The diaries for the year 1883 are shortly expected, and will
be distributed as soon as possible after arrival.

Special attention is drawn to the arrangements for the election of the new Pharmacy Board made by the returning-
officer.

The following amounts have been received for the Benevolent Fund from members who did not attend the dinner:—
Dr. J. E. Neild, £1 1s.; R. S. D. Morgan, £1 1s.; Henry
Francis, £1 1s.; Geo. Lewis and Sons, £1 1s.; W. A. Stokes,
£1 1s.; E. L. Marks, £1 1s.; C. Marston, £1 1s.; A. B. Clemes,
£1 1s.; Dr. Jas. Robertson, £1 1s.; T. H. Walton, £1 1s.;
John Jackson, 10s.; A. Wallworth, 10s.

THE C. F. COOK FUND.—Mr. Bowen desires to acknowledge
the following sums received for this fund:—J. A. Hicks,
Brighton, £1; F. Reeve, Queensland, £1 1s.; J. B. Mummery,
5s.

The last of the winter course of lectures in connection with
the Technological Museum was delivered by Mr. Dunn on the
4th December in the lecture-hall of the institution. The
course has been under the superintendence of Mr. Cosmo
Newbery, and has included classes in practical chemistry and
metallurgy for advanced pupils, and elementary chemistry for
beginners. The later lectures have been well attended.
Another course will commence in March next.

The following legally qualified medical practitioners have
been registered under the provisions of the Medical Practi-
tioners Statute, 1865:—Samuel William Bierley, Yarra Bend;
Charles Rooke, Germanton, New South Wales; John Brett,
Melbourne; William Henry Dutton, Castlemaine; Jeremiah
M'Kenna, Emerald Hill.

Mr. J. C. Goold, of Kyneton, has disposed of his business at
Kyneton to Mr. Queale. Mr. Goold is now managing for
Messrs. D. R. Long and Son, Bourke-street.

Mr. C. E. Towl has been recommended by the Board of
Examiners for the gold medal of 1882. In their report they
give him great praise for his papers.

The business for some years past carried on by Mr. T.
Norris at 70 Chapel-street, Prahran, has been transferred to
Mr. T. M. Dalton.

We are requested by Mr. Rivers Langton to state that he
has undertaken the agency of Messrs. Lynch and Co., Aldersgate-street, London, in all the Australasian colonies.

Messrs. Warner and Scott, Sturt-street, Ballarat, have purchased from Mr. J. T. Macgowan the business formerly carried
on by him at Ballarat.

Mr. Edward L. Holdsworth, son of Mr. John Holdsworth,
J.P., of Sandhurst, has commenced business on his own account
at Long Gully. Mr. Holdsworth is well known in the district,
having been with his father for a number of years.

The obituary of the month contains the names of Mr.
Charles Ogg, the esteemed and well-known chemist of Collins-
street and South Yarra; Mr. A. F. Pulling, Coburg; Mr. F. P.
Sheehy, who died at Wellington, New Zealand; and Mr.
William Cornish (formerly of Chapel-street, Prahran), who died
in Sydney from an overdose of chloral.

The business of Mr. Tom Luke at Shepparton has been purchased by Mr. Alexander A. Morrison, lately an assistant to
Mr. Wylie, of Hawthorn.

Messrs. Wm. Ford and Co. (Messrs. Swift and Reed, proprietors) have signed a contract for extensive alterations to their business premises in Swanston-street. The improvements will embrace an entire alteration to the front building, which will be considerably enlarged, and a new building at the back for the wholesale and manufacturing department.

Mr. J. W. Smith, who for some time was in charge for Mr. J. D. Evans, of Smith-street, Collingwood, has purchased from Mr. William Stephens his business at Footscray.

THE ANNUAL DINNER OF THE PHARMACEUTICAL SOCIETY OF VICTORIA.

THE annual dinner was held at Clements' Café, on Wednesday, the 13th December, 1882. There was a good attendance, and the manner in which the dinner was served reflected great credit on Mr. Clements.

The president of the society, Mr. Wm. Bowen, occupied the chair. The vice-chairs were occupied by Mr. John T. Thomas, vice-president of the society, and Mr. J. Bosisto, M.L.A., president of the Pharmacy Board. Amongst the visitors present were Messrs. Rivers Langton, Daniel Wilkie, B. C. Hartiman, W. J. Bowen, and T. Fripp.

The country districts were represented by Mr. Henry Brind, Ballarat ; Mr. John Holdsworth, Sandhurst, and Mr. A. J. Owen, Geelong. Letters of apology were received from Mr. Frank Senior, president of the Pharmaceutical Society, N.S.W; Drs. Moloney, Hewlett, and Robertson ; Mr. Geo. Lewis ; Mr. H. Wheeler, president of the Ballarat District Chemists' Association ; Mr. J. Harris, M.L.A. ; Mr. G. D. Carter, M.L.A ; Mr. C. D. Barraud, president of the Pharmacy Board, Wellington ; Mr. J. V. Ross, president of the Pharmaceutical Society, Christchurch ; Mr. Graves Aickin, Auckland, &c.

The chairman proposed the toasts of Her Majesty the Queen, their Royal Highnesses the Prince and Princess of Wales, and His Excellency the Governor, all of which were duly honoured.

Dr. William Thomson, who was received with applause, proposed "The Pharmaceutical Society of Victoria," coupled with the name of Mr. William Bowen, president. The members of the society deserved great credit for the manner in which they had raised the status of that body, and he felt highly gratified at the fact that they had made him an honorary member. In early days the chemical and drug trade was associated with that of the grocer, but through the exertions of Mr. Bosisto and others whom he saw around him that night, the connection had been severed ; they now enjoyed a separate constitution. The medical profession, he might point out, was deeply interested in the welfare of the society, for as pharmacy advanced so would physic. He wished the society a long and increasingly prosperous career. (Cheers.)

Mr. Bowen, on rising to respond, was warmly applauded, and said :—I thank you for the kind manner in which you have been pleased to respond to the last toast. In replying thereto I will endeavour briefly to refer to some of the more important events which have occurred during the past year interesting to our body as pharmaceutical chemists. You will doubtless remember that, at the last annual dinner, reference was made to the establishment of a school of pharmacy. Although during the last session lectures have been regularly delivered, and as a result of such teaching I may mention that every student from this school who presented himself for examination passed with considerable credit, yet the council of the society have felt hampered by the consideration that we had no local habitation. They therefore determined to apply to the Government for a grant of land in order to carry out their views, and I feel proud in telling you to-night that the Government have displayed their wisdom and intelligence in recognising the importance and justice of our claims by granting us a site in every way suitable for our requirements. On this land there is a building erected, which the council have purchased and paid for, and as soon as we obtain possession of the same, which will probably be in a few months, by the judicious expenditure of a few hundred pounds in restoring and rendering the same suitable for our occupation, the members of this society may well be congratulated on the establishment of the Victorian School of Pharmacy—with a splendid lecture-hall, a completely fitted laboratory, a museum, library, and classrooms—on a sound and substantial basis, and on a scale at least equal, if not surpassing, anything yet attempted in this colony. As soon as this school is complete and open I anticipate a large addition to the number of students, not only from among those who intend to pursue the calling of a pharmaceutical chemist, but from the public at large, many of whom are desirous of attending the lectures on chemistry and botany ; besides, there will probably be some of the students from the medical school, for I regret to say that, at this institution, practical pharmacy is ignored—or, at all events, if my information is correct, all that is required from the student is a certificate of having attended at some open dispensary for a short period ; and my information goes further than this—that such certificate can readily be obtained at the expense of a few pounds, a few cigars, and a pack of cards. I assure our medical friends present, the managers of that institution, and all who feel an interest in the Medical School of Victoria, that I do not refer to this matter in any carping spirit, or with any feeling of class antagonism ; but I assure them, with every feeling of regard and candour, that this school will never attain the same high position of those grand institutions of the mother-country until they have included in its curriculum an intimate knowledge of practical pharmacy. Too much importance cannot be attached to the School of Pharmacy which we are about to inaugurate, as the health of the public at large is dependent in a great degree upon the intelligence and good training of the young pharmaceutical students. On the 1st of January last a new regulation of the Pharmacy Act came into force, by which all apprentices before the registration of their indentures by the Pharmacy Board, will require to present a certificate of having passed the matriculation examination of the University, or some other examination equivalent to the same, in which Latin, English, and arithmetic are essential subjects. This I regard as a most important step, as prior to this date apprentices have been found who postponed the passing the preliminary examination until a later period ; and surely it is a much easier matter to pass such an examination when fresh from their scholastic studies. The mind of the student will thus he relieved, and entirely devoted to the study of the other essential branches of knowledge. During the past year the council considered it desirable to offer some encouragement to the students ; they therefore determined to present a gold medal to the most successful of the students after their examination in the several subjects, chemistry, materia medica, and botany ; and I have much pleasure in announcing that the first presentation was made, in the month of June, to Mr. William Lowe, a gentleman who greatly distinguished himself ; and I have every confidence in stating that if he continues his studies with the same devotion he will prove an ornament to his profession. In the month of July, at a meeting of the society, a deputation was appointed to represent the chemists before the Tariff Commission. This deputation was courteously received, and from representations from their standpoint made to that body I have much pleasure in anticipating that a more equitable arrangement of the tariff will result. In August last rules were passed by the council for the protection of the society against the improper use of their diplomas. Cases have occurred where persons have joined the society, paid their subscription for one year, obtaining the diploma, and then forfeited their position as members by non-payment of their subscription. By the new rule which is now in force any person before he is admitted as a member of the society has to sign a declaration that in the event of his ceasing to become a member from any cause that he or his representatives will return the diploma, and thus prevent the fraudulent practice now existing. On behalf of the Pharmaceutical Society I am bound to express my thanks, not only to our old friends, Mr. Blackett and Mr. Bosisto, but likewise to Mr. Zox, Mr. Laurens, and other parliamentary representatives who were familiar with the plain unvarnished statement of our position, and who have so ably represented the same to the Government. My thanks are likewise especially due to the honorary secretary, Mr. Harry Shillinglaw, for the valuable assistance and suggestions I have invariably received from him ; and I assure you, gentlemen, that with such ability and support the duties of president of this society are reduced to a mere formality. I thank you, again, for your kind response to the toast of the Pharmaceutical Society of Victoria.

Dr. Neild then proposed the "Pharmacy Board," coupled with the name of Mr. Joseph Bosisto, M.L.A. He need hardly remind the gentlemen there that night of the fact that the Pharmacy Board mainly owed its origin to the gentleman whose name was associated with the toast. The board, although only some six years in existence, had already done good service. It had brought about a closer alliance between the chemists and druggists and the medical profession, and a cordial understanding now existed which was of mutual advantage. He was sorry to say that medical students did not at present receive the same careful training in pharmacy that they did in his earlier days; but the efforts now being made by the board would lead to an improvement in that direction. The fact that it had been decided to appoint a professor of pharmacy, and to establish a laboratory, showed that the importance of communicating a thorough knowledge of practical chemistry was being recognised. He was glad that the old county court had been granted by the Government for the purpose of founding a college of pharmacy; and when such an institution was completed the authorities of the University would have to come to the Pharmaceutical Society. ("Hear, hear.") He would like to see an affiliated college, and he could not see any obstacle in the way of forming an alliance with the University. (Applause.) Before sitting down he wished to express satisfaction at seeing so many members of the Legislature present. He had been informed that they had greatly assisted the society in the efforts of that body to secure a suitable site for the proposed college, and he was sure that their efforts were fully appreciated. (Applause.) Mr. Bosisto, who had worked so long and faithfully in the interests of the chemists and druggists of the colony, both in his private and legislative capacities, was especially deserving of thanks. He was a gentleman of whom every one was proud. The chemists and druggists were proud of him and the medical profession was proud of him. (Applause.) He (Dr. Neild) had known Mr. Bosisto ever since he had come to Victoria—over thirty years—and the respect and esteem with which he had then regarded that gentleman had gone on increasing ever since. Messrs. Bosisto, Blackett, Laurens, and Zox, who were present with them that night, were each and all creditable members of Parliament, and were respected by their fellow-citizens accordingly. (Loud applause.)

The toast was drunk with much enthusiasm, and, after musical honours,

Mr. Joseph Bosisto responded. He congratulated the members of the Pharmaceutical Society on the advance made by that body during the past year. With reference to the Board of Pharmacy, he might state that its efforts had been attended with much success, and its members deserved great credit for carrying out the provisions of the Act, with the administration of which they were entrusted. Although that Act had been passed six years before, it had been found so free from defects of any kind that no amending Act had since then been found necessary. This fact proved that the pharmaceutists who had framed the Act knew their business. The Poisons Act—a measure which had been passed hurriedly—had not worked so satisfactorily. Several cases of poisoning had occurred, but the sale of the drugs could not be traced owing to the defective machinery of the Act on one point. Under that Act pharmaceutists kept a register of every poison vended, a register that was perfect in every way, but no such check was imposed on a numerous class of tradesmen who were allowed to sell compounds in the highest degree dangerous to human health and life. He alluded to the grocers, who were practically irresponsible. ("Hear, hear.") In a short time an Act would have to be passed for regulating such cases, and for preventing the indiscriminate sale of virulent poisons. The appointment of a new Board of Pharmacy would soon be necessary, and he exhorted the pharmaceutists of the colony to exercise the greatest care in the election of the members of that body, otherwise the Act would fail in its operation. He had been president of the board for six years—ever since the passing of the Act—and he had no desire to continue in the position any longer. He did not wish to take any active part in the administration of the Act, as he would prefer standing by and watching the operations of the measure. He would at all times take a deep interest in the affairs of the Pharmacy Board and Pharmaceutical Society, but he had given the best part of his lifetime to such matters, and therefore desired a little rest. In conclusion, he might state that he did not intend to stand again either for the position of president or as a member of the board. He thanked those present for their very kind expressions of regard. (Applause.)

Mr. F. S. Grimwade, president of the Melbourne Chamber of Commerce, proposed "The Parliament of Victoria." In speaking to the toast, he could conscientiously say that pharmacists need not be ashamed of the legislators who had sprung from their ranks. Amongst past legislators who had distinguished themselves was Mr. George Harker; and at present there were Messrs. Bosisto, Blackett, and M'Intyre, all four of whom were chemists. ("Hear, hear.")

Mr. E. L. Zox, M.L.A., responded, and in the course of a humorous speech alluded to the remarks made by Dr. Thomson in the early part of the proceedings concerning the investigations recently made into the rise of disinfectants. By many people those remarks might be held to be highly suggestive as bearing on the toast of the Parliament, for it was an undoubted fact that the shameful waste of time which had characterised the last few sessions caused the very name of Parliament to stink in the nostrils of the public. (Laughter.) The Government did very little work. It had delegated most of its functions to Royal Commissions, boards of inquiry, and select committees. There was a Royal Commission on the tariff, another on the Education Act, and a third on the police force, all of which were sitting, and others were in contemplation. He thought, and sincerely hoped, that the time was not far distant when the people of the colony would have cause to be more proud of their representatives than they were at present. (Applause.) There was one matter which he desired to refer to before resuming his seat. When the appeal was first made on behalf of the suffering Jews in Russia the Pharmaceutical Society generously contributed £30 or £40 to the fund; and on behalf of the Anglo-Jewish Association, with which he was connected, he desired to publicly return his thanks for the donation. (Applause.)

Messrs. C. R. Blackett and J. Laurens, M.L.A.'s, also responded. The first-named gentleman deprecated the present system of party government into which the colony had drifted, and trusted that a change into a purer political atmosphere would be speedily made. (Cheers.)

Mr. Rivers Langton said, in proposing the toast of "The Pharmaceutical Society of Great Britain, and Kindred Societies"—I have an easy task, for I carry with me, addressing as I do so intelligent a body of pharmacists, the sympathy of you all. Every one of you here present this evening must recognise the great good the Pharmaceutical Society of Great Britain has done for your business. Speaking from an experience of over thirty years, I have watched the progress of this society, and the wonderful improvement it has worked in the social status of the chemist. The *London Times*, in a recent leading article, has spoken of the chemist as "an important public servant." The compliment is well deserved; but the position is one of great responsibility and trust. It requires, sir, not only a thorough knowledge of the art of dispensing, but a perfect familiarity with the articles dispensed, that they really are of the finest quality, and such as the physician has prescribed, and Dr. Neild has only paid you a just tribute when he spoke of the services rendered by the pharmacist to the medical profession, and the sympathy existing between the two. Your president, in his remarks this evening, with a modesty which we must all admire, has alluded to "the calling of a pharmaceutical chemist." I think he might claim for you the dignity of a profession, for undoubtedly the dispensing of medicines and knowledge of drugs is a profession. Dr. Thomson has spoken of the connection in bygone days existing between the chemist and the grocer, but he never spoke more truly when he said that there was no connection whatever existing at the present time. No sooner does an article get into demand than its sale is monopolised by the grocer, and what is termed the business of a chemist and druggist is narrowed and narrowed every year. The path of the modern pharmacist is one of great difficulty, nor do I think the remuneration received has kept progress with the services rendered; nor do the public yet recognise sufficiently the great services rendered them by the pharmacist. You cannot compare the retailing of medicines with the sale of other goods forming the necessaries of every-day life, and sold in unlimited quantities. But difficulties in some form or other are ever in the path of the chemist. To-day it is the co-operative store; but I do not think the salaried assistant of one of the stores brings the heart and zeal to his work which the chemist does; the latter is entirely at the call of the public at all hours, Sunday not excepted, whilst the stores are only open from stated hours; and those people who go to them to save threepence on a bottle of medicine are the very last who would have any scruple in calling up the chemist at any hour of the night to dispense a prescription which they could not get done in the new channel. Gentlemen, I ask you to drink prosperity to the Pharmaceutical Society of Great Britain, and kindred societies.

Mr. David Jones, who responded, said that the name of England was dear to all colonists who were proud of her annals, institutions, and organisations. He was certain that the institution which they had just honoured was one which they all respected. ("Hear, hear.") The only point in which it had failed, however, was that it had not been of a sufficiently trade character, but that would doubtless be rectified in time.

Mr. C. R. Blackett, M.L.A., who proposed "The Medical Society," said that the Pharmaceutical Society had to deplore the loss of several members, amongst whom were the late Mr. Ogg and Mr. Long. He had much pleasure in proposing the toast allotted to him in the programme, the Medical Society having always worked in harmony with pharmacists whenever occasion or opportunity arose. Dr. Neild, who was closely identified with the society, had always been ready to lend a helping hand to the Pharmaceutical Society, and the latter body was much indebted to that gentleman in consequence. (Applause.)·

Dr. Neild and Baron Sir F. von Müeller, K.C.M.G., responded, the last-named gentleman alluding in a gracefully worded speech to the high objects of pharmacy.

Mr. Henry Brind proposed "Our Visitors," to which Mr. B. C. Harriman responded.

"The Press" and "The Ladies" were duly honoured, and the proceedings then terminated, the dinner having been of a thoroughly enjoyable character throughout.

SYDNEY.

THE Council of the Pharmaceutical Society held its monthly meeting on 21st November, at the board-room, Phillip-street. Present—the president (in the chair), and Messrs. Abraham, Guise, Larmer, Pratt, Watt, and M'Carthy. The minutes of last meeting were read and confirmed.

Mr. James Bowen, of Sydney, applied for the registration of his indentures, dated 23rd October, 1873. Granted.

Mr. James Foot, of Orange, applied for membership. The council directed that the applicant must pass a satisfactory examination before his admission.

The secretary laid on the table copies of the Tasmanian Pharmacy Act.

Several accounts were passed, the principal one being the sum of £40 for new books purchased since last monthly meeting.

The secretary called attention to the courteous conduct of the Victorian Pharmaceutical Society in inviting representatives to their annual dinner, and greatly regretted that he could not be present.

The meeting then closed.

SUPPOSED CASE OF POISONING.

A MAN named William Cornish, aged forty, was found dead in his bed at his residence, 2 Cook-street, Moore Park, Sydney. It appears that the deceased, who was a chemist, had come from Melbourne about twelve months ago, and had recently been in the service of Messrs. Elliott Bros., Pitt-street. The deceased was married, and leaves a widow and two children. An inquest into the circumstances attending the death was commenced at the Victoria Hotel by the coroner. Dr. Wades, who had made a post-mortem examination, said that the man had been dead for three or four hours when he was first called in. He had removed the stomach, and enclosed it in a bottle for analysis of its contents. Mr. G. A. Gaud, chemist, said that on the 20th inst. he had supplied deceased at his written request with half an ounce of chloral hydrate. This was more than sufficient to cause death, if taken in one dose. He was informed, before supplying the poison, that deceased was a chemist, and understood drugs. The widow of deceased stated that her husband had lately been out of employment, and had not done anything for a living for some time past. He was low-spirited during the past week, but never spoke of committing suicide. She last saw him alive on Saturday morning, about breakfast time, and about midday she saw him lying in his bedroom. He had several medicine bottles in his bedroom, some of which contained poison.

The inquest at this stage was adjourned for the proper analysis of the deceased's stomach.

The adjourned inquest into the circumstances in connection with the death of William Cornish, who was found dead in his bed about one o'clock on Saturday afternoon, by his wife, at his late residence, 2 Cook-street was continued on 1st December, at the Victoria Hotel, by Mr. Sbiell, J.P., city coroner. After evidence had been given by Dr. Wades, a verdict of died from natural causes was returned.

NEW ZEALAND.

PHARMACY BOARD EXAMINATIONS.

THE second modified examination under the Pharmacy Board was held simultaneously at Wellington, Auckland, Christchurch, and Dunedin on the 11th November. Five candidates presented themselves, four of whom failed to pass. Messrs. John English and Thos. M. Wilkinson conducted the examination in Dunedin.

PHARMACY BOARD.

QUARTERLY EXAMINATIONS.

THE quarterly examinations under the Pharmacy Act, 1876, were held at the rooms of the Pharmacy Board, Collins-street. At the modified examination, held before Messrs. Blackett and Johnson, on the 4th December, 1882, the following candidates passed:—

1. Reader, F. M. F., Smith-street, Fitzroy.
2. Leddin, H. J., Williamstown.
3. Fox, F. J., Collingwood.
4. Williams, Fred, Melbourne.

The examination for the School of Pharmacy (major certificate) was held on Tuesday, the 5th December. In their report the examiners state that five out of the six candidates exhibited an amount of knowledge that was highly satisfactory. The specimens of live plants for the examination in botany were kindly supplied by Mr. Guilfoyle, of the Botanical Gardens, and represented most of the natural orders of medicinal plants. In concluding their report the examiners bear testimony to the excellent manner in which the students had been taught. The following are the candidates who passed in all subjects:—

1. Towl, Charles Edward, Fitzroy.
2. Higgins, John M., South Yarra.
3. Richards, Augustus Charles, Richmond.
4. Davis, Henry, Melbourne.

In Materia Medica and Botany only.

5. Woodfull, Thomas, Melbourne.

PRELIMINARY EXAMINATION, 17TH DECEMBER.

1. Turner, Thomas Edward.
2. Henshall, Chas. L.
3. Gaffney, John.
4. Wragge, Henry G.
5. Hall, Hector E.

THE MAJOR EXAMINATION.—PRACTICAL PHARMACY.—8TH DECEMBER.—FINAL EXAMINATION.

Percy Wisewould, Melbourne.

SANDHURST SCHOOL OF MINES.

THE year just closing has been one of great success in the laboratory department; lectures in chemistry and botany by Mr. E. L. Marks have been well attended, whilst laboratory practice has been diligently pursued, the principles, once learned, enabling students to branch out into their special paths, hence working independently. As much progress may be made as can be digested. Three of the laboratory students have successfully passed their first year in medicine at the Melbourne University, and as chemistry is one of the subjects the assistance gained at the School of Mines is of practical value. Former students from Sandhurst continue to do well, and are not neglectful of the advantages they derived during their term of study. For the matriculation examination this year six of Mr. Marks' pupils in chemistry and botany are presenting themselves, in addition to others who prefer the examination of the Education Department.

NOTES ON SOME LEGUMINOUS PLANTS,

BY BARON VON MUELLER, K.C.M.G., M. & PH.D., F.R.S.

AVAILING myself of the concessions, made by the editor of this periodical for my furnishing occasional contributions for its columns, I beg to direct the attention of the pharmaceutic profession of Australia now to some of the therapeutically interesting leguminous plants, indigenous to this part of the globe and needing further chemical elucidation. The order of Leguminosæ is the leading one in Australia, numbering, so far as hitherto known, 1058 species in this part of the globe. As may be imagined, among such a host of forms, some must be of importance for medical purposes ; and as several species of Oxylobium and its sub-genus Gastrolobium, also of Isotropis of Gompholobium and its sub-genus Burtonia, as well as of Swainsona, have proved dangerous to pastoral animals, it will be worthy of inquiry, particularly where these kinds of plants abound, and thus ample material is available, in what chemically defined principle their powerful and even virulent efficacy may consist, the active matter having in no instance as yet been isolated. The well-known Abrus precatorius, which extends also to the intra-tropical regions of Australia, affords in its pretty seeds, as shown recently, likewise a very peculiar therapeutic remedy of lasting importance. The leaves of some of our native Cassias are violently drastic in their effect ; yet others need still to be tried as substitutes for Senna.

Like in the ordinary European Laburnum the powerful principle is concentrated in the seeds, which yield the Alkaloids Cytisin and Laburnin, so also may perhaps distinct chemical combinations be traced chiefly to seeds of the above-mentioned Australian plants. Thus, then, it may become understood, why Lotus australis proves at times poisonous to pastural animals and at other times not. Even the long known and widely distributed Goodia lotifolia and Indigofera australis have recently been regarded by some settlers as deleterious to stock. In the numerous country places, where now pharmaceutic establishments exist, these kind of plants, as readily and copiously at hand, might be subjected to chemical tests. If once their active principles are found out, it will be easier to institute physiologic experiments with them than with the crude plant. Subjoined is the definition of a new Bossiæa, a genus also worthy of chemical analysis of its seeds, approaching as it does in some respects Goodia, in others Oxylobium and its allies. The discovery of this new plant comparatively near a harbour, known since nearly a century, may also show, that the search for plants in Australia has nowhere yet been exhaustive.

Bossiæa Webbii.

.Glabrous ; branchlets thin, neither compressed nor angular; stipules minute, deltoid ; leaves opposite, flat, renate-semiorbicular, in front copiously denticulated ; flower-stalks extremely short ; bracts very small, rhomboid, roundish, incurved; bracteoles longer than the calyx, fugacious, lanceolar, oblong, rigid, both parallel and curved over the upper side of the flower ; calyx very small, its upper lip almost truncate, about as long as the lower lip ; upper petal evidently longer than the others ; ovary narrow-lanceolar, stalked, glabrous.

On the summit of Mount Lindsay, near King George's Sound ; W. Webb. This pretty species comes nearest in affinity to B. Aquifolium ; but it differs essentially in dwarf stature, much smaller and more rigid leaves, which are neither grey underneath nor provided with large and sharply acuminated teeth, nor is the upper lip of the calyx deeply cleft, at least not at the time of flowering. Ripe fruit as yet unknown. B. Aquifolium I noticed on the Preston-River to be a very tall almost arborescent shrub.

Obituary.

CHARLES OGG.

.It is with deep regret that we have to announce the death of Mr. Charles Ogg, one of our earliest chemists. Mr. Ogg was born at Market-Resan, in the county of Yorkshire, in the year 1827. After leaving school he was apprenticed to a chemist and druggist at Hull ; at the termination of his period of pupilage he found his way to London, and engaged as assistant to a surgeon in Oxford-street ; then went to Mr. Pope Roach's, a very respectable business. Subsequently he lived with the late John Garle, one of the examiners of the Pharmacentical Society ; then with the well-known Henry Deane, and lastly with Godfrey and Cooke, Conduit-street. In 1850 Mr. Ogg emigrated to Australia. In those days there was little employment for pharmacists, and the subject of our obituary obtained employment as a reaper to a Mr. Horatio Cooper, of the Plenty, and "was glad to get the job." Wishing to return to his own business, he applied to a chemist in Elizabeth-street, who offered him "£1 a week and his tucker." The young man who had lived with Godfrey and Cooke,

thought himself worth more than that, and left the pharmacy of *that* street with contempt. Then he went farming at Templestowe, and lost all he had, then to the "diggings," where he was successful. In 1855 he bought a small business from a Dr. Barry, at South Yarra, and for many years carried on a very successful business. In 1873 Mr. Ogg started a new business in Collins-street East, which was, we believe, flourishing at the time of his decease. It is a curious coincidence that once in former years, when our friend was reduced to less than his last sixpence, in taking a walk up Collins-street he picked up a sovereign exactly opposite the place where his shop was to be. Mr. Ogg was a member of the Pharmaceutical Society, and, until his illness, a regular attendant at the meetings of the council. His advice was always listened to with respect, and he always supported measures which had for their object the elevation of the business. It was necessary to know him intimately to fully appeciate the sterling qualities which he possessed. His death, which was long expected by his friends, took place on 10th December, in the fifty-fifth year of his age. He leaves three sons of tender age to the guardianship of his friends and executor.

EXAMINATION OF VASELINE.

THE petroleum derivatives variously called *cosmoline, saxoline, petroleum jelly,* &c., consist of those portions of petroleum which are soft or pasty at ordinary temperatures. They are obtained from the last distillate or from the undistilled portion by treatment with superheated steam, followed by filtration through animal charcoal. Vaseline is a colourless or pale yellow, translucent, slightly fluorescent, semi-solid. Under the miscroscope distinct crystals are visible, which become more numerous on application, if cold. It melts at 35 degs. to 40 degs. C., and has a density of 0·840 to 0·866 in the melted state. It is odourless, fixed at ordinary temperatures, but commences to fume at 160 degs. C., and distils under pressure with slight decomposition. It usually contains about one-half of one per cent. of moisture and a trace of ash.

The following tests for vaseline and its purity are recommended by A. H. Allen, in his excellent treatise on *Commercial organic analysis:*

Vaseline is insoluble in water, and nearly so in alcohol. In ether it dissolves freely, the solution exhibiting a strong blue fluorescence. It is also readily soluble in chloroform, benzine, carbon bisulphide, and turpentine. From these and its ethereal solution alcohol precipitates it, it is said, as a crystalline mass. Vaseline is miscible in all proportions with fixed and volatile oils. With glycerine it forms an intimate mixture which separates into its constitutents when warmed, the melted vaseline floating on the glycerine.

Vaseline is a mixture of hydrocarbons, consisting chiefly of hydrides between $C_{19} H_{16}$ and $C_{20} H_{42}$, but its behaviour with bromine shows that olefins are also present. As a true paraffine it is neutral in reaction, and but little affected by chemical reagents. It is not saponified or otherwise acted on by alkalies, and is unaffected by hydrochloric or dilute nitric acid. Some samples blacken on treatment with cold concentrated sulphuric acid, a reaction which indicates the presence of bodies other than paraffines.

Vaseline does not oxidise or turn rancid on exposure to air, and this property, together with its indifference to reagents, renders it a valuable substitute for lard in the preparation of ointments liable to change, such as those containing sulphur, iodides, and compounds of lead, zinc, and mercury. For these and similar purposes it is well suited, especially as it appears to possess decided curative powers of its own. On the other hand, considerable local irritation has been observed to be caused by vaseline in certain cases, a fact which is not improbably due to imperfect removal of the agents used in its purification.

TESTS FOR PURITY.

Good vaseline should be completely volatile when heated on platinum, without giving any smell of burning fat (acrolein), or rosin. When agitated with twice its measure of strong alcohol it should remain practically undissolved. The spirit should not acquire an acid or alkaline reaction, and should not give any notable precipitate on dilution with water. When agitated with cold concentrated sulphuric acid, diluted with one-ninth of its weight of water, vaseline gives no marked increase of temperature, and ought not to become very strongly coloured. When subjected to the saponification process employed for the determination of hydrocarbons in fixed oils, vaseline, should yield to the ether an amount of unsaponifiable matter almost equal to the original weight of vaseline used for the experiment; while on the other hand, the aqueous liquid separated from the ethereal layer should yield no notable precipitate on being acidulated.

PRESERVATION OF INDIA-RUBBER.

A GERMAN scientist named Hempel has recently made a discovery which should be of great value to patentees of soda water stoppers and others whose inventions depend upon the use of India-rubber in any form. Every one who uses vulcanised rubber finds that articles made of it get hard and brittle after a time, so as to be useless. M. Hempel, after making researches into the cause of this hardening, has come to the conclusion that it is due to the gradual evaporation of the solvents employed when it is being vulcanised. He has fortunately found a method, not only of preventing this evaporation, but of replacing the solvent by another less open to this objection. He found that if the India-rubber was put directly into the solvent it always absorbed too much of it, but the object was attained by putting the article in an atmosphere saturated with the vapour of the solvent. Rubber stoppers, etc., are protected and prevented from spoiling by being put in a desiccator, or large glass box, in which is an open vessel of ordinary *kerosene*. Hempel found that sealing India-rubber articles in a glass vessel would preserve them for a long time, but that it is useless to attempt to keep them in a wooden box. As far as practicable they should be kept in the dark. Old rubber that has become hard is softened in a very short time by putting it in a vessel with vapour of bisulphide of carbon; but owing to the intensely noxious smell of this chemical we would not recommend this process to the patentee of soda water stoppers. If, however, it is resorted to, the rubber articles should be immediately afterwards exposed to the vapour of kerosene.

REMINISCENCES OF A PHARMACIST.
(*Continued.*)
BY J. B. MUMMERY.

IT is now my intention to bring my reminiscences to a close by narrating a few cases of poisoning by design or misadventure, which caused a good deal of excitement at the time they occurred; and should these lines meet the eyes of any who were sufferers by the lamentable mishaps recorded, I trust that they will believe that I have but one object in alluding to them —that is of showing to the younger members of our profession the great need there is for constant care and watchfulness on the part of those who have the handling of deadly drugs and chemicals, and the necessity of fitting themselves, by study and attention, for the right performance of the arduous but honourable duties of their calling.

The cases to which I shall allude occurred many years ago, when a very slight amount of medical knowledge was considered necessary to allow a person to assume the title of chemist and druggist, and no law then existed to prevent any one who was in possession of sufficient cash to purchase a show-bottle or two and a small quantity of drugs from opening a shop for their sale, or even dispensing prescriptions.

Such times have, happily, passed away for ever, and any one who now seeks the honour or the emolument of our business must be able to pass such an examination as will make fatalities from ignorance eventually an impossibility. If I had been writing these papers six months ago I should probably have said that such was an impossibility then; but a recent case which occurred at Brisbane (the circumstances attending which have been made known to us through the medium of the public press) proves that the "halcyon" days of pharmacy have not fully arrived, and indeed cannot be expected to do so until time has removed from the ranks of registered pharmacists all those who, through what may be reasonably called a defect in the law, have obtained their qualification more by good luck than by evidence of practical knowledge.

A COLONIAL "PALMER."

Many of my readers will no doubt recollect the case of the notorious Doctor Palmer, who was executed in England for murder of the most atrocious kind, no less than the killing by slow degrees his wife and one or more of his most intimate friends, for the purpose of gaining possession of sums for which he had induced them to insure their lives. His crimes were of such a kind that beside them the deeds of those who

slay by knife or bullet are acts of humanity and mercy, for they in most cases bring about a speedy end; but the wretch Palmer administered his poison in small and continuous doses to the wife of his bosom, as well as his intimate friends, witnessing their agony for weeks before death put an end to their sufferings. Well, just about the time that this fiend was executed, Sydney produced an imitator in the person of one Doctor Beer. The cases were not exactly parallel, for Beer did not kill his wife, but a female with whom he seems to have been on such intimate terms as to induce her to effect an insurance on her life in his favour.

The poison chosen to end the poor creature's existence was belladonna, and it was proved at the inquest that as much as ten grains of the extract had been given for a dose. Human nature could not stand this, and the poor woman succumbed, as a matter of course, to the anxiety of her medical attendant (in whom she seemed to have placed implicit confidence to the last), not for her life, but for her death.

Certain suspicious circumstances which came to light soon after her decease led to investigation, and subsequently an inquest and trial, in which the doctor barely escaped hanging. He was convicted of manslaughter, and sentenced to ten years' penal servitude, notwithstanding a professional brother or two swore to the fact of ten grains of the extract of belladonna being a reasonable dose.

Dr. Beer did his ten years (or as much of it as the law required), and came out of gaol a sadder and, it is to be hoped, a better man. I have heard that he published a pamphlet on his release to prove that he was an innocent and ill-used individual, and the very model of what a doctor should be, but whether he succeeded in creating this impression I am unable to say; but as I believe that he practised again in Sydney after his release, it is probable that he did.

Several cases of accidental poisoning by careless or incompetent dispensers occurred in Sydney during a comparatively short period, and this was by no means to be wondered at considering the attainments of many of those who practised pharmacy in the olden days. Amongst such cases, a fatality to an infant under the care (if I recollect aright) of a Doctor Degner, was the means of bringing to light one of the grossest pieces of carelessness on the part of a dispenser that I think the world ever heard of. A 2-oz. mixture, with teaspoonful doses, was made up by the doctor himself, and handed to the messenger, and the first dose of this medicine caused the death of the child in great agony a few hours after it was administered. An investigation showed the fact that a perfectly colourless mixture, which should have been but a simple saline, consisted of dilute sulphuric acid to the extent of 90 per cent., and the way in which the mistake occurred was this:—The doctor was in the habit of making up his own medicines, assisted by his groom, who dusted and arranged the dispensary, and filled up some of the bottles. On a low shelf stood three or four square quart gin bottles, one containing dilute sulphuric acid, the others being filled with plain and simple medicated waters, no labels or marks being placed upon them to indicate what their contents were, their position on the shelf being the only guide. The idea of having bottles containing liquids precisely alike in appearance, and one of these of deadly properties, in vessels without a label of any kind to indicate what was in them, was a piece of unpardonable neglect, which led, as might have been expected, to the fatal result above mentioned by the simple fact of the man having changed the position of the bottles, and placed the acid where the water should have been, and the dispenser hurriedly laid hold of what he thought was a harmless liquid, filled up the bottle, corked, sealed, and delivered it.

No sort of punishment, I believe, was meted out to the doctor. I am under the impression that he was not even reprimanded. Probably the astute jurymen imagined that his diploma gave him a general license to kill or cure; at all events he went on doing one or the other, although probably the mishap gave him an idea that it would pay to put labels on his bottles for the future.

(*To be continued.*)

AN ANTI-NAUSEANT.—R. Creasote, 20 drops; acet. acid, 40 drops; morph. sulph., 2 grains; water, 2 ounces, M. Sig. Teaspoonful in a little water.—*Ohio Med. Journal*, April, 1882.

STICKY FLY PAPER.—Melt one part of castor oil with three parts of common resin, and spread on strong paper previously sized with a solution of glue.

PRELIMINARY EXAMINATION.

THE questions for the examination held on the 7th December, 1882, were as follows :—

Time allowed—Three hours for the three subjects.

LATIN.

(a) Translation and grammar, Cæsar, De Bello Gallico, Book I.

(b) Translation of simple sentences from English into Latin.

1. Translate closely and literally :—

(a) *Compluribus* his proeliis pulsis, ab Ocelo, quod est *citerioris* provinciæ extremum, in fines *Vocontiorum* ulterioris provinciæ die septimo *pervenit*, inde in Allobrogum fines, ab Allobrogibus in Segusianos exercitum ducit.

(b) Dumnorigem ad se vocat, fratrem adhibet; quæ in eo *reprehendat*, ostendit, quæ ipse intelligat, quæ civitas *queratur*, proponit; monet ut in reliquum *tempus* suspiciones vitet ; *præterita* se Divitiaco fratri condonare dicit.

Parse the words underlined in above extracts. N.B.—In parsing noun or adjective, give case, number, gender, and nominative and genitive case ; in parsing verbs, give person, number, tense, mood, voice, and principal parts. All Latin words should be written out in full.

2. Decline together—locus superior, commune periculum.

3. Give the principal parts and meanings of—dono, utor, mitto, cognosco, refero, speculor.

4. Translate into Latin :—

(a) Duringa 11 these days Ariovistus kept his men in the camp.

(b) Both his wives perished in that battle.

(c) The fifth day from that day was appointed for a conference.

ARITHMETIC.

First four rules, simple and compound, vulgar and decimal fractions, and simple and compound proportion. British and metrical systems of weights and measures.

1. Find the sum, difference, product, and quotient (dividing the greater by the less) of the numbers 54,989 and 618,415.

2. Multiply £19 18s. 11¾d. by 45 ; and divide £39 18s. 7d. by 30¼.

3. Simplify $(\frac{1}{2} + \frac{3}{4} + \frac{5}{6}) \div (\frac{7}{8} - \frac{2}{3})$.

4. Simplify $\frac{\cdot 5 \times 18 - \cdot 3 \times 4}{\cdot 25 \times 9 + \cdot 275 \times \cdot 9}$.

5. How many lbs. of sugar at 8d. per lb. should I get for 18 lbs. of tea at 5s. 4d. per lb.?

6. If £240 gain £16 in 16 months, what sum will gain £5 6s. 8d. in 8 months ?

7. Write out avoirdupois weight. Reduce 20 ozs. apothecaries' weight to grains.

8. (a) If the metre is equal to 39·371 inches, how many inches are there in a kilometre ?

(b) The gramme is = 15·432 grains nearly. Find how many grammes there are in 1 lb. troy.

N.B.—All the steps of the work should be neatly and clearly shown, and all results should be in their simplest form.

ENGLISH—GRAMMAR AND COMPOSITION.

1. What is a proper noun ? Give three instances.

2. Name the simple relatives used in English. Why are they so called?

3. Write out :—

(a) Past indicative active verb " drive."

(b) Comparison of—well, fine, brightly.

4. "There a *tide* in the affairs of men,
Which taken at the flood *leads on* to fortune."

(a) Parse the underlined words.

(b) Distinguish the sentences, and say what kind of sentences they are.

5. Write a short piece of composition, with careful punctuation and penmanship, on—

A Cricket Match ; or, The Value and Good Results of Perseverance.

Evidence is brought forward in the *British Medical Journal* (p. 178) that the official solution of atropine of the *British Pharmacopœia* is liable to produce glaucoma, and that a very much weaker solution would serve to produce mydriasis or dilatation of the pupil. Dr. Ringer is of opinion that a solution formed by diluting the *Pharmacopœia* liquor with two or three hundred times its bulk of water would be sufficiently strong.

Notes and Abstracts.

CONCENTRATED COMPOUND INFUSION OF GENTIAN.—The above is a preparation extensively used in England for extemporaneous making the compound infusion of gentian of the *British Pharmacopæia*. The concentration is not officinal, and is obtained in various ways, one of which is the following :—

Gentian root	... .	4½ lbs., avoirdupois.
Dried orange peel	... ...	4½ „ „
Fresh lemon peel	... ...	9 „ „
Cold water	... ...	13 quarts (imperial).
Alcohol ...	... ...	1 gallon „
Oil of lemon	... ...	1 drachm.
Oil of orange	... ...	1 „

Macerate the gentian and orange and lemon peel for fourteen days with the alcohol and water, with frequent agitation. Then express the liquid ; add to it the essential oil, shake well, and filter through paper. The result is a fine clear liquid, of pleasant flavour, and keeping well. One fluid drachm of it, mixed with seven fluid drachms of water, produces one fluid ounce of liquid possessing all the qualities of the officinal infusion.

ORANGE WINE.—The oranges must be perfectly ripe. Peel them and cut them in halves, crosswise of the cells ; squeeze into a tub. The press used must be so close that the seeds cannot pass into the mast. Add two pounds of white sugar to each gallon of sour orange juice, or one pound to each gallon of sweet orange juice ; and one quart of water to each gallon of the mixed sugar and juice. Close fermentation is necessary. The resultant wine is amber-coloured, and tastes like dry hock, with the orange aroma. Vinegar can be made from the refuse, and extract from the peels.

Karlsbad Sprudel Salt, which was formerly very improperly prepared is now obtained by heating the spring water to boiling, filtering, evaporating, and saturating the residue with carbonic acid from the springs. The composition of the salt is as follows :—Sodium bicarbonate, 35·95 ; lithium bicarbonate, ·39 ; sodium sulphate, 42·03 ; potassium sulphate, 3·25 ; sodium chloride, 18·16 ; sodium fluoride, ·09 ; sodium borate, ·07 ; silicic anhydride, ·03 ; and ferric oxide, ·01 part. One liter of sprudel water yields about 5½ grams of salt. An *artificial* salt resembling the preceding is made, according to Professor Harnack, by mixing exsiccated sodium sulphate 100 parts, sodium bicarbonate 80 parts, and sodium chloride 40 parts.—*Phar. Centralh.*, 1882, No. 21, p. 241.

Professor J. E. De Vri, the celebrated Dutch quinologist, obtained his diploma in pharmacy 6th June, 1832. On the semi-centennial anniversary thereof he received from the King of Holland the order of Knight of the Dutch Lion, and was presented, in the name of the pharmacists of the Netherlands, with a silver statue of Hippocrates, placed upon a marble base, to which was attached a medal representing the goddess Insulinda leaning against a red cinchona tree. This was accompanied by a costly album, containing an address and the signatures of 322 pharmacists of the Netherlands.

SOME REMARKS UPON MODERN PHARMACEUTICAL STUDY.

(BY H. J. MOLLER.)

(From Pharmaceutical Journal.)

FRANCE.

MY notes on the study of pharmacy in France I have myself collected from different journals, programmes, collections of laws, &c., in the Bibliothèque Nationale here in Paris. I am highly indebted to Professor Planchon for the kindness with which he has given me all further information that I desired.

France is the country possessing the largest number of special schools of pharmacy ; and pharmaceutical study is here so highly developed, that, so far as I can see, only Germany can compete with it.

The most famous school of pharmacy in France is the Ecole supérieure de pharmacie de Paris. The present school is situated in the Rue de l'Arbalète, in the old Quartier Latin, and was founded as early as the sixteenth century by the pharmacist Nicolaus Houël, but was at first a very unimportant institution. In 1777 the school was much improved, and obtained fixed professors. At length Napoleon Bonaparte issued the law of Germinal 21, of the year XI (*i.e.*, 11th April, 1803), which ordered the establishment of three large écoles supérieures de pharmacie in Paris, Strassburg,* and Montpellier. Later, Louis Phillippe issued an "Ordonnance du Roi du Septembre 27, 1840," which connected the pharmaceutical schools with the universities, and gave them the same rights as the other departments of the universities (for example : Ecole de médecine, Ecole de droit, &c.).

The above-mentioned "Ecole supérieure de pharmacie de Paris," in the Rue de l'Arbalète, is no longer sufficient for the present requirements of the science and for the great number of students.† A fine new building has herefore been erected on ground which formerly was a part of the Jardin du Luxembourg. This new school, on the corner of the Avenue de l'Observatoire and Rue Michelet, is by far the largest pharmaceutical institute in the world, and will cost between four and five millions of francs. The two amphitheatres, where the lectures are to be held, can each contain five hundred auditors, and the large building, where the laboratories are collected in three stories, is about 250 paces long ; all the other parts of the school being in proportion to these rooms, it is easy to get an idea of the large scale on which this school is built. A small part of the new school is already used, but the whole institute will not be finished before the spring, 1881.

Besides these three "Ecoles supérieures de pharmacie" in Paris, Montpellier, and Nancy, France has also three so-called "Facultés mixtes de médecine et de pharmacie" in Lille, Lyons, and Bordeaux. These six schools are higher than the preparatory pharmaceutical schools ("les écoles préparatoires de médecine et de pharmacie"), which are again divided into "Ecoles de plein exercice de médecine et de pharmacie" (in Marseilles and Nantes) and "Ecoles préparatoires secondaires." At the present time one of the last-mentioned schools is found in each of the following sixteen cities :—Alger, Amiens, Angers, Arras, Besançon, Caen, Clermont, Dijon, Grenoble, Limoges, Poitiers, Reims, Rennes, Rouen, Toulouse, and Tours.

There are two classes of pharmacists in France, but according to a decree of 31st August, 1878, there is no other difference between the education of "les pharmaciens de première classe" and "les pharmaciens de seconde classe," than that the first must be "bacheliers"—i.e., have passed the whole classical school—while the second need only to have passed "la classe de quatrième." ‡ There is in addition a higher diploma for the pharmacists of the first-class. This diploma is called "le diplôme supérieur de pharmacien de première classe" and gives the right to compete for the professorships in the pharmaceutical sciences at the "Facultés mixtes de médecine et de pharmacie."

According to the "décret du Juillet 12, 1878, relatif aux conditions à remplir pour obtenir le diplôme de pharmacien de première classe," which, as above mentioned, is now also applicable to the pharmacists of the second class, the candidate must prove that he has passed the required examinations in the classical school. Then he must stay three years in a pharmacy before he passes his first pharmaceutical examination ("un examen de validation de stage"), which corresponds to the German "Gehülfenprüfung." This examination is ordered by a decree of 30th December, 1878, and is held at the pharmaceutical schools by a professor and two pharmacists of the first class; it embraces (1) a "galenical" or chemical preparation according to the pharmacopœia ; (2) the preparation

*After the war 1870-71 this school was transferred to Nancy. The old French pharmaceutical school in Strasaburg is the same, which now, under the direction of Professor Flückiger, has the title, "Das pharmaceutische Institut der Universität zu Strassburg."

† There are now nearly six hundred pharmaceutical students at the Paris school.

‡ According to the "décret" and the "arrête" of 19th June, 1880, the French classical school ["les lycées"] consist of the following classes :—

Division élémentaire :
(1) Classe préparatoire.
(2) Classe de huitième [the lowest age of the scholar is nine years].
(3) Classe de septième [ten years].

Division de grammaire :
(4) Classe de sixième [eleven years. Here the pupil commences to learn Latin, ten hours a week].
(5) Classe de cinquième [twelve years ; ten hours of Latin a week].
(6) Classe de quatrième [thirteen years ; six hours of Latin and six hours of Greek a week. It is the final examination of this class which is demanded in order to be a pharmacist of the second class].

Division supérieure :
(7) Classe de troisième [fourteen years].
(8) Classe de seconde [fifteen years].
(9) { Classe de rhétorique } [sixteen years].
    { Classe de philosophie }

It is the final examination of this last class which is demanded in order to be a pharmacist of the first-class and it gives the right to the titles of respectively "bachelier ès lettres" or "bachelier ès sciences."

of a remedy after a prescription ; (3) the determination of ten compound remedies and of thirty plants or parts of plants, belonging to the *materia medica ;* and (4) the answering of questions upon different pharmaceutical operations.

Now the student leaves the pharmacy and spends three years in a school of pharmacy ; if he intends to be a pharmacist of the first class, he is obliged to pursue his studies at one of the six higher pharmaceutical schools. At the end of each year he passes an examination ; the first includes physics, chemistry, toxicology, and pharmacy; the second embraces botany, zoology, *materia medica,* pharmacy, and mineralogy ; the third consists of pharmaceutical and chemical preparations. At the first examination the candidate must make a chemical analysis, and at the second a microscopical preparation. At the third examination he is given four days to make the required preparations under the survey of a professor ; the oral test at this last examination is held in two sittings.

"Le diplôme supérieur de pharmacien de première classe" can be given to the pharmacists of the first class after the defence of a thesis and some new and very severe examinations.

Pharmaceutical study in France, at least in the six higher schools, and especially in the Parisian school, must be regarded as having attained as high a state of development as any in Europe. I shall not here trto the reader with a complete review of these studies, but only refer to the programmes of the respective schools.

Here I shall end these short remarks on the present state of pharmaceutical study. It is not for me to make the application of these notes to English pharmacy, since I know too little of its needs. My desire has been only to give a short report of what I have seen and learned of the important educational foundation of our profession. I could have wished to make these communications at least as complete as in the original Danish edition, but a journal is not the right place for such more comprehensive researches, and therefore I must beg my English colleagues to receive my notes as they now lie before them, and I shall be very happy if, in this abbreviated form, their interest has been preserved.

FIRE AT MESSRS. HEMMONS, LAWS AND CO.'S

ABOUT half-past two on the morning of the 21st December a very serious fire occurred on the premises occupied by Messrs. Hemmons, Laws and Co., wholesale chemists and chemical manufacturers, Russell-street. It appeared that the *employés* were working up till half-past ten o'clock on Wednesday night, and when the managers were leaving for the night the place appeared to be perfectly safe, there being not the slightest indication that any portion of the goods was on fire. Shortly after two o'clock, however, one of the men connected with the fire brigade station stated that he had seen smoke emanating from the building, and consequently a man was at once ordered to make inquiries and ascertain from what building the smoke was proceeding. He returned in a short time and gave the alarm, "Place on fire." The building being close to the station Mr. Hoad and his men were quickly on the scene, and to their great surprise on reaching the back of the premises they discovered, judging from the glare through the windows, that the upper story was in flames. Shortly after their arrival the windows began to break owing to the great heat, and the flames wildly rushed forth. Two or three streams of water were brought to bear on the back, while some of the men then proceeded to the front, and again it was evident that this division of the building was also on fire, as the same indications as those observable at the back were evident. Streams of water were at once brought to bear upon the front, and in a very short space of time from the outbreak of the fire the West End, Carlton Brewery, Albion, and Hawthorn brigades had arrived, and with this additional assistance Mr. Hoad was able to keep the flames from spreading to the adjoining houses. The flames, however, shortly made their way through the roof, which fell in with a terrible crash in about ten minutes from the commencement of the blaze. The men connected with the various brigades worked with great spirit during the night, but it was almost impossible to save anything, so rapidly did the flames spread. Owing to the valuable nature of the goods, which consisted of drugs, medicines, and other constituents only to be found in such an establishment, the damage will be enormous ; it is estimated from £15,000 to £20,000. The stock is covered by insurance to the extent of £12,000.

burg,* and Montpellier. Later, Louis Philippe issued an "Ordonnance du Roi du Septembre 27, 1840," which connected the pharmaceutical schools with the universities, and gave them the same rights as the other departments of the universities (for example : Ecole de médecine, Ecole de droit, &c.).

The above-mentioned "Ecole supérieure de pharmacie de Paris," in the Rue de l'Arbalète, is no longer sufficient for the present requirements of the science and for the great number of students.† A fine new building has herefore been erected on ground which formerly was a part of the Jardin du Luxembourg. This new school, on the corner of the Avenue de l'Observatoire and Rue Michelet, is by far the largest pharmaceutical institute in the world, and will cost between four and five millions of francs. The two amphitheatres, where the lectures are to be held, can each contain five hundred auditors, and the large building, where the laboratories are collected in three stories, is about 250 paces long ; all the other parts of the school being in proportion to these rooms, it is easy to get an idea of the large scale on which this school is built. A small part of the new school is already used, but the whole institute will not be finished before the spring, 1881.

Besides these three "Ecoles supérieures de pharmacie" in Paris, Montpellier, and Nancy, France has also three so-called "Facultés mixtes de médecine et de pharmacie" in Lille, Lyons, and Bordeaux. These six schools are higher than the preparatory pharmaceutical schools ("les écoles préparatoires de médecine et de pharmacie"), which are again divided into "Ecoles de plein exercice de médecine et de pharmacie" (in Marseilles and Nantes) and "Ecoles préparatoires secondaires." At the present time one of the last-mentioned schools is found in each of the following sixteen cities :—Alger, Amiens, Angers, Arras, Besançon, Caen, Clermont, Dijon, Grenoble, Limoges, Poitiers, Reims, Rennes, Rouen, Toulouse, and Tours.

There are two classes of pharmacists in France, but according to a decree of 31st August, 1878, there is no other difference between the education of "les pharmaciens de première classe" and "les pharmaciens de seconde classe," than that the first must be "bacheliers"—i.e., have passed the whole classical school—while the second need only to have passed "la classe de quatrième." ‡ There is in addition a higher diploma for the pharmacists of the first-class. This diploma is called "le diplôme supérieur de pharmacien de première classe" and gives the right to compete for the professorships in the pharmaceutical sciences at the "Facultés mixtes de médecine et de pharmacie."

According to the "décret du Juillet 12, 1878, relatif aux conditions à remplir pour obtenir le diplôme de pharmacien de première classe," which, as above mentioned, is now also applicable to the pharmacists of the second class, the candidate must prove that he has passed the required examinations in the classical school. Then he must stay three years in a pharmacy before he passes his first pharmaceutical examination ("un examen de validation de stage"), which corresponds to the German "Gehülfenprüfung." This examination is ordered by a decree of 30th December, 1878, and is held at the pharmaceutical schools by a professor and two pharmacists of the first class; it embraces (1) a "galenical" or chemical preparation according to the pharmacopœia ; (2) the preparation

*After the war 1870-71 this school was transferred to Nancy. The old French pharmaceutical school in Strasburg is the same, which now, under the direction of Professor Flückiger, has the title, "Das pharmaceutische Institut der Universität zu Strassburg."

† There are now nearly six hundred pharmaceutical students at the Paris school.

‡ According to the "décret" and the "arrête" of 10th June, 1880, the French classical schools ["les lycées"] consist of the following classes :—

Division élémentaire :
(1) Classe préparatoire.
(2) Classe de huitième [the lowest age of the scholar is nine years].
(3) Classe de septième [ten years].

Division de grammaire :
(4) Classe de sixième [eleven years. Here the pupil commences to learn Latin, ten hours a week].
(5) Classe de cinquième [twelve years ; ten hours of Latin a week].
(6) Classe de quatrième [thirteen years ; six hours of Latin and six hours of Greek a week. It is the final examination of this class which is demanded in order to be a pharmacist of the second class].

Division supérieure :
(7) Classe de troisième [fourteen years].
(8) Classe de seconde [fifteen years].
(9) { Classe de rhétorique } [sixteen years].
      { Classe de philosophie }

It is the final examination of this last class which is demanded in order to be a pharmacist of the first-class and it gives the right to the titles of respectively "bachelier ès lettres" or "bachelier ès sciences."

of a remedy after a prescription ; (3) the determination of ten compound remedies and of thirty plants or parts of plants, belonging to the *materia medica*; and (4) the answering of questions upon different pharmaceutical operations.

Now the student leaves the pharmacy and spends three years in a school of pharmacy ; if he intends to be a pharmacist of the first class, he is obliged to pursue his studies at one of the six higher pharmaceutical schools. At the end of each year he passes an examination ; the first includes physics, chemistry, toxicology, and pharmacy; the second embraces botany, zoology, *materia medica*, hydrology, and mineralogy ; the third consists of pharmaceutical and chemical preparations. At the first examination the candidate must make a chemical analysis, and at the second a microscopical preparation. At the third examination he is given four days to make the required preparations under the survey of a professor ; the oral test at this last examination is held in two sittings.

"Le diplôme supérieur de pharmacien de première classe" can be given to the pharmacists of the first class after the defence of a thesis and some new and very severe examinations.

Pharmaceutical study in France, at least in the six higher schools, and especially in the Parisian school, must be regarded as having attained as high a state of development as any in Europe. I shall not here tire the reader with a complete review of these studies, but only refer to the programmes of the respective schools.

Here I shall end these short remarks on the present state of pharmaceutical study. It is not for me to make the application of these notes to English pharmacy, since I know too little of its needs. My desire has been only to give a short report of what I have seen and learned of the important educational foundation of our profession. I could have wished to make these communications at least as complete as in the original Danish edition, but a journal is not the right place for such more comprehensive researches, and therefore I must beg my English colleagues to receive my notes as they now lie before them, and I shall be very happy if, in this abbreviated form, their interest has been preserved.

FIRE AT MESSRS. HEMMONS, LAWS AND CO.'S

ABOUT half-past two on the morning of the 21st December a very serious fire occurred on the premises occupied by Messrs. Hemmons, Laws and Co., wholesale chemists and chemical manufacturers, Russell-street. It appeared that the *employés* were working up till half-past ten o'clock on Wednesday night, and when the managers were leaving for the night the place appeared to be perfectly safe, there being not the slightest indication that any portion of the goods was on fire. Shortly after two o'clock, however, one of the men connected with the fire brigade station stated that he had seen smoke emanating from the building, and consequently a man was at once ordered to make inquiries and ascertain from what building the smoke was proceeding. He returned in a short time and gave the alarm, "Place on fire." The building being close to the station Mr. Hoad and his men were quickly on the scene, and to their great surprise on reaching the back of the premises they discovered, judging from the glare through the windows, that the upper story was in flames. Shortly after their arrival the windows began to break owing to the great heat, and the flames wildly rushed forth. Two or three streams of water were brought to bear on the back, while some of the men then proceeded to the front, and again it was evident that this division of the building was also on fire, as the same indications as those observable at the back were evident. Streams of water were at once brought to bear upon the front, and in a very short space of time from the outbreak of the fire the West End, Carlton Brewery, Albion, and Hawthorn brigades had arrived, and with this additional assistance Mr. Hoad was able to keep the flames from spreading to the adjoining houses. The flames, however, shortly made their way through the roof, which fell in with a terrible crash in about ten minutes from the commencement of the blaze. The men connected with the various brigades worked with great spirit during the night, but it was almost impossible to save anything, so rapidly did the flames spread. Owing to the valuable nature of the goods, which consisted of drugs, medicines, and other constituents only to be found in such an establishment, the damage will be enormous ; it is estimated from £15,000 to £20,000. The stock is covered by insurance to the extent of £12,000.

[SUPPLEMENT ONLY.]

THE

Chemist & Druggist.

WITH AUSTRALASIAN SUPPLEMENT.

(Published under direction of the Pharmaceutical Society of Victoria.)

No. 57. { Published on the 15th of every Month. } Registered for Transmission as a Newspaper. JANUARY, 188 { Subscription, 15s. per Annum, including Diary, Post Free.

Printed by Mason, Firth & M'Cutcheon, 51 & 53 Flinders Lane West, Melbourne.

The Chemist and Druggist.

WITH AUSTRALASIAN SUPPLEMENT.

OFFICE: MUTUAL PROVIDENT BUILDINGS, COLLINS STREET WEST.

Published on the 15th of each Month.

THIS Journal is issued gratis to all paid-up Members of the PHARMACEUTICAL SOCIETY OF VICTORIA, and to non-members at Fifteen Shillings per annum, payable in advance. A copy of *The Chemists and Druggists' Diary,* published annually, is forwarded post free to every subscriber.

Advertisements, remittances, and all business communications to be addressed to THE HONORARY SECRETARY OF THE PHARMACEUTICAL SOCIETY, MELBOURNE.

SCALE OF CHARGES FOR ADVERTISEMENTS:

Per annum.		Per annum.	
One Page £8 0 0	Quarter Page ..£3 0 0		
Half do. 5 0 0	Business Cards .. 2 0 0		

Special rates for wrapper and pages preceding and following literary matter. Advertisements of Assistants Wanting Situations, 2s. 6d. each. Advertisements for insertion in the current month should be sent to the office before the 10th.

COMMUNICATIONS for the EDITORIAL department of this Journal should be addressed to THE EDITOR, MUTUAL PROVIDENT BUILDINGS, COLLINS STREET WEST, MELBOURNE.

No notice can be taken of anonymous communications. Whatever is intended for insertion must be authenticated by the name and address of the writer—not necessarily for publication, but as a guarantee of good faith.

BIRTHS.

EAGLES.—On the 26th November, at Richmond, the wife of F. T. Eagles, chemist, of a son.

GOULD.—On the 2nd January, at Kyneton, the wife of James Crosbie Goold, of a son.

NELSON.—On the 12th December, the wife of W. Y. Nelson, chemist, Brunswick-street, Fitzroy, of a son (stillborn).

MARRIAGES.

PEDDINGTON—IRISH.—On the 28th December, at the residence of the bride's brother-in-law, 71 Gore-street, Fitzroy, by the Rev. P. Bailhache, W. T. Peddington, of Carlton, only son of the late James Peddington, to Alice Ruby Irish, youngest daughter of the late John Irish, Fitzroy.

JONES—BERESFORD.—On the 13th December, at the Wesleyan Church, Richmond, by the Rev. W. A. Quick, John Clark Cunliffe, the eldest son of John Clark Jones, Esq., J.P., pharmacist, Richmond, to Florance Annie, only daughter of David Henry Beresford, Esq., of Melbourne.

THE PRESCRIPTION OF PROPRIETARY MEDICINES.

THE October number of the *Therapeutic Gazette* contains an essay by Dr. Lindsley, Professor of Materia Medica at Yale College, in the United States of America, upon this subject, in which he argues that it is demoralising to the medical profession, and detrimental to the public welfare, to prescribe proprietary or secret medicines for the sick. As lovers of scientific pharmacy and strenuous opponents of all forms of nostrum-mongering quackery, we invite our readers to a serious consideration of this question. Dr. Lindsley defines proprietary medicines to be any medicines respecting which some person or persons possess an ownership, either of the method of preparation or of some element in their composition which is secret, or else of some exclusive right to the manufacture or sale, by which the medical profession is, on the one hand, kept in ignorance of their full qualities, or, on the other, deprived of such free and unlimited use of them as would be enjoyed from fair and honourable competition in their production. It is not, we suppose, objected that a medi-

cine, the composition and strength of which is known, should be prescribed—for example, Battley's sedative solution of opium, and other simple pharmaceutical preparations, the action of which is exactly established—but to such complex mixtures as chlorodyne, lacto peptine, *et hoc genus omne.* Many compounds containing unknown proportions of very active and dangerous drugs are manufactured in large quantities in America, and are prescribed by medical men "to save themselves the trouble of thinking" and the pharmacist "the exercise of any knowledge of his business." It cannot be doubted, we think, that the gradually increasing employment of these compounds threatens to destroy legitimate and scientific pharmacy, and so render nugatory the efforts which are being made to educate and elevate our calling. It will, unless efforts are made, most surely reduce the medical man to the position of a more or less respectable quack, to say nothing of the detrimental influence which it will have, directly or indirectly, upon the progress of therapeutics, materia medica, chemistry, pharmacy, and hygiene. "What," says our essayist, "will the next generation of medical men know about lacto peptine, maltine, vitalized phosphates celerina, malto-coca, hydroleine, sistenine, caulocorea, viburnum compound, and an innumerable host of mixtures? These are all of ephemeral existence, other than what they derive from the advertising pages of medical journals and the newspapers. They are for the most part the invention of tradesmen, and in no sense represent the growth and progress of medical science."

What must be thought of such stupid "remedies" as liver pads, &c.?

In Australia, the evil complained of by honest and enlightened physicians in America is not so great, but we have observed a growing tendency towards the same state of things. The ceaseless efforts and ingenious devices of enterprising agents from these great manufacturing houses will ultimately bring about a deplorable condition of pharmacy in Australia, unless efforts are earnestly made to stem the tide which would seem to be setting in.

What inducement will there be for our young men to study and become accomplished pharmaceutical chemists when any errand boy would have enough knowledge to dispense these "ready put up" medicines? Dr. Lindsley well says, in speaking from the medical man's point of view —"I doubt if any one will ever devise a process more suicidal to our professional interests or dangerous to the welfare of the sick public. There are scarcely any of the common ills of flesh that are not provided for by these shrewd manufacturing chemists, and our drug stores are stocked with remedies ready prepared for the cure of each. The druggist is just as familiar with their virtues as the physician. Both get their knowledge from the same source—viz., the wrappers and advertisements. If, then, one's wife is the victim of dysmenorrhœa, why should he go to his physician when his druggist can probably show him his own physician's certificate to the virtues of Hadyn's viburnum compound for that trouble ?" And so on, and so on.

It is to be feared that the almost absolute ignorance of our youthful medical men of pharmacy—as no adequate teaching is provided for them at our medical school—will render them peculiarly liable to fall into the same practice which has assumed such formidable dimensions among our American cousins. Our medical men in Victoria have for the most part obtained their ideas of professional ethics from the mother-country, and are not so liable to fall into the same practice as the often imperfectly educated American doctor, and if they will only bear in mind that the so-called formula of these nostrums is often, and, indeed, generally deceptive, and cannot be tested, they will hesitate to give any encouragement to their use.

Dr. Lindsley ridicules with the lash of an unsparing pen the host of quack medicines with fine semi-scientific names, and recommended by *their disinterested* makers in advertisements made up of grandiloquent jargon. It is not to be wondered at that the ignorant become easy victims to these vultures of physic ; but it is past all understanding how men of intelligence and education should, without effort, quietly take for granted the silly and unverified assumptions and assertions of these persons !

The following announcement, clipped from an American medical journal, is a sample :—" Petroleum compound is a perfect emulsion of petroleum syrup and pure cod liver oil, combined with hypophosphites of lime and soda ; is palatable and agreeable, and forms the most agreeable and sure remedy for the certain cure of consumption, asthma, bronchitis, hay fever, and all chronic lung diseases." Considering that the most eminent physicians are of opinion, after long experiment, that hypophosphites are of no real value, "comparatively if not absolutely worthless," to use the words of Dr. Quain, what must be thought of those medical professors and teachers who append their certificate to such trash. *Verb. sap.* Here follow two more which we have culled from *New Remedies.* The first is certificated by fifteen M.D.'s, and the second by fourteen ! Let any honest man of ordinary education read, and reflect as he reads, and we know what *his* feelings will be ; let him take particular notice of "formula":—"To physicians. —Bromidia. Formula.—Every fluid drachm contains 15 grs. each of pure brom. potas. and purified chloral, and ⅛ gr. each of gen. imp. ext. cannabis ind. and hyoscyam. Dose.—One-half to one fluid drachm in water or syrup every hour until sleep is produced. Bromidia is the hypnotic *par excellence.* It produces refreshing sleep, and is exceedingly valuable in sleeplessness, nervousness, neuralgia, headache, convulsions, colic, &c., and will relieve when opiates fail. Unlike preparations of opium, it does not lock up the secretions. In the restlessness and delirium of fevers it is absolutely invaluable. Iodia.— Formula.—Iodia is a combination of active principles obtained from the green roots of stillingia, helonias, saxifraga, menispermum, and aromatics. Each fluid drachm also contains 5 grs. iod. potas. and 3 grs. phos. iron. Dose.

—One or two fluid drachms (more or less, as indicated) three times a day before meals. Iodia is the ideal alterative. It has been largely prescribed in syphilitic, scrofulous, cutaneous, and female diseases, and has an established reputation as being the best alterative ever introduced to the profession."

The Month.

The last day for receiving nominations for the election of members of the Pharmacy Board is on Tuesday, the 30th January, at four o'clock p.m.

The *Pharmaceutical Register* for the year 1883 is now ready, and copies can be obtained at the office of the Pharmacy Board, or from any of the wholesale chemists.

The *Chemist and Druggist* diaries for 1883 have all been distributed. In any case where copies have miscarried notification should be sent to Mr. Shillinglaw at the rooms.

The following additional sums have been forwarded in aid of the Benevolent Fund :—Messrs. J. Barton, Nelson, New Zealand, 10s.; C. Curtis, Melbourne Hospital, 10s. 6d.; and Robert J. Ellery, the Observatory, £1 1s.

The following additional legally qualified medical practitioners have been registered under the provisions of the Medical Practitioners' Statute, 1865:—Michael Dominic Murphy, Brunswick ; Frederic Dougan Bird, Melbourne.

Tenders are invited by Messrs. Davy, Cole and Flack for the purchase of the business of Messrs. Hood and Co., Elizabeth-street, Melbourne. The tenders must be sent in by the 31st January. Full particulars will be found in our advertising columns.

The following are the nominations for the Pharmacy Board of Victoria up to the time we went to press :—C. R. Blackett, Fitzroy ; George Lewis, Melbourne ; Henry Brind, Ballarat ; John Holdsworth, Sandhurst ; William Bowen, Melbourne ; Alfred J. Owen, Geelong ; George E. Green, Geelong ; James Brinsmead, St. Kilda. There are seven members for election.

Mr. J. T. Macgowan, late of Sturt-street, Ballarat, has opened a new pharmacy on the Sandridge-road.

Mr. J. Bagley, of Queensberry-street, Hotham, has removed into new and commodious premises opposite his old place of business.

Mr. W. H. H. Lane, the representative of Messrs. Warner and Co., Philadelphia, has returned to the colonies from America.

Mr. S. H. Henshall, who for many years carried on business at Seymour in connection with Messrs. Gould Bros., has started on his own account.

Mr. S. M. Burroughs (Messrs. Burroughs, Welcome and Co.) is at present in Dunedin. Mr. Burroughs speaks in high terms of the kindness shown him in New Zealand.

Meetings.

PHARMACY BOARD OF VICTORIA.

The monthly meeting was held at 100 Collins-street on the 10th January, 1883 ; present—Messrs. Bosisto, Blackett, Bowen, Brind, Holdsworth, Lewis, and Owen ; the president, Mr. J. Bosisto, M.P., in the chair.

The minutes of the previous meeting were read and confirmed.

Applications for Registration as Pharmaceutical Chemists. —The following were approved :—J. S. Cobb, certificate from Pharmaceutical Society of Great Britain ; F. Williams, H. J. Leddin, W. M. F. Reader, passed modified examination ; Percy

Wisewould, passed major examination ; William Robinson, in business before passing of Act.

Quarterly Examinations.—The board of examiners forwarded their report, having passed—major, examination, one ; modified, four ; preliminary, five.

Additional articles to be proclaimed poisons within the meaning of the Sale and Use of Poisons Act were agreed to, and a request forwarded to the Chief Secretary that the Governor would issue a proclamation.

Permission to Continue Business.—Permission was granted, under section 23 of the Pharmacy Act, to the following persons (widows and executrixes of pharmaceutical chemists) to carry on business for a period of twelve months ending the 31st December, 1883 :—M. L. Long, Melbourne ; Sarah Jessie Obbinson, Toorak ; Elizabeth Lloyd, Chiltern ; Lavinia Imes, Emerald Hill ; H. G. Ewing, Fitzroy.

The following certificates under the Sale and Use of Posions Act, 1876, were renewed for the year ending 31st December, 1883, to persons distant four miles from a registered pharmaceutical chemist:—Godfrey Barker Berry, Taradale ; Charles Lane De Boos, Euroa ; Samuel Hart, Euroa ; Ah Sam, Swift's Creek, Omeo ; Ho Ah Yen, Swift's Creek, Omeo ; Thomas Montgomery, Mortlake ; Nam Shing, Spring Creek, Beechworth ; Henry Playford, Dookie South ; Sun Lee On, Omeo ; Edward William Worthington, Avenel ; Robert Smart, Allansford ; William John Connolly, Rupanyup.

Names Erased from the Register.—C. F. Cook, A. F. Pulling, F. P. Sheehey, C. Ogg, deceased.

Alterations of Regulations in reference to Term of Office of Members of the Board.—Mr. Lewis's resolution on this subject, providing for the retirement of two members of the board every year, was further discussed and agreed to.

Finance.—The audited balance-sheet to the 31st December, 1882, was submitted and passed.

Pharmaceutical Register of Victoria.—A copy of the *Pharmaceutical Register* for the year 1883 was laid on the table, and certified to by the board.

THE PHARMACEUTICAL SOCIETY OF VICTORIA.

THE monthly meeting of the council was held at the rooms, 100 Collins-street, on the 1st December, 1882 ; present—Messrs. Bowen, Hunstman, Hooper, Nicholls, Baker, Thomas, Best, Gamble, Swift, and Shillinglaw ; the president, Mr. Bowen, in the chair.

The minutes of the previous meeting were read and confirmed, and the following new members were duly elected :—John N. Woolcott, Echuca ; Richard C. Hill, Bothwell, Tasmania ; Walter Long and Arthur J. Lovely, Adelaide ; Richard B. Bridge, Maldon, Essex, England ; John K. Forrest, Melbourne.

Report of Land and Building Committee.—The committee reported that, after several interviews with the Hon. the Commissioner of Public Works, it had been finally decided by him to sell to the society the building, &c., known as the old county court, situated in Swanston-street, for the sum of £400. After due consideration the committee agreed to the proposal, and that sum was paid to the Public Works Department on the 13th November, 1882, and on the purchase being completed the building was insured by the society for the sum of £1250. It was resolved, on the motion of Mr. Hunstman, that the action of the committee be approved. The motion was carried unanimously.

Vacancy in the Council.—The vacancy in the council, caused by the resignation of Mr. John Ross, was filled by the appointment of Mr. Walter Jones, Bay-street, Sandridge.

Annual Balance-sheet.—The treasurer reported the balance-sheet would be ready for presentation at the next meeting.

BOOKS, &C., RECEIVED.—*Australasian Medical Gazette*, November ; *American Journal of Pharmacy*, October ; *Australian Medical Journal ; Chemical News ;* Catalogue of Optical Instruments, by Messrs. Queen and Co., Philadelphia, presented by W. and C. H. Lane; *Druggists' Circular*, October ; *European Mail*, October ; Messrs. Sleeman and Co.'s *Drug Circular*, September ; Messrs. Rocke, Tompsitt and Co.'s *Price Lists*, December ; Messrs. Felton, Grimwade and Co.'s *Price Lists*, December ; *New Remedies*, October ; *Pharmaceutical Journal*, September ; *Scientific American*, September ; *Therapeutic Gazette*, September ; *Working Bulletin*, for the Scientific Investigation of

Cheken berberis, Aquifolium, Grindelia robusta, Ustilago madis, Sierra salvia, Chlor-anodyne, Warburg's Febrifugæ tincture, Queoracho, Folia garobæ, Cascara sagrada, from Messrs. Parke, Davis and Co., Detroit ; Lecture on "Radiant Matter" and Queen's Supplementary Catalogue, presented by W. and C. H. Lane. (The preceding notice was crowded out of our last issue).

BOOKS, &C., RECEIVED.—*Chemical News ; American Journal of Pharmacy*, November ; *Therapeutic Gazette*, October ; *New Remedies*, November ; *New York Druggists' Circular*, November ; "Working Bulletin for the Scientific Investigation of Stigmata of Maize, Menthol, Convallaria Majalis, Viburnum Prunifolium, and Tomato," presented by Messrs. Parke, Davis and Co.; *Scientific American*, November ; *Analyst*, October ; *Pharmaceutical Journal*, October ; *Nature*, September and October ; *European Mail*, November and December ; Messrs. Burgoyne, Burbridges and Co.'s *Monthly Trade Report*, November ; *On Consumption of the Lungs, or Decline and its Successful Treatment*, by Geo. T. Congreve ; Reports of Mining Surveyors and Registrars, quarter ending 30th September, 1882 ; Messrs. Felton, Grimwade and Co.'s *Monthly Trade Report*, January ; Messrs. Sleeman and Co.'s *Monthly Trade Report*, November ; *Australian Medical Journal*, November ; Messrs. Rocke, Tompsitt and Co.'s *Monthly Trade Report*, January.

SYDNEY.

THE monthly meeting of the Pharmaceutical Council was held at the Board-room, Phillip-street, on Tuesday, 19th December; present—the president (in the chair), and Messrs. Abraham, Guise, Larmer, Macarthy, Watt, and the secretary.

The minutes of last meeting were read and confirmed.

Applications for membership were received from J. Bradbury (M.P.S., Vic.), J. R. Hudson (M.P.S., Vic.), J. M. Wright, A. Scowen, and J. Bowen, and were granted.

The applications of J. Doyles, of Parramatta; F. Rich, of Walgett; and A. H. Florance (M.P.S., Vic.), of Tumberumba, were postponed.

Applications for registration of indentures were received from W. H. Hudson, of Corowa, to J. R. Hudson ; from N. B. Pollard to F. Cherry, of Hay ; and from John C. Hosking, and granted.

The monthly account for books purchased from Geo. Robertson and Co., £31 2s. 6d., was ordered to be paid.

The meeting then closed.

At the pharmacy examination of the Technical College, held at the close of the year, Mr. E. Wright was awarded the first prize offered by the college committee, and Mr. A. Henry obtained the lecturers' prize. The examiners appointed were Mr. A. J. Watt and Mr. Fred. Wright.

At the quarterly examination of the Pharmacy Board, held on 4th January, three out of five applicants presented themselves, and failed to obtain the required number of marks for a pass.

Mr. Hallam, a gentleman well-known in Victoria, is opening in business as a chemist and druggist at the corner of College and Liverpool streets, Sydney.

A meeting has been called to organise monthly meetings of the trade for the discussion of topics connected with pharmacy, especially the new Act to regulate the sale of poisons.

Legal and Magisterial.

PROSECUTION UNDER THE "SALE AND USE OF POISONS ACT."

AT the Castlemaine Police Court on 12th January (before the Mayor, Messrs. Greenhill, Pearce, Bone, and Cramer, J.P.'s) Lee Sou and Charles Suey were summoned by the police for selling a preparation of opium to C. Wayne in December, the same being a poison, and they having no license from the Pharmacy Board. Mr. Merrifield appeared for defendants, and said the charge could not lie against thd storekeeper and his assistant, but only against the person who sold. He referred to the Act, and pointed out that it was not intended to restrict the sale of opium for smoking. So long as the sale was confined to Chinese it should not operate, but sales to Europeans brought defendant within the four corners of the Act, and a small fine, such as 5s. each, would meet the case. If a European went to China and found the sale of tobacco was prohibited, they would feel much aggrieved. A certificate was granted by the Pharmacy Board to chemists for the sale of poisons, but such a certificate could not be granted to Chinese storekeepers. They did not want a license to sell poisons, but merely required permission to sell opium for smoking to their countrymen. Sergeant Acton pointed out that both defendants had pleaded guilty of selling, and he handed in their depositions taken at the coroner's inquest. The majority of the bench, the chairman said, was in favour of defendants being fined 20s., and 2s. 6d. costs each, in default of payment, the amount to be levied by distress. The fine was paid.—*Mount Alexander Mail.*

BRIEF NOTES ON THE GENUS GREVILLEA.

By BARON FERD. VON MUELLER, K.C.M.G., M. & PH.D., F.R.S.

THE genus Grevillea is not only one of the most beautiful in the whole vegetation of Australia, but also one of the richest in species, 162 well-marked specific forms standing on record from our continent, irrespective of seven others peculiar to New Caledonia, as shown by Brogniart; but the genus does not extend to New Zealand, nor are as yet congeners known from New Guinea or any other country. Singularly enough only one species reaches Tasmania, though several other Proteaceæ occur there. It might be anticipated that in such a host of plants some could be found of medicinal value. Indeed Dr. Leichhardt in his first celebrated expedition noticed already that the viscid fruits of a tropical Grevillea had epispastic properties. The kernels of Grevillea annulifera are much sought by the natives near Shark-Bay as food, on account of the almond-like taste. Economically Grevillea robusta is important for its wood in cooperage, while the splendour of this tree during the long time of its yearly flowering is such as to render it one of the most magnificent for gardens in any country with a clime free of severe frosts. Indeed for this reason several walks of the Melbourne Botanical Gardens were lined with this Grevillea by me as far back as 1857, and about a dozen years afterwards they had formed by their rapid growth shade-lines, which became already adorned for some months yearly with a mass of floral gold. The mellaginous exudations of the trusses of flowers attract not only a number of honey-sucking birds, but are resorted to by bees also; hence also the rural importance of this tree. It would be of moment if the peculiarities of the tan of any of the arboreous species were rendered known through exact chemical examination; and as Grevilleas occur in all parts of Australia, from the glaciers of our Alps to the arid sands of our deserts and to the tropical jungles, no lack of material exists for the operations of any chemists who may wish to inquire into the technologic and also therapeutic properties of these plants. To show that even the long series of described species is not yet an exhaustive one, I offer the diagnosis of a new kind at this opportune occasion.

Grevillea deflexa.

Shrubby; leaves narrow or linear-lanceolate, mucronate-pointed, recurved at the margin, soon glabrous above, grey-silky beneath; racemes axillary, rather short, turned downward on a slender stalk; bracts minute, fugacious; flowers several times longer than the pedicels; petals of a reddish colour, contracted above the middle, dilated at the recurved summit, outside appressed-hairy, inside towards the middle bearded; hypogynous gland ample, anteriorly descendent; style glabrous, short-exserted; stigma nearly lateral, raised at the centre; ovary on a very short stipe, densely white-downy. In the vicinity of the Gascoyne-River; Forrest and Palak. The racemes resemble externally those of Grevillea Huegelii; but this new species requires to be inserted into the section Plagiopoda.

Much has yet to be learned concerning the regional distribution of the numerous Grevilleas and their special relation to geologic features.

REPORT ON THE ALKALOIDAL VALUE OF CULTIVATED AND WILD BELLADONNA PLANTS.

(By A. W. GERRARD, F.C.S.)

AN opportunity having occurred to obtain considerable supplies of wild-grown belladonna, I have utilised the occasion by instituting a comparative examination of the differences, if any, existing between it and the cultivated kind.

The wild belladonna, upon which my experiments have been conducted, was grown at Lastingham, near Pickering, Yorkshire, in a very poor limestone soil, incapable of producing ordinary cultivated crops, in which, however, the belladonna luxuriates, reaching 6 feet in height. For its collection and selection I am indebted to Dr. Sydney Ringer. As well as I could judge by comparison its age was three or four years.

The cultivated plant was grown by the well-known firm of W. Ransom, of Hitchin, on a chalk subsoil, with 12 inches of stiff loom on the surface. The plants were 3 to 4 feet in height, and believed to be three years of age.

The entire plants were sent me immediately after collection, the wild towards the end of September, the cultivated at the beginning of October. At this period of the year, I am informed by Mr. Ransom, it is considered less active than during July, which is the month of flowering. The wild plant, by reason of the distance it had to travel, did not arrive in such good condition as the cultivated, it having lost its green colour and freshness, but was otherwise uninjured. Both kinds were dried at a temperature of 100° F., and divided into its various parts of root, stem, leaf, and fruit, and well powdered, each part being then separately estimated for its percentage of alkaloid by the process described by the author (*Pharm. Journ.*). The result, as tabulated, shows, besides the comparative strength of the two kinds, also the distribution of the alkaloid in various parts of the plant, and it is worthy of notice that, in both cases, more is obtained from the leaf than the root, this being contrary to the general belief.

The alkaloid in each case was dried over sulphuric acid, and weighed as absolute alkaloid in nearly colourless crystals. In the residues there always appeared a small portion of alkaloid, seemingly different to atropine, being more soluble in water, and more readily volatilised. I hope to turn my attention to this observation on some future occasion.

Alkaloidal value of cultivated and wild belladonna plants :—

WILD PLANT.		CULTIVATED PLANT.	
Part used.	Per cent. yield of Alkaloid.	Part used.	Per cent. yield of Alkaloid.
Root	.45	Root	.35
Stem	.11	Stem	.07
Leaf	.58	Leaf	.4
Fruit	.34	Fruit	.2

So far this examination demonstrates that the wild plant is richest in alkaloid, and has the highest value; but it should be mentioned that the cultivated plant was of excellent quality, that is, judged by commercial belladonna leaves, three samples of which I had previously examined, yielding respectively ·07, ·11, and ·22 per cent. of alkaloid.

It would at present be only speculative to assign any reasons for the differences here shown in the two varieties, but it would appear that a soil of chalky formation favours the development of the alkaloidal principles, for it is a notable coincidence that both plants examined were grown upon chalk, and both are rich in alkaloid; but in that soil where the chalk preponderates, the plants are shown to reach the highest perfection.

As regards commercial belladonna leaves, I should infer that most of them were the growth of a soil unsuited to them; otherwise, they must undergo considerable deterioration by keeping, for in no case have I been able to obtain so good a yield of alkaloid from them as from recent leaves.

Further experiments are yet required to substantiate the above views, and to assist me I shall be glad to receive communications from gentlemen who could direct me where to obtain belladonna plants from other than chalky soils.

It is my intention to continue these observations, and estimate the amounts of alkaloid present in the leaves and root of the plant at the period of flowering, if possible up to the sixth year of its growth.

The following is a report on the Alkaloid from Wild Belladonna, by John Tweedy, F.R.C.S., Professor of Ophthalmic Surgery to University College.—"I have made a large number of comparative experiments with the two solutions of atropine you gave me some weeks ago. As the result of my observations, I may say that in every instance I found the atropine from the wild plant more prompt in its action and more energetic, that is, it dilated the pupil, and suspended the power of accommodation quicker, and its effects lasted longer. I am inclined to think that the solution of the atropine from the wild plant was, likewise, less irritating than the other. This may have been due to the greater purity of the alkaloid prepared by yourself, whereby it contained a larger proportion of hyoscyamine.

"I may add, as a curious fact, that the solution of the atropine from the wild plant has kept better than the other. This difference has been observed in three different portions preserved in separate bottles. The commercial plant already contains a large quantity of fungus, while the other is still free. "As far as I know each specimen has been preserved with equal care."—*Pharmaceutical Journal.*

FREDERICK WOHLER.

ON the last Wednesday in September there passed away at Göttingen, in his eighty-third year, one of the most illustrious chemists that the present century has yet seen, and one who in the length of his life seemed almost to form a connecting link with a time when the science of chemistry was, comparatively speaking, still in swaddling clothes. Frederick Wöhler was born in the year 1800, in Frankfort-on-the-Maine. He first studied medicine and chemistry at Marburg and afterwards at Heidelberg, where upon the advice of Gmelin he gave up the idea of practising medicine and decided to devote himself to chemistry. In 1823 he went to Stockholm and became a pupil of Berzelius. Famous as was the master, Wöhler was at that time his only scholar. As to the school, two common rooms with some simple accommodation, though without furnace, ventilation, or water supply, constituted a not very pretentious laboratory; but Wöhler had been preceded there by such men as Mitscherlich and Henry and Gustavus Rose, and was followed by Magnus. One long pine bench for the master and another for the pupil; some cases against the wall to hold reagents; a mercury trough, a glass-blowing table, a sink, and a pail used in common by the household servant, constituted the furniture of one room, and the balances and other apparatus that of the other, whilst the sand-bath was found in the kitchen. Such were the surroundings where the Swedish chemist did most of his famous work, and where his German pupil learned to follow in his footsteps. Late in life Wöhler loved to recall the memories of his earlier years, and some other interesting autobiographical details of his connection with Berzelius have already appeared in the *Pharmaceutical Journal.*

In the first few years after Wöhler's return to Germany he obtained some minor posts; but in the year 1836 he succeeded Stromeyer as Professor of Chemistry in the University of Göttingen and Director of the Chemical Institute; and he was also appointed Inspector-General of Pharmacies in the Kingdom of Hanover. His university appointments he retained until his death; the inspectorship he eventually resigned, Dr. Wiggers being chosen as his successor. But of greater importance even than his professorial work were the numerous memoirs, reporting the results of most important and diverse researches, with which he enriched chemical literature. No less than two hundred and sixty-eight communications of which he was the sole author are enumerated in the Royal Society's Catalogue, besides thirty or forty written in conjunction with such men as Justus von Liebig, Henri Ste.-Claire Deville and others. His first paper appeared in 1821, and was upon the occurrence of selenium in oil of vitriol prepared from a Bohemian mineral. Other papers followed pretty quickly, and in 1827 he announced that he had succeeded in isolating the metal aluminum by igniting the chloride in the presence of potassium. For thirty years this work appeared without adequate result, and it was Deville's successful researches upon the preparation of sodium and aluminum that first brought this metal within the reach of the manufacturer. M. Dumas, at a recent meeting of the Academy of Sciences, speaking of the joint work of Wöhler and Deville, said:—" United by a rivalry that would have caused division between less elevated minds, these two great chemists pursued in common their researches in mineral chemistry, utilised their respective labours to elucidate points still obscure in the history of boron, silicium and the platinum metals, and remained closely bound in a friendship which increased every year." Wöhler's early connection with Berzelius would appear to have influenced the direction of his work to a considerable extent, as is shown by his numerous papers on the isolation of elemental bodies—such as aluminum, glacinium, tungsten, boron, iridium, osmium,

silicium, vanadium, &c.—and on various points of mineralogical chemistry.

But, perhaps, Wöhler's most famous communication was that upon the artificial formation of urea, published in 1828, in which he took up the position of pioneer in the synthesis of organic compounds. Before that time the apparently distinctive peculiarity of the compounds found in or eliminated from animal or vegetable organisms had given rise to the idea that their formation was due to some special agency, to which the term "vital force" was applied, and the chemistry of organic compounds was treated as a branch of chemical science distinct from the chemistry of inorganic compounds. But the discovery by Wöhler, that the highly nitrogenous body, urea, could be produced by the molecular rearrangement of cyanate of ammonium made the first breach in this wall of partition, and when Fownes subsequently showed that cyanogen could be formed by the direct combination of its elements, the steps in the passage from the simple inorganic substance to the "organic" compound were complete. Since that time many other compounds occurring in animal and plant organisms have been formed synthetically, but in the words of a competent judge, M. Dumas, " La formation artificielle de l'urée reste encore l'exemple le plus net et plus élégant de ce genre de créations."

Mention might be made of Wöhler's researches in conjunction with Liebig on the benzoic compounds and on the derivatives of uric acid, as well as a number of papers on essential oils; but it would be evidently impossible to attempt in these columns to analyse the subjects of all his memoirs, and enough has been said to give some indication of their importance. Before concluding, however, a few words must be devoted to another phase of his literary and scientific work. Many of his memoirs first saw the light in the famous *Annalen der Chemie und Pharmacie*, and of that journal he was one of the principal editors from the year 1838 until the time of his death. He was also the author of several larger works, such as *Elements of Organic Chemistry* (1831), *Examples in Mineral Analysis* (1840), and *Practical Exercises in Chemical Analysis* (1853), and was co-editor of the *Handwörterbuch der Chemie.*

Notwithstanding his great age, Dr. Wöhler appears to have taken outdoor exercise within a week of his death, his final illness only lasting four days.

SOME NOTES ON FOREIGN PHARMACY AND PHARMACIES.

(By JAMES BRINSMEAD.)

THE pleasure I have experienced in reading Mr. Mummery's " Reminiscences" has led me to think that perhaps some of my own experiences (extending, as they did, over many years) of pharmacy in some continental countries might interest my brother pharmacists, and more especially those younger ones who, from curiosity or a laudable ambition to gain experience, may be tempted some day to travel.

I intend to lightly sketch the foreign pharmacist and his pharmacy, his social position, duties, and privileges, &c.; also the foreign assistant, *his* education, remuneration, and accomplishments; at the same time to point out some incidents amusing and otherwise which happen to a young Englishman when first he leaves his island home for continental Europe.

Most people learn French, sometimes from a "native," whose grammar and accent are not always reliable; at other times from some one who "has been there." I studied under a "native," with the result that when I reached Rouen and wanted a shoeblack to operate on my boots, I could only succeed by pantomime, my professor having unfortunately forgotten to teach me a sentence to be used when boots are to be blacked.

I began to think my professor (for such was his title) a fraud, and meditated when I should return to the old country giving him a call and telling him so in his own language. This I thought very unlikely, for the only words I could understand from the conversations going on around me were " oui" and " non," which led me to despair of ever acquiring French.

My destination being Paris, I spent very little time in the old Norman city of Rouen—just enough to get a glimpse of the inside of its interesting cathedral and the outside of a few chemists' shops. Very quiet and solemn these pharmacies appeared to me. No show in the windows, and a perfect absence of "sundries." Pharmacy in France being a *quasi* monopoly, I saw that the pharmacien confined himself very properly to the sale of drugs and the dispensing of prescriptions.

And here I will mention that pharmacy as practised on the Continent is strictly confined to the pharmacien. Doctors are not allowed to compound prescriptions, nor is the general public permitted to deal in drugs.

In Germany the monopoly is complete, one apotheker being allowed a certain district, with so many inhabitants, all to himself. In return for this protection he must sell all drugs according to a tariff fixed by Government, the price even of a bottle being settled for him. It is usual there to mark the price charged opposite each item, the total forming the cost of prescription, which, being marked in plain figures, is an assurance to the patient that the same price will be charged everywhere—at least in Germany. The law compels him also to supply any drug required at all hours, and he may be called upon to supply a halfpennyworth of syrup of violets at three in the morning in winter, with the thermometer far below zero.

The monopoly, however, causes the value of a pharmacy to reach a very high figure, and when one is for sale competition for its purchase is usually very keen. Once in possession the apotheker very often delegates all active duties to a competent managing assistant, the fear of a rival having no existence.

In France, Switzerland, Italy, and some other countries, there is no regulation as to the number of pharmacies, except that in the case of the first-named country no single pharmacien may own two pharmacies within a radius of one kilometre (about two-thirds of a mile). In these countries prices vary greatly, according to locality ; for instance, a 5-oz. mixture dispensed for sixty centimes (about sixpence) at Sienna, in Italy, would be charged two francs and a-half (or two shillings) at any first-rate pharmacy in Paris. Such divergencies are rather astonishing to customers, and frequently involve a little diplomatic explanation, which, though it may silence, I know observed does not always appear to satisfy ; the sufferer often retiring with a dubious look, which seems to say that " there are more mysteries in pharmacy than are dreamt of in his philosophy."

Many very old and extraordinary remedies are still in daily use in the more remote parts, and the belief in witchcraft and the power of the evil eye are indulged in by great numbers. As an instance of the latter, although beyond the region of pharmacy, I may mention that one day, whilst sitting in a *café* in a large city of central Italy, I saw a very old woman, terribly wrinkled, enter and begin to beg. Immediately, as if by common consent, every person in the room—and there could not have been fewer than forty—pointed the index and little finger towards the unfortunate woman, by which means they hoped to ward off the malefic influence of her glance.

Some pharmacies, especially in Italy, enjoy a reputation for certain drugs, customers coming or sending great distances to this particular chemist's shop. Sometimes it is oil of almonds, much used internally, and which they press fresh in the customer's presence ; at other times it may be syrup of snails, also in great repute as a specific in consumption, or some specialty popularly supposed to be obtainable nowhere else, and which has been sold nowhere else within the memory of man.

English drugs have a great reputation, and deservedly so, although a great many articles are palmed off as English that are innocent of a visit to Britain.

Such drugs as Peruvian bark, senna, myrrh, scammony, and many others, I have never been able to obtain in perfection except from London firms. Certain chemicals, also—as, for instance, the bicarbonates of soda and potash—made on the Continent would not be tolerated in any English pharmacy. Essential oils, as a rule, are far dearer in price and inferior in quality to the English makers', and although when exported in bulk they are sometimes lower in price, such is not the case when purchased in small quantities on the spot.

On the other hand, all foreign pharmacies of any importance possess a good laboratory, with at least one still ; and in general I have observed that the preparations are turned out with skill, and the work carried on with a due regard to economy. Great cleanliness is the rule. In many pharmacies all lozenges, pâtes, syrups, and a great many extracts are made on the premises ; and here I will observe that the French are remarkable skillful in the preparation of pâtes

and syrups, the consumption of which amongst them is enormous. Beetroot sugar is used, which does not taste nearly so sweet as that extracted from the cane.

Their fluid extracts also deserve notice, some of them—as, for instance, the extracts of antiscorbutic plants—retaining the characteristic flavour and qualities of the herbs from which they are obtained in a remarkable degree.

Very frequently a lady may be observed sitting at the head of the counter and acting as clerk, but I have never seen them act in any other capacity in pharmacy.

Somewhere near the centre of the pharmacy a table, with writing materials, is commonly placed for the convenience of medical men who may wish to write prescriptions. At this table, in small towns, congregate all the idlers and gossipers, making the pharmacy a general centre for news and scandal. Here politics and the news of the day are freely discussed, and all the small talk of a country town gets thoroughly threshed out.

Notes and Abstracts.

TO CLEAN BRASS.—The Government method prescribed for cleaning brass, and in use at all the United States arsenals, is claimed to be the best in the world. The plan is to make a mixture of one part common nitric acid and one-half part sulphuric acid, in a stone jar, having also ready a pail of fresh water and a box of sawdust. The articles to be treated are dipped into the acid, then removed into the water, and finally rubbed with sawdust. This immediately changes them to a brilliant colour. If the brass has become greasy, it is first dipped in a strong solution of potash and soda in warm water ; this cuts the grease, so that the acid has free power to act.

MANUFACTURE OF STRONG PARCHMENT-PAPER IMPERVIOUS TO WATER.—According to the *Journ. Soc. of Arts*, a strong impervious parchment-paper is obtained by thoroughly washing woollen or cotton fabrics, so as to remove gum, starch, and other foreign bodies, then to immerse them in a bath containing a small quantity of paper pulp. The latter is made to penetrate the fabric by being passed between rollers. Thus prepared, it is afterwards dipped into sulphuric acid of suitable concentration, and then repeatedly washed in a bath of aqueous ammonia until every trace of acid has been removed. Finally, it is pressed between rollers to remove the excess of liquid, dried between two other rollers which are covered with felt, and lastly calendered.

POISONOUS COLOURS.—The German Government has just laid before the Reichstag the following decree, bearing date 1st May, 1882, concerning the prohibition of poisonous colours for the colouring of certain alimentary substances and articles of food. 1. The use of poisonous colours for the manufacture of food-products or articles of food intended for sale is prohibited. Those which contain the following materials or compositions are considered as poisonous colours within the meaning of this enactment:—Antimony (oxide of antimony), arsenic, barium (except sulphate of baryta), lead, chromium (except pure chromic oxide), cadmium, copper, mercury (except cinnabar), zinc, tin, gamboge, picric acid. 2. The preserving and packing of food-stuffs or food-products intended for sale in wrappers coloured with the above-cited poisonous colours, or in barrels in which the poisonous colour is so employed that the poisonous colouring matter can pass into the contents of the barrel, is prohibited. 3. The employment of poisonous colours enumerated in Art. 1. is prohibited for the manufacture of playthings, with the exception of varnish and oil-paints made of zinc-white and chrome-yellow (chromate of lead). 4. The use of colours prepared with arsenic, for the manufacture of paper-hangings, as well as that of pigments containing copper prepared with arsenic, and of matters containing similar colours for the manufacture of materials of dress, is prohibited. 5. The putting on sale, and the sale, wholesale or retail, of food-stuffs and food-products preserved or packed contrary to the regulations of Articles 1 and 2, as well as playthings, paper-hangings, and dress-materials manufactured in contravention of the directions in Articles 3 and 4, are prohibited. 6. This law will come into operation on 1st April, 1883.—*Br. Med. Journ.*

REMINISCENCES OF A PHARMACIST.

(By J. B. MUMMERY.)

(Continued.)

THOSE who have read these papers will not be surprised to find that the proprietor of the Camperdown Apothecaries' Hall made himself famous in a case of poisoning. Fatal mistakes in dispensing have occurred from time immemorial, even by competent hands, and where every precaution appeared to have been taken to prevent them; but when such fatalities are brought about by the sheer incompetency of those who have assumed a calling which they know nothing about, from greed or any other unworthy motive, they assume another shape than mere inadvertence, at least so thinks the writer.

THE NEW SHOP.

Amongst the many improvements made in the city of Sydney about the year 1856 was the conversion of a part of the old dull market wall facing George-street into a row of attractive shops; and as this part of the city was about its best business portion, it is not to be wondered at that the shops let readily; and amongst the successful applicants for occupancy was the gentleman who owned the establishment I have already described as "Apothecaries' Hall." The shop was duly opened as a chemist's, and over the window appeared in gold letters the name of the *quondam* dealer in chamois bags and gold-diggers' belts. Whether he succeeded in attracting any amount of business to his establishment or not I cannot say; but I think his career was too limited for that; for one Saturday night, shortly after opening, a person came in for a given quantity of the harmless, old-fashioned mixture of syrup of squills and oil of almonds. Of course, any apprentice of a month's standing would have known the kind of oil indicated, but J. D. did not, for he gave the essential oil of bitter almonds with syrup of squills, the first dose of which was fatal to the child. The defence at the inquest was that the chemist (?) imagined that the mixture was required for flavouring; but, seeing that syrup of squills is not considered a flavouring agent generally, it will not need a very imaginative person to think that J. D. (like the young man at Brisbane, of whose fatal mistake we have recently had an account) was not aware that there was any difference between the distilled oil of bitter almonds and the expressed oil of sweet.

In this case, as in Doctor Degner's, no punishment was awarded. The Attorney-General of the day, indeed, refused to file a bill; but punishment came as a matter of course. The shop was marked as a dangerous establishment, and a week or two afterwards the shutters were up.

A SAD CASE.

I now come to a case which presented peculiar features, and which ended in fatal result to a personal friend of my own, a Mr. Charles Goddard. This gentleman was an engraver in a good way of business in Sydney, and had only been married a few weeks at the time of his melancholy death, which occurred through a mistake of a chemist's assistant.

The unfortunate man suffered dreadfully from hœmorrhoids, for the relief of which he was in the habit of taking a decoction of "Tormentilla root."

On leaving business one day he called at a chemist's shop in King-street and requested to be supplied with a portion of the root named, and which having received he carried home and boiled in the usual way, and put aside to cool. He then sat down to partake of his tea. Just before going to rest he swallowed the dose which was fated to cause his death, and had no sooner done so than he said to his wife, "I am poisoned! I am sure there must be some mistake; this is not the medicine which I usually take." A medical man was immediately sent for, but before his arrival unmistakable evidence of aconite poisoning had set in, and in spite of the most vigorous efforts to counteract its effects, poor Goddard never saw the morning light.

This case, as may be expected, created a great commotion in Sydney, for the victim was not only well known, but greatly respected.

On examining the drawer at the chemist's from which the root had been taken, which was labelled "Tormentilla," it was found that all the upper portion of its contents were aconite, and it came out that the mistake was caused by the senior assistant having carelessly examined a parcel which had been brought to him by a junior from a back store, which the latter had been cleaning and arranging, who, having found a parcel without a label, or with an indistinct superscription, took it into the shop to his superior, and this individual, either from ignorance or carelessness, pronounced it "Tormentilla," and shot it into the drawer accordingly; and, by that act, signed the death-warrant of the gentleman whose sad fate I have just narrated. The business of the shop (which had formerly been a very good one) fell off to such an extent as to cause the ruin of the proprietor, and I am not sure whether the business exists at all at the present day; but if it does I expect that it will take generations to effectually wipe out the stain which by this one fatality became attached to it.

ONLY A CHILD.

One other case of poisoning by negligence and then, I think, I shall pretty nearly have exhausted the patience of my readers. It occurred to the child of a next door neighbour of mine at Camden, a country town about forty miles from Sydney where for some years previously to my coming to Melbourne I kept a chemist's shop. The affair occurred shortly before I went there, and was caused by one of the local storekeepers.

A child of a Mrs. H. was taken ill with some infantile ailment for which the mother deemed a dose of tincture of rhubarb an expedient remedy, and sent to the store for some accordingly (there was no chemist in the place at that time), administered a dose, and put the child to bed. Some time afterwards the anxious mother, becoming alarmed at certain symptoms which had developed themselves, sent in haste to the doctor, who at once pronounced the case one of opium poisoning, from which the poor little sufferer died, in spite of the most strenuous efforts on the part of the medical attendant to save it. The cause of the painful affair will be anticipated by my readers. The storekeeper had given laudanum instead of tincture of rhubarb—a mistake which, I think, did not cause him a very great amount of remorse, judging by the persistent and careless way in which he dabbled in drugs and chemicals, even after he was relieved of the absolute necessity of doing so by the establishment of a chemist's shop in the town.

(To be concluded in our next.)

BACILLI AS ETIOLOGICAL FACTORS IN DISEASE.

IF there has been any one feature more prominent than another in medicine during the past two or three years more particularly, that feature has been the inquiry into the causation of disease. This inquiry may be said to be characterised by a species of materialism—that is, the search has been for demonstrable germs, which, being taken into the system, give rise to the particular diseases; or, in other words, the tendency has been to regard disease as the fruitage of certain seeds, sown in the soil of the system. This conception is, we say, somewhat materialistic as opposed to the somewhat vague hypotheses of telluric and other intangible influences, which have for many years dominated the professional mind.

Our readers are doubtless familiar with the experiments which Pasteur, Koch, Klebs, Tommasi-Crudeli, Sternberg, Wood, and Formad have reported within the past year. The activity of investigation in this direction is clearly manifested by this array of names, and the expectant medical mind looks longingly towards the east for the appearance of the day-star of hope for deliverance from the uncertainty which has, ever since medicine started on its history, so perplexed the searcher into the causes of diseases. As yet, however, although hope has been buoyant and full of lively anticipation, it has not had much that it can plant its foot upon, as upon a solid foundation. Pasteur, it is true, has discovered the *fons et origo malis* of the splenic fever and cholera which have been wont to decimate the herds and chicken coops of France; but although his discoveries have raised us up to where we can well-nigh isolate the bacillus which works death in the form of diphtheria and scarlatina, we have not yet been quite able to do so. When this greatest among modern savants discovered the germ of these diseases which deal death to these lower animals, and by cultivating them, robbed them sufficiently of their virulence to permit of their inoculation into the well beast, which it thoroughly protected against the spontaneous and fatal form of the disease, the heart of humanity gave an exultant throb. Was it too much to hope from these experiments that the germs of diphthcria and scarlatina might soon be detected and isolated, and that they too, by cultivation, might be sufficiently mitigated in their virulence to permit of their injection in the prophylaxis of two of the most fatal diseases of the nursery, after the same manner that we now prevent small-pox? A year has, however, passed without a realisation of the hope. Will it ever be realised?

Koch has detected, or at least has flattered himself that he has detected, the bacillus which on infesting the system causes consumption, the most fatal of the diseases to which human flesh is heir. This discovery has, however, not borne any fruit in practical results in either man or animal; and granting that he has not deceived himself, as some observers claim that he has, it is somewhat difficult to see wherein any such result is to accrue.

Tommasi-Crudeli, in Europe, and Sternberg, under the direction of the National Board of Health, in this country, have been investigating the bacillus malariæ, with, however, no harmony of result, the former claiming to have found the bacillus, and the latter either denying or doubting its existence. Any fruit that these experiments might settle for ever the vexed question of the material nature of the cause of fever and ague has not yet been justified, and although the investigations and speculations of these gentlemen are interesting from a scientific point of view, their fruit in practical results is as yet problematical.

The investigations and experiments of Drs. Wood and Formad, into the origin and causation of diphtheria, have been extremely interesting. Their only practical result thus far has been in the direction of establishing the fact of the local origin of the disease—that is, that it originates on the mucous membrane of the throat and afterwards becomes systemic, instead of vice versa, as many have held. These experiments have moreover been decidedly in support of the view of the unity as opposed to the duality of diphtheria and croup.

In the midst of the activity above indicated, and in spite of the fact that the practical outcome is as yet little or nothing, it will be seen that when such outcome is developed, if haply it ever is, it will not surprise us or find us unprepared to avail ourselves of the immense possibilities which they have in store.—*Therapeutic Gazette.*

DETERMINATION OF ALUM IN BREAD.

WE take the following from *Allen's Commercial Organic Analysis*, Vol. II., 399, which work should be on the shelves of every library :—

Of the constituents of alum, the only one which is of service for its determination in bread is the aluminium. Pure wheat grain appears to be wholly destitute of aluminium compounds, but commercial wheat flour, to which no alum has been added, is apt to contain small, but sensible traces of aluminium derived from extraneous mineral matter. Such aluminium is present as silicate, and gives no blue colour with the logwood test. On the other hand, all the ordinary methods of quantitatively estimating the alum are incapable of distinguishing between the aluminium present as silicate and that existing in a soluble form. Hence, it is usual to make a correction for the aluminium present as silicate. This is difficult to do with any approach to accuracy, but it may be taken as a rule that from the amount of alum calculated from the total aluminium in the bread should be subtracted a weight equal to the silica found, when the difference will be approximately the true amount of alum added.

The following method should be employed for the determination of the total alumina and silica in bread—100 grams' weight of the sample is dried at 100° C., and then incinerated. This is best done by heating it in a platinum tray (about five inches by three) in a gas-muffle, but may also be effected in a platinum dish or large crucible placed over a Bunsen's burner. The heat should be moderate, so as to avoid fusion of the ash. The process is completed by adding pure sodium carbonate and a little nitre, and heating the mixture to fusion. The product is rinsed out with water into a beaker, acidulated with hydrochloric acid, and evaporated to dryness. The residue is taken up with dilute acid, and the liquid filtered from the silica, which is washed, dried, and weighed. To the solution dilute ammonia is added, till the precipitate barely redissolves on stirring, when a slightly acid solution of ammonium acetate is added, and the whole allowed to stand in the cold for twelve hours. The liquid is then filtered, the precipitate washed, and dissolved in the smallest quantity of hydrochloric acid. The solution so obtained is poured into an excess of an aqueous solution of *pure* caustic soda contained in a large platinum crucible. After heating for some time, the liquid is considerably diluted and filtered. The filtrate is acidulated with hydrochloric acid, a few drops of sodium phosphate added, and then a slight excess of ammonia. The liquid is kept hot till all smell of ammonia is lost, when it is filtered, and the precipitated aluminium phosphate washed, ignited, and weighed. Its weight, multiplied by 3·686, gives the ammonium alum, or by 3·873, the potassium alum in the 100 grams of bread taken. The amount so found requires a correction equal to the percentage of silica obtained. By multiplying the percentage of alum by 280, the number of grains of alum per four-pound loaf will be obtained. The number of miligrams of AlPO$_4$ per 100 grams of the bread gives, without calculation, a close approximation to the number of grains of ammonium alum per four-pound loaf.

Throughout the foregoing process the use of porcelain vessels should be wholly avoided, and care should be taken that the alkaline liquids are not beated in glass. The caustic soda employed should be scrupulously free from alumina.

Are Improvements in Pharmacy Profitable to the Drug Trade ?

THE question is sometimes raised as to which is the more profitable for the Drug Trade generally—the sale of drugs and medicines in the ordinary or crude forms by measure or weight, or in the shape of modern improvements in pharmacy as compressed tablets, capsuled pills, &c.

Any one who has been familiar with the drug trade for, say, ten or twenty years past will, we believe, admit that it is now a much larger business, and supports and enriches a far greater number than formerly. This is undoubtedly owing to the multiplied number of drugs and preparations in demand, and also to the more varied, elegant, and palatable forms in which even the old drugs are prepared, leading to their extensive employment by delicate patients who had previously rejected them. And more than this : are not the increase of business and profits to be still more attributed to the fact that drugs prepared so as to be elegant in appearance and agreeable in taste bring far better prices, and so are much more profitable than the same drugs in less desirable forms.

Let us for instance estimate the respective profits on such drugs as chlorate of potash or ammonium chloride, or bi-carbonate of potash or soda in crude form, and in the shape of the compressed tablets.

A gross of bottles of the compressed tablets, small or medium size, will realise a profit to the retailer of from £2 or £3 to £25 sterling, and sometimes more, according to prices in different places, whereas the profit on the crude drug sold by the pound or ounce would perhaps average as many shillings. For a gross of the tablets, small size, contain about 4 lbs. of drug only, medium size, say 10 lbs. drug. The customer or patient is at the same time pleased to get, say thirty or sixty doses of the medicine for from 1s. to 4s., especially as it is prepared in a highly-convenient and effective, as well as agreeable form. The medical profession and public generally are always ready to appreciate and pay well too for any real improvements in pharmacy that the trade bring to their notice by circular or by showing the goods.

Of course there are some exceptions in cases of the very poor and of those very close-fisted people who go to the leading doctors when they are ill and pay a guinea or more for a prescription and then grumble at paying three or four shillings for as many dozen doses of medicine, no matter how well prepared, and want to get cured of the gout for a sixpence.

Let us also compare the respective profits to the retail and wholesale trade on drugs, in the form of the " McK. & R." Pills, and the same sold by the pound or ounce. The wholesale druggists profit of say 10 per cent, or so on a gross of bottles of the "McK. & R." pills at 288s. would be say 25s. or 30s., while on the crude drugs of which they are composed his average profit would be, perhaps, as many pence. But the retailers' and dispensers' profit shows a far wider margin, for the gross of bottles containing 100 pills each, costing say 2s. or 2s. 6d. per bottle and retailed or dispensed at from 1s. per dozen to 3s. per dozen pills, realise a profit of from £45 to £180 sterling on one gross bottles of pills at the usual retail prices. The crude drugs of which the pills are made, sold by the ounce or pound at retail would not pay a twentieth part as much profit nor give the customer anything like as much satisfaction. Both the "McK. & R." Pills and the Compressed Tablets are now, by the aid of elaborate machinery, prepared and sold at such reasonable prices to the trade that they are now more profitable to dispense than the old way of making all pills by hand by which the delivery of the medicine is delayed and profit-

able customers are often neglected or lost, while the head dispenser is messing over a prescription for a few pills—a penny-wise and pound-foolish policy if a man's time is worth anything to his business.

The Compressed Tablets and the " McK. & R." Pills being ready for immediate dispensing, much economy of time and annoyance of delay to the patient is effected by their employment, and on account of their elegant appearance and freedom from offensive taste and smell, they are preferred by the medical profession, and are readily taken by patients who cannot or will not take the same drugs in any other form. In the tablets the customer gets 30 doses for say 1s. to 2s. 9d. In the pills a dozen doses for say 1s. 6d. to 3s., which is certainly very cheap if we consider the quality and style and the skill and machinery required in manufacturing.

The Kepler Extract of Malt may be regarded as a sort of addition, and the profit on it a clear gain to the drug trade as it is most largely used for the diastase which it contains (the starch digesting principle), and which is not permanent in isolated form. The Kepler Extract is also much more than a substitute for Beer and other malt liquors as a medicine, for its nutritive properties are not converted into alcohol by fermentation nor its digestive properties destroyed by the heat which is always employed in brewing.

The Kepler Extract is therefore highly appreciated by abstainers from alcoholic beverages, but who desire the benefit of the digestive tonic and nutritive properties of malt. A delicious beverage can be prepared from it by mixing a tablespoonful of the Extract with half a glass of milk and filling the tumbler with soda water. This is about the best way of taking the Extract at mealtimes.

The Kepler Extract is also largely used where its virtues become once known by persons who cannot take or digest Cod Liver Oil ; and this remark applies equally to the Kepler Extract with Cod Liver Oil, in which the nutritive powers of the oil are greatly increased through its minuted subdivision and consequent easy digestion. Compare the profit on 5 gallons Cod Liver Oil at 5s. gall., = 25s., with the profit on the same quantity of oil in the form of the Kepler Emulsion —viz., profit on15 dozen Kepler Oil and Extract at 9s. dozen, = 135s.—£6 15s. We have high authorities for giving the opinion that greater benefit to the patient will usually be derived from five pounds of the Kepler Emulsion of Cod Liver Oil with Extract of Malt than from twenty-five pounds of unemulsified oil ; and even more than this in cases of weak digestion where the plain oil is liable to aggravate, but which the "Kepler" Emulsion will usually relieve, the Extract of Malt being a most valuable aid to digestion as well as perfect emulsifying agent for oils.

The Beef and Iron preparation recommends itself to the trade, both on account of its popularity with the medical profession and public where it is introduced, but also because it is a profitable addition to stock.

The old way for a patient requiring such a tonic stimulant has been for the patient requiring such a stimulant to be told to stew some beef and soak some rusty nails in wine, or perhaps buying the citrate of iron at a profit of a few pence or shillings to the chemist, instead of which the chemist now supplies a highly approved pharmaceutical preparation at a profit per gross of from £3 12s. to £8 8s.

The trade on Hazeline is being worked up from nothing to a good sale and profit, and has effected cures in a variety of cases where all other remedies have proved ineffectual.

One retail chemist assures us that the profit resulting from his sale of this elegant Distillate of Witch Hazel is more than equal to the rent of his business premises located in the principal street of a large town ; and there should be no difficulty in any progressive chemists realising a sum equal to rent with our full line of new improvements in pharmacy at his command ; each of which is capable of a very large sale, if merely kept before the attention of the medical profession and public. To chemists who will take an interest in these goods, illustrated chromo-cards and circulars for free distribution, bearing name and address, also samples and medical reports will be presented on application to Burroughs, Wellcome & Co., Snow Hill, London.

FELTON, GRIMWADE & CO.'S
PRICE LIST OF PROPRIETARIES & MANUFACTURES.

	Price per dozen.	Price per case.	Price of assortment of £2 worth.	Price of assortment of £50 worth, net.
KRUSE'S FLUID MAGNESIA—				
No. 1 (½-pint, in 6 doz. cases ; retail 1/6)	9/-	... 8/6	... 8/3	... 8/-
No. 2 (pint, in 3 doz. cases ; retail 2/6) ...	16/-	... 15,-	... 13/6	... 12/10
No. 3 (quart, in 2 doz. cases ; retail 3/6)...	20/-	... 19/-	... 17/3	... 16/-
Dispensing, in 2 doz. cases	18/-	... 17/-	... 15/6	... 14/5

KRUSE'S INSECTICIDE—				
No. 1 (retail 1/-)	per dozen 8/-	... per gross 7/6	... per 5 gross 7/-	
No. 2 (retail 1/6)	„ 12/-	... ½ „ 11/3	... 3 „ 10/6	
No. 3 (retail 2/6)	„ 20/-	... ¼ „ 18/6	... 1 „ 17/6	
No. 4 (retail 5/-)	„ 40/-	... ⅛ „ 37/-	... ½ „ 35/-	
No. 5 (retail 10/-)	„ 80/-	... ¼ „ 74/-	... ½ „ 70/-	

BLOOR'S FOOD—				
No. 1	8/- per doz. ...	per gross, 7/6 per doz.	... per 3 gross, 7/. per doz.	
No. 2	15/- „ ...	½ „ 14/- „	... 2 „ 13/- „	
No. 3	48/- „ ...	¼ „ 45/- „	... 1 „ 42/- „	

WILLIAMS'S AUSTRALIAN YEAST POWDER, in ½-lb. canisters, 60/- per gross ; 1-lb. do., [10/- per doz.

„	Egg Powder, in boxes containing 3 doz. canisters	per doz., 4/6
„	Curry Powder, in boxes containing 6 doz. 1-oz.	per doz., 2/-
„	„ „ „ „ 2-oz.	per doz., 4/-
„	„ „ „ 3 doz. 4-oz	per doz., 7/-

DAY'S FARMER'S FRIEND, in 6-doz. cases ... ... per doz., 9/-; per gross, 8/6

WORMALD'S CARBOLIC TOILET SOAP, Bars, ½-lbs. and 1-lbs., in 12-lb. boxes, per box, 9/-; [6 boxes, 8/-; 12 boxes, 7/6

„	„ „ Tablets, No. 1, in 6-doz. boxes, per doz., 4/-; 1 gross, [42/-; 3 gross, 36/-
„	„ „ „ No. 2, in 3 doz. boxes, per doz., 8/-; 3 doz., 7/6; [1 gross, 72/-
„	„ „ „ small sizes, in 3-doz. boxes ... per gross, 18/-
„	Dog Soap, Tablets, No. 1 ... ... per doz., 4/-; 6 doz., 3/6 .
„	„ „ „ No. 2 ... ... per doz., 8/-; 6 doz., 7/-
„	Household Carbolic Soap, Flea Brand, in 1-cwt. cases ... ... 32/- per cwt.

VINCENT'S FULLERS' EARTH SOAP, in 3-doz. boxes, per doz., 4/-; per gross, 42/-; 3 gross, 36/-

CLARKE'S AUSTRALIAN EYE LOTION ... ... per doz., 10/-; per gross, 108/-

CARBOLIC POWDER, No. 1	per doz., 8/-; per gross, 90/-
„ „ No. 2	per doz., 12/-; per gross, 126/-

SEIDLITZ POWDERS, No. 1, Howard's Chemicals, full weights, in hinged boxes, labelled or unlabelled, [in 1-gross cases ... per doz., 9/-; per gross, 102/-
No. 2, Howard's Chemicals, in plaid boxes per doz., 8/ ; per gross, 90/-

THOMPSON'S BENZINE, 2-oz.	per doz., 4/-; in 3-doz. boxes, 45/- gross
„ „ 6-oz.	per doz., 8/-; in 3-doz. boxes, 90/- gross
„ Ess. Smoke	per doz., 12/-; 3 doz., 11/-
„ Glycerine, 4-oz.	per doz., 8/-; 3 doz., 7/6
„ Essence Rennet, concentrated, pints	per doz., 12/-

FELTON, GRIMWADE & CO., 31 & 33 Flinders Lane West.

INDEX

Australasian Supplement to Chemist and Druggist.

VOL. V.

FROM JUNE, 1882, TO MAY, 1883.

All letters to the Editor will be found arranged under the head of Correspondence.

INDEX, Vol. V.—(Continued).

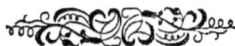

Casuarina macphlora 92.

[SUPPLEMENT ONLY.]

THE
Chemist & Druggist.

WITH AUSTRALASIAN SUPPLEMENT.

(Published under direction of the Pharmaceutical Society of Victoria.)

No. 48. { PUBLISHED ON THE 15TH OF EVERY MONTH. }
Registered for Transmission as a Newspaper.

APRIL, 1882.

{ SUBSCRIPTION, 15s. PER ANNUM, INCLUDING DIARY, POST FREE.

BOTANIC GARDENS

Printed by Mason, Firth & M'Cutcheon, 51 & 53 Flinders Lane West, Melbourne.

PEARCE'S LAVENDER

With Musk.

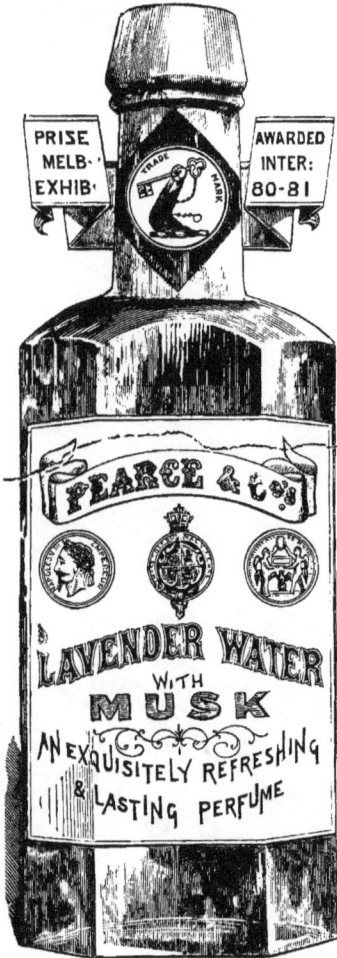

PRISE
MELB·
EXHIB·

AWARDED
INTER:
80-81

THIS is a well-known fragrant Perfume, and from its cheapness may be used lavishly.

Sprinkled about the Room, or used in a Bath, it will be found most refreshing and invigorating.

As a perfume for the handkerchief, its peculiar fragrance and exquisitely penetrating odour, so delightfully refreshing in hot climates and grateful to the invalid, render it one of the Standard Perfumes of the day.

PROPRIETORS:

HEMMONS, LAWS & Cº

WHOLESALE DRUGGISTS,

RUSSELL ST., MELBOURNE.

which we are quite sure will be equally welcomed. The Juvenile Telescope Company having received their telescope from England have accepted the kind offer of Mr. Wall to give them two evenings per month on astronomical science, also at his school, so that the council seem to be thoroughly alive to the desirability of popularising their well conducted institution.

NOTE ON AN HITHERTO IMPERFECTLY KNOWN CALLISTEMON,

BY BARON FERD. VON MUELLER, K.C.M.G., M. & PH.D., F.R.S., &c.

THOUGH the Australian vegetation has become gradually unfolded in most of its features, yet much remains to be closer observed, and even in the vicinity of larger settlements new or rare plants remain to be traced, as will be exemplified on this occasion. It was early in the year 1853 when the writer noticed on one of the rivulets of the Buffalo-Range a myrtaceous peculiar tall then fruiting shrub, which in the absence of flowers was referred to the genus Melaleuca, and for which, in allusion to its pine-like habit, the name M. pityoides was chosen (First General Report, 12). Six years later Dr. Miquel in an essay on various Australian plants received from me, suggested that this Melaleuca might be transferable to the closely allied genus Callistemon (Nederlandisk Kruidkundig Archief, IV., 142). In 1863, when occasion arose, to revise the species of Callistemon, I ventured to refer this doubtful plant (Fragm. Phytogr. Austr., IV, 64) as a form to C. salignus, a species singularly variable in its ascent from the lowlands to the highest Alps. To this Mr. Bentham (Flor. Austr., III., 121) somewhat demurred, pointing to Melaleuca nodosa and M. pungens as very similar in foliage. Matters concerning this plant remained in doubt till last spring, when I received flowering specimens, gathered far upon the Ovens-River by Mr. C. Falk, and when other samples, also in flower, were collected by the Rev. B. Scortechini, who obtained his material at the sources of the Bremarcsque-River, on the boundary line between New South Wales and Queensland. By these means it is now clearly proved, that the plant should be referred to Callistemon; indeed, its flowers show such close resemblance to those of the small blossomed variety of C. salignus, as perhaps to render it desirable to regard it merely as an extreme form of that species. If specific value is to be attributed to it, the diagnosis would be as follows :—

Callistemon pityoides.

F. v. M., Systematic Census of Australian Plants, 140 (1882).

Leaves short, thinly cylindrical, somewhat awlshaped, slightly compressed or sometimes semi-cylindrical, soon glabrous; bracts lanceolate-linear or narrow, or some ovate-lanceolar; rachis and often also the calyces short veiny; lobes of the calyx semi ovate-roundish or some almost sorbi-lar, membranous, about half as long as the tube, considerably shorter than the petals, finally deciduous; stamens comparatively short; filaments pale yellowish, glabrous, also at twice as long as the petals, or some three times as long; anthers yellow; style glabrous; fruits truncate-ovate, rarely depressed-globular, more or less contracted at the summit; valves silky at the surface.

In its external aspect this plant resembles more the larger forms of Melaleuca ericifolia than even the smaller of Callistemon salignus. To the pharmaceutic profession it is of particular interest as the quality of the oil of the foliage and its percentage remain to be ascertained yet. After Mr. Bosisto's enterprising and successful efforts, to give to the distillation of oils from our myrtaceous trees large commercial dimensions, local pharmaceutists should feel encouraged in effecting additional tests of the Myrtaceæ in this respect, the number of species on record from Australia having reached to 650, whereby this order of plants stands with us second only to Leguminoseæ, but surpassing far the latter in technical importance.

PHARMACY IN THE FRENCH ACADEMIES.

A VISITOR to the new School of Pharmacy in Paris will readily perceive that French pharmacists are by no means disposed to forget the past history of their art. Good reason have they indeed to be proud of the parts played in the world of science by their predecessors, and M. Lefort needs no justification for taking the opportunity afforded by a recent meeting of the Paris Pharmaceutical Society to call attention specially to the extent to which pharmacy has been represented in the scientific academies of France.

The first Academy of Sciences in France was founded in the year 1666, by Louis XIV., at the instigation of his famous finance minister, Colbert. It was intended to be devoted to practical science rather than to the reading of papers, and with this object laboratories were maintained at the royal expense at the place of meeting, in which experiments and observations were made and the results obtained were discussed by the members in common. Animal and vegetable products, minerals, and especially mineral waters, were submitted to such analysis as was then possible, and it was only natural that after a few years pharmacists should be called to take part in the work. The first pharmacist admitted into the Academy of Sciences, in 1686, was Moses Charras, the author of a Pharmacopée galénique et chimique and next, in 1699, came Nicholas Lémery, the author of the Cours de Chimie. Then followed Boulduc, Geoffroy, Rouelle, and Cadet de Gassicourt. But the revolutionary wave that swept away men did not spare institutions, and a few months before Lavoisier was sent to the guillotine the academies in France were suppressed as useless. In 1795, however, the Convention established a new "Institut des Sciences et des Arts," which included all the academies as they now exist. In the new Academy of Sciences, as in the old, pharmacists have taken an honourable place, as will be seen from the following roll of names:—Bayen, the two Pelletiers, Vauquelin, Parmentier, Baumé, Deyeux, Proust, Serullas, Robiquet, Lesson, Gaudichaud, Balard, Bussy, Gerhardt, Lecoq, Planchon, Berthelot, Chatin, Girardin, and Milne-Edwards. Each of these men was a legally qualified pharmacist ; but there have been others also who commenced their scientific career in a pharmacy, among whom may be mentioned Dumas, Frémy, and Trecul.

The Academy of Medicine was founded in the year 1820, by a decree of Louis XVIII., and one of its duties was to be to reply to questions of the Government on all subjects affecting the public health, and particularly in respect to new and secret remedies, and natural and artificial mineral waters. Originally the academy was divided into three sections—medicine, surgery and pharmacy—and the first nine nominations to the pharmacy section were—Boullay, Deyeux, Fabre, Henri, Laugier, Pelletier, Planche, Robiquet, and Vauquelin. Amongst the earlier elections by the academy itself were—Boudet, Derome, Caventou, Guibourt, Labarraque, Bussy, Chevallier, Derosne, Frémy, and Serullas. Since the year 1829 the Academy of Medicine has been divided into sections, of which that devoted to pharmacy is the eleventh, but pharmacists frequently figure in other sections. The list given by M. Lefort, of eminent pharmacists who have been connected with this academy as members, associates or correspondents, is too long for quotation here, and this is the less necessary since it includes many names that have already been mentioned. At present there is only the one class of members, limited to one hundred, and amongst them are included many whose names have frequently appeared at the head of articles published in these pages.—Pharmaceutical Journal.

PERUVIAN AND WATTLE BARKS.

PART of the following letter appeared recently in the columns of the Argus, respecting the production of Cinchona bark in Ceylon :—" Enquiries of a most important nature are now being made with regard to the growth of wattle bark for tanning purposes. It appears there is a demand for Mimosa seed in Ceylon for the dual purpose of growing it for its bark, as well as a shelter for young Cinchona trees. Connected therewith a discovery has been made that the medicinal properties of Peruvian bark resides in the outer cuticle, which can be excised from the tree without causing its destruction. Now, if the same holds good with regard to wattle bark, an annual crop can be obtained from it, whilst still affording shelter to the others. Since the above appeared in print, a letter has been received from Baron Von Mueller on the subject, in which he expresses an opinion favourable to the hypothesis,and if labour was as cheap in Victoria as it is in Ceylon, there is not the slightest doubt that the discovery would be of vast importance both to the growers and users of wattle bark, and remove one of the causes of anxiety with regard to its produc-

LANGTON, EDDEN, HICKS & CLARK

WHOLESALE

Export Chemists and Druggists,

230, 231, 232 UPPER THAMES STREET,

LONDON.

Indents executed on the best possible terms, both as regards
Quality and Price.

LANGTON'S COD LIVER OIL, in 10-oz. and 20-oz. Bottles.

LANGTON'S DECOCTION JAMAICA SARSAPARILLA, in 10-oz.
and 20-oz. Bottles.

SPECIAL QUOTATIONS FOR LARGE BUYERS.

Letters and Orders to be addressed to—

MR. RIVERS LANGTON,

16 Vaughan's Chambers, 48 Queen Street,

MELBOURNE.

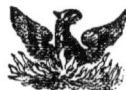

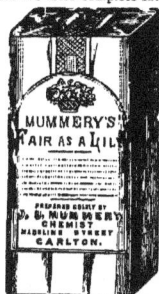

J. BOSISTO

Desires to direct the Medical Profession and Pharmaceutical Chemists to his

Special Chemical and Pharmaceutical Preparations from Australian Vegetation.

OL. EUCALYPTI ESS.

Obtained from the Amygdalina Odorata species : the Eucalyptus Oil of Commerce.

For External Use. — A valuable remedy for Rheumatism, Lumbago, Sciatica, Sprains, Chilblains, Whooping Cough, Croup, Asthma, Bronchitis, Sore Throat, Chronic Hepatitis, and all other painful affections where a stimulating application is required.

Mode of Application for rapid effect. — Apply the Oil with much friction, until a glow of warmth is established.

For a Soothing & Steady Action. — Shake well together a tablespoonful of the Oil with half-a-pint of warm water, saturate a cloth with this and apply over the painful part — repeating, if necessary, in half-an-hour.

For Internal Use. — For Coughs, Asthmatic and Throat Affections — 5-drop doses on loaf-sugar occasionally.

This Oil is a thorough **Deodorant and Disinfectant**, and an antiseptic of great power. A few drops sprinkled on a cloth and suspended in a sick room renders the air refreshing ; and for disinfecting and deodorising, a tablespoonful of the Oil added to two or three pounds' weight of sawdust, well mixed and distributed, will speedily produce a purifying effect.

Bosisto's Eucalyptus Oil is the genuine Essence of the Tree, and all labels bearing the name of Bosisto and the Parrot Brand may be relied on.

☞ NOTE.—To ensure the certainty of obtaining this Oil is by purchasing it from the Wholesale Houses in packages or bottles, bearing the certificate and signed "J. Bosisto and Co.," together with the trade mark—Parrot Brand, yellow ground.

SYRUPUS ROSTRATI.

Prepared from the Inspissated Juice of the Red Gum Tree of Victoria.

A delicate mucilaginous astringent in combination with tonic properties. Employed with benefit in all affections of the mucous membrane of the Stomach and Bowels, and is a valuable remedy in the treatment of Chronic Dysentery and Diarrhœa. As a topical astringent in relaxation of the Uvula and Tonsils, either in the form of a Gargle, Syrup, or Lozenge, it forms one of the most useful remedies. Soluble in Alcohol, Cold or Boiling Water. Incompatibles—the Alkalies and the Metallic Salts.

OL. EUCALYPTI GLOBULI ESS. $C_{12}H_{20}O.$

Anthelmintic—By Enema 30 to 60 minims in mucilage of starch.

Internally—Dose 3 to 5 minims in gum mucilage, syrup, or glycerine.

Tonic, Stimulant, and Antiseptic.

A small dose promotes appetite ; a large one destroys it. In stronger doses of 10 to 20 minims it first accelerates the pulse, produces pleasant general excitement (shown by irresistible desire for moving about) and a feeling of buoyancy and strength. Intoxicating in very large doses, but, unlike alcohol or opium, the effects are not followed by torpor, but produce a general calmness and soothing sleep. A strong cup of Coffee will at once remove any unpleasantness arising from an over-dose.

EUCALYPTOL. $C_{12}H_{20}O.$

From Eucalyptus Globulus. Therapeutic use. For Inhalation in Bronchial Affections. Quantity employed —From half to one teaspoonful with half a pint of hot water in the Inhaler.

TINCT. EUCALYPTI GLOBULI (BOSISTO'S).

Tonic, Antiperiodic, and Antiseptic.—An important remedial agent in Intermittent and Remittent Fevers, also successfully employed in affections of the respiratory Organs— Bronchitis, Asthma, Ephysema, Whooping Cough—relieving Fits of Coughing, and allaying the irritation of the Bronchi by promoting expectoration.

Dose. — 20 to 30 minims in Syr. Aurantii, Wine, or on Loaf-sugar. For Children, the dose in proportion to age.

Employed also in purulent Catarrhal Affections of the Urethra and Vagina in dilution ; and as an Antiseptic in dressing wounds.

TINCT. EUCALYPTI ROSTRATI (BOSISTO'S).

This species of the Eucalypti (Red Gum) possesses a delicate mucilaginous astringent and is a safer and more effective remedy than either Kino or Catechu.

Dose. — Adult, one fluid drachm ; generally in combination with Conf.; Arom.;

CIGARETTES OF EUCALYPTUS GLOBULUS.

Recommended for Bronchial and Asthmatic Affections, and also for the Disinfecting and Antiseptic Properties.

EUCALYPTENE : from Eucalyptus Globulus.

The Tonic or bitter principle in an amorphous condition ; employed in Low Fevers in doses of one to three grains.

LIQUOR EUCALYPTI GLOBULI.

The Fever and Ague Remedy. Dose—For Ague and Dengue Fever, 30 to 60 minims in half a wineglassful of mucilage and water, or glycerine and water, with the occasional addition of two minims of Eucalyptol every two or three hours during the paroxysms of Ague. Incompatibles—the Mineral Salts.

UNG. EUCALYPTI VIRIDIS.

Antiseptic Emollient ; rapidly sets up a healthy action, In 1lb. jars.

OL. ATHEROSPERMA MOSCHATA ESS.

The physiological effects of this Oil, in small doses, are Diaphoretic, Diuretic, and Sedative, and it appears to exert a specific lowering influence upon the heart's action. As a medicine it has been introduced into the European Hospitals, and employed successfully in cases of Heart Disease. Administered in one or two drop doses at intervals of six or eight hours.

LIQUOR ATHEROSPERMA MOSCH.

Employed in Asthma and all affections of the respiratory organs.

The following Articles are prepared ready for the Counter Trade :—

EUCALYPTUS OIL, in Bottles, 1s. and 2s. each.
———————— OINTMENT, in Pots, 1s. each.
———————— PILLS, in Bottles, 2s. each.
———————— CIGARETTES, in Boxes, 2s. each.
———————— LOZENGES, RED GUM, in Boxes, 1s. & 2s. each.
———————— SYRUP, RED GUM, in Bottles, 1s. 6d. and 2s. 6d. each.
ATHEROSPERMA, in Bottles, 1s. 6d. and 2s. 6d. each.

Each bears the Trade Mark—Parrot Brand.

J. BOSISTO, Manufacturing Pharmaceutical Chemist

(LABORATORY: RICHMOND, MELBOURNE),

By whom the Eucalyptus preparations were first introduced, both in Australia and in Europe, and to whom has been awarded the Silver Medal of the Society of Arts, London ; the Gold Medal of the Sydney International, the Gold Medal of the Melbourne International Exhibitions, and prize medals from the various European, American, and other Australian Exhibitions, dating from the first of his investigations of this vegetation in 1853, and published in the Transactions of the Royal Society of Victoria, Exhibition Reports, &c.

NOTE.—The Medical Profession and Pharmaceutical Chemists are requested when ordering through Wholesale Houses to state distinctly that Bosisto's Preparations are wanted.

BURGOYNE, BURBIDGES, CYRIAX & FARRIES,

WHOLESALE AND

EXPORT DRUGGISTS,

𝕸𝖆𝖓𝖚𝖋𝖆𝖈𝖙𝖚𝖗𝖎𝖓𝖌 𝕮𝖍𝖊𝖒𝖎𝖘𝖙𝖘,

AND DRUGGISTS' SUNDRIESMEN,

COLEMAN ST., LONDON.

SOLE AGENT FOR THE COLONIES—

T. LAKEMAN,

24 O'CONNELL STREET, SYDNEY.

INDEX TO LITERARY CONTENTS.

The Chemist and Druggist.
WITH AUSTRALASIAN SUPPLEMENT.

OFFICE: MUTUAL PROVIDENT BUILDINGS, COLLINS STREET WEST.
Published on the 15th of each Month.

THIS Journal is issued gratis to all paid-up Members of the PHARMACEUTICAL SOCIETY OF VICTORIA, and to non-members at Fifteen Shillings per annum, payable in advance. A copy of *The Chemists and Druggists' Diary*, published annually, is forwarded post free to every subscriber.

Advertisements, remittances, and all business communications to be addressed to THE HONORARY SECRETARY OF THE PHARMACEUTICAL SOCIETY, MELBOURNE.

SCALE OF CHARGES FOR ADVERTISEMENTS:
Per annum.		Per annum.
One Page £8 0 0	Quarter Page ..£3 0 0	
Half do. 5 0 0	Business Cards .. 2 0 0	

Special rates for wrapper and pages preceding and following literary matter. Advertisements of Assistants Wanting Situations, 2s. 6d. each. Advertisements for insertion in the current month should be sent to the office before the 10th.

COMMUNICATIONS for the EDITORIAL department of this journal should be addressed to THE EDITOR, MUTUAL PROVIDENT BUILDINGS, COLLINS STREET WEST, MELBOURNE.

No notice can be taken of anonymous communications. Whatever is intended for insertion must be authenticated by the name and address of the writer—not necessarily for publication, but as a guarantee of good faith.

ANNUAL SUBSCRIPTIONS TO THE SOCIETY.

ALL annual subscriptions are now due.
Member's subscription	...	...	...£1 1 0
Associate's	...	...	... 0 10 6
Apprentice's	...	...	... 0 5 0

Cheques and Post-office orders should be forwarded to the Honorary Secretary, No. 4 Mutual Provident Buildings, Collins-street, Melbourne.

THE LIBRARY.

THE Library is open daily (Saturdays excepted), from 9.30 a.m. to 4.30 p.m. Catalogue of the books can be obtained on application.

BIRTH.

LONGMORE.—On the 29th March, at Kensington, the wife of Francis Longmore, chemist, of a son.

MARRIAGE.

CATTACH—HEWS.—On the 5th April, at the residence of the bride's parents, by the Rev. Thos. Porter, Alexander M. Cattach, son of the late James Cattach, to Eliza, fifth daughter of James Hews, Ryrie-street, Collingwood.

DEATHS.

MURRAY.—On the 3rd April, at the Alfred Hospital, Robt. D. Murray, dispenser, son of the late Andrew Murray, Prince's-street, Edinburgh. Beloved and regretted.

COWL.—On the 31st March, at Walhalla, of phthisis, Gertrude, the beloved wife of R. H. Cowl; aged 23 years.

KERNOT.—On the 26th March, at Milton-house, Newtown, Geelong, Charles Kernot, M.L.A., aged 62 years.

M. YVON ON THE PURITY OF CHLOROFORM.

M. YVON has suggested a new and delicate method of testing the purity of chloroform for anæsthetic purposes. At a meeting of the Paris Société de Pharmacie he read a paper upon this subject, which has been published in the *Journal de Pharmacie et de Chimie*, a résumé of which is given in the *Pharmaceutical Journal* (pp 711, 12), and may be consulted with advantage. We transcribe the following as containing the proposed mode of testing, which would appear worthy of attention :—

Referring to the characteristics requisite for chloroform that is to be used for anæsthetic purposes, as described by Professor

Regnault—viz., that it should have a mild odour, be neutral to test paper, give no precipitate when shaken with solution of argentic nitrate, not acquire a brown colour when heated to the boiling point with caustic potash, not blacken when mixed with concentrated sulphuric acid, nor dissolve or consequently become coloured by certain aniline derivatives such as rosaniline or aniline blue—M. Yvon is of opinion that these characters do not constitute a sufficient guarantee of purity unless the boiling point of the liquid has previously been found correct. That he considers to be an absolute necessity, having examined many samples which were not quite pure, although they bore the tests above mentioned. In seeking for further tests of purity, M. Yvon first tried the determination of the boiling point, and by that means was able to classify the samples operated upon under two heads. The first commenced to distil about 59·4° C., the temperature rising gradually to 60·4°, 61·2°, and 63·4° by the time three-fourths had passed over and then rising to 64·4° and even 65·5°. The samples of the second class began to distil at 61°, and nearly eight-tenths passed over at that temperature, after which the temperature rose up to 66°.

Making due allowance for the difficulty of obtaining absolutely precise results by this means, M. Yvon nevertheless felt justified in concluding that the samples examined by him contained substances rather more volatile, and others rather less volatile than chloroform, without, however, affecting the reactions which are accepted as characteristic of the purity of chloroform.

After some further trials of a mixture of bichromate of potash and sulphuric acid M. Yvon finally decided to employ permanganate of potash, as he found that salt was not reduced by pure chloroform. He first used an aqueous solution containing ·025 per cent. of the salt, shaking half a cubic centimetre with 5 cub. cent. of the chloroform to be tested and found that the greater the impurity of the sample the more rapid was the reduction of the permanganate. Subsequently a greater sensibility was given to the permanganate by applying it in the presence of a free alkali. A solution containing 1 part permanganate with 10 parts caustic potash in 250 parts of water has a fine violet colour, which is instantly changed to green by contact with impure chloroform. In testing a great number of samples of chloroform from various sources, M. Yvon did not find any that were free from impurity. With ordinary commercial chloroform the passage from violet to green was almost instantaneous; with chloroform described as pure it took place within ten or fifteen seconds, and with anæsthetic chloroform within from thirty to fifty seconds.

The Month.

WE may remind our readers that the Royal Society of New South Wales offer a series of prizes, of the value of £25 each, for the best communication, the result of original research, upon eight subjects of colonial interest, one of which, "The Chemistry of the Australian Gums and Resins," must be sent in not later than 31st August, 1883.

The Pharmacy Board have resolved to enforce the fourteenth clause of the Pharmacy Act, and to prosecute persons who neglect to comply with its provisions. The first case brought forward was that of W. F. G. Nettleton, at Warrnambool, who was fined £2 and £1 1s. costs.

At the City Police Court, Adelaide, on the 29th March, a woman was fined for selling milk after the Board of Health had ordered her to desist, in consequence of her having lost two of her sons by typhoid fever. She continued selling milk, and infected some of her customers.

for three days. Having filtered it, pour it on 1 lb. (avoirdupois weight) of sugar contained in an evaporating dish or other suitable vessel, and allow the alcohol to evaporate spontaneously. When dry dissolve in half-pint of water in which, if orange syrup is to be made, 1½ ounces of citric acid—if lemon, 2 ounces of the acid and 2 drachms—are to be dissolved. This mixture, added to 11 pints of simple syrup, will produce fine flavoured syrups, which keep well.

SECRET REMEDIES.

IN considering the subject a distinction should be made between "secret remedies" and "specialties." A "specialty" may be defined as any substance or product which, prepared according to an official formula, realises an improvement in the art of pharmacy, and presents special therapeutic advantages. A "secret remedy" is any simple or compound substance or medicine employed in the treatment of disease, which has not received official sanction or publication, and which has not been prepared for a particular case upon a medical prescription. One is the product of the professional skill and practical sense of the pharmacist, and is generally met with in competitions and industrial exhibitions. The other is a product of charlatanism and an inordinate desire to acquire a fortune rapidly; it makes itself known especially by advertisements in the public prints. Even if the remedies of which neither the basis nor the proportions are known ought to be rejected from therapeutics, genuine specialties, which mark a progress in the pharmaceutic art, or are intended to facilitate the administration of certain medicines, might, up to a certain point, be admitted. The distinction between a specialty and a secret remedy is not, however, always easy to establish.

The public has acquired a taste for secret remedies, and will continue to take them; secret remedies enjoy a prestige that imposes upon the public, and it will be difficult to fight against this infatuation. The word public is here used in the widest sense, as including the learned as well as the ignorant. And it is certain the public will have secret remedies as long as it has incurable invalids haunted by the hope of being healed or having their pains assuaged. The medicine that would appear without any value if it were given simply under the cover of the pharmacist, with his label, becomes a panacea, and imposes upon the public as soon as it is noisily advertised and covered with a stamp and a specious prospectus; if, in addition, it be prescribed by a medical man, the confidence becomes unlimited.—*Pharmaceutical Journal.*

INQUEST.

MR. MAUNSELL held an inquest on 6th March, at the Travellers' Rest Hotel, Gerogery, on the body of William Francis Wilkes, chemist. The following evidence was taken :—James E. Britton deposed : I first met the deceased in Albury on the 20th February, when he informed me he was hard up ; that he was a chemist by profession, and had been managing a shop in Chiltern. He told me his father was a medical man in England, and that he was expecting money from home. I saw the deceased the last time alive about a quarter of a mile from Brown's Springs Station. He used to eat large quantities of salt and drink a great deal of water. He had a good appetite. Jesse Young, boundary rider, deposed : I found deceased lying dead on a rock about a mile from the station on Tuesday last. He was lying on his face, and there was no appearance of any struggle. There was no blood on him. Henry Lucas, manager of Brown's Springs Station, corroborated the evidence of last witness. His hat and clothes were found half a mile from the place where he was found. Deceased had only his trousers on ; no shirt. Dr. J. Leonard, duly qualified medical practitioner, deposed : I find nothing to account for death, but from the evidence given I believe him to have died from exhaustion consequent on exposure. I think he must have had delirium, and, probably, had been drinking heavily recently. The jury found the cause of death was exhaustion and exposure.

VICTORIA PHARMACEUTICAL SOCIETY'S MEDAL IN GOLD.

SCHOOL of pharmacy prizes presented by the Council—Chemistry ("elementary and practical"), botany, *materia medica*, and pharmacy.

At the end of each term a gold medal will be offered for competition. Students who have attended more than one term will be ineligible to compete. The medals can only be taken by students who have worked in the laboratory for not less than 75 per cent. of their period of study, and who are connected with the Society as registered apprentices of the same. On receiving the report of the examiners, the Council will award the prizes.

Notes and Abstracts.

FOWLER'S SOLUTION.—Dannenberg does not regard the algaceous growth, occasionally observed in this liquid, as being of any importance concerning the arsenic present ; but he directs attention to the gradual oxidation, in partly filled bottles, of the arsenious to arsenic acid, as was shown by Fresenius many years ago. According to Frerichs and Wœhler arsenic acid is far less poisonous than arsenious acid, and it is obvious that it cannot be immaterial which of the two compounds is present. Fowler's solution should be prepared only in small quantities and preserved in well-stopped vials.—*Phar. Centralhalle,* 1881, p. 319.

PREPARATION OF SODIUM ETHYLATE.—Hager gives the following directions:—100 grams absolute alcohol are placed into a glass flask of 350 ccm. (about 12 ozs.) capacity ; small pieces of the metallic sodium of the size of a pea or bean are then gradually added, and the flask is closed with a cork, through which a long open glass tube passes for the purpose of condensing the alcoholic vapours evolved during the reaction. The addition of sodium is continued, until 12 grams of the metal have been used, repeated agitation being required towards the end of the process. The hot thickish liquid is now poured into a porcelain dish, the flask is rinsed out with a little hot alcohol, any undissolved sodium is carefully removed, and the liquid is heated until, after cooling, it will completely solidify, when the mass is rubbed into a fine powder and carefully preserved. Thus prepared, it contains some alcohol in combination, which may be expelled by heating it to 200° C. In contact with water it is decomposed into alcohol and sodium hydrate. Its action is milder than that of caustic soda, and it is more conveniently applied than the latter. Richardson's sodium ethylate is a clear solution of 1 part of the above compound in three parts of absolute alcohol. Freshly prepared it is colourless ; but brown yellow if made from old ethylate.—*Ibid.,* p. 359.

ELASTIC ADHESIVE PLASTER.—Dr. W. P. Morgan, in a communication to the Boston *Medical and Surgical Journal,* states that he has been trying to obtain an elastic adhesive plaster that, when attached to the skin, should yield to the movement of the muscles and parts beneath without the sensation of stiffness or an uncomfortable wrinkling. Not being able to obtain an article of this description, he procured some india-rubber, and, giving it a coat of plaster such as is recommended in Griffith's *Formulary* under the name of "Boynton's Adhesive Plaster" (lead plaster 1 lb., resin 6 drachms), he found the material he wished. After using it as a simple covering for cases of psoriasis, intertrigo, &c., he extended its use to incised wounds, abscesses, &c., and found it invaluable. Placing one end of the strip of plaster upon one lip of the wound, and then stretching the rubber and fastening the other end to the opposite lip of the wound there is perfect apposition of the several parts, the elastic rubber acting continually to draw and keep the parts together. When unable to get the sheets of rubber, one may use broad letter-bands (sold by stationers), by giving them a coat of plaster.—*Ohio Medical Journal,* September, 1881, p. 136.

A valuable paper, by M. Paul Bert, on the administration of anæsthetics, has recently been read before the Academy of Sciences (*Comptes Rendus,* Vol. xciii., p. 768). M. Bert finds by experiment that if an anæsthetic be mixed with variable quantities of atmospheric air there comes a point at which an animal made to breathe such an atmosphere exhibits anæsthesia, and that this point bears a definite relation to the point at which the anæsthetic proves fatal. In experiments made upon dogs, mice, and sparrows, using chloroform, ether, amylene, and bromide and chloride of ethyl, it was found that the fatal dose was double that required to produce insensibility. In the case of protoxide of nitrogen the ratio is one to three. The result shows that chloroform acts not by the quantity inhaled, but by the amount of air mixed with it. This important result, although the experiments had not then been made upon mankind, shows that in all probability careful observation made by those who have the administration of chloroform in their hands may reduce its use to a minimum of risk and that in the future it may be employed with scientific precision. An instrument by which the amount of admixture of air and chloroform could be easily regulated before inhalation seems therefore to be a desideratum.

RABBIT EXTERMINATION.

Bisulphide of Carbon.

THE undersigned are now prepared to supply **BISULPHIDE OF CARBON** in one gallon and five gallon packages, in quantities to suit purchasers.

The Manufacturers would call the attention of purchasers to the report of the Government Analyst on the samples of Bisulphide of Carbon manufactured at their works, and submitted to him for analysis; also, to his suggestions as to the mode of applying the Bisulphide of Carbon for the destruction of Rabbits or other Vermin.

GOVERNMENT ANALYST'S REPORT.

12th June, 1879.

I have examined Felton, Grimwade & Co.'s BISULPHIDE OF CARBON. There are two varieties, viz, the crude and the rectified. The former is, in my opinion, quite sufficient for Destroying Rabbits or other Vermin, and for ordinary manufacturing purposes. The best way to use it for Rabbits is to place the requisite amount in a shallow tin dish of any convenient size, and place in it some very absorbent substance of the nature of sponge, so as to draw it up and expose a very extensive surface for speedy evaporation. In the absence of sponge, a handful of wool, tow, or even sawdust may be used. Unless some absorbent material of the nature of those named is used, the evaporation is liable in cold weather to proceed too slowly, and so much of its effects become lost.

The samples of Bisulphide imported from Europe possess no advantages over the colonial-made article.

WM. JOHNSON,
Government Analytical Chemist.

FELTON, GRIMWADE & CO.,

MANUFACTURING CHEMISTS, &c.,

SANDRIDGE CHEMICAL WORKS,

AND AT

31 and 33 FLINDERS LANE WEST,

MELBOURNE.

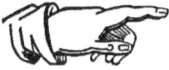